**Proteins are essential to life—prime players
in your health, fitness, and weight control.**

How can you maximize your protein intake?

If you're thinking about using protein supplements,
snacking on energy bars, or eating more soy foods,
Nolan & Heslin, the nutrition experts, will help you
determine your individual protein requirements and design
the best meal plan to optimize your fitness and your health.

***THE PROTEIN COUNTER,* Third Edition**

provides all the information you need, with more than
15,000 food listings—alphabetized for quick, easy
reference—giving the portion size, protein, calorie,
carbohydrate, and fat values for each food. Everything
you need to know about protein is at your fingertips!

Pack it in your gym bag!

The
PROTEIN
COUNTER
Third Edition

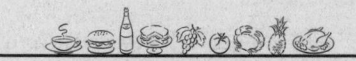

Karen J. Nolan, Ph.D.
and Jo-Ann Heslin, M.A., R.D.

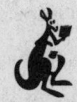

POCKET BOOKS
New York   London   Toronto   Sydney

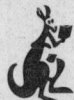

Pocket Books
A Division of Simon & Schuster, Inc.
1230 Avenue of the Americas
New York, NY 10020

This Pocket Books paperback edition January 2011

POCKET and colophon are registered trademarks of Simon & Schuster, Inc.

For information about special discounts for bulk purchases, please contact Simon & Schuster Special Sales at 1-866-506-1949 or business@simonandschuster.com.

The Simon & Schuster Speakers Bureau can bring authors to your live event. For more information or to book an event, contact the Simon & Schuster Speakers Bureau at 1-866-248-3049 or visit our website at www.simonspeakers.com.

Cover photo by Adam Gault/Getty Images

Manufactured in the United States of America

10 9 8 7 6 5 4 3 2 1

ISBN 978-1-4165-0984-4

For
Our families
Who support us through every project

ACKNOWLEDGMENTS

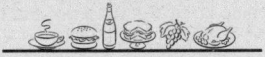

For all her continuous support and help, our agent, Nancy Trichter.

For her suggestions and editing skills, Sara Clemence.

For all her patience, comments, and questions, our favorite reviewer, Jean Schwarsin.

Without the tireless cooperation of Stephen Llano and the production department at Pocket Books, *The Protein Counter,* Third Edition, would never have been completed.

A special thank you to our editor, Micki Nuding.

And we would like to thank all of our readers for their suggestions and questions. Your input helps us to provide you with the most useful information.

The fact that protein food is both a fuel and a building material makes its place in the diet confusing.

Mary Swartz Rose, Ph.D.
Feeding the Family
The Macmillan Company, 1919

CONTENTS

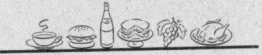

INTRODUCTION

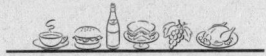

We count fat. We count carbs. But what about protein?

Protein is a substance that helps form everything from your toenails to your heart muscle. It is part of your immune system and a source of energy. It can even help you lose weight.

Protein is part of every cell inside you. It's needed in thousands of chemical reactions and holds our bodies together structurally. But it's a very misunderstood nutrient.

Bombarded with information about the benefits and hazards of high protein diets, and faced with dozens of choices for protein bars, it's no wonder you are confused. How much protein do you need? What are the best ways to get it? What does protein actually do?

Keep reading.

Protein is important because:

- It helps form the structure of your body—skin, organs, bones, hair, and muscles.

- It provides the raw material to build and repair your body.

- It is part of your immune system, fighting infections and viruses.

- It is a major part of every enzyme in the body.

1

- It is part of many important hormones.
- It helps keep the body's fluids stable.
- It transports needed substances and nutrients around the body.
- It helps maintain the body's neutrality, which is vital to life.
- It helps you lose weight and maintain weight loss.
- It offers protection against chronic disease.
- It is a source of energy (calories).

WHAT IS PROTEIN, EXACTLY?

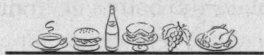

A more accurate question might be, What are proteins? After all, there are thousands of different proteins, all with a specific function in our bodies. Protein is found in every cell, tissue, and substance in the body except for urine and bile.

Collagen, for example, is the protein that gives your skin and bones their strength. Hair and nails are made of keratin. Actin and myosin make up muscle.

Proteins are made up of long strings of amino acids. And, just as the 26 letters in the alphabet can be combined to make up a tremendous variety of words, the 20 amino acids can be combined to make an infinite variety of proteins. There are even some proteins that are made up of hundreds of amino acids strung together.

Amino acids are the building blocks of protein. Eleven of the 20 amino acids are called nonessential, even though they are important, because they can be made in the body. The remaining 9 are called essential because your body cannot manufacture them. You need to get them from the protein foods you eat. Your body uses food proteins to manufacture body proteins.

That is why eating protein foods every day is so important. Your body builds and repairs itself out of proteins. Some of the protein used to maintain your body comes from recycled amino acids when old cells are broken down, and some comes from a pool of extra amino acids stored in the body. But the rest comes from food. Your body counts on you to eat protein daily to replace its supply.

PROTEIN POINT

Your body makes about 300 grams of protein every day.
Almost two-thirds are made from recycled body protein.
This efficient recycling system is one reason why we do not need to eat very large amounts of protein every day.

Amino acids are small protein fragments. Proteins, on the other hand, are very large molecules made up of long strings of amino acids.

As the protein chain is formed, it becomes three-dimensional. Its shape determines its function and how it acts in the body. Proteins are far more varied and complicated than fats or carbohydrates.

The first step in digestion is to break down, or denature, food proteins. This uncoils the protein strand so that the individual amino acids can be broken apart and reused by your body to build, repair, and replace worn-out cells. Your body efficiently recycles the food protein and turns it into body parts.

Proteins are found in both animal and vegetable foods.

FOOD SOURCES OF PROTEIN

Animal Sources	Plant Sources
Beef	Dry beans
Bison	Cereals
Cheese	Lentils
Chicken	Meat substitutes
Duck	Nut Butter
Eggs	Nuts
Finfish	Peanut Butter
Game	Peanuts
Ham	Peas
Lamb	Seeds
Milk	Soybeans
Ostrich	Soycheese
Pork	Soymilk
Shellfish	Texturized soy protein
Turkey	Tofu
Veal	Wheat gluten (seitan)
Wild poultry	
Yogurt	

PROTEIN POINT
You Denature (Uncoil) Proteins
When You Cook.

*Vinegar, wine, and juice marinades are acidic enough
to break apart food proteins and make meat, poultry,
and fish more tender and tasty.*

*Heat cooks an egg and breaks apart proteins,
turning the egg from a liquid to a solid.*

HOW MUCH PROTEIN DO YOU NEED?

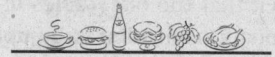

This is the simple question, but the answer is more complex. It depends on your weight, age, sex, and state of health.

The Institutes of Medicine's Dietary Reference Intakes (DRIs) for adults in the United States and Canada recommends 0.8 grams of protein per kilogram of body weight (1 kilogram = 2.2 pounds). Many experts disagree with this recommendation. Here's what the experts are saying.

The average American eats about 66 grams of protein a day. Most of us eat less red meat and more fish and poultry. The amount we normally eat exceeds the recommendation of 56 grams of protein a day for men and 46 grams of protein a day for women. But even though we are eating more than the DRI protein recommendations, it actually may not be enough protein for good health. Here's why.

Americans are heavier today. The current protein recommendation is based on a reference body weight for men of 154 pounds (70 kilograms) and for women of 125 pounds (57 kilograms). But the average American woman now weighs slightly more than 164 pounds, and the average man, 191 pounds. Many experts believe that the current recommendations are underestimates, based on what most adults actually weigh.

In early 2010, researchers challenged the studies used to define our current protein recommendations and concluded that the average protein intake should be raised. The researchers felt that the old studies used to define our protein recommendations needed to be updated with more precise measurement techniques. Based on the newer research methods, the following chart provides an updated set of recommendations for your daily protein need. Select your age, level of activity, or current condition to determine how much protein you need daily.

HOW MUCH PROTEIN YOU NEED EACH DAY

Age or Condition	Grams Protein per Kilogram of Weight*
Adults, 19 to 50 years old	0.9 to 1.2
Adults over 50	1.0 to 1.5
For weight loss	1.0 to 1.8
Recreational athletes	1.2 to 1.4
Endurance athletes	1.2 to 1.7
For strength training	1.7 to 1.8
For rheumatoid arthritis	1.5 to 2.0
For infections, fractures, fever, surgery	2.0
For severe trauma, wound healing, burns	2.5 to 3.0

* Recommendations are based on normal kidney function

Making the Research Practical

You're probably wondering, how do I use all those grams and kilograms to make daily food choices? It really is easy. We'll show you how.

FIGURING OUT YOUR
DAILY PROTEIN REQUIREMENT

1. Determine your daily protein factor.

Go to the table How Much Protein You Need Each Day and select the category that is right for you.

For example, if you are a recreational athlete, your protein factor is 1.2 to 1.4 grams of protein. You can select the lower, upper, or average range for this group. For the example, we will select the average of 1.3.

Your daily protein factor is: _____

2. Convert your weight in pounds to kilograms.

Divide your weight in pounds by 2.2.

For example, if you weigh 185 pounds:

$$185 \text{ pounds} \div 2.2 = 84 \text{ kilograms}$$

Your weight in kilograms: _____

3. Determine your daily requirement for protein.

Multiply your protein factor by your weight in kilograms.

Continuing to use our example, our recreational athlete, who weighs 84 kilograms, selected a protein factor of 1.3.

1.3 (protein factor) × 84 kilograms (weight) =
109 grams of protein/day
**Protein Factor × Weight in Kilograms =
Grams Protein/Day**

Your daily protein requirement is: _____ grams of protein per day

Now that you know how much protein you need each day, use *The Protein Counter* to select the best choices to meet your needs. Every listing gives you the grams of protein in a serving of food. Simply add up your protein intake over the day to reach your goal. If your situation changes, you can recalculate your needs based on these three easy steps.

Your Daily Protein Record will help you keep track. You don't need to track carbohydrate and fat every day—or at all, unless you wish. Many athletes and dieters track all 3 nutrients because it helps them plan healthy meals.

YOUR DAILY PROTEIN RECORD

Daily Protein Goal _____   **Daily Fat Goal** _____

Daily Carbohydrate Goal _____   **Date** _____

FOOD	PORTION	CALORIES	PROTEIN	CARB	FAT
AM					
AM Totals		_____	_____	____	____
MIDDAY					
Midday Totals		_____	_____	____	____
PM					
PM Totals		_____	_____	____	____
Daily Totals		_____	_____	____	____

PROTEIN'S HEALTH BENEFITS

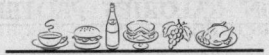

*Muscle can keep you healthy, lower your risk
for disease, and help you lose weight.*

A growing body of research is now suggesting that muscle not only builds strength but also promotes a long, active life. It may also help prevent many chronic diseases such as type 2 diabetes, heart disease, and osteoporosis.

Confused? You thought we were talking about protein and health. But muscles are made up of protein. They are the body's primary protein reserves. So when you have adequate muscle mass, you have excellent protein reserves to draw on as needed. Experts are now suggesting that maintaining and preserving our body's muscle mass throughout life is a key step in achieving good health and living a long life.

Let's see what the experts are suggesting.

- A high protein, lowfat diet helps reduce the risk of heart disease for women.

- A higher protein intake helps control blood sugar levels for people with type 2 diabetes.

- A modest substitution of carbohydrate-rich foods for protein-rich foods helps reduce blood pressure in those with high blood pressure.

- Vegetable proteins—rice, pasta, cereals, tofu, soybeans—help lower high blood pressure.

- Body muscles (your protein reserves) help you cope with stress.

- Body muscles (your protein reserves) aid in effective cancer treatment and lower the risk for recurrence.

- Eating enough protein prevents sarcopenia—the loss of muscle mass, strength, and function—as you age.

- Eating enough protein helps prevent osteoporosis— adult bone thinning. Muscles exert physical force on your bones, which stimulates the body to make more bone and prevents age-related thinning.

- Middle-aged people who eat adequate protein have a lower risk for hip fracture as they age.

- Eating potassium-rich fruits and vegetables helps prevent muscle loss as you age.

And, if all this evidence isn't convincing enough, protein can help you lose weight and keep it off.

THE SKINNY ON PROTEIN
AND WEIGHT LOSS

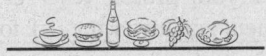

There is a connection between protein and weight loss, and
it has to do with muscle.

Most people don't appreciate the role muscle plays in
preventing obesity and losing weight. Muscle is very active
tissue—it twitches and moves even while you are sleeping.
Because of this almost constant motion, muscle uses more
calories than fat tissue does. So the more muscle in your
body, the more calories you will burn.

Picture a healthy, young man with an average muscle
mass. He has anywhere from 77 to 110 pounds of muscle
in his body. In contrast, an older woman can have as little as 28 pounds of muscle. The young man will burn close to
500 calories a day just supporting his muscle, but the older
women uses barely 120 calories because she has so much
less muscle.

The same logic goes for someone who is heavy but not
very fit. They have a lot more fat than active muscle mass,
and their bodies burn fewer calories.

If you increase your muscle mass with exercise and diet,
you will burn more calories and can lower your risk for obesity. That goes for children, adults, and the elderly. We begin

to lose muscle in our 30s and 40s, not coincidentally the same time that people commonly report packing on pounds. If you continue to exercise and do resistance training, you can prevent muscle loss and protect yourself from gaining extra weight over your lifetime.

PROTEIN POINT

Resistance training and eating adequate protein can build muscle at any stage in life.
Nursing home residents in their 90s who started to exercise built muscle.

Studies have shown that people who add extra protein and exercise to a diet plan in order to build muscle tend to lose weight faster and maintain their weight loss over time.

But the connection between protein and weight loss goes even further.

- Dieters who eat at least 1 gram of protein per kilogram of body weight each day lose more fat and less muscle while they are losing weight. Some experts feel an even higher protein intake might be better.

- Including some protein at every meal and snack makes you feel satisfied longer and less hungry.

- Drinking nonfat milk (high in protein) in the morning makes you feel fuller longer and can reduce the number of calories you eat at lunch.

- Dieters find high protein diets tastier and more satisfying than lowfat diets, which means they are more likely to stick to their diet plans.

PROTEIN POINT
Protein Uses More Calories
*The body uses 20% to 35% of the energy (calories)
found in protein foods just to break down and reuse
the amino acids.
To break down and use carbohydrates
and fats, only 5% to 15% of the energy
(calories) found in the food is used.*

But don't get carried away. As we explain in the next section, when you eat too much protein—more than you need to build and repair cells—the leftover is converted into fat and stored. Taking extra protein supplements or eating very large portions of protein foods can result in unwanted weight gain.

Are high protein, low carb diets good for weight loss?

These diets come and go. You will lose weight quickly, but a good deal of the initial weight loss is water weight. The real problem with a very low carb, high protein diet is that you eat little or no fruits, breads, cereals, and pasta. Protein and carb work together. Without carb, protein is burned for calories and not used to maintain the well-being of your body. Long term, these diets are hard to stick to.

Very high protein diets also are very high in fat because they rely heavily on meat, cheese, and poultry. Long term, this is not the healthiest approach. Many people who try these diets may experience constipation, nausea, weakness, dehydration, and fatigue. Diets that contain 50% or more protein are not recommended.

High protein diets that are successful for weight loss contain 25% to 30% protein, 40% carb, and 30% to 35% fat.

THE FACTS ABOUT PROTEIN AND ATHLETES

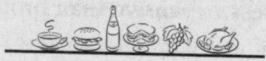

True or false?
Eating large amounts of protein builds muscle.

The answer is false. Surprised? Many people drink protein shakes and eat protein bars, thinking that the more protein they eat, the more they'll build muscle and enhance their performance.

The truth is that athletes do need more protein than the average person—but they do not need huge amounts.

What builds muscles is exercise, carbohydrates for fuel, and a small amount of extra protein to build and repair muscles after exercise. Let's see why.

About 40% to 45% of your body weight is made up of muscle. For athletes, that ratio may be slightly higher. About one quarter of muscle by weight is protein. The rest is made up of water, fat, stored glucose, and some minerals.

Some argue that when exercise stresses and breaks down your muscle, you need extra protein to repair the damage and build up new tissue. But the more you exercise, the more efficient your body becomes at recycling and reusing the amino acids that are the result of muscle breakdown.

Experts estimate that 10 to 14 grams of extra protein per day is enough to build one pound of muscle in a week. You can easily get that amount by eating an extra 1½ ounces of meat, fish, or poultry, 1½ glasses nonfat milk, or ½ cup cottage cheese each day. All of these choices are a lot more familiar, tasty, and less expensive than protein supplements, bars, and powders.

PROTEIN POINT

A quarter cup of canned tuna packed in water (a 2-ounce serving) has 16 grams of protein.

Well-trained athletes do need a small additional amount of protein after a workout—about 10 to 20 grams. That is more than enough, along with healthy meals, to repair any damage caused during a strenuous workout.

You get even better results by eating 20 grams of carbohydrate after a workout along with the extra protein. That way, you're replacing your body's supply of both amino acids (protein) and glucose (calories). Studies have shown that this carbohydrate-protein, post-exercise supplement increases performance and reduces fatigue.

Other studies have shown that adding 4 extra ounces of high protein foods a day increased muscle buildup by 50%. Keep in mind that high protein foods are not totally protein. A 4-ounce hamburger contains only one ounce of protein. So if you added a 4-ounce hamburger to your daily intake, you would be adding 1 additional ounce of protein daily. This once again shows that we only need a little extra protein a day to build muscle.

Protein buildup seems to hit a ceiling at 30 grams of protein per meal. If you eat more than that, the protein is likely to be stored as fat. So, if you eat a 16-ounce steak for dinner, most of the extra protein will be stored as fat and not be used to make muscle. If, however, you eat 4 extra ounces of protein a day spread across breakfast, lunch, and dinner, muscle buildup is optimized.

PROTEIN POINT

Want to Boost Your Morning Protein?

Add an egg white or quarter cup of egg substitute to your scrambled egg.

If you are still committed to your protein bars or protein supplement, read the label carefully. Keep your post-exercise portion below 20 grams of protein. If you use it with meals, keep the portion below 15 grams. If you snack on protein bars throughout the day, buy those with less protein per bar. Keep in mind that all these bars and supplements do have extra calories. Do you need them? Though most experts feel that protein supplements are not needed, if taken in the right amounts with enough fluids they also do little harm. Just remember: too much of a good thing isn't always good for you.

How much protein is too much?

Protein amounts up to 40% of total calories each day do not seem to cause a problem as long as kidney function is good. Your kidneys excrete the nitrogen that results from protein breakdown, and this puts some stress on that organ.

Most of us eat 10% to 15% of our calories as protein. Athletes and dieters may increase this amount to 20% to 25% of total calories. We'd recommend no more than 30% at the upper limit. Above this amount, it is hard to eat enough carbohydrates, and meals become more difficult to plan and they are not as tasty. At very high protein levels, if you try to keep fat to a reasonable amount, 30% to 35% of calories, it becomes even harder to plan meals with a healthy variety of foods.

How do I figure out the percentages of protein, carbohydrate, and fat I should eat each day?

First pick how much protein you wish to eat each day. For this example we'll pick 25%. If you eat 2500 calories a day, 25% of 2500 would be 625 protein calories.

$$2500 \text{ calories} \times 25\% = 625 \text{ protein calories}$$

That leaves 75% of your remaining calories each day to divide between carbohydrate and fat. If you eat 25% of your calories as fat, which would be considered a lowfat diet, then 50% of your calories are left for carbohydrate.

For fat:
$$2500 \text{ calories} \times 25\% = 625 \text{ calories}$$
For carbohydrate:
$$2500 \text{ calories} \times 50\% = 1250 \text{ calories}$$

If you would like to take this one step further and figure out the grams of protein, fat, and carbohydrate to eat each day, it is quite easy to do. All you need to know is that every gram of protein and carbohydrate equals 4 calories, and every gram of fat equals 9 calories.

For protein: $625 \text{ protein calories} \div 4 =$
156 grams protein
For carbohydrate: $625 \text{ carbohydrate calories} \div 4 =$
156 grams of carbohydrate
For fat: $1250 \text{ fat calories} \div 9 = 139 \text{ grams of fat}$

On the Daily Protein Record, page 10, you can record your daily protein, fat, and carbohydrate goals and keep track of the foods you eat to see if you meet your target goals.

PROTEIN POINT

Checking Your Protein Math

See the chart How Much Protein You Need Each Day, page 7, to see if the percentage of protein you have selected is in line with your needs.

Example: If you are a 190-pound man who regularly does strength training, you should eat 1.7 to 1.8 grams of protein per kilogram of weight.

190 pounds ÷ 2.2 = 86 kilograms
86 × 1.7 = 146 grams of protein a day
86 × 1.8 = 154 grams of protein a day

Many athletes regularly eat energy bars and energy drinks. Don't confuse energy needs with protein needs. Both energy bars and drinks can fit into a healthy eating plan; just think about your reason for using them and make sure the brand you are buying is meeting your needs.

Which are the best energy bars to buy?

What are you looking for? Do you want a protein replacement post-exercise? Are you looking for a meal replacement? Are you dieting? Do you need a mental pick-me-up? Do you need energy during a long run?

First, let's sort the bars into general categories:

- Energy bars—tend to have more carbohydrates for a quick energy boost. A good choice on a long run.

- Diet bars—have less carbohydrate and fewer calories. A good choice if you are trying to lose weight or you're watching calories.

- Meal replacement bars—have more protein, fat, and carbohydrate, are often larger and have more calories. A good choice when you have no time to eat.

- Protein bars—simply have more protein, often between 10 and 30 grams per bar. At the lower end of protein, they could be a good post-exercise snack.

When buying energy bars, first consider why you are using them, and then read the label. Many are high in sugar, others are very low in protein. Also look at calories and the size of the bar. Some 1.5-ounce bars—about 2 bites—pack a wallop of calories.

Eating an energy bar occasionally is fine. Even eating one daily as a snack or meal replacement is okay. But many of these expensive treats are little more than fortified candy bars. And some taste downright dreadful in the name of being healthy. *The Protein Counter* lists over 100 energy bars to make it easy for you to compare brands by protein amounts.

PROTEIN POINT

That old standby, peanut butter on whole wheat bread, offers quick energy, high quality protein, fiber, and essential nutrients at a fraction of the cost of highly fortified energy bars.

Which are the best energy drinks to buy?

As with energy bars, first, what is your reason for using energy drinks? Few, if any, contain protein. Most are high in sugar and stimulants like caffeine for a mental pick-me-up. Most have more sugar or carb than is needed in a given volume of liquid to make them a good fluid/energy replacement during performance. Serious athletes usually dilute drinks like Gatorade, because a high sugar intake during performance can be dehydrating.

Once again, read labels carefully to make the best choices for your purposes. *The Protein Counter* lists over 100 energy drinks, so it is easy for you to compare brands.

PROTEIN POINT

Common Foods Are Better
Than Sports Supplements

*Gold medal winner Michael Phelps drank Carnation
Instant Breakfast between races at the Olympics.
Lowfat chocolate milk provides as good or even better
recovery after strenuous exercise than sports drinks.
Cereal plus nonfat milk is as good as sports
drinks for post-exercise muscle recovery.*

WHAT IF I DON'T EAT MEAT?

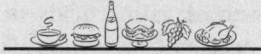

Many people don't eat meat, and they can still get adequate protein every day. Some don't eat red meat, but they eat fish and poultry and perhaps even pork. Others eat no meat, fish, or poultry, but may still use eggs, milk, and cheese. Still others eliminate all animal foods from their diet. In every case, you can meet your protein needs.

All of the following foods contain about the same amount of protein as 1 ounce of meat.

PROTEIN EQUIVALENTS

1 ounce of protein = 6 to 8 grams protein

1 ounce fish or poultry	½ cup cooked beans
1 egg	½ cup cooked lentils
¼ cup cottage cheese (2 ounces)	¼ cup cooked soybeans
¾ cup yogurt	2 tablespoons roasted soynuts
1 cup milk	
2 tablespoons dry milk powder	1 cup soy milk
2 tablespoons peanut butter	1 cup cooked pasta
¼ cup nuts	1 cup cooked green peas
¼ cup seeds	¼ cup (1.5 ounces) tofu

If I am a vegetarian, do I have to combine vegetable proteins to be sure I get enough amino acids in my diet?

What you are referring to is protein complementation: combining 2 or more proteins to be sure that you get the entire complement of essential amino acids (see below). Many plant proteins are missing or low in one or more essential amino acids, but if you combine them—rice and beans, for instance—the amino acid profile becomes stronger and more similar to that found in animal protein.

If you use dairy products, cereal and milk are a great complement to one another, as is adding a small amount of cheese to a meal. But even if you are a vegan, you can get all the protein you need from vegetable sources. It was once believed that you needed to complement vegetable proteins in the same meal, but this belief is no longer current. Eating different vegetable proteins throughout the day will complement your overall intake of amino acids. Below are some typical complementary protein combinations.

COMPLEMENTARY PROTEIN COMBINATIONS

Bean burritos

Hummus (made of chickpeas + sesame seed paste)

Pasta and beans

Peanut butter sandwich

Rice and beans

Rice and lentils

Split pea soup with bread or crackers

Trail mix (nuts and seeds)

Is it true that some proteins are better than others?

You might have heard people say that some foods have a "higher quality" protein than others. All protein foods contain amino acids. What they are referring to is called the biological value of a specific protein food. Biological value is determined by the number and amount of amino acids that a food provides. Eggs are the gold standard, supplying all the amino acids the body needs in the right amounts.

Meat, fish, dairy products, and soy also have high biological values. Grains, beans, nuts, and seeds have intermediate biological value because they do not have enough of one or more of the essential amino acids. These foods can be complemented by a small amount of animal protein or another vegetable protein to make their amino acid amounts stronger (see the question above about complementing proteins). Fruits and vegetables are entirely lacking one or more amino acids, and are considered incomplete proteins or foods of low biological value for protein. It doesn't mean that fruits and vegetables are not the best choices; they are simply not your best protein choices. We don't rely on them for our protein needs.

WHY PROTEINS ARE
A REALLY BIG DEAL

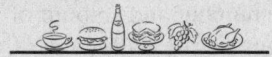

Every day, you lose millions of cells. They are used up, worn out, rubbed off—or even cut off, like your beard or fingernails. You build up, break down, and replace cells around the clock. Your body uses protein constantly.

When you see how many functions proteins have in your body, you'll start to understand why you can't live without them.

Structure and Movement

Proteins help form the architecture of your body. Every structural part of the body—hair, bones, muscles, teeth—contains different proteins.

Other proteins act like tiny motors helping you do physical work. When you get up off a chair, walk across a room, or pick up a heavy box, tiny proteins slide past each other to power your muscles. These microscopic motor proteins also help new cells to divide and sperm to swim.

Immunity

If you don't eat enough good quality protein, your immune response could be weakened and your risk of illness and infection goes up. That's because you rely on blood protein, known as antibodies, to fight against bacteria and viruses that could cause infection.

Each antibody is specific to a certain bacteria or virus. Once your immune system learns to make a certain antibody, your body can protect itself more quickly the next time you are exposed to that germ.

Enzymes

Your body contains thousands of enzymes. These are proteins that set off or speed up necessary chemical reactions in your body. Digestive enzymes help you break down food to use in the body (some of it protein!). Some enzymes help your cells release energy (calories) to be burned as fuel to keep the body moving and functioning. Enzymes also trigger reactions that build muscles, tissues, and body structures.

Hormones

These are chemical messengers that are made in one part of the body but act on cells in another part of the body.

SOME IMPORTANT HORMONES

Hormone	Number of Amino Acids	Function
Angiotensin II	8	Helps regulate blood pressure
Vasopressin	9	Increases water recycling in the kidney
Gastrin	14	Aids in digestion
Insulin	51	Controls glucose in the blood
Leptin	167	Suppresses hunger
Growth hormone	191	Regulates the body's development
Prolatin	198	Aids breastfeeding
Luteinizing hormone	204	Aids testosterone

Blood Neutrality

Remember learning about pH levels in science class? The body works very hard to keep the pH of the blood as close to neutral as possible. The pH scale goes from 1 to 14 (lower is more acid, higher is more alkaline). The pH of the blood is 7.4—close to neutral, which is the spot where your body works the best. Blood values above 8.0 or below 6.8, for just a few hours, can cause death. Blood proteins act as buffers, keeping your blood in that safe neutral range.

Transportation

Many substances need to move around the complex system that is your body, as well as into and out of cells. Proteins help move things around. Proteins can act as channels to allow materials to pass through cell membranes easily. Sometimes the proteins act as pumps, driving vital elements into cells.

Proteins also act as carriers, transporting needed substances through the bloodstream and delivering them where they're needed. The blood is mainly water, so it is difficult for fat and fat soluble vitamins (like A, D, E, and K) to move through the bloodstream without a carrier. Protein carries them along. Iron is moved by the protein transferrin. And fats are ferried through the blood as lipoproteins. You may recognize that one, because your doctor measures some of these lipoproteins when testing cholesterol levels—HDLs (high density lipoproteins) and LDLs (low density lipoproteins).

Fluid Balance

Your body is full of fluids, both inside and outside the cells. In order for your body to work properly, these fluids levels need to be in balance.

Proteins in the blood help maintain the correct level of fluid in the bloodstream. When your heart beats, the force pushes fluid out of tiny capillaries. Blood proteins, such as albumin and globulin, are too big to pass through capillary walls, so they stay inside, attracting water back to replace what has been pushed out. If there isn't enough protein to keep the levels normal, fluids leak into the body's tissues, causing swelling, which is called edema.

Source of Nitrogen

Protein, fat, and carbohydrate are all made of carbon, hydrogen, and oxygen. But protein also contains nitrogen—and in fact, it is your body's only source of nitrogen, which is one of the 6 essential elements for life. When proteins are broken down in the body, nitrogen is excreted through the urine, stools, sweat, hair, and other body fluids. This nitrogen must be replaced by eating protein foods.

During growth, we use more protein than we break down, and we hold onto nitrogen in the body. This is called positive nitrogen balance. In illness, dieting, or starvation, we break down more protein and get rid of more nitrogen— negative nitrogen balance. Healthy adults want to be *in* nitrogen balance: taking in the same amount of protein that they break down every day.

It is now believed that inflammation, a symptom of many chronic diseases, causes nitrogen loss, and eating more protein might help reduce your risk for heart disease and other chronic inflammatory illnesses.

Energy (Calories)

It might seem odd that we list calories as the last function of protein, but this is where it belongs. The body does not want to use protein as calories, because protein has too many other important jobs to perform in the body.

Using carbohydrate and fat as fuel first spares protein to build and repair the body. It's only when your body does not have enough energy to perform vital functions that it will burn up protein. This can happen on a diet or during starvation. The body sacrifices its own muscle to use for fuel.

Bottom Line

- Protein's primary job in the body is to build and repair cells.

- Using protein as fuel is wasteful.

- We all need protein to live, but no one needs to eat very large amounts.

- Extra protein by itself does not build muscles—protein, carbohydrate, and extra exercise are the key factors in stimulating muscle growth.

USING YOUR PROTEIN COUNTER

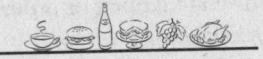

The Protein Counter lists the portion size, calories, protein, carbohydrate, and fat values for more than 15,000 foods. Now you can compare the values in your favorite foods and, when necessary, choose substitutes before you go out to shop or eat. This will save you time and help you decide what to buy.

The counter section of the book is divided into two parts: Part One: Brand Name, Nonbranded (Generic), and Take-Out Foods (page 37); and Part Two: Restaurant Chains (page 435). Each part lists the foods or restaurant chains alphabetically.

In Part One for each category, you will find nonbranded (generic) foods listed first, in alphabetical order, followed by an alphabetical listing of brand name foods. The nonbranded listings will help you estimate calorie, protein, carbohydrate, and fat values when you don't see your favorite brands. They can also help you evaluate store brands. Large categories are divided into subcategories, such as canned, fresh, frozen, and ready-to-eat, to make it easier to find what you're looking for. Some categories have "see" and "see also" references, to help you find related items.

Because we eat out so often, more than 800 take-out foods are listed in Part One. These are found in the take-out subcategory in many categories throughout this section. Look there for foods you take out or order in, because these foods are not nutrition labeled.

Most foods are listed alphabetically, but in some cases foods are grouped by category. For example, a tuna sandwich is found in the SANDWICH category. Other group categories include:

ASIAN FOOD   **Page 45**
  Includes all types of Asian foods
  except egg rolls and sushi, which
  are found in the egg rolls and sushi
  categories.

DELI MEATS/COLD CUTS   **Page 178**
  Includes all sandwich meats except
  chicken, ham, and turkey, which have
  their own separate categories.

DINNER   **Page 179**
  Includes all prepared dinners listed
  by brand name, except pasta dinners,
  which are found in the pasta dinner
  category.

LIQUOR/LIQUEUR   **Page 254**
  Includes all alcoholic beverages and
  mixed drinks except beer and ale,
  champagne, and wine, which are
  found in their own separate categories.

NUTRITION SUPPLEMENTS   **Page 278**
Includes all dieting aids, meal
replacements, and drinks, except
energy bars and energy drinks, which
are found in their own separate
categories.

SANDWICHES   **Page 348**
Includes popular sandwich, calzone,
and panini choices.

SNACKS   **Page 365**
Includes a variety of snack items, such
as pork rinds and cheese puffs.

SPANISH FOOD   **Page 386**
Includes all types of Spanish and
Mexican foods except salsa and
tortillas, which are found in their own
separate categories.

In Part Two, Restaurant Chains, 82 national and regional restaurant, coffee, doughnut, frozen yogurt, ice cream, pizza, sandwich, soup, and sushi chains are listed. Brand name foods are required by federal law to have nutrition information on labels, but in most areas of the country, restaurants provide this information only voluntarily.

With *The Protein Counter* as your guide, you will never again wonder how much protein is in the foods you eat.

DEFINITIONS

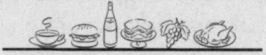

as prep (as prepared): refers to food that has been prepared according to package directions

lean and fat: describes meat with some fat on its edges that is not cut away before cooking, or poultry prepared with skin and fat as purchased

lean only: refers to lean meat that is trimmed of all visible fat, or poultry without skin

not prep (not prepared): refers to food that has not been cooked and may require the addition of other ingredients to prepare

shelf stable: refers to prepared products found on the supermarket shelf that are not canned or frozen, but are packaged and ready-to-eat, or are ready to be heated and do not require refrigeration

take-out: describes prepared dishes that you purchase ready-to-eat; those serve as a guide to the calories, protein, fat, and carbohydrates in products you may purchase

ABBREVIATIONS

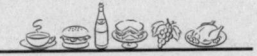

avg	=	average
diam	=	diameter
fl	=	fluid
frzn	=	frozen
g	=	gram
in	=	inch
lb	=	pound
lg	=	large
med	=	medium
mg	=	milligram
oz	=	ounce
pkg	=	package
pt	=	pint
prep	=	prepared
qt	=	quart
reg	=	regular
sec	=	second
serv	=	serving
sm	=	small
sq	=	square
tbsp	=	tablespoon
tr	=	trace
tsp	=	teaspoon
w/	=	with
w/o	=	without
<	=	less than

NOTES

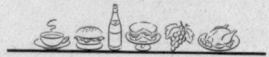

cals = calories
prot = protein
fat = fat
carb = carbohydrates
All protein, fat, and carbohydrate values are given
  in grams.
– (dash) indicates that values are not available
tr (trace) = less than 1 gram of protein, fat, or
  carbohydrate
0 (zero) indicates there are no calories, protein, fat,
  or carbohydrate in that food

Discrepancies in figures are due to rounding of values, product reformulation, and reevaluation. The current labeling law allows rounding. Some of the data listed are analysis data, obtained directly from manufacturers, not from labels; therefore, some values may differ slightly from labels because the values have not been rounded.

PART ONE

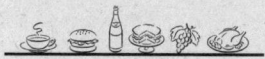

Brand Name, Nonbranded (Generic), and Take-Out Foods

PROTEIN POINT

The word *protein* comes from the Greek word
protos, meaning "of prime importance."
You cannot live without protein.

FOOD	PORTION	CALS	PROT	FAT	CARB
ABALONE					
breaded & fried	1 serv (3 oz)	162	17	6	9
steamed	1 serv (3 oz)	127	17	3	6
ACAI JUICE					
Arthur's					
Acai Plus	1 bottle (11 oz)	230	2	5	45
Bossa Nova					
Acai Juice Blueberry	8 oz	89	0	0	21
Acai Juice Mango	8 oz	89	0	0	23
Acai Juice Original	8 oz	94	0	0	21
Acai Juice Passion Fruit	8 oz	89	0	0	23
Acai Juice Raspberry	8 oz	89	0	0	23
O.N.E.					
Amazon Acai	1 bottle (11 oz)	157	1	3	32
Zola					
100% Juice	1 box (11 oz)	170	2	2	30
ACEROLA					
fresh	1 (5 g)	2	tr	tr	tr
ACEROLA JUICE					
juice	1 cup	56	1	1	12
ADZUKI BEANS					
canned sweetened	½ cup	351	6	tr	81
dried cooked w/o salt	½ cup	147	9	tr	28
Arrowhead Mills					
Organic Dried not prep	¼ cup	130	8	0	26
AKEE					
fresh	3.5 oz	223	5	20	5
ALCOHOL (see BEER AND ALE, CHAMPAGNE, LIQUOR/LIQUEUR, MALT, WINE)					
ALE (see BEER AND ALE)					
ALFALFA					
sprouts	½ cup	40	1	tr	1
ALLIGATOR					
cooked	3 oz	126	28	2	0

FOOD	PORTION	CALS	PROT	FAT	CARB
ALLSPICE					
ground	1 tsp	5	tr	tr	1
ALMONDS					
almond butter w/ salt	2 tbsp	203	5	19	7
almond butter w/o salt	2 tbsp	203	5	19	7
almond extract	1 tsp	38	5	tr	–
almond paste	¼ cup	260	5	16	27
chocolate covered	6 pieces (0.6 oz)	102	3	8	6
dry roasted w/ salt	¼ cup	206	8	18	7
dry roasted w/o salt	¼ cup	206	8	18	7
honey roasted	¼ cup	214	7	18	10
jordan almonds	6 (0.7 oz)	99	2	4	14
oil roasted w/ salt	¼ cup	238	8	22	7
oil roasted w/o salt	¼ cup	238	8	22	7
praline	17 pieces (1.4 oz)	210	5	12	21
yogurt covered	6 pieces (0.8 oz)	122	3	8	10
American Almond					
Marzipan	2 tbsp	130	2	5	19
Arrowhead Mills					
Organic Almond Butter Creamy	2 tbsp	200	7	17	6
Back To Nature					
California Sea Salt Roasted	1 oz	160	6	14	6
Diamond					
Slivered	¼ cup (1 oz)	170	7	15	6
Fisher					
Roasted & Salted	¼ cup (1 oz)	170	6	15	5
Godiva					
Dark Chocolate Almonds	1 pkg (2 oz)	310	8	24	23
Justin's					
Almond Butter Classic	2 tbsp (1.1 oz)	200	7	18	6
Almond Butter Maple	2 tbsp (1.1 oz)	190	6	16	8
Love'n Bake					
Almond Paste	2 tbsp	140	4	9	13
Almond Schmear	2 tbsp	140	4	8	14
Roasted Butter	2 tbsp	180	6	16	6
Mrs. May's					
Almond Crunch	1 oz	156	5	13	8

FOOD	PORTION	CALS	PROT	FAT	CARB
Naturally More					
Almond Butter	2 tbsp	190	9	16	8
Planters					
Chocolate Lovers Dark Chocolate	11 pieces (1.4 oz)	220	4	17	18
Dry Roasted	23 pieces (1 oz)	160	6	14	6
Sunkist					
Accents Italian Parmesan	1 tbsp	40	1	4	1
Accents Original Oven Roasted	1 tbsp	40	1	4	1
AMARANTH					
leaves cooked	½ cup	14	1	tr	3
uncooked	½ cup (3.4 oz)	365	14	6	65
Arrowhead Mills					
Organic Whole Grain not prep	¼ cup	180	7	3	31
ANCHOVY					
boneless	1 oz	60	8	3	0
canned in oil drained	1 can (2 oz)	94	13	4	0
fresh	1 (4 g)	8	1	tr	0
fresh fillets	3 (0.4 oz)	21	2	1	tr
Polar					
Rolled Fillets w/ Capers In Olive Oil	7 pieces (0.6 oz)	40	4	3	0
ANGLERFISH					
raw	3.5 oz	72	15	1	0
ANISE					
seed	1 tsp	7	tr	tr	1
ANTELOPE					
roasted	4 oz	215	41	4	0
APPLE					
CANNED					
sliced sweetened	½ cup	68	tr	1	17
Glory					
Fried Apples	½ cup	80	0	0	21
Polar					
Fuji	½ cup	50	0	0	12

FOOD	PORTION	CALS	PROT	FAT	CARB
DRIED					
chopped	½ cup	104	tr	tr	28
cooked w/o sugar	½ cup	73	tr	tr	20
rings	5	78	tr	tr	21
Bare Fruit					
Chips Cinnamon	1 pkg (0.6 oz)	43	0	0	12
Chukar Cherries					
Cherry Apple Slices	10 (1 oz)	110	0	0	28
Crispy Green					
Freeze-Dried	1 pkg (0.35 oz)	40	0	0	8
Fruit Ripples					
Cinnamon Apple	1 pkg	50	0	0	13
Strawberry Apple	1 pkg	50	0	0	13
Mrs. May's					
Fruit Chips	1 pkg	35	0	0	8
Nature's Envy					
Apple Chips Original	1 pkg (0.8 oz)	80	0	0	20
Stoneridge Orchards					
Green Wedges	⅓ cup (1.4 oz)	140	0	0	32
Sun-Maid					
Apples	¼ cup (1.4 oz)	120	1	0	29
FRESH					
apple	1 sm	55	tr	tr	15
apple	1 med	72	tr	tr	19
apple	1 lg	110	1	tr	29
candied	1 sm (4.9 oz)	179	2	3	40
candied	1 med (6.5 oz)	234	2	4	52
candied	1 lg (9.8 oz)	357	3	6	79
w/ skin sliced	1 cup	57	tr	tr	15
w/o skin sliced	1 cup	53	tr	tr	14
Chiquita					
Apple	1 (6.4 oz)	95	0	0	25
Apple Bites	1 pkg (2.5 oz)	30	0	0	8
Apple Bites w/ Caramel	1 pkg (2.5 oz)	70	0	0	17
Earthbound Farms					
Organic Slices	1 pkg (2 oz)	30	0	0	7
Eastern Select					
Gala	1 (5.5 oz)	80	0	0	22

FOOD	PORTION	CALS	PROT	FAT	CARB
Mrs. Prindable's					
Caramel Triple Chocolate	¼ apple (1.7 oz)	120	1	6	17
Caramel Walnut	¼ apple (2 oz)	160	2	10	17
Sullivan					
McIntosh	1 (5.4 oz)	80	0	1	22
FROZEN					
sliced w/o sugar	½ cup	42	tr	tr	11
REFRIGERATED					
Country Crock					
Cinnamon Apples	½ cup (4.4 oz)	130	0	3	26
TAKE-OUT					
baked	1 (6 oz)	128	tr	tr	42
baked no sugar	1 (5.6 oz)	136	tr	tr	24
fried apple rings	1 serv (2.7 oz)	91	tr	4	15
APPLE JUICE					
cider	1 cup	117	tr	tr	29
juice + vitamin C & calcium	1 cup	117	tr	tr	29
mulled cider	1 serv	265	1	1	42
unsweetened w/o vitamin C	1 cup	117	tr	tr	29
Apple & Eve					
100% Juice	8 oz	110	1	0	26
Back To Nature					
100% Juice	1 pkg (6 oz)	80	0	0	21
Fizz Ed.					
Green Apple	1 can (8.4 oz)	100	0	0	25
Izze					
Sparkling Fortified Apple	1 can (8.4 oz)	90	0	0	23
Land O' Lakes					
Juice	1 cup (8 oz)	120	0	0	29
Mott's					
100% Natural	1 bottle (14 oz)	200	1	0	48
Nantucket Nectars					
100% Juice Pressed Apple	8 oz	120	0	0	30
Organic Cloudy Apple	8 oz	120	0	0	29
Old Orchard					
Cider 100%	8 oz	120	0	0	29
Healthy Balance Apple	8 oz	30	0	0	6
Organic 100% Juice	8 oz	128	0	0	29

FOOD	PORTION	CALS	PROT	FAT	CARB
Santa Cruz					
Organic	8 oz	120	tr	0	30
Snapple					
100% Juiced Green Apple	8 oz	160	0	0	41
Juice Drink Apple	8 oz	110	0	0	27
Tree Ripe					
Organic 100% Juice	6 oz	80	0	0	21
Tropicana					
Orchard Style	1 bottle (14 oz)	200	tr	0	50
Walnut Acres					
Organic Juice	8 oz	110	0	0	29
APPLESAUCE					
sweetened	½ cup	97	tr	tr	25
unsweetened	½ cup	52	tr	tr	14
GoGo Squeez					
Apple	1 pkg (3 oz)	60	0	1	14
Apple Banana	1 pkg (3 oz)	60	0	tr	14
Apple Cinnamon	1 pkg (3 oz)	50	0	tr	10
Apple Peach	1 pkg (3 oz)	60	0	tr	13
Mott's					
Healthy Harvest Granny Smith No Sugar Added	1 pkg (3.9 oz)	50	0	0	13
Organic Original	½ cup (4.5 oz)	110	0	0	27
Organic Unsweetened	½ cup (4.3 oz)	50	0	0	14
Single-Serve Cinnamon	1 pkg (4 oz)	100	0	0	25
Musselman's					
Unsweetened	1 pkg (4 oz)	50	0	0	12
Revolution Foods					
Organic Unsweetened	1 pkg (4 oz)	50	0	0	13
Santa Cruz					
Organic	½ cup (4.5 oz)	60	0	0	13
Organic Apple Apricot	1 pkg (4 oz)	60	0	0	14
Organic Apple Blueberry	1 pkg (4 oz)	60	0	0	14
Organic Apple Cherry	½ cup (4.5 oz)	60	0	0	15
APRICOT JUICE					
nectar	6 oz	106	1	tr	27
Santa Cruz					
Organic Nectar	8 oz	120	0	0	29

FOOD	PORTION	CALS	PROT	FAT	CARB
APRICOTS					
canned heavy syrup	½ cup	91	1	tr	23
canned in juice	½ cup	59	1	tr	15
canned in water	½ cup	33	1	tr	8
canned light syrup	½ cup	80	1	tr	21
dried halves	6	51	1	tr	13
dried halves cooked w/o sugar	½ cup	106	2	tr	28
fresh	1	17	tr	tr	4
fresh sliced	½ cup	40	1	tr	9
frozen sweetened	½ cup	119	1	tr	30
Elizabeth's Natural					
Turkish Dried	5 (1.8 oz)	90	1	0	22
Harvest Bay					
Dried	5 (1.4 oz)	60	2	0	15
Mariani					
Ultimate Dried	¼ cup (1.4 oz)	100	1	0	24
S&W					
Whole In Heavy Syrup	½ cup (4.5 oz)	120	tr	0	29
Sunsweet					
Dried	6 pieces (1.4 oz)	100	1	0	25
ARROWHEAD					
corm boiled	1 med	9	1	tr	2
ARROWROOT					
raw	1 root (1.2 oz)	21	1	tr	4
raw root sliced	1 cup	78	5	tr	16
Bob's Red Mill					
Starch	¼ cup	110	0	0	28
ARTICHOKE					
CANNED					
hearts in oil	1 serv (3 oz)	100	3	7	9
Cento					
Hearts Quartered Marinated	2 pieces	20	0	2	2
Gertie's Finest					
Tapenade	2 tbsp	29	1	3	2
Native Forest					
Organic Hearts Quartered	1 serv (4 oz)	35	2	0	6
Polar					
Hearts	2	18	2	0	3
Hearts Quartered Marinated	1 oz	25	1	2	5

FOOD	PORTION	CALS	PROT	FAT	CARB
Progresso					
Hearts	2 (4.6 oz)	30	1	0	7
Hearts Marinated	2 (1.1 oz)	60	0	5	2
Roland					
Hearts	½ cup (4.6 oz)	50	3	0	9
The Gracious Gourmet					
Artichoke Parmesan Tapenade	2 tbsp (1 oz)	30	1	2	3
FRESH					
cooked	1 med	60	4	tr	13
hearts cooked	½ cup	42	3	tr	9
Ocean Mist					
Lemon	1 (4.2 oz)	60	4	0	13
FROZEN					
cooked	1 cup	42	3	tr	9
cooked w/o salt	1 pkg (9 oz)	108	7	1	22
C&W					
Hearts	12 pieces (3 oz)	40	2	1	7
TAKE-OUT					
stuffed	1 (8.8 oz)	397	15	14	54

ASIAN FOOD (*see also* CURRY, DINNER, EGG ROLLS, SAUCE, SOY SAUCE, SUSHI)

FOOD	PORTION	CALS	PROT	FAT	CARB
CANNED					
chow mein chicken w/o noodles	1 cup	194	20	8	10
La Choy					
Chow Mein Beef	1 cup	90	8	2	11
Chow Mein Chicken	1 cup (9.3 oz)	100	8	3	10
Sweet & Sour Noodles	1 cup	150	6	2	29
Teriyaki Chicken	1 cup (8.6 oz)	120	7	4	16
FRESH					
wonton wrapper	1 (0.3 oz)	23	1	tr	5
FROZEN					
Amy's					
Asian Noodle Stir Fry	1 pkg	290	9	7	50
Indian Mattar Paneer	1 pkg (10 oz)	320	11	8	54
Indian Palak Paneer	1 pkg (9.9 oz)	270	10	9	38
Indian Paneer Tikka	1 pkg (9.4 oz)	320	8	18	36
Indian Vegetable Korma	1 pkg (9.4 oz)	310	9	12	41
Thai Stir Fry	1 pkg (9.4 oz)	310	8	11	45
Contessa					
Chow Mein Chicken w/ Sauce not prep	1¾ cups	320	16	3	55

FOOD	PORTION	CALS	PROT	FAT	CARB
Curry Chicken w/ Sauce not prep	1¾ cups	240	12	8	29
Fried Rice Chicken w/ Sauce not prep	1¾ cups	260	17	4	49
General Tsao Shrimp w/ Sauce not prep	1¾ cups	270	10	4	49
Kung Pao Shrimp w/ Sauce not prep	1¾ cups	200	10	4	30
Lo Mein Shrimp w/ Sauce not prep	1¾ cups	250	11	10	29
Stir-Fry Beef w/ sauce not prep	1¾ cup	190	13	3	28
Stir-Fry Chicken w/ Sauce not prep	1¾ cups	160	16	3	18
Stir-Fry Shrimp w/ Sauce not prep	1¾ cups	120	9	3	16
Sweet & Sour Shrimp w/ Sauce not prep	1½ cups	180	9	0	40
Tandoori Chicken w/ Sauce not prep	1⅓ cups	200	15	4	27
Ethnic Gourmet					
Bhartha Eggplant	1 pkg (11 oz)	300	8	9	47
Dal Bahaar	1 pkg (11 oz)	360	13	8	61
Kaeng Kari Kai	1 pkg (10 oz)	390	20	11	54
Korma Chicken	1 pkg (10 oz)	340	21	9	44
Korma Vegetable	1 pkg (11 oz)	300	8	6	52
Kotopoulo Domato Ke Feta	1 pkg (10 oz)	340	20	11	41
Pad Thai Chicken	1 pkg (10 oz)	410	20	7	66
Pad Thai Shrimp	1 pkg (10 oz)	410	17	7	70
Tandoori Chicken w/ Spinach	1 pkg (10 oz)	170	14	5	19
French Meadow Bakery					
Vegetarian Dal Makhani	1 pkg (12 oz)	370	8	19	39
Gluten Free Cafe					
Asian Noodles	1 pkg (9.2 oz)	340	8	10	53
Glutino					
Gluten Free Chicken Pad Thai Peach	1 pkg (7 oz)	370	17	5	65
Healthy Choice					
Five Spice Beef & Vegetables	1 pkg (10 oz)	310	15	5	49
General Tso's Spicy Chicken	1 pkg (10.7 oz)	310	18	4	50

FOOD	PORTION	CALS	PROT	FAT	CARB
Helen's Kitchen					
Thai Yellow Curry w/ Tofu Steaks & Vegetables & Basmati Rice	1 pkg (9 oz)	280	12	5	30
Joy Of Cooking					
Lo Mein Vegetable	1 cup (7.7 oz)	220	9	3	40
Kahiki					
Beef & Broccoli	1 pkg (10.9 oz)	360	23	10	42
Chicken Fried Rice	1 pkg (10.9 oz)	460	16	10	75
General Tso's Chicken	1 pkg (10 oz)	400	12	10	66
Naturals General Tso's Chicken	1 pkg (10 oz)	330	18	5	52
Naturals Mandarin Orange Chicken	1 pkg (10 oz)	340	17	5	58
Naturals Szechuan Peppercorn Beef	1 pkg (10 oz)	350	19	14	35
Naturals Teriyaki Mixed Vegetables	1 pkg (10 oz)	260	8	2	51
Sesame Orange Chicken	1 pkg (10.9 oz)	420	15	12	60
Soothing Lettuce Wraps	4 tbsp (2 oz)	90	5	4	9
Tempura Chicken Nuggets	¾ cup (3.5 oz)	230	13	14	10
Tropical Sweet & Sour Chicken	1 pkg (10.9 oz)	490	14	11	82
Organic Classics					
Thai Chicken Curry	1 pkg (10 oz)	420	19	17	50
Tyson					
Meal Kit Chicken Fried Rice	2½ cups	440	27	6	69
MIX					
Nissin					
Chow Mein Chicken as prep	½ pkg (2 oz)	240	6	9	34
Chow Mein Thai Peanut as prep	½ pkg (2 oz)	270	6	12	35
SHELF-STABLE					
Healthy Choice					
Fresh Mixers Sesame Teriyaki Chicken	1 pkg (7.9 oz)	380	13	6	69
Fresh Mixers Sweet & Sour Chicken	1 pkg (7.9 oz)	390	12	3	78
Fresh Mixers Szechwan Beef w/ Asian Noodles	1 pkg (6.9 oz)	370	14	6	65
TAKE-OUT					
beef & broccoli	1 cup	221	18	12	10

FOOD	PORTION	CALS	PROT	FAT	CARB
beef w/ black bean sauce	1 serv (7 oz)	288	35	14	6
buddha's delight w/ cellophane noodles fat choi jai	1 serv (7.6 oz)	211	7	4	44
bun baked red bean	1 (1.1 oz)	102	3	3	16
cha siu bao steamed buns w/ chicken filling	1 (2.3 oz)	160	5	3	26
chicken masala	1 serv (8 oz)	430	44	25	8
chicken tandoori	1 serv (4 oz)	156	19	8	2
chicken tikka	1 serv (2.5 oz)	173	24	8	1
chinese garlic chicken	1 cup (5.7 oz)	290	22	19	8
chinese style fried egg noodles w/ seafood & lettuce	1 serv (14 oz)	694	27	37	63
chow mein beef w/o noodles	1 cup	271	22	15	12
chow mein chicken w/ noodles	1 cup (7.7 oz)	273	19	14	20
chow mein noodles	1 cup	237	4	14	26
chow mein pork w/o noodles	1 cup	284	22	16	12
chow mein shrimp w/o noodles	1 cup	154	16	5	11
chow mein vegetable w/o noodles	1 cup	224	5	15	16
dim sum deep fried beancurd w/ shrimp	1 (1.1 oz)	77	5	6	2
dim sum deep fried yam	1 (2.4 oz)	201	3	12	23
dim sum meat filled	3 pieces (4 oz)	124	13	3	11
dim sum steamed chives & prawns	1 (1.2 oz)	48	3	2	5
egg foo yung beef	1 patty (6 oz)	243	17	16	7
egg foo yung chicken	1 patty (3 oz)	121	8	8	4
egg foo yung pork	1 patty (3 oz)	125	8	8	4
egg foo yung shrimp	1 patty (3 oz)	153	8	12	3
filipino chicken adobo	1 serv (15 oz)	555	33	26	45
foochow fish ball	1 (1 oz)	36	2	2	3
fried rice	1 cup	333	12	12	42
fried rice beef	1 cup	346	12	14	42
fried rice chicken	1 cup	329	12	12	42
fried rice pork	1 cup	335	12	13	42
fried rice shrimp	1 cup	323	11	12	42
general tsao's chicken	1 cup (5 oz)	296	19	17	16
green beans szechuan style	1 cup	176	4	12	16
indian style fried egg noodles w/ eggs tomato sauce & lime	1 serv (15 oz)	721	29	31	80

FOOD	PORTION	CALS	PROT	FAT	CARB
korean spicy shredded chicken	1 serv (5 oz)	258	23	16	5
kung pao beef	1 cup	410	28	30	9
kung pao chicken	1 cup (5.7 oz)	434	29	31	12
kung pao pork	1 cup	460	26	34	12
kung pao shrimp	1 cup	345	30	20	11
lemon chicken w/o vegetables	1 serv (6.6 oz)	503	34	28	26
lo mein beef	1 cup	286	14	11	31
lo mein chicken	1 cup (7 oz)	280	16	9	33
lo mein meatless	1 cup	234	8	6	38
lo mein pork	1 cup	314	13	14	34
lo mein shrimp	1 cup	236	11	7	33
moo goo gai pan chicken	1 cup (7.6 oz)	272	15	19	12
moo shu pork w/o pancake	1 cup	512	19	46	5
pakhoras	1 (2.5 oz)	163	8	8	16
paneer pakhora	1 (2.2 oz)	183	8	13	8
peking duck w/ pancakes & seafood sauce	1 serv (14 oz)	1871	39	121	157
phad thai w/ chicken	1 cup (7 oz)	358	18	15	39
pork w/ chinese cabbage	1 serv (4 oz)	120	11	8	1
sesame seed paste bun	1 (2.5 oz)	220	5	6	39
shrimp chips banh phong tom	6 med	214	3	14	20
shrimp w/ lobster sauce	1 cup	298	35	12	8
shu mai chicken & vegetable dumplings	6 (3.6 oz)	160	10	5	18
sukiyaki beef	1 cup	165	19	7	6
sukiyaki chicken	1 serv (18 oz)	436	71	8	19
sweet & sour chicken w/o rice	1 cup	670	45	37	36
sweet & sour pork w/ rice	1 cup	268	13	6	40
sweet & sour pork w/o rice	1 cup	231	15	8	25
sweet & sour shrimp	1 cup	480	12	30	46
szechuan chicken	1 cup (5.7 oz)	180	16	9	9
szechuan shrimp & vegetables	1 cup	159	14	7	10
tempura vegetable	8 pieces	90	2	6	8
tempura hawaiian fish tofu vegetable	2 cups	285	11	22	13
teriyaki beef	1 cup	454	51	19	13
teriyaki chicken	¾ cup	399	30	27	7
teriyaki chicken w/ rice	1 serv (11 oz)	430	19	6	77
teriyaki shrimp	1 cup	271	39	3	14

FOOD	PORTION	CALS	PROT	FAT	CARB
thai style pineapple rice w/ ham & pork floss	1 serv (7.7 oz)	408	13	14	60
wonton fried meat filled	1 (0.7 oz)	54	3	3	5
wonton meat & shrimp boiled	1 (0.5 oz)	19	1	1	2

ASPARAGUS
CANNED

FOOD	PORTION	CALS	PROT	FAT	CARB
spears	1 cup	46	5	2	6
spears	1	3	tr	tr	tr
Del Monte					
Spears Extra Long	½ cup	20	2	0	3
Gertie's Finest					
White	1 oz	15	1	0	3
Green Giant					
Spears Extra Long	5	20	2	0	3
McSweet					
Pickled Spears	6 (1 oz)	25	0	0	6
Native Forest					
White	1 serv (4 oz)	20	2	0	3
S&W					
Spears	½ cup (4.4 oz)	20	2	0	3
FRESH					
cooked	½ cup	20	2	tr	4
cooked	4 spears	13	1	tr	2
spears raw	4	10	1	tr	2
Alpine Fresh					
Fresh Green	5 spears (3.3 oz)	20	2	0	5
Ocean Mist					
Spears	5 (3.3 oz)	25	2	0	4
FROZEN					
cooked	1 pkg (10 oz)	53	9	1	6
cooked	4 spears	11	2	tr	1
C&W					
Spears	7 (3 oz)	20	2	0	3
Joy Of Cooking					
Tender	½ cup (3.3 oz)	70	2	5	4

ATEMOYA

FOOD	PORTION	CALS	PROT	FAT	CARB
fresh	½ cup	94	1	1	24

FOOD	PORTION	CALS	PROT	FAT	CARB
AVOCADO					
california mashed	¼ cup	96	1	9	5
california peeled & pitted	1	289	3	27	15
florida mashed	¼ cup	69	1	6	5
florida peeled & pitted	1	365	7	31	24
Cabilfrut					
Hass fresh	⅕ med (1.1 oz)	55	tr	3	3
Chiquita					
Fresh	1 (7 oz)	322	4	29	17
Earthbound Farms					
Organic Fresh	⅕ med (1 oz)	55	1	5	3
Simply Avo					
Hass Avocado Pulp	2 tbsp	50	1	5	3
Hass Halves	⅙ pkg (1.1 oz)	50	1	5	3
Wholly Guacamole					
Classic	2 tbsp	50	1	4	2
Organic	2 tbsp	50	1	5	2
Pico De Gallo Style	2 tbsp	40	1	3	2
TAKE-OUT					
guacamole	1 serv (2.2 oz)	105	1	10	5
BACON					
bacon grease	1 tbsp	116	0	13	0
beef breakfast strips cooked	3 strips	153	11	12	tr
gammon lean & fat grilled	4.2 oz	274	35	15	0
pan fried	3 strips	109	6	9	tr
turkey	2 (0.8 oz)	84	7	6	1
Applegate Farms					
Natural Dry Cured Cooked	2 slices (0.5 oz)	60	4	5	0
Organic Turkey	1 slice (1 oz)	35	6	2	0
Boar's Head					
Fully Cooked Slices	3 (0.5 oz)	70	4	6	0
Butterball					
Turkey Bacon	1 slice (0.5 oz)	25	2	2	0
Hormel					
Microwave Ready	2 slices (0.5 oz)	80	5	7	0
Real Bits	1 tbsp (7 g)	25	3	2	0
Jimmy Dean					
Lower Sodium	1 slice (0.3 oz)	50	4	4	0
Original	1 slice (0.3 oz)	50	4	4	0
Thick Slice	1 slice (0.5 oz)	80	5	6	0

FOOD	PORTION	CALS	PROT	FAT	CARB
Oscar Mayer					
Bacon Bits	1 tbsp (7 g)	25	3	2	0
Hardwood Smoked	2 slices (0.5 oz)	70	4	6	0
Lower Sodium	3 slices (0.5 oz)	70	4	6	0
Ready To Serve	3 slices	70	5	5	0
Uncured	3 slices (0.5 oz)	60	7	5	1
Tyson					
Hickory Thick Cut	2 pieces (0.8 oz)	140	8	11	0
BACON SUBSTITUTES					
bacon bits meatless	1 tbsp	33	2	2	2
meatless	1 strip	16	1	1	tr
Bob's Red Mill					
Bac'Ums	4 tsp	25	3	1	2
Worthington					
Stripples	2 strips (0.5 oz)	60	2	5	2
BAGEL					
cinnamon raisin	1 lg (4 in)	244	9	2	49
cinnamon raisin	1 mini	71	3	tr	14
egg	1 lg (4.5 in)	364	14	3	69
low carb	1 (4 oz)	216	12	0	42
mini onion	1 (1.4 oz)	100	4	0	20
oat bran	1 lg (4 in)	227	10	1	47
plain	1 med (3.5 in)	289	11	2	56
plain	1 sm (3 in)	190	7	1	37
plain	1 lg (4.5 in)	360	14	2	70
Enjoy Life					
Nut Gluten Free Classic Original	1 (3 oz)	270	5	7	46
Finagle A Bagel					
Cinnamon Raisin	1 (4 oz)	300	8	1	67
Everything	1 (4 oz)	310	9	3	62
Onion	1 (4 oz)	300	9	1	65
Plain	1 (4 oz)	290	8	1	63
Poppy Seed	1 (4 oz)	310	11	4	60
Sesame	1 (4 oz)	310	10	5	60
French Meadow Bakery					
100% Spelt	1 (3.4 oz)	270	11	2	52
Hemp	1 (3.4 oz)	280	19	8	35
Sprouted Cinnamon Raisin	1 (3.5 oz)	270	15	2	50

FOOD	PORTION	CALS	PROT	FAT	CARB
Natural Ovens					
Blueberry	1 (3 oz)	250	11	2	47
Brainy	1 (3 oz)	230	11	3	40
Whole Wheat	1 (3 oz)	230	10	3	40
New York Style					
Crisps Natural Whole Wheat	6	120	4	6	16
Crisps Plain	7	140	3	6	17
Pepperidge Farm					
100% Whole Wheat	1	250	11	2	49
100% Whole Wheat Mini	1 (1.4 oz)	100	4	1	20
Everything	1	260	9	2	53
Plain Mini	1	110	4	1	22
Thomas'					
100% Whole Wheat Mini	1 (1.5 oz)	110	5	1	22
Bagel Holes Plain	3 (1.6 oz)	120	4	1	24
Bagelbread Mini Squares 100% Whole Wheat	1 (2 oz)	150	7	1	30
BAKING POWDER					
baking powder	1 tsp	2	0	0	1
low sodium	1 tsp	5	tr	tr	2
Bob's Red Mill					
Baking Powder	1 tsp	5	0	0	1
Calumet					
Double Acting	⅛ tsp	0	0	0	0
Davis					
Baking Powder	1 tsp	0	0	0	tr
BAKING SODA					
baking soda	1 tsp	0	0	0	0
Bob's Red Mill					
Baking Soda	¼ tsp	0	0	0	0
BALSAM PEAR (BITTER GOURD)					
leafy tips cooked w/o salt	1 cup	20	2	tr	4
leafy tips raw	1 cup	14	3	tr	2
pods raw sliced	1 cup	16	1	tr	3
pods sliced cooked w/ salt	1 cup	24	1	tr	5
BAMBOO SHOOTS					
canned sliced	½ cup	12	1	tr	2
fresh sliced cooked w/ salt	½ cup	7	1	tr	1
raw sliced	½ cup	20	2	tr	4

FOOD	PORTION	CALS	PROT	FAT	CARB
La Choy					
Bamboo Shoots	½ cup	10	tr	0	2
Polar					
Sliced	½ cup	25	1	0	3
BANANA					
baked	1 (4.5 oz)	163	2	tr	42
banana chips	1 oz	147	1	10	17
fresh	1 sm (6 in)	90	1	tr	23
fresh	1 lg (8 in)	121	1	tr	31
fresh	1 med (7 in)	105	1	tr	27
fresh baby	1 extra sm (<6 in)	72	1	tr	19
fresh mashed	½ cup	100	1	tr	26
fresh sliced	1 cup	134	2	1	34
green fried	1 (3.1 oz)	152	1	8	21
green pickled	½ cup	240	1	22	11
green sliced fried	1 cup	323	2	18	45
powder	1 tbsp	21	tr	tr	5
red ripe	1 (7 in)	93	1	tr	24
red ripe sliced	1 cup	134	2	1	34
whole dried	1 piece (1.2 oz)	130	1	1	33
Bob's Red Mill					
Chips	25 (1.4 oz)	210	0	11	26
Brothers-All-Natural					
Crisps	1 pkg (0.58 oz)	66	1	0	16
Chiquita					
Fresh	1 med (4.1 oz)	105	1	0	27
Crispy Green					
Freeze-Dried	1 pkg (0.5 oz)	55	1	0	13
Kopali					
Organic Dark Chocolate Covered	½ pkg (1 oz)	120	1	6	19
Nana Flakes					
100% Natural	1 tbsp (0.2 oz)	22	0	0	6
Tree Of Life					
Dried Sweetened	½ cup (1.6 oz)	240	1	15	27
TAKE-OUT					
batter dipped fried	1 sm (4 oz)	266	3	15	32
batter dipped fried sliced	1 cup	335	4	19	40

FOOD	PORTION	CALS	PROT	FAT	CARB
fried dwarf w/ cheese	1 (1.4 oz)	84	1	5	10
fritter	1 (2.3 oz)	197	1	5	36

BANANA JUICE
Snapple
Juice Drink Go Bananas	8 oz	110	0	0	28

BARBECUE SAUCE
barbecue	2 tbsp	52	0	tr	13
low sodium	2 tbsp	52	0	tr	13

Bear-Man
Black Bear Boogie	2 tbsp	40	0	1	8
Growlin' Grizzly	2 tbsp	60	1	1	12

Bone Suckin'
Sauce	2 tbsp	40	0	0	10

Cattlemen's
Classic	2 tbsp	60	tr	0	15
Smokehouse	2 tbsp	60	tr	0	14

Chef Hymie Grande
Cascabel Express Barbecue Glaze	2 tbsp (1.2 oz)	30	tr	0	7
Polapote Barbecue Glaze	2 tbsp (1.2 oz)	30	tr	0	7

Dave's Gourmet
Badlands BBQ	2 tbsp (1.1 oz)	40	1	1	8

Naturally Fresh
BBQ	2 tbsp	40	0	0	10

OrganicVille
Original No Added Sugar	2 tbsp (1 oz)	50	0	0	13

Ribber City
Kansas City	2 tbsp (1.1 oz)	40	0	0	11

The Gracious Gourmet
Spicy Barbeque Glaze	2 tbsp (1 oz)	35	1	1	7

World Harbors
Bar-B	2 tbsp (1.2 oz)	70	0	0	16
Buccaneer Blends Fra Diavlo	2 tbsp (1.2 oz)	45	1	0	11
Buccaneer Blends Honey Mango	2 tbsp (1.3 oz)	60	0	0	13
Buccaneer Blends Sticky Rum	2 tbsp (1.2 oz)	50	0	0	13

BARLEY
flour	1 cup	511	16	2	110
pearled cooked	1 cup (5.5 oz)	193	4	1	44
pearled uncooked	¼ cup	176	5	1	39

FOOD	PORTION	CALS	PROT	FAT	CARB
Arrowhead Mills					
Organic Pearled not prep	¼ cup	160	5	1	32
BARRACUDA					
broiled	4 oz	239	27	14	tr
cooked flaked	1 cup	287	32	16	1
poached	4 oz	227	29	11	0
TAKE-OUT					
breaded & fried	4 oz	282	26	17	5
BASIL					
fresh chopped	2 tbsp	1	tr	tr	tr
ground	1 tsp	4	tr	tr	1
leaves fresh	5	1	tr	tr	tr
BASS					
breaded baked	4 oz	205	25	7	10
pickled mero en escabeche	2 oz	156	7	14	tr
striped baked	3 oz	105	19	3	0
striped bass farm raised	4 oz	110	20	3	0
BAY LEAF					
crumbled	1 tsp	2	tr	tr	tr
BEAN SPROUTS (see ALFALFA, SPROUTS)					
BEANS (see also individual names)					
CANNED					
baked beans plain	½ cup	119	6	tr	27
baked beans vegetarian	½ cup	119	6	tr	27
baked beans w/ franks	½ cup	184	9	9	20
baked beans w/ pork	½ cup	134	7	2	25
baked beans w/ pork & tomato sauce	½ cup	119	7	1	24
refried beans	½ cup	134	8	1	23
Allens					
Original Baked	½ cup	150	6	1	29
Refried Black Beans No Fat Added	½ cup	120	7	0	23
Amy's					
Organic Refried	½ cup	140	8	3	21
Organic Refried Light In Sodium	½ cup (4.6 oz)	140	7	3	21

FOOD	PORTION	CALS	PROT	FAT	CARB
B&M					
Baked Original	½ cup (4.6 oz)	180	7	3	31
Barbeque Baked	½ cup (4.6 oz)	190	8	1	39
Country Style	½ cup (4.6 oz)	170	7	1	35
Vegetarian	½ cup (4.6 oz)	160	7	1	31
Bush's					
Honey	½ cup	160	6	1	32
Vegetarian Fat Free	½ cup	130	6	0	29
Campbell's					
Pork & Beans	½ cup	140	6	2	25
Gebhardt					
Refried	½ cup	90	6	2	16
Refried Fat Free	½ cup	80	6	0	17
Refried Jalapeno	½ cup	100	6	2	17
Green Giant					
Three Bean Salad	½ cup	80	3	0	18
Hormel					
Kid's Kitchen Microwave Meals Beans & Wieners	1 pkg (7.7 oz)	310	12	13	37
Old El Paso					
Refried Fat Free Spicy	½ cup	100	6	0	18
Pace					
Refried Salsa	½ cup	70	4	0	14
Read					
3 Bean Salad	⅓ cup	60	1	0	13
Rosarita					
Refried	½ cup	120	7	2	18
Refried Black Beans No Fat	½ cup	110	7	0	19
Refried Fat Free	½ cup	100	7	0	19
Refried Vegetarian	½ cup	120	7	2	19
Van Camp's					
Baked Beans Homestyle	½ cup	170	7	1	33
Beanee Weenee BBQ	1 can	260	15	8	35
Beanee Weenee Original	1 can	240	14	8	29
Beanee Weenee w/ Chili	1 can	240	14	9	26
Pork And Beans	½ cup	110	6	1	23
Wagon Master					
Pork & Beans	½ cup	130	7	1	23
TAKE-OUT					
baked beans	½ cup	191	7	7	27

FOOD	PORTION	CALS	PROT	FAT	CARB
barbecue beans	3.5 oz	120	4	tr	26
frijoles a la charra w/ pork tomatoes & chili peppers	1 cup	341	14	22	23
refried beans	½ cup	43	2	2	5
three bean salad	1 cup	114	4	5	15
BEAR					
simmered	3 oz	220	28	11	0
BEAVER					
roasted	4 oz	240	39	8	0
BEE POLLEN					
bee pollen	1 tsp (5 g)	16	1	tr	2
Tree Of Life					
Bee Pollen	1 tsp (7 g)	30	tr	1	3
BEECHNUTS					
dried	1 oz	163	2	14	10
BEEF (*see also* BEEF DISHES, JERKY, MEATBALLS, VEAL)					
CANNED					
corned beef	1 oz	71	8	4	0
Hormel					
Dried Beef	1 oz	50	8	2	1
Libby's					
Corned Beef	2 oz	120	14	7	0
Corned Beef Hash	1 cup	420	19	24	33
Potted Meat	¼ cup	120	9	9	0
Roast Beef w/ Gravy	⅔ cup	140	25	4	3
FRESH					
arm pot roast trim 0 fat braised	3.5 oz	297	29	19	0
arm pot roast trim ⅛ in fat braised	3.5 oz	302	30	19	0
beef crumbles 70% lean pan browned	3 oz	230	22	15	0
bottom round roast trim 0 fat braised	4 oz	253	38	10	0
bottom round roast trim 0 fat roasted	3.5 oz	187	27	8	0
bottom round roast trim ½ in fat braised	4 oz	337	22	22	0

FOOD	PORTION	CALS	PROT	FAT	CARB
bottom round roast trim ⅛ in fat braised	4 oz	280	37	13	0
bottom round roast trim ⅛ in fat roasted	4 oz	247	30	13	0
bottom sirloin butt roast trim 0 fat roasted	3.5 oz	182	27	8	0
brisket flat half trim ⅛ in fat braised	3.5 oz	298	29	19	0
brisket flat trim 0 fat braised	3.5 oz	221	32	9	0
brisket point half trim 0 fat braised	3.5 oz	358	24	29	0
brisket point half trim ¼ in fat braised	3.5 oz	404	22	22	0
brisket point half trim ⅛ in fat braised	3.5 oz	349	24	27	0
chuck boston cut roast trim 0 fat roasted	3.5 oz	207	26	11	0
chuck boston cut roast trim ¼ in fat roasted	3.5 oz	242	24	15	0
chuck bottom roast trim 0 fat braised	3.5 oz	334	27	24	0
chuck bottom roast trim ¼ in fat braised	3.5 oz	345	27	26	0
chuck fillet steak trim 0 fat broiled	4 oz	181	29	6	0
chuck top roast trim 0 fat broiled	4 oz	245	29	13	0
club steak trim ½ in fat broiled	4 oz	384	28	29	0
corned beef brisket cooked	3 oz	213	15	16	tr
crosscut shank trim ¼ in fat stewed	1 serv (6.8 oz)	510	60	28	0
delmonico steak trim ¼ in fat broiled	4 oz	409	27	33	0
entrecote steak trim ½ in fat broiled	4 oz	413	27	33	0
eye round roast trim 0 fat roasted	4 oz	190	33	5	0
eye round roast trim ¼ in fat roasted	4 oz	283	31	17	0

FOOD	PORTION	CALS	PROT	FAT	CARB
filet mignon roast trim ¼ in fat roasted	4 oz	376	27	29	0
filet mignon roast trim ⅛ in fat roasted	4 oz	367	27	28	0
filet mignon trim 0 fat broiled	4 oz	247	31	13	0
filet mignon trim ⅛ in fat broiled	4 oz	303	30	19	0
ground 70% lean broiled	3.5 oz	273	25	18	0
ground 75% lean broiled	2.5 oz	195	18	13	0
ground 80% lean broiled	3 oz	234	22	15	0
ground 85% lean pan fried	3 oz	197	21	12	0
ground 90% lean pan fried	3 oz	173	21	9	0
ground 95% lean pan fried	3 oz	139	22	5	0
ground lowfat w/ carrageenan raw	4 oz	160	20	7	tr
london broil trim 0 fat broiled	3.5 oz	188	28	8	0
london broil trim ¼ in fat broiled	4 oz	260	35	12	0
new york strip steak trim 0 fat broiled	4 oz	219	33	9	0
oxtails cooked	6 pieces (6.3 oz)	472	56	26	0
porterhouse steak trim 0 fat broiled	1 lb	1252	109	87	0
porterhouse steak trim ¼ in fat broiled	1 lb	1492	102	117	0
porterhouse steak trim ⅛ in fat broiled	4 oz	337	27	25	0
porterhouse steak trim ⅛ in fat broiled	1 lb	1324	107	99	0
rib eye roast trim ¼ in fat roasted	3.5 oz	365	23	30	0
rib eye steak trim ⅛ in fat broiled	4 oz	221	34	9	0
rib roast trim ¼ in fat roasted	4 oz	406	26	33	0
rib steak trim ¼ in fat broiled	4 oz	388	25	31	0
round tip roast trim 0 fat roasted	4 oz	213	30	9	0
sandwich steaks thinly sliced	1 serv (2 oz)	173	9	15	0
shell steak trim ¼ in fat broiled	4 oz	366	29	27	0

FOOD	PORTION	CALS	PROT	FAT	CARB
shortribs lean & fat braised	1 serv (7.8 oz)	1060	49	94	0
skirt steak trim 0 fat broiled	4 oz	289	27	19	0
t-bone steak trim 0 fat broiled	4 oz	280	27	18	0
t-bone steak trim ¼ in fat broiled	1 lb	1388	106	103	0
t-bone steak trim ⅛ in fat broiled	1 lb	804	70	56	0
tip round roast trim ⅛ in fat roasted	4 oz	248	31	13	0
top loin steak boneless trim ⅛ in fat broiled	4 oz	299	30	19	0
top round roast trim 0 fat braised	4 oz	237	40	7	0
top round roast trim ¼ in fat braised	4 oz	281	38	13	0
top round roast trim ¼ in fat roasted	4 oz	265	31	15	0
top round steak trim ¼ in fat pan fried	4 oz	314	37	17	0
top sirloin steak trim ⅛ in fat broiled	4 oz	275	31	16	0
top sirloin steak trim ⅛ in fat pan fried	4 oz	355	33	24	0
tri-tip roast trim 0 fat roasted	3.5 oz	218	26	12	0
tri-tip steak trim 0 fat broiled	4 oz	300	34	17	0
Laura's Lean					
Eye Of Round	4 oz	135	25	4	0
Ground Beef 92% Lean	4 oz	160	21	9	0
Ground Beef Patties	1 (4 oz)	160	21	9	0
Ground Round 96% Lean	4 oz	140	24	5	0
Sirloin Tip	4 oz	130	24	4	0
Top Round	4 oz	135	25	4	0
Organic Prairie					
90% Lean Ground	4 oz	250	30	13	0
Rumba					
Cheekmeat	4 oz	300	18	25	0
Crosscut Hind Shank	4 oz	190	23	10	0
Marrow Bones	4 oz	290	21	22	0
Oxtail	4 oz	260	21	21	0
Short Ribs	4 oz	400	17	36	0

FOOD	PORTION	CALS	PROT	FAT	CARB
FROZEN					
patty broiled medium	3 oz	240	21	17	0
Organic Prairie					
Rib Eye Steak	1 (6 oz)	470	47	31	0
READY-TO-EAT					
dried beef smoked chopped	1 oz	37	6	1	1
roast beef spread	¼ cup	127	9	9	2
Applegate Farms					
Organic Roast Beef	2 oz	80	12	3	0
Healthy Ones					
Deli Roast Beef	2 oz	70	9	2	1
Laura's Lean					
Beef Pot Roast Au Jus	3 oz	110	17	4	3
Oscar Mayer					
Slow Roasted Shaved	¼ pkg (1.8 oz)	60	10	3	0
Tyson					
Beef Strips Seasoned	1 serv (3 oz)	130	18	6	1
TAKE-OUT					
roast beef rare	2 oz	70	12	2	0
BEEF DISHES					
CANNED					
corned beef hash	3 oz	155	10	10	9
Hormel					
Beef Stew	1 pkg (7.5 oz)	150	10	6	15
Corned Beef	1 serv (2 oz)	120	15	6	0
Corned Beef Hash	1 cup (8.3 oz)	390	21	24	22
Corned Beef Hash 50% Reduced Fat	1 cup (8.3 oz)	290	21	12	24
Roast Beef Hash	1 cup (8.3 oz)	390	21	24	22
Roast Beef In Gravy	1 serv (5.8 oz)	130	18	3	8
Libby's					
Hawaiian Corned Beef	2 oz	120	14	7	0
FROZEN					
Quaker Maid					
Sandwich Steaks Pure Beef	1 serv (1.8 oz)	120	8	10	0
Tyson					
Steak Country Fried	1 (3.2 oz)	310	10	23	15
MIX					
Hamburger Helper					
Beef Pasta as prep	1 cup	270	4	10	24

FOOD	PORTION	CALS	PROT	FAT	CARB
Cheddar Cheese Melt as prep	1 cup	310	3	12	30
Cheesy Baked Potato as prep	1 cup	310	2	11	30
Chili Cheese as prep	1 cup	340	4	13	33
Double Cheesy Quesadilla as prep	1 cup	350	3	11	36
Italian Sausage as prep	1 cup	290	4	10	29
Microwave Singles Cheesy Lasagna	1 pkg	210	8	5	33
Philly Cheesesteak as prep	1 cup	320	4	13	27
Salisbury as prep	1 cup	260	4	10	27
Tomato Basil Penne as prep	1 cup	300	4	10	31
REFRIGERATED					
Hormel					
Beef Tips & Gravy	1 serv (4 oz)	170	21	8	4
Laura's Lean					
Meatloaf w/ Tomato Sauce	1 serv (5 oz)	230	19	8	27
Shredded Beef w/ Barbecue Sauce	1 serv (5 oz)	245	22	5	27
Tyson					
Chuck Roast w/ Vegetables	1 serv (4 oz)	320	18	21	14
Seasoned Meatloaf	1 serv (5 oz)	320	14	23	16
Steak Tips In Bourbon Sauce	1 serv (5 oz)	180	20	5	12
TAKE-OUT					
beef bourguignonne	1 cup	339	36	12	10
beef satay + peanut sauce	2 skewers	253	25	16	6
bool kogi korean marinated beef ribs	4 oz	190	18	10	6
bracciola	1 roll (4.7 oz)	276	27	14	8
bubble & squeak	5 oz	186	2	13	16
bulgoghi korean grilled beef	1 serv (5.2 oz)	256	23	15	5
chipped beef on toast	1 slice (5 oz)	226	11	10	22
cornish pasty	1 (8 oz)	847	20	52	79
goulash w/ potatoes	1 cup	298	27	12	19
greek moussaka	1 serv (8.5 oz)	450	24	33	12
irish stew	1 cup (7 oz)	280	23	16	10
kebab indian	1 (5.4 oz)	553	47	40	2
kheena	6.7 oz	781	34	71	1
koftas	5	280	18	22	3
meatloaf	1 lg slice (5 oz)	294	23	17	9

FOOD	PORTION	CALS	PROT	FAT	CARB
pepper steak	1 cup	317	28	20	5
pot roast w/ gravy	1 serv (6 oz)	320	54	10	4
samosa	2 (4 oz)	652	6	62	20
shepherd's pie	1 serv (7 oz)	282	16	16	20
sloppy joes	1 serv (9 oz)	398	39	6	48
steak & kidney pie w/ top crust	1 slice (5 oz)	400	21	26	23
stew w/ potatoes & vegetables	1 cup	199	16	5	22
stroganoff	1 cup	394	26	25	15
swiss steak w/ sauce	1 serv (8 oz)	234	26	10	8
toad in the hole	1 (4.7 oz)	383	10	29	23

BEEFALO

roasted	4 oz	213	35	7	0

BEER AND ALE

alcohol free beer	7 fl oz	50	1	tr	11
ale brown	10 oz	77	1	0	8
ale pale	10 oz	88	1	0	12
beer cooler	1 (16 oz)	194	1	0	34
beer light	12 oz can	103	1	0	6
beer regular	12 oz can	153	2	0	13
black & tan	1 serv (12 oz)	146	1	0	13
black velvet	1 (10 oz)	160	1	0	8
boilermaker	1 serv	216	1	0	13
lager	10 oz	80	1	0	4
lager & black	1 (14 oz)	241	1	0	39
mead	1 serv	250	1	0	13
pilsener lager	7 oz	85	1	tr	13
shandy	1 serv	125	1	0	12
stout	10 oz	102	1	0	6
trojan horse	1 (16 oz)	189	1	0	35

Michelob

Ultra	1 bottle (12 oz)	95	1	0	3

BEET JUICE

juice	7 oz	72	2	0	16

BEETS
CANNED

harvard	½ cup	90	1	tr	22
pickled	½ cup	74	1	tr	18
sliced	½ cup	37	1	tr	9

FOOD	PORTION	CALS	PROT	FAT	CARB
Freshlike					
Pickled Sliced	4 slices (1 oz)	20	0	0	4
Greenwood					
Harvard	1 serv (4.4 oz)	100	1	0	27
Pickled	1 oz	25	0	0	6
S&W					
Sliced	½ cup (4.3 oz)	35	1	0	8
Sliced Pickled	1 oz	15	0	0	4
FRESH					
greens cooked w/o salt	½ cup	19	2	tr	4
sliced cooked	½ cup	37	1	tr	8
whole cooked	2 med (3.5 oz)	44	2	tr	10

BEVERAGES (*see* BEER AND ALE, CHAMPAGNE, COFFEE, DRINK MIXERS, ENERGY DRINKS, FRUIT DRINKS, ICED TEA, LIQUOR/LIQUEUR, MALT, MILKSHAKE, SMOOTHIES, SODA, TEA/HERBAL TEA, WATER, WINE, YOGURT DRINKS)

BISCUIT
FROZEN

FOOD	PORTION	CALS	PROT	FAT	CARB
Jimmy Dean					
Snack Size Sausage On A Biscuit	2	400	9	30	24
MIX					
plain as prep	1 (2 oz)	190	4	7	27
Bisquick					
Heart Smart	⅓ cup	140	3	3	27
REFRIGERATED					
plain baked	1 (1 oz)	93	2	4	13
Pillsbury					
Buttermilk	3 (2.2 oz)	150	4	2	29
Flaky Layers	3 (2.2 oz)	160	4	4	28
Grands! Butter Tastin'	1 (2 oz)	190	4	9	24
Grands! Buttermilk Reduced Fat	1 (2 oz)	170	4	6	26
Grands! Golden Wheat Reduced Fat	1 (2.1 oz)	180	4	7	27
Grands! Original	1 (2 oz)	190	4	9	24
Grands! Original Reduced Fat	1 (2 oz)	170	4	6	26
Perfect Portions Butter Tastin'	1 (1.9 oz)	190	4	9	23
TAKE-OUT					
buttermilk	1 lg (2.7 oz)	280	5	13	37
oatcakes	2 (4 oz)	115	3	5	16
plain	1 sm (1.2 oz)	127	2	6	17

FOOD	PORTION	CALS	PROT	FAT	CARB
tea biscuit	1 (3 oz)	210	5	3	30
w/ egg	1 (4.8 oz)	373	12	22	32
w/ egg & bacon	1 (5.3 oz)	458	17	31	29
w/ egg & ham	1 (6.7 oz)	442	20	27	30
w/ egg & sausage	1 (6.3 oz)	581	19	39	11
w/ egg & steak	1 (5.2 oz)	410	18	28	21
w/ egg cheese & bacon	1 (5.1 oz)	477	16	31	33
w/ ham	1 (4 oz)	386	13	18	44
w/ sausage	1 (4.4 oz)	485	12	32	40

BLACK BEANS
dried cooked	1 cup	227	15	1	41
Allens					
Black Beans	½ cup	100	6	1	19
Goya					
Black Beans	½ cup (4.3 oz)	90	7	1	19
Tree Of Life					
Organic	½ cup (4.6 oz)	130	8	1	24

BLACKBERRIES
canned in heavy syrup	½ cup	118	2	tr	30
fresh	½ cup	31	1	tr	7
unsweetened frzn	½ cup	48	1	tr	12
Cascadian Farm					
Organic frzn	1 cup	80	1	1	22
Oregon					
In Light Syrup	½ cup	120	1	0	29

BLACKBERRY JUICE
canned	6 oz	65	1	1	13
Izze					
Sparkling Esque Blackberry	1 bottle (12 oz)	50	0	0	12

BLACKEYE PEAS
catjang dried cooked	1 cup (2.9 oz)	200	14	1	35
cooked	1 cup	198	13	1	36
cowpeas canned	1 cup	184	11	1	33
cowpeas frozen cooked	½ cup	112	7	tr	20
cowpeas leafy tips chopped cooked	1 cup	12	2	tr	1
cowpeas leafy tips raw chopped	1 cup	10	1	tr	2
w/pork	½ cup	199	7	4	40

FOOD	PORTION	CALS	PROT	FAT	CARB
TAKE-OUT					
blackeye peas & pork	1 cup	236	24	5	25
BLINTZE					
Golden					
Cheese	1 (2.1 oz)	80	6	2	13
Ratner's					
Cheese	1 (2.2 oz)	100	5	2	16
TAKE-OUT					
cheese	1 (2.7 oz)	160	5	9	15
BLUEBERRIES					
canned in heavy syrup	½ cup	113	1	tr	28
fresh	1 pt	229	3	1	58
fresh	½ cup	41	1	tr	11
frzn unsweetened	½ cup	40	tr	1	9
C&W					
Ultimate	¾ cup	70	0	0	16
Chukar Cherries					
Puget Sound Dried	¼ cup	160	tr	0	38
White Chocolate Covered	3 tbsp (1.4 oz)	223	2	12	26
De-Lite					
Dried Sweetened	1 oz	86	1	1	23
Emily's					
Dark Chocolate Covered	¼ cup (1.4 oz)	170	1	8	27
LiteHouse					
Glaze	3 tbsp	70	0	0	17
Marie's					
Glaze	2 tbsp	40	0	0	10
Stoneridge Orchards					
Organic Dried Wild Whole	⅓ cup (1.4 oz)	130	1	0	33
Whole Dried	⅓ cup (1.4 oz)	130	0	0	33
Sunsweet					
Dried	¼ cup (1.4 oz)	140	1	0	33
Tree Of Life					
Dried	¼ cup (1.5 oz)	150	4	0	38
BLUEBERRY JUICE					
Izze					
Sparkling Blueberry	1 bottle (12 oz)	120	0	0	33
Tart Is Smart					
Wild Blueberry Concentrate	0.5 oz	35	0	0	9

FOOD	PORTION	CALS	PROT	FAT	CARB
Walnut Acres					
Organic	8 oz	130	0	0	31
BLUEFIN					
fillet baked	4.1 oz	186	30	6	0
BLUEFISH					
fresh baked	3 oz	135	22	5	0
BOAR					
wild roasted	3 oz	136	24	4	0
Natural Frontier Foods					
Wild Boar Steaks	1 (4 oz)	170	25	8	0
BOK CHOY (see CABBAGE)					
BONITO					
dried	1 oz	50	8	2	0
fresh	3 oz	117	20	4	0
BORAGE					
fresh chopped	1 cup	19	2	tr	3
BOTTLED WATER (see WATER)					
BOYSENBERRIES					
frzn unsweetened	½ cup	33	1	tr	8
in heavy syrup	½ cup	113	1	tr	29
BRAINS					
beef pan fried	3 oz	167	11	13	0
beef simmered	3 oz	123	10	9	0
lamb braised	3 oz	123	11	9	0
lamb fried	3 oz	232	14	19	0
pork braised	3 oz	117	10	8	0
veal braised	3 oz	116	10	8	0
veal fried	3 oz	181	12	14	0
BRAN					
corn	1 cup (2.7 oz)	170	6	1	65
oat	½ cup (1.6 oz)	116	8	3	31
oat cooked	½ cup (3.8 oz)	44	4	1	13
rice	½ cup (2.1 oz)	187	8	12	29
wheat	½ cup (2 oz)	63	5	1	19

FOOD	PORTION	CALS	PROT	FAT	CARB
Bob's Red Mill					
Rice Bran	2 tbsp	60	2	3	8
Quaker					
Unprocessed	⅓ cup (0.6 oz)	35	3	1	11
Tree Of Life					
Oat Bran	½ cup (1.6 oz)	120	3	4	31
Organic Wheat Bran	¼ cup (1.1 oz)	190	4	18	4
BRAZIL NUTS					
dried unblanched	1 oz	186	4	19	4
BREAD					
CANNED					
boston brown	1 slice (1.6 oz)	88	2	1	19
B&M					
Raisin Brown Bread	½ in slice (2 oz)	130	3	1	29
FROZEN					
Cedarlane					
Organic Mediterranean Stuffed Focaccia	1 piece (4 oz)	295	13	10	37
Pepperidge Farm					
Garlic	1 slice (2.5 in)	170	4	7	24
Texas Toast Five Cheese	1 slice	150	4	7	18
Whole Grain Texas Toast	1 slice	150	4	8	14
MIX					
cornbread	1 piece (2 oz)	188	4	6	29
READY-TO-EAT					
anadama	1 piece (1.1 oz)	87	2	1	16
baguette whole wheat	2 oz	140	6	0	29
cassava	1 piece (3.5 oz)	299	3	1	71
challah	1 slice (1.4 oz)	115	4	2	19
cinnamon	1 slice (0.9 oz)	69	2	1	13
cracked wheat	1 slice (1.1 oz)	78	3	1	15
cuban bread	1 slice (1.1 oz)	83	3	1	16
french	1 slice (1.1 oz)	88	3	1	17
italian	1 loaf (1 lb)	1255	41	4	256
navajo fry	1 piece	281	6	10	41
oat bran	1 slice (1.1 oz)	71	3	1	12
oatmeal	1 slice (0.9 oz)	73	2	1	13

FOOD	PORTION	CALS	PROT	FAT	CARB
pan criollo	1 piece (0.9 oz)	69	2	1	13
pannetone	1 slice (0.9 oz)	86	2	2	15
pita	1 sm (1 oz)	77	3	tr	16
pita	1 lg (2 oz)	165	5	1	33
pita whole wheat	1 lg (2.2 oz)	170	6	2	35
pita whole wheat	1 sm (1 oz)	74	3	1	15
pumpernickel	1 slice (0.9 oz)	65	2	1	12
raisin	1 slice (1.1 oz)	88	3	1	17
rye	1 slice (1.1 oz)	83	3	1	15
seven grain	1 slice (1.1 oz)	80	3	1	15
wheat berry	1 slice (0.9 oz)	65	2	1	12
wheat bran	1 slice (1.3 oz)	89	3	1	17
wheat germ	1 slice (1 oz)	73	3	1	14
white cubed	1 cup	93	3	1	18
whole wheat	1 slice (1 oz)	69	3	1	13
Alvarado Street Bakery					
Sprouted Soy Crunch	1 slice (1.2 oz)	90	5	1	15
Sprouted Whole Wheat	1 slice	90	4	1	19
Arnold					
100% Natural Soft Honey Wheat	2 slices (2 oz)	150	6	2	28
Grains & More Double Omega	1 slice	110	5	2	19
Jewish Rye	1 slice	90	2	2	17
Sandwich Thins Multi-Grain	1 (1.5 oz)	100	4	1	22
Sandwich Thins Whole Grain White	1 (1.5 oz)	100	4	1	22
Whole Grains 100% Whole Wheat Double Fiber	1 slice	100	4	2	21
Whole Grains 12 Grain	1 slice	110	5	2	21
Whole Grains 15 Grain	1 slice	110	5	2	21
Whole Grains 7 Grain	1 slice	110	4	2	22
Aunt Gussie's					
Gluten Free Focaccia Bread Kalamata Olive	1 piece (2.7 oz)	180	3	2	37
Gluten Free Focaccia Bread Rosemary	1 piece (2.7 oz)	180	3	2	38
Baker's Inn					
9 Grain	1 slice	100	5	2	18
Cracked Wheat	1 slice	100	4	2	18

FOOD	PORTION	CALS	PROT	FAT	CARB
Honey White Made w/ Whole Grain	1 slice	110	4	2	19
Honey Whole Wheat	1 slice	100	4	2	19
Potato Made w/ Whole Grain	1 slice	100	4	2	18
Comfort Care					
Cabin Hearth Whole Wheat	1 oz	170	9	3	31
Ecce Panis					
Classic Ciabatta	⅛ loaf (2 oz)	180	6	2	36
Freihofer's					
100% Whole Wheat	1 slice	90	4	2	17
French Meadow Bakery					
100% Rye Salt Free	1 slice (1.6 oz)	90	2	0	23
100% Spelt	2 slices (2.4 oz)	170	6	1	33
European Sourdough Rye	1 slice (1.7 oz)	90	2	0	22
Gluten Free Multigrain	1 slice (1.8 oz)	150	4	5	23
Hemp	2 slices (2.4 oz)	200	13	5	24
Kamut	2 slices (3 oz)	170	8	1	31
Men's Bread	2 slices (2.4 oz)	200	15	8	17
Our Daily Bread	2 slices (2.4 oz)	160	10	3	24
Sprouted Cinnamon Raisin	1 slice (1.5 oz)	100	2	1	19
Summer	1 slice (1.2 oz)	90	4	0	17
Gillian's Foods					
Gluten Free Cinnamon Raisin	1 slice (2 oz)	130	5	1	25
La Tortilla Factory					
Wraps Smart & Delicious Gluten Free Dark Teff	1 (2.3 oz)	180	2	5	31
Wraps Smart & Delicious Gluten Free Ivory Teff	1 (2.3 oz)	180	2	5	30
Mrs. Baird's					
Acti-Fiber Wheat	2 slices (2.2 oz)	160	5	3	30
Whole Grain Wheat Sugar Free	1 slice (1.1 oz)	70	4	2	13
Natural Ovens					
100% Sweet Whole	1 slice	90	4	2	16
Carb Conscious Original	1 slice	80	8	2	9

FOOD	PORTION	CALS	PROT	FAT	CARB
Healthy Beginnings Better White	1 slice	110	5	2	20
Healthy Beginnings Honey Wheat	1 slice	120	4	2	21
Hunger Filler Whole Grain	1 slice	100	5	2	15
Organic Plus Whole Grain & Flax	1 slice	120	4	2	22
Whole Grain Oat Nut Crunch	1 slice	100	5	3	15
Nature's Own					
100% Whole Wheat	1 slice	50	4	1	10
9 Grain	1 slice	120	4	2	24
Hearty Oatmeal	1 slice	100	5	2	18
Wheat Double Fiber	1 slice	10	4	1	10
Wheat Light	2 slices	80	5	1	19
Wheat N' Fiber	1 slice	60	6	1	7
Whole Wheat w/ Organic Flour	1 slice	100	5	2	21
Nature's Pride					
100% Whole Wheat	1 slice (1.5 oz)	110	5	1	20
100% Whole Wheat Double Fiber	1 slice (1.5 oz)	100	4	1	20
Country Buttermilk	1 slice (1.5 oz)	110	4	2	21
Healthy Multi-Grain	1 slice (1.5 oz)	110	5	9	20
Honey Wheat	1 slice (1 oz)	70	3	1	13
Nutty Oat	1 slice (1.5 oz)	110	5	2	19
Oroweat					
100% Whole Wheat	1 slice (1.3 oz)	100	41	1	19
Country Potato	1 slice (1.3 oz)	100	3	1	20
Country Whole Grain White	1 slice (1.3 oz)	90	4	2	17
Double Fiber	1 slice (1.3 oz)	70	4	1	16
Honey Fiber Whole Grain	1 slice (1.3 oz)	80	4	1	18
Russian Rye	1 slice (1 oz)	80	3	1	13
Seven Grain	1 slice (1.3 oz)	100	3	1	20
Whole Grain & Flax	1 slice (1.3 oz)	100	4	2	17
Pepperidge Farm					
100% Natural Whole Grain German Dark Wheat	1 slice	100	4	2	20
Breakfast Apple & Grains	1 slice	90	4	2	18
Canadian White	1 slice	100	3	2	18
Carb Style 7 Grain	1 slice	60	5	2	8
Farmhouse Hearty White	1 slice	120	4	2	22
Farmhouse Honey Wheatberry	1 slice	120	4	2	22

FOOD	PORTION	CALS	PROT	FAT	CARB
Farmhouse Whole Grain White	1 slice (1.5 oz)	110	4	2	21
Fruit & Grain Cranberry Orange	1 slice (1.4 oz)	90	4	2	19
Honey Flax Whole Grain	1 slice (1.5 oz)	100	5	2	19
Hot & Crusty Italian	1 slice (2 in thick)	150	5	2	29
Jewish Rye Whole Grain Seeded	1 slice	70	3	1	14
Light Style 7 Grain	1 slice	45	2	0	9
Light Style Oatmeal	3 slices	140	7	1	27
Party Pumpernickel	5 slices	130	5	2	23
Very Thin White	3 slices	120	4	1	24
Vitality Oats & Barley	1 slice (1.5 oz)	120	4	2	21
Whole Grain 100% Soft Whole Wheat Double Fiber	1 slice	100	4	2	21
Whole Grain Soft Honey Oat	1 slice (1.5 oz)	100	5	2	19
Whole Grain Swirl Cinnamon w/ Raisins	1 slice (1 oz)	80	3	1	13
Roman Meal					
Muesli	1 slice (1.5 oz)	110	5	2	19
Original Whole Grain	2 slices (2 oz)	130	5	2	25
Rudi's Organic Bakery					
100% Whole Wheat	1 slice	100	4	1	19
14 Grain	1 slice	90	4	1	19
Artisan Country French	1 slice	100	4	1	20
Artisan Rosemary Olive Oil	1 slice	100	3	1	19
Low Carb Right Choice	1 slice	45	4	1	7
Spelt Ancient Grain	1 slice	120	4	3	20
Whole Grain Apple N Spice	1 slice	110	4	1	24
S. Rosen's					
Hawaiian	1 slice	110	3	2	21
Rye Black Bavarian	1 slice	100	3	2	19
Sara Lee					
Soft & Smooth 100% Whole Wheat	1 slice	70	3	1	12
Soft & Smooth Whole Grain White	2 slices	150	6	2	28
Sonoma					
Wraps Organic Multi Grain	1 (2.4 oz)	180	6	7	27
Wraps Organic Wheat	1 (2.4 oz)	190	5	7	30
Wraps Original White Whole Wheat	1 (2.4 oz)	200	6	5	33

FOOD	PORTION	CALS	PROT	FAT	CARB
Stroehmann					
Dutch Country Twelve Grain	1 slice	100	4	2	18
Potato	1 slice	100	3	2	18
Soft Rye Seeded	1 slice	90	3	2	16
Sun-Maid					
Raisin Cinnamon Swirl	1 slice (1.2 oz)	100	3	2	18
The Baker					
Yoga Bread	1 slice	70	3	1	13
Thomas'					
Breakfast Original	1 slice	90	4	1	17
Sahara Pita Pockets Mini Whole Wheat	1 (1 oz)	70	3	1	13
Swirl Cinnamon Raisin	1 slice	120	3	2	21
Tumaro's					
Wraps Chipotle Chili & Peppers	1 (2.3 oz)	170	4	2	34
Wraps Sun Dried Tomato & Basil	1 (2.3 oz)	170	5	2	34
Wonder					
Classic White	1 slice (1 oz)	70	4	1	2
Classic White Sandwich	1 slice (0.9 oz)	60	2	1	13
REFRIGERATED					
Pillsbury					
Italian	⅛ pkg (1.6 oz)	110	4	2	21
TAKE-OUT					
banana	1 slice (2 oz)	196	3	6	33
chapati as prep w/ fat	1 (1.6 oz)	95	3	2	18
chapati as prep w/o fat	1 (2.5 oz)	141	5	1	31
cornbread	1 piece (2.3 oz)	183	4	6	27
cornstick	1 (1.4 oz)	118	3	4	18
focaccia onion	1 piece (4.6 oz)	282	6	10	43
focaccia rosemary	1 piece (3.5 oz)	251	6	7	40
focaccia tomato olive	1 piece (4.7 oz)	270	6	8	42
garlic bread	1 slice (1 oz)	96	2	4	13
irish soda bread	1 slice (3 oz)	247	6	4	48
italian garlic	1 loaf (11 oz)	990	23	38	137
naan	1 bread (3.5 oz)	286	7	9	43

FOOD	PORTION	CALS	PROT	FAT	CARB
papadum fried	1 (6 g)	30	1	2	2
paratha plain	1 (1.6 oz)	136	3	5	19
poori indian puffed bread	1 piece (1.3 oz)	112	3	4	16
zucchini	1 slice (1.4 oz)	150	2	7	19

BREAD COATING
Zatarain's
Crispy Seasoned Fish-Fri	2 tbsp	50	1	0	11

BREADCRUMBS
dry seasoned	¼ cup	115	4	2	21
fresh	¼ cup	30	1	tr	6
plain	¼ cup	107	4	1	19

Edward & Sons
Organic Lightly Salted	⅓ cup	110	7	1	21
Organic Panko	⅓ cup	110	2	1	21

Gillian's Foods
Plain Gluten Free	¼ cup (1.2 oz)	60	2	1	14

Krasdale
Seasoned	¼ cup	120	4	2	21

Progresso
Garlic & Herb	¼ cup (1 oz)	110	4	2	19
Plain	¼ cup (1 oz)	110	4	2	20

Southern Homestyle
Corn Flake Crumbs	2 tbsp	40	1	0	9
Tortilla Crumbs	2 tbsp	40	1	0	9

BREADFRUIT
fresh	1 sm (13.5 oz)	396	4	1	104
fried	1 cup	379	2	21	52
raw	1 cup	227	2	1	60

BREADNUTTREE SEEDS
dried	1 oz	104	2	tr	23

BREADSTICKS
plain	1 sm	21	1	tr	3
plain	1 lg	41	1	1	7

Fattorie & Pandea
Fornini w/ Sea Salt	5 (1.2 oz)	140	4	5	21

Ferrara
Slim Thin Torinese Style	6 (0.5 oz)	60	2	1	11

FOOD	PORTION	CALS	PROT	FAT	CARB
Pepperidge Farm					
Garlic frzn	1	160	5	5	25
Pillsbury					
Cornbread Twists	1 (1.4 oz)	140	3	6	18
Original Soft	2 (1.8 oz)	140	4	3	25
Stella D'Oro					
Original	1 (0.3 oz)	40	1	1	6
Roasted Garlic	1	45	1	1	7
Sesame	1 (0.4 oz)	50	2	3	6
Sodium Free	1 (0.3 oz)	40	1	1	6

BREAKFAST BARS (see CEREAL BARS, ENERGY BARS)

BROCCOFLOWER

fresh raw	½ cup (1.8 oz)	16	1	tr	3

BROCCOLI

FRESH					
chinese broccoli (gai lan) cooked	½ cup	10	1	tr	2
raab cooked	½ cup	28	3	tr	3
raw	1 bunch (1.3 lbs)	207	17	2	40
raw flower	1 piece	3	tr	tr	1
raw flowers	1 cup	20	2	tr	4
BroccoSprouts					
Broccoli Sprouts	½ cup	16	1	0	2
Mann's					
Broccoli Wokly	1 serv (3 oz)	25	3	0	4
Broccolini	8 stalks (3 oz)	35	3	0	6
Ocean Mist					
Rapini Broccoli Rabe Chopped Raw	1 cup	9	1	0	1
FROZEN					
chopped cooked	½ cup	26	3	tr	5
spears cooked	½ cup	26	3	tr	5
spears cooked	1 pkg (10 oz)	70	8	tr	13
Birds Eye					
Broccoli & Cheese Sauce	½ cup	90	3	5	8
Steamfresh Cuts	1 cup (3.1 oz)	30	2	0	4
Steamfresh Florets	1 cup (2.3 oz)	30	1	0	4

FOOD	PORTION	CALS	PROT	FAT	CARB
C&W					
Broccoli & Cheddar Cheese Sauce	1⅓ cups	70	4	3	7
Florets	1 cup	30	1	0	4
Cascadian Farm					
Organic Florets	⅔ cup	20	2	0	4
Dr. Praeger's					
Broccoli Bites	2 (2 oz)	110	3	4	17
Green Giant					
Broccoli & Cheese Sauce	⅔ cup	60	2	3	7
Cuts as prep	⅔ cup	25	1	0	4
Pasta Broccoli & Alfredo Sauce as prep	1 cup	210	9	4	34
TAKE-OUT					
batter dipped & fried	4 pieces	77	2	5	6
w/ cheese sauce	1 cup	242	12	15	16
BROWNIE					
brownie	1 (2 oz)	227	3	9	36
butterscotch	1 (1.2 oz)	151	2	8	19
Arrowhead Mills					
Gluten Free as prep	1	160	1	8	21
Betty Crocker					
Dark Chocolate as prep	1	170	1	7	25
Dark Chocolate as prep	1	160	1	7	24
Fudge Low Fat as prep	1	140	1	3	28
Original Supreme as prep	1	160	1	6	26
Triple Chunk as prep	1	180	1	8	25
Walnut as prep	1	170	1	9	22
Warm Delights Hot Fudge	1 pkg (3 oz)	370	5	12	61
Bob's Red Mill					
Gluten Free as prep	1	140	2	5	27
Duncan Hines					
Chocolate Fudge frzn	1/12 pkg (1.4 oz)	170	2	8	23
Dark Chocolate Chunk Mix as prep	1/16 pkg	170	2	7	25
Milk Chocolate Mix as prep	1/20 pkg	180	2	9	23
Peanut Butter Cup Mix as prep	1/16 pkg	170	2	8	23
Turtle Mix as prep	1/16 pkg	160	2	7	23
Walnut Mix as prep	1/16 pkg	180	2	8	24

FOOD	PORTION	CALS	PROT	FAT	CARB
Erin Baker's					
Organic Bites	1 (1 oz)	100	2	3	18
Organic Bites Double Chocolate Chip	1 (1 oz)	90	2	2	19
Foxy's Bake Shop					
Milk Chocolate	½ (1.7 oz)	200	3	11	23
White Chocolate	½ (1.7 oz)	200	3	12	23
French Meadow Bakery					
Gluten Free Fudge Bites	2 (1.3 oz)	170	2	7	26
Glenny's					
100 Calorie 75% Organic	1 (1.45 oz)	100	4	4	12
Hershey's					
Brownie	½ pkg (1.5 oz)	190	2	9	28
Pillsbury					
Traditional Chocolate Fudge	1 (1.4 oz)	150	2	6	24
Turtle Supreme Bars	1 (1.4 oz)	180	2	9	23
VitaBrownie					
Dark Chocolate Pomegranate	1 (2 oz)	100	3	2	21
Deep Velvety Chocolate	1 (2 oz)	100	4	3	23
BRUSSELS SPROUTS					
FRESH					
cooked	6 pieces	45	3	1	9
Ocean Mist					
Brussels Sprouts	4 (2 oz)	40	2	1	6
Select Gourmet					
Fresh	½ cup	35	3	0	8
FROZEN					
cooked	1 cup	65	6	1	13
Birds Eye					
Steamfresh Baby	10 (2.9 oz)	45	3	0	8
Steamfresh Singles Baby	1 pkg (3.2 oz)	50	3	0	9
C&W					
Petite	10 (3 oz)	45	3	0	8
Green Giant					
Baby & Butter Sauce as prep	½ cup	60	3	1	9
BUCKWHEAT					
groats roasted cooked	1 cup (6 oz)	155	7	1	33
groats roasted uncooked	½ cup	292	11	3	61

FOOD	PORTION	CALS	PROT	FAT	CARB
Bob's Red Mill					
Organic Kernels	¼ cup	142	5	1	31
BUFFALO (*see also* JERKY)					
burger	3 oz	202	20	13	0
chuck braised	4 oz	205	36	6	0
top round steak broiled	3 oz	313	54	9	0
water buffalo roasted	3 oz	111	23	2	0
Natural Frontier Foods					
Burgers	1 (5 oz)	170	22	9	0
Ground	4 oz	170	22	9	0
Steaks	1 (4 oz)	160	28	3	0
BULGUR					
cooked	½ cup	76	3	tr	17
uncooked	½ cup	239	9	1	53
Bob's Red Mill					
From Soft White Wheat	¼ cup	150	4	1	32
Near East					
Whole Grain Wheat Pilaf as prep	1 cup	200	7	4	40
TAKE-OUT					
tabbouleh	1 cup	198	3	15	16
BURBOT (FISH)					
fresh baked	3 oz	98	65	1	0
BURDOCK ROOT					
cooked w/o salt	1 root (5.8 oz)	146	3	tr	35
cooked w/o salt	1 cup	110	3	tr	26
BUTTER					
clarified butter	1 tbsp (0.4 oz)	112	tr	13	0
clarified butter	¼ cup (1.8 oz)	449	tr	51	0
honey butter	¼ cup (2.5 oz)	338	tr	23	36
honey butter	1 tbsp (0.6 oz)	85	tr	6	9
light butter whipped salted	1 tbsp (0.3 oz)	48	tr	5	0
stick salted	1 (4 oz)	810	1	92	tr
stick salted	1 tbsp (0.5 oz)	102	tr	12	tr
stick salted	¼ cup (2 oz)	407	tr	46	tr
stick unsalted	1 (4 oz)	810	1	92	tr
stick unsalted	¼ cup (2 oz)	407	tr	46	tr
stick unsalted	1 tbsp (0.5 oz)	102	tr	12	tr
whipped salted	¼ cup (1.3 oz)	271	tr	31	tr
whipped salted	1 tbsp (0.3 oz)	67	tr	8	tr

FOOD	PORTION	CALS	PROT	FAT	CARB
Cabot					
Salted	1 tbsp	100	0	11	0
Country Crock					
Spreadable Butter w/ Canola Oil	1 tbsp (0.4 oz)	80	0	9	0
Deerfield					
Creamy	1 tbsp	100	0	11	0
Earth Balance					
Butter Blend Unsalted	1 tbsp	100	0	11	0
Horizon Organic					
European	1 tbsp	100	0	12	0
Land O' Lakes					
Light Salted	1 tbsp (0.5 oz)	50	0	6	0
Light Whipped Salted	1 tbsp (0.4 oz)	45	0	5	0
Salted	1 tbsp (0.5 oz)	100	0	11	0
Spreadable w/ Canola Oil	1 tbsp (0.5 oz)	100	0	11	0
Whipped Salted	1 tbsp (0.2 oz)	50	0	6	0
Organic Valley					
European Style	1 tbsp	110	0	12	0
Straus					
Organic European Style Lightly Salted	1 tbsp (0.5 oz)	110	0	12	0
Organic European Style Sweet Butter	1 tbsp (0.5 oz)	110	0	12	0

BUTTER SUBSTITUTES

stick	1 stick	811	1	91	1
Butter Buds					
Granules	1 pkg (2 g)	5	0	0	2
Sunsweet					
Lighter Bake	1 tbsp	35	0	0	9

BUTTERBUR

canned fuki chopped	1 cup	3	tr	tr	tr
fresh fuki	1 cup	13	tr	tr	3

BUTTERNUTS

dried	1 oz	174	7	16	3

BUTTERSCOTCH (see also CANDY)

E. Guittard					
Baking Chips	33 (0.5 oz)	80	tr	5	10

FOOD	PORTION	CALS	PROT	FAT	CARB
Hershey's					
Chips	1 tbsp (0.5 oz)	80	1	4	9
CABBAGE (*see also* COLESLAW)					
chinese bok choy shredded cooked w/o salt	1 cup	20	3	tr	3
chinese pe-tsai shredded cooked w/o salt	1 cup	17	2	tr	3
green raw shredded	1 cup	19	1	tr	4
green shredded cooked w/o salt	1 cup	34	2	tr	8
japanese pickled	½ cup	22	1	tr	4
red raw shredded	1 cup	22	1	tr	5
red shredded cooked w/o salt	1 cup	44	2	tr	10
savoy shredded cooked w/o salt	1 cup	35	3	tr	8
Aunt Nellie's					
Sweet & Sour Red	¼ cup	40	0	0	10
Glory					
Country Cabbage	½ cup	25	1	0	6
TAKE-OUT					
creamed	1 cup	158	5	10	13
kimchee	1 cup	32	2	tr	6
stuffed cabbage w/ rice & beef	1 (3.6 oz)	117	9	5	9
sweet & sour red cabbage	4 oz	61	1	3	8
CACAO					
Kopali					
Organic Dark Chocolate Covered Cacao Nibs	½ pkg (1 oz)	140	2	10	15
Navitas Naturals					
Butter	1 tbsp	120	0	14	0
Nibs	1 oz	130	4	12	10
Powder	1 oz	120	5	3	18
Sunfood					
Organic Cacao Beans	1 oz	171	4	13	8
Organic Cacao Nibs	1 oz	171	4	13	8
CACTUS					
fresh cooked w/ fat	1 pad (1 oz)	11	tr	1	1
fresh cooked w/o fat	1 cup (5.2 oz)	22	2	tr	5
pricklypear	1 (3.6 oz)	42	1	1	10
pricklypear fresh	1 cup (5.2 oz)	61	1	1	14

FOOD	PORTION	CALS	PROT	FAT	CARB
CAKE (see also CAKE MIX)					
battenburg cake	1 slice (2 oz)	204	3	10	28
cream puff shell	1 (2.3 oz)	239	6	17	15
crumpet	1 (2.3 oz)	131	4	1	31
dutch honey cake	1 slice (0.8 oz)	70	1	0	17
eccles cake	1 slice (2 oz)	285	2	16	36
madeira cake	1 slice (1 oz)	98	1	4	15
sponge	1 piece (1.3 oz)	110	2	1	23
sponge cake dessert shell	1 (0.8 oz)	70	1	2	12
treacle tart	1 slice (2.5 oz)	258	3	10	42
Amy's					
Organic Chocolate	1 slice	170	2	6	27
Toaster Pops Apple	1 (2.1 oz)	150	3	4	27
Aunt Trudy's					
Organic Baklava Soy Nut	1 (1.8 oz)	190	4	6	29
Balocco					
Il Panettone	1 serv (3.5 oz)	380	7	15	54
Bellino					
Pandoro	1 (2.8 oz)	330	7	16	39
Betty Crocker					
Warm Delights Cinnamon Swirl	1 (3.3 oz)	390	4	10	72
Earth Cafe					
Cheesecake Vegan Blueberry Thrill	1 slice (2 oz)	193	3	15	12
Cheesecake Vegan Coconut Carob	1 slice (2 oz)	206	3	16	13
Cheesecake Vegan Rockin' Raspberry	1 slice (2 oz)	194	3	15	12
El Monterey					
Cheesecake Bites Caramel	1 (2 oz)	180	2	10	23
Cheesecake Bites Raspberry	1 (2 oz)	200	3	11	21
Entenmann's					
Cheese Cake Deluxe French	⅙ cake (3.8 oz)	390	6	24	39
Fillo Factory					
Organic Apple Strudel	1 (4.4 oz)	290	3	10	47
Organic Apple Turnovers	1 (3 oz)	180	2	6	30
French Meadow Bakery					
Gluten Free Cupcake Chocolate	1 (2 oz)	220	24	8	35
Gluten Free Cupcake Yellow	1 (2 oz)	230	20	9	35
Vegan Carrot	¼ cake (2.6 oz)	13	2	0	38

FOOD	PORTION	CALS	PROT	FAT	CARB
Glenny's					
Blondie 100 Calorie 75% Organic	1 (1.45 oz)	100	4	3	12
Gourmet Pastries					
Baklava Walnut	1 piece (1.8 oz)	240	3	11	30
Guiltless Gourmet					
Dessert Bowl Bananas Foster Cake	1 pkg (2 oz)	200	3	2	42
Dessert Bowl Black Velvet Cake	1 pkg (2 oz)	200	4	3	42
Hostess					
100 Calorie Pack Mini Carrot Cake	1 pkg (1.2 oz)	100	2	3	20
100 Calorie Pack Mini Chocolate Cupcakes	1 pkg (1.3 oz)	100	2	3	22
100 Calorie Pack Mini Coffee Cake Cinnamon Streusel	1 pkg (1.2 oz)	100	2	3	21
100 Calorie Pack Mini Golden Cupcakes	1 pkg (1.2 oz)	100	2	3	20
Cup Cakes Chocolate	1 (1.8 oz)	170	1	6	30
Ho Hos	1	120	1	6	18
Twinkies	1 (1.5 oz)	150	1	5	27
Lance					
Honey Bun	1 (3 oz)	320	4	13	47
Mrs. Freshley's					
Golden Cupcakes Creme Filled	1 pkg (1.3 oz)	100	2	3	24
Mrs. Smith's					
Carrot	⅙ cake (2.9 oz)	300	3	16	37
Cobbler Blackberry	1 serv (4 oz)	260	2	10	43
Singles Heavenly 100 New York Cheesecake	1 (0.9 oz)	100	2	6	9
Neuman's					
Date Nut Bread	1 oz	90	2	2	17
Pepperidge Farm					
Chocolate Coconut 3 Layer	⅛ cake	240	2	10	33
Devil's Food 3 Layer	⅛ cake	220	2	9	34
Golden 3 Layer	⅛ cake	230	2	9	34
Lemon 3 Layer	⅛ cake	240	2	11	34
Turnover Apple	1	290	4	15	36
Turnover Peach	1	290	4	15	35

FOOD	PORTION	CALS	PROT	FAT	CARB
Pillsbury					
Caramel Rolls	1 (1.7 oz)	170	2	7	24
Cinnamon Rolls w/ Icing	1 (3.5 oz)	310	5	9	54
Cinnamon Rolls w/ Icing Reduced Fat	1 (1.5 oz)	140	2	4	24
Toaster Strudel	1 (2 oz)	200	3	9	28
Toaster Strudel Blueberry	1 (2 oz)	190	3	9	26
Toaster Strudel Cream Cheese	1 (2 oz)	200	3	11	23
Toaster Strudel Raspberry	1 (2 oz)	190	3	9	26
Toaster Strudel Wildberry	1 (2 oz)	190	3	9	25
Turnovers Cherry	1 (2 oz)	180	2	8	24
TAKE-OUT					
angelfood	1 slice (2 oz)	143	3	tr	33
apple crisp	1 serv (8.6 oz)	384	4	8	76
apple turnover	1 (6.6 oz)	661	7	34	83
baklava	1 piece (2.7 oz)	334	5	23	29
basbousa namoura	1 piece (1 oz)	60	2	3	10
bean cake	1 cake (1.1 oz)	130	2	7	16
black forest chocolate cherry	1 piece (2.5 oz)	187	2	9	27
boston cream pie	1 slice (3.2 oz)	232	2	8	39
cannoli w/ cannoli cream	1	369	6	21	42
carrot w/ icing	1 slice (4.7 oz)	543	5	28	70
cheesecake	1 slice (4.5 oz)	410	11	25	37
cheesecake chocolate	1 slice (4.5 oz)	489	8	32	49
chinese moon cake	1 (4.8 oz)	458	9	6	92
coconut mochiko filipino cake	1 piece (2.7 oz)	252	3	12	35
coffeecake iced	1 piece (1.6 oz)	175	3	8	24
cream puff custard filled chocolate frosted	1 (3.9 oz)	293	7	18	27
eclair	1 (3.5 oz)	262	6	16	24
french apple tart	1 (3.5 oz)	302	4	15	37
fruitcake	1 slice (1.5 oz)	139	1	4	26
funnel cake	1 (3.2 oz)	276	7	14	29
gingerbread	1 piece (2.4 oz)	213	3	7	35
jelly roll	1 slice (1.8 oz)	146	3	2	28

FOOD	PORTION	CALS	PROT	FAT	CARB
jelly roll lemon filled	1 slice (3 oz)	210	3	2	48
napoleon	1 mini (1 oz)	123	2	9	9
napoleon	1 (3 oz)	348	5	25	25
panettone	½ cake (2.9 oz)	300	6	12	43
petit fours	2 (0.9 oz)	120	1	7	15
pineapple upside down	1 piece (4.2 oz)	387	4	15	61
pound	1 slice (1 oz)	120	2	5	15
pound fat free	1 slice (2 oz)	160	3	1	35
sacher torte	1 slice (2.2 oz)	240	4	11	30
strawberry shortcake	1 serv (4.1 oz)	211	4	5	40
strudel apple	1 piece (2.2 oz)	175	2	7	26
strudel cheese	1 piece (2.2 oz)	195	6	8	24
strudel cherry	1 piece (2.2 oz)	179	3	6	29
sweet potato w/ glaze	1 piece (2.7 oz)	275	4	12	39
tiramisu	1 cake (4.4 lbs)	5732	101	421	439
tiramisu	1 piece (5.1 oz)	409	7	30	31
torte chocolate ganache	1 slice (3.5 oz)	400	7	26	40
trifle w/ cream	6 oz	291	4	16	34
white w/ coconut icing	1 slice (3.9 oz)	399	5	12	71
zucchini bread	1 slice (1.4 oz)	150	2	7	19

CAKE ICING

FOOD	PORTION	CALS	PROT	FAT	CARB
chocolate	¼ cup	269	1	7	53
vanilla	¼ cup	322	tr	8	64
Betty Crocker					
HomeStyle Mix Fluffy White as prep	6 tbsp	100	tr	0	24
Rich & Creamy Butter Cream	2 tbsp (1.3 oz)	140	0	5	15
Rich & Creamy Chocolate	2 tbsp (1.2 oz)	130	0	5	21
Rich & Creamy Creamy White	2 tbsp (1.2 oz)	140	0	5	23
Rich & Creamy Lemon	2 tbsp (1.2 oz)	140	0	5	23
Rich & Creamy Vanilla	2 tbsp (1.2 oz)	140	0	5	23
Whipped Fluffy White	2 tbsp (0.8 oz)	100	0	5	15

FOOD	PORTION	CALS	PROT	FAT	CARB
Duncan Hines					
Chocolate Butter Cream	2 tbsp (1.2 oz)	140	0	6	22
Chocolate Fudge	2 tbsp (1.2 oz)	130	tr	6	21
Classic Vanilla	2 tbsp	140	0	6	23
Cream Cheese	2 tbsp (1.2 oz)	140	0	6	23
Milk Chocolate	2 tbsp (1.2 oz)	140	0	6	22
Manischewitz					
Dairy Free Chocolate	2 tbsp (1.2 oz)	138	0	5	22
Naturally Nora					
Frosting Mix Chocolate as prep	½12 pkg	150	1	7	24
Frosting Mix Vanilla as prep	½12 pkg	170	tr	8	25
CAKE MIX					
Betty Crocker					
Gingerbread as prep	1	220	2	6	39
Pineapple Upside Down as prep	⅙ cake	390	2	13	66
Pound Cake as prep	⅛ cake	260	2	8	45
SuperMoist Carrot as prep	½12 cake	260	1	12	35
SuperMoist Chocolate as prep	½12 cake	250	2	11	35
SuperMoist Devil's Food as prep	½12 cake	260	2	12	35
SuperMoist Lemon as prep	½12 cake	240	1	9	35
SuperMoist Milk Chocolate as prep	½12 cake	240	2	9	35
SuperMoist Spice as prep	½12 cake	270	2	13	34
SuperMoist Vanilla as prep	½12 cake	230	2	9	35
SuperMoist White as prep	½12 cake	220	2	8	35
SuperMoist Yellow as prep	½12 cake	230	1	9	35
Bisquick					
Heart Smart	⅓ cup	140	3	3	27
Duncan Hines					
Angel Food as prep	½12 pkg	140	31	0	31
Cupcake Mix Classic Yellow as prep	1	130	2	6	17
Decadent Carrot as prep	½12 pkg	260	4	11	37
Golden Butter Recipe as prep	½12 pkg	270	3	14	35
Lemon Supreme as prep	½12 pkg	270	3	12	36
Red Velvet as prep	½12 pkg	270	4	13	35
Yellow Classic as prep	½12 pkg	270	3	12	36
Naturally Nora					
Cheerful Chocolate as prep	½12 pkg	300	3	14	39
Sunny Yellow as prep	½12 pkg	280	2	12	39
Surprising Stars as prep	½12 pkg	300	3	12	42

FOOD	PORTION	CALS	PROT	FAT	CARB
CALABAZA					
fresh	½ cup	32	1	tr	8
CALZONE (*see* SANDWICHES)					
CANADIAN BACON					
grilled	2 slices (1.6 oz)	87	11	4	1
Applegate Farms					
Natural	2 slices (2 oz)	90	12	4	1
Celebrity					
98% Fat Free	3 slices (1.8 oz)	60	10	1	1
Organic Prairie					
Hardwood Smoked	1 oz	40	7	1	1
CANADIAN BACON SUBSTITUTES					
Yves					
Meatless Canadian Bacon	2 slices (2 oz)	80	17	1	2
CANDY					
butterscotch	1 piece (6 g)	24	0	tr	6
candied cherries	1 (4 g)	12	0	tr	3
candied citron	1 oz	89	tr	tr	23
candied lemon peel	1 oz	90	tr	tr	23
candied orange peel	1 oz	90	tr	tr	23
candied pineapple slice	1 slice (2 oz)	179	tr	tr	45
candy corn	1 oz	105	tr	0	27
caramels	1 piece (8 g)	31	tr	1	6
caramels chocolate	1 piece (6 g)	22	tr	tr	6
carob bar	1 (3.1 oz)	453	11	28	42
dark chocolate	1 oz	150	1	10	16
fondant	1 piece (0.6 oz)	57	0	0	15
fondant chocolate coated	1 piece (0.4 oz)	40	tr	1	9
fondant mint	1 oz	105	tr	0	27
fruit pastilles	1 tube (1.4 oz)	101	2	0	25
fudge brown sugar w/ nuts	1 piece (0.5 oz)	56	tr	1	11
fudge chocolate marshmallow	1 piece (0.7 oz)	84	1	3	14
fudge chocolate marshmallow w/ nuts	1 piece (0.8 oz)	96	1	4	15
fudge chocolate w/ nuts	1 piece (0.7 oz)	81	1	3	14
fudge peanut butter	1 piece (0.6 oz)	59	1	1	13
fudge vanilla w/ nuts	1 piece (0.5 oz)	62	tr	2	11
gumdrops	10 lg (3.8 oz)	420	0	0	108

FOOD	PORTION	CALS	PROT	FAT	CARB
gumdrops	10 sm (0.4 oz)	135	0	0	35
hard candy	1 oz	106	0	0	28
jelly beans	10 lg (1 oz)	104	0	tr	26
jelly beans	10 sm (0.4 oz)	40	0	tr	10
lollipop	1 (6 g)	22	0	0	6
marzipan	1 oz	128	3	7	15
milk chocolate	1 bar (1.55 oz)	226	3	14	26
milk chocolate crisp	1 bar (1.45 oz)	203	3	11	28
milk chocolate w/ almonds	1 bar (1.45 oz)	215	4	14	22
nougat nut cream	0.5 oz	49	1	4	8
organic dark chocolate w/ raisins & pecans	1.4 oz	220	2	14	22
peanut bar	1 (1.4 oz)	209	6	14	19
peanut brittle	1 oz	128	2	5	20
peanuts chocolate covered	1 cup (5.2 oz)	773	19	50	74
peanuts chocolate covered	10 (1.4 oz)	208	5	13	20
praline	1 piece (1.4 oz)	177	1	10	24
pretzels chocolate covered	1 (0.4 oz)	50	1	2	8
pretzels chocolate covered	1 oz	130	2	5	20
sesame crunch	20 pieces (1.2 oz)	181	4	12	18
sweet chocolate	1 bar (1.45 oz)	201	2	14	25
sweet chocolate	1 oz	143	1	10	17
taffy	1 piece (0.5 oz)	56	0	1	14
toffee	1 piece (0.4 oz)	65	tr	4	8
truffles	1 piece (0.4 oz)	59	1	4	5
3 Musketeers					
Bar	1 (2.1 oz)	260	2	8	46
Fun Size	3 bars (1.6 oz)	190	1	6	34
Minis	7 (1.4 oz)	170	1	5	32
Mint	1 bar (1.2 oz)	150	1	5	26
5th Avenue					
Bar	1 (2 oz)	260	4	12	37
Almond Joy					
Bar	1 (1.6 oz)	220	2	13	26
Andes					
Dark Chocolate Covered Cherries	2 (1 oz)	110	1	5	19
Thins Cherry Jubilee	8 pieces (1.3 oz)	200	2	13	22

FOOD	PORTION	CALS	PROT	FAT	CARB
Thins Creme De Menthe	8 pieces (1.3 oz)	200	2	13	22
Annabelle's					
Skinny Hunk Chewy Nougat	1 bar (1 oz)	100	0	1	24
Baby Ruth					
Fun Size	2 bars (1.3 oz)	170	2	8	24
Snack Bars	2 (1.3 oz)	170	2	8	24
Bartons					
Cashew Toppers	1 (1 oz)	140	3	9	14
Benecol					
Smart Chews Caramel	1 piece	20	0	0	4
Benedetto					
Cubetti Mini Caramel Mint Protein 1st	5 pieces (1.7 oz)	178	19	5	17
Cupola Mini Mint Protein 1st	5 pieces (1.7 oz)	122	11	3	15
Betty Crocker					
Fruit Gushers Rockin' Blue Raspberry	1 pkg (0.9 oz)	90	0	1	20
Blow Pop					
Regular	1 (0.6 oz)	60	0	0	16
Brach's					
Mellowcreme Pumpkins	6 pieces (1.5 oz)	150	0	0	38
Breath Savers					
Peppermint	1 (1.8 g)	5	0	0	2
Bubble Chocolate					
Dark Chocolate	1 bar (1.41 oz)	200	2	15	22
Milk Chocolate	1 bar (1.41 oz)	220	3	15	21
Cadbury					
Caramello	1 (1.6 oz)	220	3	10	29
Dairy Milk	7 blocks (1.4 oz)	200	3	11	23
Milk Chocolate Fruit & Nut	10 blocks (1.4 oz)	200	4	10	24
Milk Chocolate Roast Almond	7 blocks (1.4 oz)	210	4	13	21
Royal Dark	7 blocks (1.4 oz)	170	2	12	23

FOOD	PORTION	CALS	PROT	FAT	CARB
Cella's					
Milk Chocolate Covered Cherries	2 (1 oz)	120	1	5	20
Charleston Chews					
Chocolate	1 bar (1.9 oz)	230	2	6	43
Vanilla	1 bar (1.9 oz)	230	2	8	44
Charms					
Fluffy Stuff Cotton Candy	1 pkg (0.6 oz)	70	0	0	17
Sour Balls	1 (5 g)	20	0	0	5
Squares	2 pieces	20	0	0	6
Chew-ets					
Peanut Chews Original Dark	3 pieces	170	3	9	22
Choward's					
Mints All Flavors	3 (5 g)	20	0	0	5
Chuao Chocolatier					
Choco Pod Banana	1 (0.4 oz)	50	tr	3	6
Choco Pod Passion	1 (0.4 oz)	50	0	4	5
CocoaVia					
Dark Chocolate Blueberry & Almond Bar	1 (0.8 oz)	100	1	6	12
Dark Chocolate Covered Almonds	1 pkg (1 oz)	140	3	11	12
Dark Chocolate Crispy Bar	1 (0.7 oz)	90	2	5	11
Dark Chocolate Original Bar	1 (0.8 oz)	80	1	6	12
Milk Chocolate Almond Bar	1 (0.8 oz)	110	2	7	12
Milk Chocolate Bar	1 (0.8 oz)	110	1	6	13
Milk Chocolate Covered Raisins	1 pkg (1 oz)	150	2	6	22
Crispy Cat					
Roasted Peanut	1 bar (1 oz)	220	4	10	29
Dare					
RealFruit Gummies All Flavors	8 pieces (1.4 oz)	120	2	0	28
Dots					
All Flavors	12 (1.5 oz)	140	0	0	35
Dove					
Dark Chocolate Cranberry Almond	⅓ pkg (1.2 oz)	170	2	10	20
Milk Chocolate Roasted Almond	⅓ bar (1.2 oz)	180	3	12	18

FOOD	PORTION	CALS	PROT	FAT	CARB
E. Guittard					
Bar Quevedo Bittersweet 65% Cacao	1 (2 oz)	290	3	23	29
Bar Sur Del Lago Bittersweet 65% Cacao	1 (2 oz)	290	3	23	29
Emily's					
Espresso Beans Dark Chocolate Covered	26 (1.4 oz)	220	2	19	24
Enjoy Life					
Boom Choco Boom Dark Chocolate Dairy Nut Soy Free	1 bar (1.4 oz)	200	2	15	22
Equal Exchange					
Organic Chocolate Espresso Bean	1 bar (1.4 oz)	216	2	15	22
Organic Milk Chocolate	1 bar (1.4 oz)	230	4	16	19
Organic Very Dark Chocolate	1 bar (1.4 oz)	220	3	17	18
Ferrero					
Rocher	3 pieces (1.3 oz)	220	3	16	16
Rondnoir	3 pieces (1.4 oz)	220	3	14	21
Frooties					
Chewy Candy Fruit Flavored	12 pieces (1.3 oz)	104	0	3	29
Ghirardelli					
Luxe Milk Chocolate	4 sq (1.5 oz)	220	3	13	26
Squares Milk Chocolate w/ Caramel Filling	3 (1.6 oz)	220	2	12	27
Squares Mint Indulgence	3 (1.6 oz)	210	1	11	30
Squares 60% Cacao Dark Chocolate	4 (1.5 oz)	220	2	17	23
Squares 60% Cacao Dark Chocolate w/ Caramel	3 (1.6 oz)	220	2	15	25
Godiva					
Truffles Assorted	2 pieces (1.4 oz)	210	3	13	20
Good & Plenty					
Licorice	33 (1.4 oz)	140	tr	0	35
Guylian					
Twists Milk Chocolate Truffle	5 pieces (1.2 oz)	230	2	19	15

FOOD	PORTION	CALS	PROT	FAT	CARB
Twists Original Praline	4 pieces (1.2 oz)	200	3	13	19
Hammond's					
Root Beer Drops	3 (0.6 oz)	60	0	0	14
Heath					
Bar	1 (1.4 oz)	210	1	13	24
Hershey's					
Bar Milk Chocolate w/ Almonds	1 (1.4 oz)	210	4	14	21
Bar Special Dark	1 (1.4 oz)	180	2	12	25
Bliss Dark Chocolate Bar	1 (1.3 oz)	160	2	12	21
Bliss Milk Chocolate	6 (1.5 oz)	210	3	14	24
Bliss Milk Chocolate Meltaway	6 (1.5 oz)	220	3	15	24
Bliss Milk Chocolate Raspberry Meltaway	6 (1.5 oz)	220	3	14	24
Cacao Reserve 35% Cacao Milk Chocolate w/ Hazelnuts	3 sq (1.3 oz)	220	3	15	18
Cacao Reserve 65% Cacao Dark	3 blocks (1.3 oz)	180	4	15	18
Kisses Cherry Cordial	9 (1.5 oz)	180	2	7	30
Kisses Hugs	9 (1.4 oz)	210	3	12	23
Kisses Milk Chocolate	9 (1.4 oz)	230	3	13	24
Kisses Special Dark	9 (1.4 oz)	180	2	12	25
Milk Chocolate Bar	1 (1.5 oz)	210	3	13	26
Milk Chocolate w/ Almonds Bar	1 (1.5 oz)	210	3	13	25
Nuggets Milk Chocolate	4 (1.4 oz)	200	3	12	25
Nuggets Milk Chocolate w/ Almonds	4 (1.3 oz)	200	4	13	20
Pieces All Flavors	51 (1.4 oz)	190	4	9	25
Ice Breakers					
Coolmint	1 (0.8 g)	0	0	0	tr
Jay's					
Cotton Candy	1 pkg (2 oz)	220	3	0	56
Jolly Rancher					
Gummies	9 (1.4 oz)	120	2	0	28
Original Assortment	3 (0.5 oz)	50	0	0	13
Junior					
Caramels	1 box (1.4 oz)	170	1	3	35
Mints	1 box (1.4 oz)	170	1	3	35
KitKat					
Bar	1 (1.5 oz)	210	3	11	28

FOOD	PORTION	CALS	PROT	FAT	CARB
Kopali					
Organic Dark Chocolate Covered Espresso Beans	½ pkg (1 oz)	120	1	7	17
Lance					
Chewz Strawberry	1 pkg (1.1 oz)	120	0	1	28
Peanut Bar	1 (2.3 oz)	340	13	19	29
Let's Do Organic					
Black Licorice Bars	1 (0.9 oz)	80	1	0	20
Black Licorice Chews	8 (1.4 oz)	130	2	0	30
Gummi Bears	1 pkg (0.9 oz)	80	0	0	22
Lindt					
Lindor Truffles 60% Extra Dark	3 pieces (1.3 oz)	210	2	19	15
Lindor Truffles Swiss Dark Chocolate	3 (1.4 oz)	240	2	18	17
Petits Desserts Assorted	4 (1.3 oz)	210	2	15	20
Love Candy					
Dark Chocolate	1 bar (1.5 oz)	190	2	11	21
Milk Chocolate	1 bar (1.5 oz)	200	1	11	22
Yogurt Supreme	1 bar (1.5 oz)	190	1	11	23
Mama's Goodies					
Butter Nut Crunch Almond	1 piece (1.33 oz)	220	3	15	20
Butter Nut Crunch Sesame Seed	1 piece (1.33 oz)	220	2	14	20
Nut Butter Crunch Macadamia & Coconut	1 piece (1.33 oz)	220	1	17	20
Mamba					
Fruit Flavor	6 (0.9 oz)	170	0	3	36
Sour	6 (0.9 oz)	100	0	2	22
Mike & Ike					
All Flavors	1 pkg (2 oz)	200	0	0	50
Milk Duds					
Chocolate	13 (1.4 oz)	170	1	6	28
Milkfuls					
Candy	6 (1.4 oz)	170	tr	3	35
Milky Way					
Fun Size	2 bars (1.2 oz)	150	1	6	24
Mounds					
Bar	1 (1.7 oz)	230	2	13	29

FOOD	PORTION	CALS	PROT	FAT	CARB
Mr.Goodbar					
Bar	1 (1.7 oz)	250	5	17	26
Necco					
Banana Splits	4 (1.4 oz)	150	0	2	36
Clark Junior Bar	1 (0.5 oz)	60	1	3	10
Conversation Hearts Tiny	40 (1.4 oz)	160	0	0	39
Double Dipped Peanuts	15 (1.4 oz)	200	3	11	25
Junior Assorted Wafers	1 roll (0.5 oz)	50	0	0	13
Mary Janes	5 (1.4 oz)	160	1	4	32
Mint Juleps	4 (1.4 oz)	150	0	2	36
Nonpareils	10 (1.4 oz)	190	1	9	29
Squirrel Nut Caramel	5 (1.6 oz)	170	1	3	37
Nestle					
Crunch Stix	1 (0.6 oz)	90	tr	5	12
PayDay					
Peanut Caramel	1 (1.8 oz)	240	7	13	27
Pot Of Gold					
Nut Assortment	4 (1.4 oz)	210	3	13	23
Pecan Caramel Clusters	4 (1.4 oz)	200	2	12	23
Truffle Assortment	3 (1.5 oz)	200	2	9	27
Pure Fun					
Organic Vegan Barrels Of Fun Root Beer Float	2 (0.5 oz)	60	0	0	13
Organic Vegan Candy Canes	1 (0.5 oz)	62	0	0	14
Organic Vegan Chocolate Meltdowns All Flavors	3 (0.6 oz)	70	0	0	16
Organic Vegan Citrus Slices All Flavors	3 (0.6 oz)	60	0	0	15
Organic Vegan Cotton Candy All Flavors	¼ pkg (0.5 oz)	60	0	0	15
Organic Vegan Jaw Boulders All Flavors	2 (0.5 oz)	58	0	0	13
Organic Vegan Pure Pops All Flavors	3 (0.6 oz)	60	0	0	15
Raisinets					
Candy	3 pkg (1.7 oz)	200	2	8	34
Reese's					
Crispy Crunchy Bar	1 (1.7 oz)	250	5	14	29
FastBreak	1 (2 oz)	260	5	12	35
NutRageous	1 (1.8 oz)	260	6	16	28
Pieces Peanut Butter	1 pkg (1.5 oz)	210	5	10	26

FOOD	PORTION	CALS	PROT	FAT	CARB
ReeseSticks					
Wafer Bar Chocolate & Peanut Butter	1 (1.5 oz)	210	4	13	23
Riesen					
Candy	4 (1.3 oz)	170	1	4	28
Rolo					
Chewy Caramels In Milk Chocolate	3 pkg (1.7 oz)	220	2	10	33
Russell Stover					
Private Reserve Triple Chocolate Mousse	3 pieces (1.3 oz)	220	2	17	19
Private Reserve Vanilla Bean Brulee	3 pieces (1.3 oz)	180	3	13	19
See's					
Assorted Chocolates	2 (1.2 oz)	160	2	9	20
Nuts & Chews	3 (1.6 oz)	240	4	16	25
Soft Centers	2 (1.4 oz)	170	1	9	25
Sencha Naturals					
Green Tea Mints All Flavors	3	5	0	0	1
Shaman Chocolates					
Organic Extra Dark Chocolate 82% Cacao	½ bar (1 oz)	158	2	14	7
Organic Milk Chocolate w/ Macadamia Nuts & Hawaiian Pink Sea Salt	½ bar (1 oz)	91	1	1	13
Skittles					
Original Fruit	1 pkg (2.2 oz)	250	0	3	56
Sour	1 pkg (1.8 oz)	200	0	0	44
Skor					
Toffee & Milk Chocolate	1 (1.4 oz)	200	1	12	25
Slim-Fast					
Protein Snack Chews Peanut Butter	1 pkg (0.9 oz)	100	6	4	12
Smile Chocolatiers					
Choclatea Ginger Tea Milk Chocolate 37% Cacao	½ bar (1.5 oz)	230	3	15	23
Choclatea Herbal Chai Tea Dark Chocolate 64% Cacao	½ bar (1.5 oz)	220	2	17	22
Choclatea Pistachio Green Tea White Chocolate	½ bar (1.5 oz)	240	5	16	22

FOOD	PORTION	CALS	PROT	FAT	CARB
Choclatea Pomegranate White Tea Very Dark Chocolate 72% Cacao	½ bar (1.5 oz)	220	3	16	16
Choclatea White Tea Very Dark Chocolate 72% Cacao	½ bar (1.5 oz)	220	2	17	22
Sour Patch					
Kids Soft & Chewy	1 pkg (1 oz)	100	0	0	25
Starbucks					
Truffles Caffe Mocha	3 (1.3 oz)	200	3	14	19
Sugar Babies					
Candy	30 pieces (1.5 oz)	180	0	2	41
Chocolate	19 pieces (1.4 oz)	180	1	5	33
Sugar Daddy					
Pop	1 lg (1.7 oz)	200	1	3	43
Symphony					
Almonds & Toffee	1 (1.5 oz)	220	4	14	23
Take 5					
Original	1 pkg (1.5 oz)	200	4	11	25
Thorntons					
Chocolates Summer Collection	1	65	1	4	7
Toblerone					
Bittersweet w/ Honey & Almond Nugget	⅓ bar (1.2 oz)	170	1	9	20
Milk Chocolate w/ Honey & Almond Nougat	⅓ bar (1.2 oz)	170	2	9	21
White w/ Honey & Almond Nougat	⅓ bar (1.2 oz)	180	2	10	20
Toffifay					
Candy	5 (1.4 oz)	200	2	11	25
Tootsie Roll					
Midgees	6	140	0	3	28
Mini Chews	30 pieces (1.4 oz)	170	2	7	27
Pops	1 (0.6 oz)	60	0	0	15
Pops Caramel Apple	1 (0.6 oz)	60	0	1	15
Twix					
Fun Size	1 (0.6 oz)	80	1	4	10

FOOD	PORTION	CALS	PROT	FAT	CARB
Twizzlers					
Licorice	4 (1.6 oz)	150	1	1	35
Strawberry	4 (1.6 oz)	160	1	1	36
Werther's					
Caramel Milk Chocolate	6 (1.3 oz)	230	2	16	18
Original	3 (0.5 oz)	60	0	1	13
Original Sugar Free	5 (0.5 oz)	40	0	1	14
Whoppers					
Malted Milk Balls	18 (1.4 oz)	190	1	7	31
Wolfgang					
Blueberries Dipped In Dark Chocolate	2 (0.7 oz)	80	0	4	13
Cranberries Dipped In Dark Chocolate	2 (1 oz)	130	1	6	18
Raspberries Dipped In Dark Chocolate	2 (1.1 oz)	130	1	6	21
York					
Peppermint Patty	1 (1.4 oz)	140	tr	3	31
Young & Smylie					
Licorice Black	11 (1.5 oz)	140	tr	2	32
Licorice Strawberry	11 (1.5 oz)	150	1	2	33
Zagnut					
Peanut Butter & Coconut	3 (1.5 oz)	200	3	8	31
Zero					
Bar	1 (1.8 oz)	230	3	8	37
CANTALOUPE					
dried	3.5 pieces (1.4 oz)	140	0	0	34
fresh cubed	1 cup	57	1	tr	13
fresh half	½	94	2	1	22
Chiquita					
Fresh Cup Up	1 cup (6.2 oz)	60	1	0	16
CAPERS					
capers	1 tbsp	2	tr	tr	tr
CARAWAY					
seed	1 tbsp	22	1	1	3
CARDAMOM					
ground	1 tsp	6	tr	tr	1

FOOD	PORTION	CALS	PROT	FAT	CARB
CARDOON					
fresh cooked w/o salt	1 serv (3.5 oz)	22	1	tr	5
fresh shredded	1 cup (6.2 oz)	30	1	tr	7
Ocean Mist					
Cardone Fresh Shredded	1 cup (6.2 oz)	36	1	tr	9
CARIBOU					
roasted	3 oz	142	25	4	0
CARISSA					
fresh	1	12	tr	tr	3
CAROB					
carob mix	3 tsp	45	tr	0	11
carob mix as prep w/ whole milk	9 oz	195	8	8	23
flour	1 cup	185	5	1	92
flour	1 tbsp	14	tr	tr	7
Bob's Red Mill					
Powder Toasted	2 tsp	25	1	0	11
Tree Of Life					
Chips Malt Sweetened	50 (0.5 oz)	70	1	4	9
CARP					
fresh cooked	1 fillet (6 oz)	276	39	12	0
fresh cooked	3 oz	138	19	6	0
fresh raw	3 oz	108	15	5	0
roe raw	1 oz	37	7	tr	tr
CARROT JUICE					
canned	6 oz	73	2	tr	17
Hollywood					
100% Juice	1 can (12 oz)	120	2	1	27
Lakewood					
Organic	6 oz	73	2	0	17
Odwalla					
100% Juice	8 oz	70	2	0	15
CARROTS					
CANNED					
slices	½ cup	17	tr	tr	4
slices low sodium	½ cup	17	tr	tr	4

FOOD	PORTION	CALS	PROT	FAT	CARB
Allens					
Tiny Sliced	½ cup	35	0	0	8
Del Monte					
Savory Sides Honey Glazed	½ cup	70	1	0	18
S&W					
Julienne	½ cup (4.3 oz)	35	0	0	8
FRESH					
baby raw	1 (0.5 oz)	6	tr	tr	1
raw	1 (2.5 oz)	31	1	tr	7
raw shredded	½ cup	24	1	tr	6
slices cooked	½ cup	35	1	tr	8
Chiquita					
Carrot Bites w/ Ranch Dressing	1 pkg (2.5 oz)	50	1	3	7
Earthbound Farms					
Organic Tops On	1 (2.7 oz)	35	1	0	8
Organic w/ Organic Ranch Dip	1 pkg (2.2 oz)	90	1	8	5
FROZEN					
slices cooked	½ cup	26	1	tr	6
Birds Eye					
Steam & Serve Carrots & Cranberries	1 cup	130	1	5	20
C&W					
Whole Baby	⅔ cup	35	tr	0	7
Green Giant					
Honey Glazed	1 cup	90	1	3	15
Joy Of Cooking					
Bite Size	½ cup (3.3 oz)	70	1	3	12
CASABA					
cubed	1 cup (6 oz)	46	2	tr	11
melon fresh	¼ (14 oz)	115	5	tr	27
CASHEW JUICE					
O.N.E.					
Cashew Fruit	1 bottle (11 oz)	140	tr	0	34
CASHEWS					
cashew butter w/o salt	1 tbsp	94	3	8	4
dry roasted w/ salt	18 nuts (1 oz)	160	4	13	9
dry roasted w/ salt	1 oz	163	4	13	9
oil roasted w/ salt	1 oz	163	5	14	8
oil roasted w/o salt	1 oz	163	5	14	8

FOOD	PORTION	CALS	PROT	FAT	CARB
Arrowhead Mills					
Organic Cashew Butter	2 tbsp	160	4	13	9
Back To Nature					
Jumbo Sea Salt Roasted	1 oz	160	5	13	9
Lance					
Cashews	1 pkg (1.5 oz)	270	8	22	11
Navitas Naturals					
Cashews	1 oz	160	5	12	9
Peeled Snacks					
Nut Picks Cashew Later	1 pkg (1 oz)	180	4	14	9
Planters					
Chocolate Lovers Milk Chocolate	10 pieces (1.5 oz)	230	5	16	20
Dry Roasted	19 pieces (1 oz)	160	5	12	9
Organic	23 pieces (1 oz)	170	5	13	8
Sunfood					
Organic	1 oz	164	5	12	9
Tree Of Life					
Cashew Butter Creamy	2 tbsp	180	4	15	9
Yumnuts					
Chili Lime	¼ cup (1 oz)	170	6	13	7
Chocolate	¼ cup (1 oz)	160	4	11	12
Honey	¼ cup (1 oz)	170	5	12	10
Toasted Coconut	½ cup (1 oz)	170	5	13	9
CASSAVA					
diced cooked w/o fat	1 cup (4.6 oz)	213	2	tr	51
root raw	1 (14.3 oz)	653	6	1	155
TAKE-OUT					
fritter crab meat stuffed	1 (4.4 oz)	341	12	16	38
CATFISH					
channel breaded & fried	3 oz	194	15	11	7
wolffish atlantic baked	3 oz	105	19	3	0
Simmons					
Farm Raised	4 oz	140	17	6	0
CAULIFLOWER					
flowerets fresh	1 (0.5 oz)	3	tr	tr	1
flowerets fresh cooked w/o salt	3 (2 oz)	12	1	tr	2

FOOD	PORTION	CALS	PROT	FAT	CARB
fresh	1 cup	25	2	tr	5
fresh cooked w/o salt	1 cup	29	2	1	5
fresh head small	1 (9.2 oz)	66	5	tr	14
frzn cooked w/o salt	1 cup	34	3	tr	7
green fresh	1 cup	20	2	tr	4
green fresh small head	1 (11.4 oz)	101	10	1	20
pickled	¼ cup	14	tr	tr	3
pickled chow chow	¼ cup	74	1	1	16
Birds Eye					
Steamfresh Garlic Cauliflower	1 cup (2.4 oz)	40	1	2	5
Mann's					
Cauliettes Fresh	1 serv (3 oz)	20	2	0	4
TAKE-OUT					
batter dipped fried	1 cup	178	3	13	12
batter dipped fried	1 piece (0.9 oz)	55	1	4	4
w/ cheese sauce	1 cup	249	12	18	12
CAVIAR					
black or red	2 tbsp	81	8	6	1
CELERY					
fresh	1 lg stalk (2.2 oz)	9	tr	tr	2
pickled	½ cup	10	tr	tr	2
raw diced	½ cup	8	tr	tr	2
seed	1 tsp	1	tr	tr	tr
strips	1 cup	17	1	tr	4
Dole					
Stalks	2 med (3 oz)	20	1	0	5
Earthbound Farms					
Organic Hearts	2 stalks (3.9 oz)	20	1	0	5
TAKE-OUT					
creamed	½ cup	87	3	6	7
stir fried	½ cup	30	1	2	3
stuffed w/ cheese	1 (5 inch)	38	1	3	1
CELERY JUICE					
juice	1 cup	42	2	tr	9
CELERY ROOT					
fresh cooked w/o salt	1 cup (5.4 oz)	42	1	tr	9
fresh cut up	1 cup (5.5 oz)	66	2	tr	14

FOOD	PORTION	CALS	PROT	FAT	CARB
CELTUCE					
raw	3.5 oz	22	1	tr	4
CEREAL					
bran flakes	¾ cup	90	4	1	22
corn flakes	1¼ cups	110	2	tr	24
farina as prep w/ water	¾ cup	88	2	tr	19
granola	½ cup	285	9	15	32
oatmeal instant as prep w/ water	1 cup (8.2 oz)	138	6	2	24
oatmeal regular & quick as prep w/ water	¾ cup (6.1 oz)	149	5	2	19
oatmeal regular & quick not prep	⅓ cup (0.9 oz)	104	4	2	18
puffed rice	1 cup	56	1	tr	13
puffed wheat	1 cup	44	2	tr	10
shredded mini wheats	1 cup	107	3	1	24
shredded wheat rectangular	1 biscuit (0.8 oz)	85	3	tr	19
Alti Plano Gold					
Instant Quinoa Hot Cereal Spiced Apple Raisin	1 pkg	160	3	2	35
Instant Quinoa Organic Hot Cereal Oaxacan Chocolate	1 pkg	170	6	3	30
Amy's					
Bowls Organic Cream Of Rice	1 pkg (8.9 oz)	170	2	1	39
Bowls Organic Multigrain	1 pkg (8.9 oz)	190	4	2	40
Arrowhead Mills					
Organic Amaranth Flakes	1 cup	140	4	2	26
Organic Kamut Flakes	1 cup	120	4	1	25
Organic Multigrain Flakes	1 cup	170	5	2	33
Organic Nature O's	1 cup	130	4	2	25
Organic Puffed Corn	1 cup	60	2	1	12
Organic Puffed Millet	1 cup	60	2	1	11
Organic Puffed Wheat	1 cup	60	3	0	12
Organic Rice Flakes Sweetened	1 cup	180	3	1	40
Organic Shredded Wheat	1 cup	190	7	1	38
Organic Spelt Flakes	1 cup	120	4	1	24
Back To Nature					
Granola Apple Blueberry	½ cup (1.8 oz)	200	6	3	39

FOOD	PORTION	CALS	PROT	FAT	CARB
Granola Chocolate Delight	½ cup (1.75 oz)	220	5	6	37
Granola Classic	½ cup (1.8 oz)	200	6	3	39
Granola Sunflower & Pumpkin Seed	½ cup (1.6 oz)	290	6	7	31
Granola To Go Ginger Roasted Almonds w/ Flax Seed	1 serv (1.5 oz)	190	5	7	29
Granola To Go Wild Blueberry Walnut w/ Flax Seed	1 serv (1.5 oz)	190	5	6	30
Bakery On Main					
Granola Apple Cinnamon Walnut	½ cup (2 oz)	240	6	12	29
Granola Fiber Power Cinnamon Raisin	½ cup (2 oz)	230	7	6	40
Granola Maple Raisin Almond	½ cup (2 oz)	240	6	12	30
Granola Super Fruit & Nut	½ cup (2 oz)	250	6	13	29
Barbara's Bakery					
Alpen No Sugar Added	⅔ cup	200	7	3	40
Organic Breakfast O's Fruit Juice Sweetened	1 cup	120	4	2	22
Organic Brown Rice Crisps Fruit Juice Sweetened	1 cup	120	2	1	25
Organic Corn Flakes Fruit Juice Sweetened	1 cup	110	2	1	25
Organic Wild Puffs	1 cup	100	2	1	23
Organic Wild Puffs Fruity Punch	1 cup	110	2	1	26
Organic Ultima High Fiber	½ cup	90	3	1	24
Organic Ultima Pomegranate	½ cup	100	3	1	24
Puffins Cinnamon	⅔ cup	100	2	1	26
Puffins Originals	¾ cup (0.9 oz)	90	2	1	23
Shredded Oats Bite Size	1¼ cups (2 oz)	220	6	3	46
Shredded Wheat	2 biscuits (1.4 oz)	140	4	1	31
Bob's Red Mill					
Farina Creamy Brown Rice not prep	¼ cup	150	3	1	32
Muesli Old Country	¼ cup	110	4	3	21
Natural Granola No Fat	½ cup	180	5	3	35
Organic Right Stuff Hot Cereal 6 Grain not prep	¼ cup	140	6	2	27

FOOD	PORTION	CALS	PROT	FAT	CARB
Rolled Oats Gluten Free not prep	½ cup	160	7	3	27
Cascadian Farm					
Organic Clifford Crunch	1 cup	100	2	1	25
Organic Granola Oats & Honey	⅔ cup	230	5	6	42
Chappaqua Crunch					
Original Granola	⅓ cup	115	4	2	20
Simply Granola w/ Raisins	⅓ cup	120	4	2	22
Simply Granola w/ Raspberries	⅓ cup	110	4	2	21
Chia Goodness					
Apple Almond Cinnamon	2 tbsp (1 oz)	130	4	6	16
Cranberry Ginger	2 tbsp (1 oz)	130	4	7	16
Original	2 tbsp (1 oz)	140	6	8	14
Country Choice Organic					
Multigrain Hot Cereal not prep	½ cup	130	5	1	29
Oats Old Fashioned not prep	½ cup	150	5	3	27
Oats Quick not prep	½ cup	150	5	3	27
Dorset Cereals					
Berries & Cherries	½ cup	150	4	1	40
Simply Delicious Muesli	½ cup	200	6	5	37
Super Cranberry Cherry & Almond	½ cup	200	5	5	39
Earthbound Farms					
Organic Granola Maple Almond	½ cup	260	6	14	31
Enjoy Life					
Allergen Gluten Free Granola Cinnamon	½ cup	160	3	3	31
Erin Baker's					
Granola Fruit & Nut	½ cup (1.6 oz)	190	4	8	27
Granola Oatmeal Raisin	½ cup (1.6 oz)	180	4	6	30
Granola Ultra Protein Power Crunch	½ cup (1.6 oz)	200	8	6	25
Farina					
Original as prep	1 cup	120	3	0	22
General Mills					
Cheerios Crunch Oat Cluster	¾ cup	100	2	1	22
Chex Whole Grain Chocolate	¾ cup	130	2	3	26
Curves	¾ cup	100	2	1	22
Fiber One Raisin Bran Clusters	1 cup (2 oz)	170	4	1	45
Total Whole Grain	¾ cup (1 oz)	100	2	1	23
Trix	1 cup (1.1 oz)	120	1	2	28

FOOD	PORTION	CALS	PROT	FAT	CARB
Glucerna					
Crunchy Flakes 'N Raisins	1 bowl (1.6 oz)	140	4	1	36
Crunchy Flakes 'N Strawberries	1 bowl (1.5 oz)	150	4	1	37
Glutino					
Gluten Free Apple Cinnamon	½ cup	120	1	2	24
Gluten Free Honey Nut	½ cup	130	2	3	24
Health Valley					
Empower	1 cup	200	6	3	42
Granola Low Fat Tropical Fruit	⅔ cup	180	5	1	43
Heart Wise	1 cup	200	11	3	37
Organic Cherry Lemon Blast Ems	¾ cup	120	2	1	25
Organic Golden Flax	¾ cup	190	6	3	38
Organic Multigrain Apple Cinnamon Square Ems	1¼ cup	210	5	3	44
Organic Oat Bran O's	¾ cup	100	3	0	23
Rice Crunch-Ems	1 cup	110	4	0	26
Honest Foods					
Granola Planks Maple Almond Crunch	½ bar (2 oz)	250	6	10	37
Kashi					
7 Whole Grain Flakes	1 cup	180	6	1	41
7 Whole Grain Honey Puffs	1 cup	120	3	1	25
7 Whole Grain Nuggets	½ cup	210	7	2	47
7 Whole Grain Pilaf as prep	½ cup	170	6	3	30
GoLean	1 cup	140	13	1	30
GoLean Crunch Honey Almond Flax	1 cup	200	9	5	34
GoLean Crunch!	1 cup	190	9	3	36
GoLean Instant Hot Cereal Creamy Truly Vanilla	1 pkg	150	9	2	25
GoLean Instant Hot Cereal Hearty Honey & Cinnamon	1 pkg	150	8	2	26
Good Friends	1 cup	170	5	2	43
Granola Mountain Medley	½ cup	220	6	7	37
Heart To Heart Instant Oatmeal Golden Brown Maple	1 pkg	160	4	2	33
Heart To Heart Instant Oatmeal Raisin Spice	1 pkg	150	3	2	33

FOOD	PORTION	CALS	PROT	FAT	CARB
Heart To Heart Oat Flakes & Blueberry Clusters	1¼ cups	200	6	3	42
Heart To Heart Toasted Oat	¾ cup	110	4	2	25
Honey Sunshine	¾ cup (1.1 oz)	100	2	2	25
Mighty Bites All Flavors	1 cup	110	5	2	23
Organic Promise Autumn Wheat	1 cup	190	5	1	45
Organic Promise Cinnamon Harvest	1 cup	190	4	1	44
Organic Promise Strawberry Fields	1 cup	120	2	0	28
Vive Probiotic Digestive Wellness	1¼ cups	170	4	3	43
Lundberg					
Purely Organic Hot'n Creamy Rice	⅓ cup	190	4	2	43
Malt-O-Meal					
Balance	¾ cup	120	3	1	26
Cinnamon Toasters	¾ cup	130	1	4	24
Colossal Crunch	¾ cup	120	1	2	26
Creamy Hot Wheat not prep	3 tbsp	130	4	0	27
Crispy Rice	1¼ cups	130	2	0	29
Frosted Flakes	¾ cup	120	2	0	28
Frosted Mini Spooners	1 cup	190	5	1	45
Honey & Oat Blenders	¾ cup	120	2	2	25
Honey Buzzers	1¼ cups	110	1	1	26
Instant Oatmeal Apple & Cinnamon	1 pkg	130	3	2	27
Instant Oatmeal Cinnamon & Spice	1 pkg	170	4	2	36
Instant Oatmeal Maple & Brown Sugar	1 pkg	160	4	2	33
Original Hot Wheat not prep	3 tbsp	130	5	1	27
Puffed Rice	1 cup	60	1	0	13
Raisin Bran	1 cup	220	5	1	47
McCann's					
Irish Oatmeal Instant Apples & Cinnamon not prep	1 pkg (1.2 oz)	130	3	2	27
Irish Oatmeal Instant Maple & Brown Sugar not prep	1 pkg (1.5 oz)	160	4	2	32

FOOD	PORTION	CALS	PROT	FAT	CARB
Irish Oatmeal Instant Regular not prep	1 pkg (1 oz)	100	4	2	18
Irish Oatmeal Quick Cooking not prep	½ cup (1.4 oz)	150	4	2	26
Irish Oatmeal Steel Cut not prep	¼ cup (1.4 oz)	150	4	2	26
Mom's Best Naturals					
Oatmeal Instant	1 pkg	160	4	2	33
Raisin Bran	1 cup	230	5	2	49
Toasted Wheat-fuls	1 cup	200	8	1	44
Toasty O's	1 cup	120	4	2	23
Natural Ovens					
Great Granola	½ cup	250	6	9	38
Nature's Path					
Organic Flax Plus Pumpkin Raisin Crunch	¾ cup	200	6	4	41
Organic Smart Bran	⅔ cup	90	3	1	24
Organic Granola Pomegran Plus	½ cup	140	2	5	21
Nature's Plus					
Organic Oatmeal Hemp Plus	1 pkg	160	5	3	30
Newman's Own					
Sweet Enough Honey Flax Flakes	¾ cup	100	3	1	24
Sweet Enough Honey Nut O's	¾ cup	110	3	2	22
Sweet Enough Wheat Puffs	¾ cup	100	3	1	22
Post					
100% Bran	½ cup (0.8 oz)	80	4	1	22
Bran Flakes	1 cup	100	3	1	24
Cocoa Pebbles	¾ cup (1 oz)	110	1	2	26
Golden Crisp	¾ cup (1 oz)	110	1	0	25
Grape-Nuts	2 oz	200	7	1	47
Grape-Nuts O's	1 cup (1 oz)	120	2	0	28
Grape-Nuts Trail Mix Crunch	1 cup (1.7 oz)	170	4	2	37
Great Grains Raisins Dates & Pecans	¾ cup (2 oz)	210	4	5	40
Honey Bunches Of Oats	¾ cup	130	2	2	25
Honey Bunches Of Oats Peaches	1 cup	120	2	2	26
Honeycomb	1⅓ cups (1 oz)	120	2	1	28
LiveActive Mixed Berry Crunch	1 cup	190	4	2	43
LiveActive Nut Harvest Crunch	1 cup	220	5	6	39

FOOD	PORTION	CALS	PROT	FAT	CARB
Oreo O's	1 cup	110	1	2	22
Raisin Bran	1 cup (2 oz)	190	4	1	46
Selects Banana Nut Crunch	1 cup (2 oz)	240	5	6	44
Selects Blueberry Morning	2 oz	220	3	3	45
Shredded Wheat Frosted	2 oz	180	4	1	43
Shredded Wheat 'N Bran	2 oz	200	6	1	49
Shredded Wheat Original	2 biscuits (1.6 oz)	160	5	1	37
Shredded Wheat Spoon Size	1 cup	170	6	1	40
Toasties Corn Flakes	1 cup (1 oz)	100	2	0	24
Quaker					
Instant Oatmeal Cinnamon & Spice	1 pkg	170	4	2	35
Instant Oatmeal Cinnamon Roll	1 pkg	160	4	2	33
Instant Oatmeal Crunch Maple & Brown Sugar	1 pkg	190	4	3	39
Instant Oatmeal Crunch Mixed Berry	1 pkg	190	4	3	39
Instant Oatmeal Express Baked Apple	1 pkg	200	4	3	42
Instant Oatmeal For Kids Dinosaur Eggs	1 pkg	190	4	4	37
Instant Oatmeal Lower Sugar Maple & Brown Sugar	1 pkg	120	4	2	24
Instant Oatmeal Maple Brown Sugar w/ Pecans	1 pkg	160	4	4	30
Instant Oatmeal Nutrition For Women Golden Brown Sugar	1 pkg	170	5	2	32
Instant Oatmeal Organic Regular	1 pkg	100	4	2	19
Instant Oatmeal Regular	1 pkg	100	4	2	19
Instant Oatmeal Simple Harvest Apples w/ Cinnamon	1 pkg	150	4	2	32
Instant Oatmeal Strawberries & Cream	1 pkg	130	3	3	27
Instant Oatmeal Supreme Apple Raisin	1 pkg	150	4	2	32
Instant Oatmeal Supreme Cinnamon Pecan	1 pkg	180	4	4	33

FOOD	PORTION	CALS	PROT	FAT	CARB
Instant Oatmeal Take Heart Golden Maple	1 pkg	160	4	3	33
Instant Oatmeal Weight Control Banana Bread	1 pkg	160	7	3	29
Oat Bran Hot Cereal not prep	½ cup	150	7	3	25
Quick Oats Sun Country Iron Fortified	1 pkg	150	5	3	27
Ralston					
Corn Flakes	1 cup (1 oz)	100	2	0	24
Raisin Bran	1 cup (2 oz)	190	4	1	46
Roman Meal					
Cream Of Rye not prep	⅓ cup (1.4 oz)	130	6	0	27
Elements Cranberry Passion	1 cup (1.6 oz)	160	5	3	33
Hot Cereal not prep	⅓ cup (1.3 oz)	120	6	2	26
Silhouette Solution					
Oatmeal Cinnamon Apple	1 pkg. (1.39 oz)	150	15	2	17
South Beach					
Crunch Strawberry Harvest	1 cup	170	7	2	37
Crunch Vanilla Almond	1 cup	180	8	4	35
Granola Clusters Cherry Almond	1 pkg (1 oz)	130	6	4	18
Granola Clusters Mixed Berry	1 pkg (1 oz)	130	6	4	18
Stark Sisters					
Granola Lo-Fat Raspberry Blueberry	½ cup	230	4	7	38
Granola Nutty Maple	½ cup	250	6	11	32
Granola Original Maple Almond	½ cup	240	6	10	33
Sunbelt					
Granola Low Fat Cinnamon & Raisins	½ cup	250	4	3	52
Udi's					
Granola BanaBerry	¼ cup (1.1 oz)	120	3	4	19
Granola Hawaiian	¼ cup (1.1 oz)	120	3	5	19
Granola Muesli	¼ cup (1.1 oz)	120	4	4	18
Granola Nuggets	¼ cup (1.1 oz)	150	3	6	22
Granola Original	¼ cup (1.1 oz)	130	3	5	18
Uncle Sam					
Original	¾ cup (1.9 oz)	190	7	5	38

FOOD	PORTION	CALS	PROT	FAT	CARB
Weetabix					
Organic	2 biscuits (1.2 oz)	120	4	1	28
Organic Crispy Flakes	¾ cup	110	3	1	24
Wheatena					
Toasted Wheat	⅓ cup	160	5	1	33
YogActive					
Probiotic High Fibre Wheat Strawberry Raspberry	⅔ cup	160	5	3	29
Probiotic Kiwi	⅔ cup	120	3	2	23
Probiotic Strawberry	⅔ cup	130	3	2	25
Probiotic Strawberry Dark Chocolate	⅔ cup	130	3	3	26

CEREAL BARS (see also ENERGY BARS)

FOOD	PORTION	CALS	PROT	FAT	CARB
Aristo					
Acai Blueberry Lime	1 (1.3 oz)	130	3	4	22
Pomegranate & Cranberry	1 (1.3 oz)	140	3	5	21
Attune					
Wellness Yogurt & Granola Lemon Creme	1 (1.4 oz)	180	5	7	24
Wellness Yogurt & Granola Strawberry Bliss	1 (1.4 oz)	180	5	7	24
Bakery On Main					
Granola Gluten Free Extreme Trail Mix	1 (1.3 oz)	140	3	5	23
Granola Gluten Free Peanut Butter Chocolate Chip	1 (1.2 oz)	140	2	5	24
Barbara's Bakery					
Fruit & Yogurt Cherry Apple	1	150	3	3	29
Nature's Choice Blueberry	1 (1.3 oz)	150	2	2	29
Organic Crunchy Granola Cinnamon Crisp	2 (1.5 oz)	190	4	8	27
Cascadian Farm					
Organic Chewy Granola Fruit & Nut	1 (1.2 oz)	140	2	4	24
CocoaVia					
Dark Chocolate Almond	1 (0.8 oz)	90	1	2	13
Country Choice Organic					
Oatmeal Squares Apple Cinnamon	1 (2 oz)	210	4	3	41
Oatmeal Squares Maple	1 (2 oz)	210	4	3	41

FOOD	PORTION	CALS	PROT	FAT	CARB
Enjoy Life					
Allergen Gluten Free Caramel Apple	1 (1 oz)	110	2	3	21
Glenny's					
Organic Muesli Chocolate Chip	1 (1.6 oz)	170	3	3	34
Organic Muesli Raisins & Dates	1 (1.6 oz)	170	3	3	34
Slim Carb Bars Brownie Cheesecake	1 (1.3 oz)	130	12	3	19
Slim-1 w/ Acai Very Berry Blast	1 (1.1 oz)	100	2	3	21
Slim-1 w/ GreenTea Double Fudge	1 (1.1 oz)	100	3	3	20
Slim-1 w/ Hoodia Peanut Butter Caramel	1 (1.1 oz)	100	2	4	20
Glutino					
Gluten Free Breakfast Bar Apple	1 (1.4 oz)	120	2	1	25
Gluten Free Breakfast Bar Chocolate	1 (1.4 oz)	110	2	1	25
Gluten Free Organic Chocolate & Peanut	1 (1 oz)	110	2	3	19
Gluten Free Organic Wildberry	1 (1 oz)	100	1	1	21
Granola Gourmet					
Brownie	1 (1.25 oz)	150	4	6	20
Chocolate Espresso	1 (1.25 oz)	150	4	6	20
Spiced Orange Cranberry	1 (1.25 oz)	140	4	5	20
Health Valley					
Cafe Creations Cinnamon Danish	1 (1.4 oz)	130	2	3	27
Date Almond Low Fat	1 (1.5 oz)	150	1	3	32
Granola Chocolate Chip Low Fat	1 (1.5 oz)	160	2	3	32
Granola Moist & Chewy Dutch Apple	1 (1 oz)	100	1	2	20
Granola Trail Mix Cranberries Nuts & Yogurt Chips	1 (1.2 oz)	140	3	4	23
Organic Fig Cobbler	1 (1.4 oz)	130	2	3	26
Organic Raspberry Tarts	1 (1.4 oz)	150	2	3	30
Organic Strawberry Cobbler	1 (1.3 oz)	130	2	3	26
Peanut Butter & Grape	1 (1.3 oz)	130	2	3	26
Hershey's					
Sweet & Salty Granola Bar Reese's w/ Chocolate	1 (1.2 oz)	160	4	9	18

FOOD	PORTION	CALS	PROT	FAT	CARB
Sweet & Salty Granola Bar w/ Pretzels	1 (1.2 oz)	140	3	5	22
Honest Foods					
Cran Lemon Zest	1 (2.2 oz)	240	6	9	35
Farmer's Trail Mix	1 (2.2 oz)	240	6	9	35
Jungle Grub					
Berry Bamboozle w/ Vanilla Icing Gluten Free	1 (0.9 oz)	100	4	4	14
Chocolate Chip Cookie Dough w/ Chocolate Coating Gluten Free	1 (0.9 oz)	100	4	4	13
Peanut Butter Groove w/ Vanilla Icing Gluten Free	1 (0.9 oz)	100	4	4	13
Kashi					
TLC Chewy Granola Dark Mocha Almond	1 (1.2 oz)	130	6	4	21
TLC Chewy Granola Honey Almond Flax	1 (1.2 oz)	140	5	5	19
TLC Soft Baked Apple Spice	1 (1.2 oz)	110	2	3	21
TLC Soft Baked Blackberry Graham	1 (1.2 oz)	110	2	1	21
TLC Soft Baked Ripe Strawberry	1 (1.2 oz)	110	2	3	21
Kellogg's					
FiberPlus Antioxidants Chocolate Chip	1 (1.2 oz)	120	2	4	26
FiberPlus Antioxidants Dark Chocolate Almond	1 (1.2 oz)	130	2	5	24
KeriBar					
Vegan Apple Peanut Butter	1 (1.4 oz)	140	6	6	21
Vegan Cherry Almond	1 (1.4 oz)	140	8	6	21
Vegan Strawberry Chocolate Chip	1 (1.4 oz)	130	6	5	23
Kind					
Almond & Coconut	1	193	4	14	14
Almonds & Apricot In Yogurt	1	208	4	13	19
Banana & Oatbran	1	160	2	7	23
Nut Delight	1	203	7	15	12
Walnut & Date	1	150	2	7	22
Kudos					
Granola Chocolate Chip	1 (1 oz)	120	1	4	20

FOOD	PORTION	CALS	PROT	FAT	CARB
Lean Body					
Hi-Protein Granola Peanuts 'N Chocolate	1 (2.8 oz)	340	20	11	39
Natural Ovens					
Great Granola Mixed Fruit	1 (1.4 oz)	150	4	3	27
Post					
Honey Bunches Of Oats Banana Nut	1 (1.2 oz)	140	2	4	24
Honey Bunches Of Oats Oatmeal Raisin	1 (1.2 oz)	130	2	3	25
Quaker					
Breakfast Bar Apple Crisp	1 (1.3 oz)	130	1	3	27
Breakfast Bar Iced Raspberry	1 (1.3 oz)	130	1	3	26
Breakfast Bites Iced Raspberry	1 pkg (1.3 oz)	130	1	3	28
Breakfast Bites Strawberry	1 pkg (1.3 oz)	130	1	3	27
Chewy Chocolate Chip	1 (0.8 oz)	100	1	3	18
Chewy Cookies & Cream	1 (0.8 oz)	90	1	3	18
Chewy 90 Calorie Cinnamon Sugar	1 (1 oz)	90	1	2	19
Chewy 90 Calorie Honey Nut	1 (0.8 oz)	90	1	2	19
Chewy Dipps Peanut Butter	1 (1 oz)	150	3	7	18
Chewy Granola w/ Protein Peanut Butter & Chocolate	1 (1 oz)	110	5	3	18
Chewy Low Fat S'mores	1 (1 oz)	110	1	2	22
Crunchy Granola Oats & Berries	1 (1 oz)	130	2	4	23
Oatmeal To Go Oatmeal Raisin	1 (2.1 oz)	220	4	4	43
Oatmeal To Go Raspberry Streusel	1 (2.1 oz)	220	4	4	43
Q-Smart Cranberry Vanilla Almond	1 (1 oz)	120	10	6	9
Trail Mix Cranberry Raisin & Almond	1 (1.2 oz)	150	2	5	24
Reese's					
SnackBarz Peanut Butter	1 (0.9 oz)	120	2	5	16
Revolution Foods					
Jammy Sammy Apple Cinnamon & Oatmeal	1 (1 oz)	100	1	2	21
Organic Jammy Sammy PB & Grape	1 (1 oz)	110	2	3	19

FOOD	PORTION	CALS	PROT	FAT	CARB
Organic Jammy Sammy PB & Strawberry	1 (1 oz)	110	2	3	19
Roman Meal					
Whole Grain & Fruit	1 (2 oz)	190	4	2	43
Silhouette Solution					
Blueberry Pomegranate	1 (1.3 oz)	130	15	3	14
Peanut Passion	1 (1.3 oz)	130	15	4	14
South Beach					
Fiber Fit Granola Mocha	1 (1.2 oz)	120	2	4	25
Fiber Fit Granola S'Mores	1 (1.2 oz)	120	2	4	25
Wings Of Nature					
Organic Apple Cinnamon	1 (1.2 oz)	119	3	4	21
Organic Cafe Mocha Coffee	1 (1.2 oz)	153	3	9	18
Organic Cappuccino Coffee	1 (1.2 oz)	153	3	9	17
Yotta					
Apple Cinnamon	1 (1.2 oz)	120	2	1	25
Cherry	1 (1.2 oz)	120	2	1	26
Orange	1 (1.2 oz)	120	2	1	26
CHAMPAGNE					
champagne	1 serv (3.5 oz)	84	tr	0	3
mimosa	1 serv	117	1	tr	12
punch	1 serv (4 oz)	73	tr	tr	8
sekt german champagne	1 serv (3.5 oz)	84	tr	0	5
CHAYOTE					
fresh cooked	1 cup	38	1	1	8
raw	1 (7 oz)	49	2	1	11
raw cut up	1 cup	32	1	tr	7
CHEESE (*see also* CHEESE DISHES, CHEESE SUBSTITUTES, COTTAGE CHEESE, CREAM CHEESE, NEUFCHATEL)					
american	1 oz	93	6	7	2
american cheese spread	1 oz	82	5	6	2
beaufort	1 oz	115	8	9	tr
bel paese	1 oz	112	7	9	0
blue	1 oz	100	6	8	1
blue crumbled	1 cup (4.7 oz)	477	29	39	3
bocconcini smoked	1 oz	90	6	6	1
brick	1 oz	105	7	8	1
brie	1 oz	95	8	8	tr

FOOD	PORTION	CALS	PROT	FAT	CARB
cacio di roma sheep's milk cheese	1 oz	130	8	10	0
caerphilly	1.4 oz	150	9	13	0
camembert	1 oz	85	6	7	tr
cantal	1 oz	105	7	9	tr
caraway	1 oz	107	7	8	1
chabichou	1 oz	95	6	8	tr
chaource	1 oz	83	5	7	tr
cheddar	1 oz	114	7	9	tr
cheddar low sodium	1 oz	113	7	9	1
cheddar lowfat	1 oz	49	9	2	1
cheddar reduced fat	1.4 oz	104	13	6	0
cheddar shredded	1 cup	455	28	37	1
cheshire	1 oz	110	7	9	1
cheshire reduced fat	1.4 oz	108	13	6	tr
colby	1 oz	112	7	9	1
colby low sodium	1 oz	113	7	9	1
colby lowfat	1 oz	49	9	2	1
comte	1 oz	114	8	9	tr
coulommiers	1 oz	88	6	7	tr
crottin	1 oz	105	6	9	tr
derby	1.4 oz	161	10	14	0
edam reduced fat	1.4 oz	92	13	4	tr
emmentaler	1 oz	115	8	9	tr
feta	1 oz	75	4	6	1
fontina	1 oz	110	7	9	tr
frais	1.6 oz	51	3	3	3
gjetost	1 oz	132	3	8	12
gloucester double	1.4 oz	162	10	14	0
goat fresh	1 oz	23	1	2	tr
goat hard	1 oz	128	9	10	1
gorgonzola	1 oz	107	5	9	tr
gouda	1 oz	101	7	8	1
grana padano parmesan shaved	1 tbsp	20	2	2	0
gruyere	1 oz	117	8	9	tr
lancashire	1.4 oz	149	9	12	0
leicester	1.4 oz	160	10	14	0
limburger	1 oz	93	8	8	tr
lymeswold	1.4 oz	170	6	16	tr
maroilles	1 oz	97	6	8	tr

FOOD	PORTION	CALS	PROT	FAT	CARB
monterey	1 oz	106	7	9	tr
morbier	1 oz	99	7	8	tr
mozzarella	1 oz	80	6	6	1
mozzarella fresh	1 oz	80	6	6	tr
mozzarella part skim	1 oz	72	7	5	1
muenster	1 oz	104	7	9	tr
parmesan grated	1 tbsp	23	2	2	tr
parmesan hard	1 oz	111	10	7	1
picodon	1 oz	99	6	8	tr
pimento	1 oz	106	6	9	tr
pont l'eveque	1 oz	86	6	7	tr
port du salut	1 oz	100	7	8	tr
provolone	1 oz	100	7	8	1
pyrenees	1 oz	101	6	8	tr
quark 20% fat	1 oz	33	4	1	1
quark 40% fat	1 oz	48	3	3	1
quark made w/ skim milk	1 oz	22	4	tr	1
queso anejo	1 oz	106	6	9	1
queso asadero	1 oz	101	6	8	1
queso chihuahua	1 oz	106	6	8	2
queso fresco	1 oz	41	4	2	1
queso manchego	1 oz	107	8	8	tr
queso panela	1 oz	74	6	5	1
raclette	1 oz	102	7	8	tr
reblochon	1 oz	88	6	7	tr
ricotta part skim	½ cup (4.4 oz)	171	14	10	6
ricotta whole milk	½ cup (4.4 oz)	216	14	16	4
romadur 40% fat	1 oz	83	7	6	tr
romano	1 oz	110	9	8	1
roquefort	1 oz	105	6	9	1
rouy	1 oz	95	7	8	tr
saint marcellin	1 oz	94	5	8	tr
saint nectaire	1 oz	97	6	8	tr
saint paulin	1 oz	85	7	6	tr
sainte maure	1 oz	99	6	8	tr
selles sur cher	1 oz	93	5	8	tr
stilton blue	1.4 oz	164	9	14	0
stilton white	1.4 oz	145	8	13	0
swiss	1 oz	107	8	8	1
swiss processed	1 oz	95	7	7	1

FOOD	PORTION	CALS	PROT	FAT	CARB
tilsit	1 oz	96	7	7	1
tome	1 oz	92	6	7	tr
triple creme	1 oz	113	3	11	tr
vacherin	1 oz	92	5	8	tr
wensleydale	1.4 oz	151	9	13	0
whey cheese	1 oz	126	4	8	9
yogurt cheese	1 oz	80	6	7	0
Alpine Lace					
Reduced Fat Provolone	1 slice (0.8 oz)	70	6	5	1
Reduced Fat Swiss	1 slice (0.8 oz)	70	7	5	1
Reduced Fat White American	1 slice (0.8 oz)	70	5	5	1
Reduced Sodium Muenster	1 slice (0.8 oz)	90	6	7	0
Applegate Farms					
Organic Cheddar Milk	1 slice (0.7 oz)	85	5	6	0
Organic Muenster Kase	1 slice (0.8 oz)	85	5	7	0
Yogurt Cheese w/ Probiotics	1 slice (0.7 oz)	80	5	6	tr
Athenos					
Traditional	¼ cup	90	7	7	2
Traditional Reduced Fat	¼ cup	70	7	5	1
Bel Gioioso					
Mozzarella Fresh	1 in cube (1 oz)	80	5	6	0
Cabot					
Cheddar	1 oz	110	7	9	tr
Cheddar Horseradish	1 oz	110	6	9	1
Cheddar Tomato Basil	1 oz	110	7	9	tr
Cheddar Light 50% Reduced Fat	1 oz	70	8	5	tr
Cheddar Light 50% Reduced Fat Omega-3	1 oz	70	8	5	tr
Cheddar Light 75% Reduced Fat	1 oz	60	9	3	tr
Cheddar Shake	2 tsp	25	1	2	1
Monterey Jack	1 oz	110	7	9	tr
Pepper Jack 50% Reduced Fat	1 oz	70	8	5	tr
Swiss Slices	1 (1 oz)	110	8	8	1
Connoisseur					
Asiago Spread	1 tbsp	90	5	7	2
Brie Spread	2 tbsp	90	4	7	2
Gorgonzola Spread	1 tbsp	90	5	7	2
Wheel Asiago Pesto	2 tbsp	90	5	6	4
Wheel Swiss Bacon	2 tbsp	90	5	7	2

FOOD	PORTION	CALS	PROT	FAT	CARB
Cracker Barrel					
Fontina	1 slice (0.7 oz)	80	6	7	tr
Sharp Cheddar 2% Milk	1 oz	90	7	6	tr
DiGiorno					
Shredded Three Cheese Parmesan Romano & Asiago	¼ cup (1 oz)	110	9	8	1
Dragone					
Mozzarella Whole Milk	1 oz	90	6	7	tr
Parmesan Wedge	1 oz	100	9	7	tr
Ricotta Part Skim	¼ cup (2.2 oz)	90	6	6	4
Easy Cheese					
American	2 tbsp (1.1 oz)	90	5	6	2
Cheddar	2 tbsp (1.1 oz)	90	5	6	2
Finlandia					
Swiss Thin Sliced	1 slice (0.5 oz)	55	4	4	0
Fresh Made					
Farmers Cheese Nonfat	2 tbsp	15	5	0	1
Friendship					
Farmer	2 tbsp (1 oz)	50	5	3	0
Farmer No Salt Added	2 tbsp (1 oz)	50	5	3	0
Frigo					
Mozzarella Part Skim	1 oz	80	7	6	tr
Parmesan Shredded	¼ cup (1 oz)	100	9	7	1
Ricotta Whole Milk	¼ cup (2.2 oz)	110	7	8	2
Romano Shredded	¼ cup (1 oz)	100	8	7	1
Haolam					
Cheddar Sliced	1 slice (1 oz)	114	7	9	1
Horizon Organic					
American	1 slice (0.7 oz)	60	4	5	1
Cheddar	1 oz	110	7	9	tr
Monterey Jack	1 oz	100	7	8	0
Shred Mexican	¼ cup	110	7	9	tr
Shred Parmesan	1 tbsp	20	2	2	0
Slice Provolone	1 slice (0.7 oz)	70	5	6	0
Sticks Colby	1 (1 oz)	110	7	9	tr
String Mozzarella	1 stick (1 oz)	80	8	5	tr
J.L. Kraft					
Spreadable Feta & Spinach	2 tbsp	80	3	7	1

FOOD	PORTION	CALS	PROT	FAT	CARB
Kraft					
Cheddar Sharp Shredded 2% Milk	¼ cup	80	7	6	tr
Crumbles Three Cheese	¼ cup (1 oz)	110	6	9	tr
LiveActive 1% Milk Cheddar Cubes	7 (1 oz)	90	8	6	tr
LiveActive 2% Milk Marbled Colby & Monterey Jack	1 stick (1 oz)	90	8	6	tr
LiveActive Cheddar Cheese Sticks	1 (1 oz)	120	6	10	0
LiveActive Colby & Monterey Jack Cubes	7 (1 oz)	110	7	9	tr
LiveActive Mozzarella Sticks	1 (1 oz)	80	8	5	tr
Shredded Mexican Style Cheddar & Monterey Jack	¼ cup	110	6	9	1
Land O' Lakes					
American	1 slice (0.7 oz)	70	4	5	2
Chedarella	1 oz	110	7	9	0
Cheddar	1 oz	110	7	9	0
Snack 'N Cheese To Go Cheddar Mild	1 serv (0.7 oz)	80	7	7	0
Snack 'N Cheese To Go Cheddar Mild Reduced Fat	1 serv (0.5 oz)	60	5	5	0
Snack 'N Cheese To Go Co-Jack	1 serv (0.7 oz)	80	5	7	0
Snack 'N Cheese To Go Co-Jack Reduced Fat	1 serv (0.7 oz)	60	5	5	0
Swiss	1 oz	110	8	8	1
Lifeway					
Farmer's Kefir	2 tbsp	25	3	2	4
Farmer's Kefir Lite	2 tbsp	25	3	1	2
Sweet Kiss Peach	1 oz	45	3	1	6
Organic Valley					
Blue Crumbles	1 oz	100	6	8	1
Cheddar Mild	1 oz	110	7	9	0
Feta	1 oz	60	5	4	tr
Monterey Jack Shredded	¼ cup	80	8	5	1
Muenster	1 slice (0.7 oz)	80	5	6	0
Provolone	1 slice (0.7 oz)	70	5	6	0
Swiss	1 oz	110	7	9	0

FOOD	PORTION	CALS	PROT	FAT	CARB
Rosenborg					
Danish Camembert	1 oz	80	5	7	0
Rouge Et Noir					
Breakfast	1 oz	90	6	7	0
Brie Garlic	1 oz	90	6	7	0
Brie Pesto	1 oz	90	6	7	0
Brie Tomato Basil	1 oz	90	6	7	0
Brie Triple Creme	1 oz	110	4	10	0
Camembert	1 oz	90	6	7	0
Le Petit Bleu	1 oz	110	4	10	0
Le Petit Chevre	1 oz	90	5	6	0
Marin French Blue	1 oz	110	4	10	0
Marin French Gold	1 oz	110	4	10	0
Schlosskranz	1 oz	85	5	7	0
Saladena					
Goat Crumbles	¼ cup	80	5	7	tr
Sap Sago					
Fat Free Cheese Grated	1 tsp	10	2	0	0
Sargento					
4 Cheese Italian Shredded	¼ cup	80	8	5	1
4 Cheese Mexican Reduced Fat Shredded	¼ cup (1 oz)	80	8	6	tr
American Burger	1 slice (0.7 oz)	70	4	6	tr
Bistro Blends Shredded Mozzarella w/ Sun Dried Tomato & Basil	¼ cup	90	7	6	1
Blue Crumbled	¼ cup (1 oz)	100	6	8	1
Cheddar Chipotle Shredded	¼ cup	100	6	8	1
Cheddar Chipotle Sticks	1 (0.7 oz)	80	5	6	1
Cheddar Mild Cubes	7 (1 oz)	120	7	10	tr
Cheddar Mild Shredded Reduced Fat	¼ cup (1 oz)	80	7	6	tr
Cheddar White Vermont Sharp	1 slice (0.7 oz)	80	5	7	0
Cheddar White Vermont Sharp Shredded	¼ cup (1 oz)	110	7	9	1
Cheese Dips Cheddar & Buttery Pretzels	1 pkg (3.8 oz)	360	9	16	47
Cheese Dips Cheddar & Tortilla Chips	1 pkg (3 oz)	320	7	21	26
Colby-Jack Shredded	¼ cup (1 oz)	110	6	9	1
Jarlsberg	1 slice (0.8 oz)	80	6	6	tr

FOOD	PORTION	CALS	PROT	FAT	CARB
Monterey Jack Shredded	¼ cup (1 oz)	110	7	9	1
Mozzarella Reduced Fat Shredded	¼ cup (1 oz)	80	8	5	tr
Mozzarella Shredded	¼ cup (1 oz)	80	7	6	1
Muenster	1 slice (0.7 oz)	80	5	6	0
Nacho & Taco Shredded	¼ cup (1 oz)	110	7	9	1
Parmesan Grated	2 tsp (5 g)	25	2	2	0
Parmesan Shredded	2 tsp	20	2	2	0
Pepper Jack	1 slice (0.7 oz)	80	6	6	0
Provolone	1 slice (0.7 oz)	70	5	5	0
Provolone Reduced Fat	1 slice (0.7 oz)	50	5	4	0
Ricotta Fat Free	¼ cup	50	5	0	5
Ricotta Light	¼ cup	60	5	3	3
Ricotta Whole Milk	¼ cup	90	7	8	3
String	1 piece (1 oz)	80	8	6	tr
String Light	1 piece (0.7 oz)	50	6	3	tr
Swiss Reduced Fat	1 slice (0.7 oz)	80	7	4	1
Swiss Shredded	¼ cup (1 oz)	110	8	8	tr
Swiss Thick Slice	1 slice (1 oz)	110	8	8	1
Swiss Thin Sliced	1 slice (0.6 oz)	70	5	5	0
Stella					
3 Cheese Italian Shredded	¼ cup	100	8	7	1
Asiago Wedge	1 oz	110	6	9	tr
Gorgonzola Wedge	1 oz	100	6	9	tr
Kasseri Wedge	1 oz	110	6	9	tr
The Greek Gods					
Kefir Cheese	2 tbsp (1 oz)	80	2	5	2
Treasure Cave					
Blue Cheese Crumbled	¼ cup (1 oz)	100	6	8	tr
Feta Crumbled	¼ cup (1 oz)	60	4	5	tr
Gorgonzola Crumbled	¼ cup (1 oz)	100	6	8	tr
Weight Watchers					
String Light	1 stick (0.8 oz)	50	6	3	tr
Wholesome Valley					
Organic American	1 slice (0.7 oz)	50	3	4	tr
CHEESE DISHES					
Banquet					
Mozzarella Nuggets	7	270	10	16	21
Farm Rich					
Cheese Sticks Breaded	2 (2.1 oz)	210	9	12	17

FOOD	PORTION	CALS	PROT	FAT	CARB
Mozzarella Bites Breaded	4 (2.2 oz)	150	8	7	13
Original Cheese Bites Breaded	7 (2.1 oz)	180	9	11	13
Fillo Factory					
Tyropita Cheese Fillo Appetizers	3 (3 oz)	230	7	14	19
Stouffer's					
Welsh Rarebit	¼ pkg (2.5 oz)	140	6	10	6
TAKE-OUT					
fondue	½ cup (3.8 oz)	247	15	15	4
fried mozzarella sticks	3 (4.6 oz)	503	33	32	20
souffle	1 serv (7 oz)	504	23	38	18
welsh rarebit	1 slice	228	8	16	14

CHEESE SUBSTITUTES

FOOD	PORTION	CALS	PROT	FAT	CARB
mozzarella	1 oz	70	3	3	7
soya cheese	1.4 oz	128	7	11	tr
Playfood					
Cheesey Cheese	1 oz	60	2	5	4
Rice					
American Flavor Vegan	1 slice (0.7 oz)	45	1	3	0
American Flavor	1 slice (0.7 oz)	50	4	3	tr
Shreds Mozzarella Flavor	⅓ cup (1 oz)	70	6	4	3
Sheese					
Blue Style	1 oz	100	4	8	3
Cheddar Style Medium	1 oz	100	4	8	3
Creamy Mexican	2 tbsp	80	2	7	2
Creamy Original	2 tbsp	80	2	7	2
Super Stix					
Mozzarella Flavor	1 (1 oz)	70	6	5	0
Vegan Gourmet					
Cheese Alternative Cheddar	1 oz	50	2	4	2
Cheese Alternative Monterey Jack	1 oz	70	1	7	2
Cheese Alternative Mozzarella	1 oz	70	1	8	1
Cheese Alternative Nacho	1 oz	45	2	4	2
Veggie					
American Flavor	1 slice (0.6 oz)	40	3	3	tr
Grated Parmesan Flavor	2 tsp	15	2	1	0
Pepper Jack Flavor	1 oz	60	6	4	2
Shreds Cheddar Flavor	1 oz	70	6	4	0
Veggy					
Mozzarella Flavor	1 slice (0.7 oz)	40	4	3	tr

FOOD	PORTION	CALS	PROT	FAT	CARB
CHERIMOYA					
fresh	1	515	7	2	131
CHERRIES					
CANNED					
maraschino	1 (4 g)	7	tr	tr	2
maraschino	¼ cup (1.4 oz)	66	tr	tr	17
sour in heavy syrup	½ cup	116	1	tr	30
sour in light syrup	½ cup	94	1	tr	24
sour water packed	½ cup	44	1	tr	11
sweet juice pack	½ cup	68	1	tr	17
sweet pitted in heavy syrup	½ cup	105	1	tr	27
sweet water pack	½ cup	57	1	tr	15
Chukar Cherries					
Cherry Jubilee Dessert Sauce	1 tbsp	40	0	0	10
Del Monte					
Sweet Dark Pitted In Heavy Syrup	½ cup (4.2 oz)	100	tr	0	24
S&W					
Sliced	½ cup (4.7 oz)	140	1	0	34
The Gracious Gourmet					
Spiced Sour Cherry Spread	1 tbsp (0.5 oz)	15	0	0	4
DRIED					
bing unsulfured	¼ cup	130	0	0	31
montmorency tart pitted	⅓ cup	160	2	1	36
tart	½ cup	200	2	1	49
yogurt covered	¼ cup	170	1	6	29
Bob's Red Mill					
Tart	⅓ cup	140	1	0	33
Chukar Cherries					
Bing	3 tbsp	130	1	1	33
Bing Chocolate Covered	3 tbsp (1.4 oz)	180	2	9	24
Cabernet Dark Chocolate Covered	2 tbsp (1.5 oz)	180	2	9	26
Columbia River Tart	⅓ cup	120	2	1	36
Rainier	3 tbsp	130	tr	1	33
Totally Tart	⅓ cup	140	1	1	33
De-Lite					
Tart	1 oz	95	1	tr	23
Emily's					
Dark Chocolate Covered	11 (1.4 oz)	180	1	9	27

FOOD	PORTION	CALS	PROT	FAT	CARB
Peeled Snacks					
Fruit Picks Cherry-Go-Round	1 pkg (1.5 oz)	130	2	0	30
Stoneridge Orchards					
Bing	⅓ cup (1.4 oz)	130	1	0	32
Organic Montmorency Whole	⅓ cup (1.4 oz)	135	0	1	33
Sunsweet					
Tart & Sweet	¼ cup (1.4 oz)	100	1	0	30
FRESH					
sour	1 cup	52	1	tr	13
sour pitted	1 cup	78	2	tr	19
sweet	20	86	1	1	22
Chiquita					
Cherries	1 cup (4.8 oz)	87	1	0	22
FROZEN					
sour unsweetened	½ cup	36	1	tr	9
sweet sweetened	½ cup	115	2	tr	29
CHERRY JUICE					
tart cherry concentrate	1 cup	140	1	0	34
Froose					
Cheerful Cherry	1 box (4.2 oz)	80	0	0	19
HP					
Tart Montmorency Concentrate	1 oz	80	tr	0	19
Old Orchard					
100% Pure Tart Cherry	8 oz	140	0	0	34
Santa Cruz					
Organic 100% Juice Red Tart	8 oz	120	0	0	30
Smart Juice					
Organic 100% Juice Tart Cherry	8 oz	130	1	0	32
Tart Is Smart					
Tart Cherry Concentrate	1 oz	80	1	0	19
CHERVIL					
seed	1 tsp	1	tr	tr	tr
CHESTNUTS					
chinese steamed	3 (1 oz)	43	1	tr	10
creme de marrons	1 oz	73	1	tr	18
japanese roasted	1 oz	57	1	tr	13
ready-to-eat vacuum packed	5 (1 oz)	40	tr	0	8
roasted	3 (1 oz)	70	1	1	15

FOOD	PORTION	CALS	PROT	FAT	CARB
Gefen					
Whole Roasted & Peeled	¼ cup (1.4 oz)	52	1	0	11
CHEWING GUM					
bubble gum	1 block	20	0	tr	5
stick	1 piece	7	0	tr	2
sugarless	1 piece	5	0	tr	2
Bubble Yum					
Original	1 piece (8 g)	25	0	0	6
Sugarless	1 piece (5 g)	10	0	0	3
Choward's					
Scented Gum	3 pieces	10	0	0	3
Dubble Bubble					
Gumball	1 piece	10	0	0	2
Extra					
Sugar Free All Flavors	1 piece	5	0	0	2
Flare					
Warming Cinnamon	1 piece	5	0	0	2
Orbit					
Sugarfree Citrusmint	1 piece	<5	0	0	1
White Melon Breeze	2 pieces	5	0	0	2
Trident					
Extra Care	1 piece	<5	0	0	1
Splash Strawberry Lime	1 piece	<5	0	0	2
Winterfresh					
Gum	1 stick	10	0	0	2
CHIA SEEDS					
dried	1 oz	134	5	7	14
CHICKEN (see also CHICKEN DISHES, CHICKEN SUBSTITUTES, DINNER, HOT DOG)					
CANNED					
chicken spread	1 serv (2 oz)	88	10	10	2
meat drained	1 can (5 oz)	230	32	10	1
w/ broth	½ can (2.5 oz)	117	15	6	0
Hormel					
Chunk White & Dark	2 oz	70	10	3	0
Premium Chunk Breast	2 oz	60	12	2	0
Swanson					
Chunk Breast In Water	2 oz	50	9	1	1
Tyson					
Premium Chunk	½ can (2 oz)	60	10	3	0
Premium Chunk Breast	½ can (2 oz)	60	13	1	0

FOOD	PORTION	CALS	PROT	FAT	CARB
FRESH					
back w/ skin roasted bones removed	1 (3.7 oz)	318	28	22	0
back w/o skin roasted bones removed	1 (2.8 oz)	191	23	11	0
breast roasted diced	1 cup (5 oz)	231	43	5	0
breast w/ skin battered fried bones removed	½ breast (4.9 oz)	364	35	18	13
breast w/ skin floured fried bones removed	1 (3.4 oz)	218	31	9	2
breast w/ skin roasted bones removed	½ breast (3.4 oz)	193	29	8	0
breast w/ skin stewed bones removed	½ breast (3.9 oz)	202	30	8	0
breast w/o skin fried bones removed	½ breast (3 oz)	161	29	4	tr
breast w/o skin roasted bones removed	½ breast (3 oz)	142	27	3	0
breast w/o skin stewed bones removed	1 (3.3 oz)	143	28	3	0
broiler/fryer w/ skin roasted bones removed	½ (10.5 oz)	715	82	41	0
capon meat & skin roasted bones removed	½ (1.4 lbs)	1459	184	74	0
cornish hen w/ skin roasted	½ (4.5 oz)	335	29	23	0
cornish hen w/ skin roasted	1 (9 oz)	668	57	47	0
cornish hen w/o skin roasted	1 (7.7 oz)	295	51	9	0
cornish hen w/o skin roasted	½ (4 oz)	147	26	4	0
dark meat w/o skin roasted diced	1 cup (5 oz)	287	38	14	0
drumstick w/ skin battered floured & fried bones removed	1 (1.7 oz)	120	13	7	1
drumstick w/ skin battered fried bones removed	1 (2.5 oz)	193	16	11	6
drumstick w/ skin roasted bones removed	1 (1.8 oz)	112	14	6	0
drumstick w/ skin stewed bones removed	1 (2 oz)	116	14	6	0
drumstick w/o skin fried bones removed	1 (1.5 oz)	82	12	3	0

FOOD	PORTION	CALS	PROT	FAT	CARB
drumstick w/o skin roasted bones removed	1 (1.5 oz)	76	12	2	0
drumstick w/o skin stewed bones removed	1 (1.6 oz)	78	13	3	0
feet cooked	1 (1.2 oz)	73	7	5	tr
ground crumbled fried	3 oz	161	20	9	0
ground patty cooked	1 lg (2.8 oz)	190	22	11	0
ground patty cooked	1 med (2.1 oz)	142	16	8	0
ground patty cooked	1 sm (1.7 oz)	114	13	6	0
meat & skin stewed bones removed	¼ chicken (4.6 oz)	372	35	25	0
neck w/ skin battered fried	1 (1.8 oz)	172	10	12	5
neck w/ skin fried	1 (1.3 oz)	120	9	9	2
neck w/ skin simmered	1 (1.3 oz)	94	7	7	0
roaster meat & skin roasted bones removed	¼ chicken (8.4 oz)	535	58	32	0
skin battered fried from ½ chicken	6.7 oz	749	20	55	44
skin floured fried from ½ chicken	2 oz	281	11	24	5
skin roasted from ½ chicken	2 oz	254	11	23	0
skin stewed from ½ chicken	2.5 oz	261	11	24	0
tail cooked	1 (1 oz)	84	7	5	3
thigh w/ skin battered & fried bones removed	1 (3 oz)	238	19	14	8
thigh w/ skin floured fried bones removed	1 (2.2 oz)	162	17	9	2
thigh w/ skin roasted bones removed	1 (2.2 oz)	153	16	10	0
thigh w/ skin stewed bones removed	1 (2.4 oz)	158	16	10	0
thigh w/o skin fried bones removed	1 (1.8 oz)	113	15	5	1
thigh w/o skin roasted bones removed	1 (1.8 oz)	109	13	6	0
thigh w/o skin stewed bones removed	1 (1.9 oz)	107	14	5	0
wing w/ skin battered fried bones removed	1 (1.7 oz)	159	10	11	5

FOOD	PORTION	CALS	PROT	FAT	CARB
wing w/ skin floured fried bones removed	1 (1.1 oz)	103	8	7	1
wing w/ skin roasted bones removed	1 (1.4 oz)	100	9	7	0
wing w/o skin fried bones removed	1 (0.7 oz)	42	6	2	0
wing w/o skin roasted bones removed	1 (0.7 oz)	43	6	2	0
wing w/o skin stewed bones removed	1 (0.8 oz)	43	7	2	0
Perdue					
Breast Boneless Herb & Pepper	1 piece (4.8 oz)	140	29	2	0
Breast Boneless Roasted Garlic w/ White Wine	1 piece (4.8 oz)	110	29	2	1
Breast Boneless Skinless cooked	3 oz	100	23	1	0
Breast Boneless Skinless cooked	3 oz	110	25	1	0
Breast Perfect Portions Boneless Skinless	1 (4.8 oz)	130	19	2	0
Ground cooked	3 oz	170	18	11	0
Ground Breast cooked	3 oz	80	19	1	0
Oven Ready Cornish Hen Seasoned	4 oz	160	16	10	1
Oven Stuffer Drumstick	1 (3.6 oz)	190	25	11	0
Patties cooked	1 (3 oz)	170	19	11	0
Roaster Oven Ready Seasoned	4 oz	210	17	15	1
Thigh Filets Boneless Skinless	4 oz	150	22	8	0
Thighs Tender & Tasty Boneless Skinless cooked	3 oz	150	17	9	0
Whole Dark Meat cooked	3 oz	210	18	15	0
Whole White Meat cooked	3 oz	170	21	9	0
Whole Chicken Tender & Tasty cooked	3 oz	150	20	8	0
Wingettes cooked	3 oz	170	20	10	0
Wings cooked	3 oz	170	20	10	0
Tyson					
Breasts Boneless Skinless	4 oz	110	23	3	0
Cornish Hen	1 serv (4 oz)	200	19	14	0

FOOD	PORTION	CALS	PROT	FAT	CARB
Drumsticks	4 oz	150	18	9	0
Thigh Cutlets Boneless Skinless	4 oz	130	18	7	0
Whole Cut Up	4 oz	220	19	16	0
Wings	4 oz	220	17	17	0
FROZEN					
breast roll roasted	2 oz	75	8	4	1
fajita strips	1 (0.3 oz)	13	2	1	tr
patty cooked	1 (3.5 oz)	287	15	20	13
Banquet					
Wings Hot & Spicy	¼ pkg (3 oz)	260	19	17	8
Barber					
Buffalo Fingers	1 (3.3 oz)	160	15	4	18
Nuggets 4 Cheese Stuffed	3 (3 oz)	230	14	16	9
Nuggets Cheddar & Bacon Stuffed	3 (3 oz)	240	14	17	8
Potato Chip Sticks	2 pieces (4.5 oz)	350	18	24	16
Health Is Wealth					
Nuggets	4 (3 oz)	130	13	4	11
Organic Prairie					
Ground	4 oz	200	21	12	1
Whole Young Small	4 oz	260	21	17	0
Perdue					
Breast Chunks Breaded BBQ Glazed	3 oz	190	11	8	17
Breast Chunks Breaded General Tso's Glazed	3 oz	190	12	8	16
Breast Chunks Breaded Honey BBQ Glazed	3 oz	180	12	8	17
Breast Chunks Breaded Honey Dijon Glazed	3 oz	200	12	11	16
Tyson					
Any'tizers Barbeque Style Wings	3 (3.2 oz)	200	19	13	7
Any'tizers Homestyle Chicken Fries	7 (3.2 oz)	230	13	11	19
Any'tizers Popcorn Chicken	6 (2.8 oz)	220	12	10	19
Breast Pattie	1 (2.6 oz)	180	10	11	12
Cordon Bleu	1 piece (5.9 oz)	380	22	24	20

FOOD	PORTION	CALS	PROT	FAT	CARB
Diced Strips	1 serv (3 oz)	90	20	1	0
Kiev	1 piece (5.9 oz)	480	17	37	19
READY-TO-EAT					
Applegate Farms					
Organic Roasted	2 oz	60	10	2	1
Butterball					
Breast Oven Roasted Thin Sliced	4 slices (2 oz)	50	11	1	1
Breast Strips Oven Roasted	½ pkg (3 oz)	90	18	2	1
Carl Buddig					
Chicken Sliced	2 oz	85	10	5	1
Healthy Ones					
Oven Roasted 97% Fat Free	4 slices (2 oz)	60	9	2	2
Hormel					
Natural Choice Carved Breast Grilled	½ pkg (2 oz)	60	12	1	0
Oscar Mayer					
Breast Oven Roasted Thin Sliced	⅓ pkg (2 oz)	60	10	2	1
Breast Strips Breaded	½ pkg (3 oz)	170	15	6	14
Breast Strips Grilled	½ pkg (3 oz)	110	19	3	1
Perdue					
Breast Bites Popcorn Breaded	12 (3 oz)	190	10	12	14
Breast Strips Breaded Original	2 (2.6 oz)	160	9	10	12
Cutlets Breaded Original	1 (3 oz)	200	10	13	13
Nuggets Original	5 (2.9 oz)	200	10	13	13
Nuggets w/ Whole Grain Breading	4 (2.8 oz)	160	11	8	13
Short Cuts Carved Chicken Breast Original Roasted	½ cup (2.5 oz)	90	16	2	1
Short Cuts Chicken Breast Grilled	½ cup (2.5 oz)	90	16	2	1
Sara Lee					
Breast Oven Roasted	4 slices (2 oz)	45	10	1	0
Tyson					
Chicken Strips Fajita	1 serv (3 oz)	110	19	2	3
Honey Roasted Breast	2 slices (1.6 oz)	50	8	1	3
Hot Wings Buffalo Style	4	220	20	15	1
Roasted Whole Chicken Lemon Pepper	1 serv (3 oz)	120	17	6	1
Salad Kit Chunk Chicken	1 pkg (3.4 oz)	210	18	9	15

FOOD	PORTION	CALS	PROT	FAT	CARB
TAKE-OUT					
chicken tenders	4 (2.2 oz)	180	11	10	11
CHICKEN DISHES					
FROZEN					
Banquet					
Boneless Popcorn Chicken	11 pieces	180	8	9	18
Wings Honey BBQ	¼ pkg (3 oz)	270	17	17	12
Barber					
Broccoli & Cheese Reduced Fat	1 piece (5.5 oz)	250	25	13	11
Cordon Bleu	1 piece (6 oz)	370	28	23	14
Cordon Bleu Reduced Fat	1 piece (5.5 oz)	260	27	13	11
Creme Brie & Apple	1 piece (6 oz)	350	25	21	18
Kiev	1 piece (6 oz)	430	27	29	15
Mashed Potato Stuffed	1 piece (6 oz)	340	21	18	21
Skinless Breast Stuffed	1 piece (6 oz)	280	21	11	24
MIX					
Chicken Helper					
Asian Chicken Fried Rice as prep	1 cup	250	3	8	22
Classic Creamy Chicken & Noodles as prep	1 cup	280	3	8	24
Jambalaya as prep	1 cup	280	3	8	15
REFRIGERATED					
Tyson					
Chicken Breast Medallions In White Wine & Garlic Sauce	1 serv (5 oz)	140	19	6	3
Ventera					
Rollatini w/ Rice Stuffing & Marsala Wine Sauce	1 serv + sauce (6 oz)	230	24	10	9
TAKE-OUT					
arroz con pollo	1 serv (16 oz)	579	48	14	62
barbecued pulled chicken	1 serv (9 oz)	312	36	2	37
boneless breast w/ apple stuffing	1 serv (5 oz)	260	32	9	10
breast & wing breaded & fried	2 pieces (5.7 oz)	494	36	30	20
buffalo wing + sauce	2 (1.7 oz)	147	12	10	tr
cacciatore breast + sauce	1 serv (5.9 oz)	323	29	18	9

FOOD	PORTION	CALS	PROT	FAT	CARB
cacciatore drumstick + sauce	1 serv (3.2 oz)	172	15	9	5
cacciatore thigh + sauce	1 serv (3.8 oz)	204	18	11	6
cacciatore wing + sauce	1 serv (2.1 oz)	113	10	6	3
chicharrones de pollo	3 (2.6 oz)	289	16	18	14
chicken & dumplings	1 cup (8.6 oz)	368	26	19	22
chicken & noodles in cream sauce	1 cup (8 oz)	323	22	11	32
chicken a la king	1 cup (8.5 oz)	465	24	34	16
chicken cordon bleu + sauce	1 roll (8 oz)	504	44	29	11
chicken meatloaf	1 lg slice (5 oz)	243	29	9	11
chicken pie w/ top crust	1 slice (5.6 oz)	472	19	31	32
chicken satay + peanut sauce	2 skewers	239	27	12	6
chicken breast parmigiana	1 serv (5.8 oz)	278	25	14	13
chicken creole w/o rice	1 cup (8.6 oz)	187	29	4	8
chicken kiev breast meat	1 serv (9 oz)	653	72	34	11
creamed chicken	1 cup (8.5 oz)	388	30	23	14
croquette	1 (2.2 oz)	159	10	9	8
curry	1 cup (8.3 oz)	288	27	16	9
curry breast half + sauce	1 (7 oz)	244	23	14	8
curry drumstick + sauce	1 (3.7 oz)	129	12	7	4
curry thigh + sauce	1 (4.4 oz)	154	14	9	5
curry wing + sauce	1 (2.4 oz)	84	8	5	3
drumstick & thigh breaded & fried	2 pieces (5.2 oz)	431	30	27	16
fricassee	1 cup (8.6 oz)	322	29	18	8
groundnut stew hkatenkwan	1 serv (15.7 oz)	576	38	40	18
jamaican jerk wings	4 wings (9.9 oz)	709	57	51	3
jambalaya w/ sausage & rice	1 cup (8.6 oz)	393	26	21	23
sancocho de pollo dominican chicken stew	1 serv	702	71	30	34
stew	1 cup (8.8 oz)	176	15	5	19
tetrazzini	1 cup (8.6 oz)	369	20	18	29

CHICKEN SUBSTITUTES
Chicken Free Chicken

Country Smoked	2 oz	80	11	2	5

Gardenburger

Chik'n Grill	1 (2.5 oz)	100	13	3	5

FOOD	PORTION	CALS	PROT	FAT	CARB
Health Is Wealth					
Chicken-Free Nuggets	3 pieces (2.9 oz)	120	14	2	14
Loma Linda					
Fried Chik'n w/ Gravy	2 pieces (2.8 oz)	150	12	10	5
Morningstar Farms					
Chik'n Roasted Herb	1 pattie (2.2 oz)	110	13	3	9
Meal Starters Chik'n Strips	12 pieces (3 oz)	140	23	4	6
Veat					
Chick'n Free Nuggets	1 serv (2.5 oz)	140	21	5	5
Vegetarian Breast	1 (1.8 oz)	90	11	3	5
Worthington					
FriChik Original	2 pieces (3.2 oz)	140	12	8	3
Meatless Chicken Style	1 slice (2 oz)	90	9	5	2
Yves					
Meatless Chicken Burger	1 (2.6 oz)	100	15	3	5
Meatless Smoked Chicken Slices	4 (2.2 oz)	100	14	2	5

CHICKPEAS
CANNED
chickpeas	1 cup	285	12	3	54
Allens					
Garbanzo Beans	½ cup	120	5	3	19
Green Giant					
Garbanzo Beans	½ cup	100	5	2	17
Progresso					
ChickPeas	½ cup	100	5	2	17

DRIED
cooked	1 cup	269	15	4	45
Arrowhead Mills					
Organic Dried Chickpeas not prep	¼ cup	160	9	3	27

CHICORY
endive fresh chopped	½ cup	4	tr	tr	1
greens raw chopped	½ cup	21	2	tr	4

FOOD	PORTION	CALS	PROT	FAT	CARB
root raw	1 (2.1 oz)	44	1	tr	11
roots raw cut up	½ cup (1.6 oz)	33	1	tr	8
witloof head raw	1 (1.9 oz)	9	tr	tr	2
witloof raw	½ cup (1.6 oz)	8	tr	tr	2

CHILI
powder	1 tbsp	24	1	1	4
Ahh!Gourmet					
Wriggly Sambal Chili Sauce Paste	4 tbsp	170	7	9	15
Allergaroo					
Gluten Free Chili Mac	1 pkg (8 oz)	240	5	4	50
Amy's					
Organic Black Bean Medium	1 cup	200	13	2	31
Whole Meals Chili & Cornbread	1 pkg	340	11	6	59
Comfort Care					
Vegetarian White	1 cup (8 oz)	150	11	2	26
Dennison's					
Con Carne	1 cup	350	22	15	31
Fat Free w/ Beans	1 cup	210	20	2	29
Turkey	1 cup	210	16	3	29
Vegetarian	1 cup	190	9	2	34
Dynasty					
Thai Chili Garlic Paste	1 tsp (5 g)	0	0	0	0
Health Valley					
Chunky Spicy Vegetarian No Salt Added	1 cup	150	9	1	31
Vegetarian Spicy	1 cup	150	9	1	31
Heinz					
Chili Sauce	1 tbsp (0.6 oz)	20	0	0	5
Hormel					
Chili Mac	1 pkg (9.9 oz)	270	17	7	34
Chili No Beans	1 pkg (7.3 oz)	190	14	8	16
Chili No Beans Less Sodium	1 serv (8.3 oz)	220	16	9	18
Chili w/ Beans	1 serv (8.7 oz)	260	16	7	33
Chili w/ Beans Less Sodium	1 serv (8.7 oz)	260	16	7	33
Turkey Chili w/ Beans	1 serv (8.7 oz)	210	17	3	28
Vegetarian Chili w/ Beans	1 serv (8.7 oz)	190	11	1	35
Master Chili					
Chipotle Chicken No Bean	1 serv (8.3 oz)	230	18	10	18
Roasted Tomato w/ Bean	1 serv (8.7 oz)	210	14	6	25

FOOD	PORTION	CALS	PROT	FAT	CARB
McIlhenny					
Original Recipe	½ cup	50	2	1	10
Mimi's Gourmet					
Organic Vegan Gluten Free 3 Bean w/ Rice	1 pkg (11.5 oz)	270	10	6	46
Organic Vegan Gluten Free Black Bean & Corn	1 pkg (10.5 oz)	250	10	6	40
Organic Vegan Gluten Free White Bean	1 pkg (10.5 oz)	230	10	6	35
Spice Hunter					
Powder Blend Salt Free	¼ tsp	0	0	0	0
Thai Kitchen					
Roasted Red Chili Paste	1 tbsp (0.5 oz)	50	1	3	6
Worthington					
Vegetarian	1 cup	280	24	10	25
TAKE-OUT					
chiles rellenos cheese filled	1 (5 oz)	365	17	30	8
chili con carne w/ beans	1 cup	264	21	11	22
chili con carne w/ beans & chicken	1 cup (8.9 oz)	218	19	7	19
con carne w/ beans & rice	1 cup	298	11	9	45
vegetarian con carne	1 cup	272	19	7	35

CHILI PEPPER (see PEPPERS)

CHINESE FOOD (see ASIAN FOOD)

CHINESE PRESERVING MELON

cooked	½ cup	11	tr	tr	3

CHIPS (see also SNACKS)

apple chips	10 (0.8 oz)	101	tr	5	16
banana	1 oz	147	1	10	17
carrot	28 (1 oz)	95	2	tr	22
corn	1 oz	147	2	8	18
plantain	1 oz	158	tr	10	16
potato salted	1 oz	155	2	11	14
potato sticks	½ cup (0.6 oz)	94	1	6	10
potato sticks	1 pkg (1 oz)	148	2	10	15
potato unsalted	1 oz	152	2	10	15
potato unsalted reduced fat	1 oz	138	2	6	19
soy	1 oz	107	8	2	15

FOOD	PORTION	CALS	PROT	FAT	CARB
sweet potato	1 oz	141	1	7	18
taro	10 (0.8 oz)	115	1	6	16
tortilla lowfat baked	1 oz	118	3	2	23
tortilla lowfat unsalted	1 oz	118	3	2	23
tortilla white corn	1 oz	139	2	7	19
tortilla yellow corn	1 oz	139	2	6	19
Athenos					
Pita Chips Original	11 (1 oz)	120	3	4	19
Beanitos					
Pinto Bean & Flax	10 (1 oz)	150	4	8	14
Boulder Canyon					
Potato 50% Reduced Salt	14 (1 oz)	150	2	8	17
Potato Sour Cream & Chive	14 (1 oz)	150	2	8	15
Potato Spinach & Artichoke	14 (1 oz)	150	2	8	17
Brothers-All-Natural					
Potato Crisps Fresh Onion & Fresh Garlic	1 pkg	45	1	0	10
Potato Crisps Original w/ Sea Salt	1 pkg	45	1	0	10
Burger King					
Potato Flame Broiled	16 (1 oz)	150	1	8	19
Potato Ketchup & Fries	16 (1 oz)	150	1	8	19
Butterfield					
Potato Sticks Shoestring	1 pkg (1.7 oz)	250	3	15	26
Corazonas					
Tortilla Jalapeno Jack	1 oz	140	3	7	16
Tortilla Original	1 oz	140	2	7	16
Tortilla Salsa Picante	1 oz	140	2	7	16
Flat Earth					
Baked Fruit Crisps Apple Cinnamon Grove	14 (1 oz)	130	1	5	21
Baked Fruit Crisps Peach Mango Paradise	14 (1 oz)	130	1	5	21
Baked Fruit Crisps Wild Berry Patch	14 (1 oz)	130	1	5	21
Baked Veggie Crisps Farmland Cheddar	14 (1 oz)	130	2	5	19
Baked Veggie Crisps Garlic & Herb Field	14 (1 oz)	130	2	5	19

FOOD	PORTION	CALS	PROT	FAT	CARB
Baked Veggie Crisps Tangy Tomato Ranch	14 (1 oz)	130	2	5	19
FoodShouldTasteGood					
Tortilla Buffalo	10 (1 oz)	130	2	6	18
Tortilla Chocolate Gluten Free	1 pkg (1 oz)	140	2	7	19
Tortilla Multigrain Gluten Free	1 pkg (1 oz)	140	3	7	18
Tortilla Sweet Potato Gluten Free	10 (1 oz)	130	2	6	18
French's					
Potato Sticks Barbecue	¾ cup	160	2	10	16
Potato Sticks Original	¾ cup	190	2	12	16
Fritos					
Original	32	160	2	10	16
Glenny's					
Organic Soy Barbeque	1 oz	110	8	3	13
Organic Soy Creamy Ranch	1 oz	110	9	3	12
Soy Crisps Apple Cinnamon	½ pkg (0.6 oz)	70	5	2	10
Soy Crisps Caramel	½ pkg (1.3 oz)	70	5	2	9
Soy Crisps Low Fat Lightly Salted	½ pkg (0.6 oz)	70	5	1	9
Soy Crisps No Salt	½ pkg (0.6 oz)	70	5	1	9
Soy Crisps Salt & Pepper	½ pkg (0.6 oz)	70	5	1	9
Soy Crisps White Cheddar	½ pkg (0.6 oz)	70	5	2	9
Spud Delites Sea Salt	1 pkg (1.1 oz)	100	2	1	21
Veggie Fries	½ pkg (0.6 oz)	70	1	1	13
Zen Health Tortilla Crisps Original	1 oz	110	9	3	12
Guiltless Gourmet					
Tortilla Blue Corn	18 (1 oz)	120	3	3	23
Tortilla Chili Lime	18 (1 oz)	120	2	3	19
Tortilla Chipotle	18 (1 oz)	123	2	3	22
Tortilla Yellow Corn	18 (1 oz)	120	2	3	22
Tortilla Yellow Corn Unsalted	18 (1 oz)	120	3	2	22
Hippie Chips					
Baked Potato Chive-Talkin' Sour Cream	1 pkg (0.7 oz)	90	2	3	14
Baked Potato Haight-AshBerry Jalapeno	1 pkg (0.7 oz)	90	1	3	15
Baked Potato Memphis Blues Barbecue	1 pkg (0.7 oz)	90	1	3	15

FOOD	PORTION	CALS	PROT	FAT	CARB
Baked Potato Sea Of Love Salt	1 pkg (1 oz)	125	2	4	21
Baked Potato Woodstock Ranch	1 pkg (0.7 oz)	90	2	3	14
Jay's					
Potato	1 oz	150	2	10	14
Little Wings					
Multi Grain Hot Buffalo Wing w/ Bleu Cheese Drizzle	1 pkg (0.5 oz)	60	1	3	10
Lundberg					
Rice Chips Original Sea Salt	1 oz	140	2	7	18
Rice Chips Sesame Seaweed	1 oz	140	2	7	18
Rice Chips Wasabi	1 oz	140	2	6	18
Madhouse Munchies					
Potato Sea Salt	16	150	2	9	16
Potato Sea Salt & Vinegar	16	150	2	9	16
Tortilla White	9	140	2	6	19
Mexi-Snax					
Tortilla Multi-Grain Blue	15 (1 oz)	140	2	7	17
Tortilla Pico De Gallo	15 (1 oz)	140	2	7	18
Tortilla Salted	15 (1 oz)	140	2	7	18
Tortilla Tamari	15 (1 oz)	130	2	6	17
Michael Season's					
Potato Crisps Thin Baked Low Fat	14	120	2	2	23
Potato Kettle Style Reduced Fat	18	130	2	6	18
Potato Reduced Fat	20	140	2	7	17
Potato Reduced Fat Unsalted	20	140	2	7	17
Poore Brothers					
Original	14 (1 oz)	140	2	9	15
Salt & Vinegar	15 (1 oz)	150	2	9	15
Sweet Maui Onion	14 (1 oz)	140	2	9	15
Popchips					
Corn Hint Of Butter	23 (1 oz)	120	2	5	17
Potato Barbeque	19 (1 oz)	120	1	5	20
Potato Original	22 (1 oz)	120	1	5	20
Rice Sea Salt	19 (1 oz)	120	2	5	17
Rice Wasabi	20 (1 oz)	120	2	5	17
Pringles					
Jalapeno	15 (1 oz)	150	1	10	14
Loaded Baked Potato	15 (1 oz)	150	1	10	14
Minis Cheddar Cheese	1 pkg	120	1	7	12

FOOD	PORTION	CALS	PROT	FAT	CARB
Minis Original	1 pkg	120	1	7	13
Original	14 (1 oz)	160	1	11	14
Pizza	15 (1 oz)	150	1	10	14
Select Cinnamon Sweet Potato	28 (1 oz)	150	1	9	16
Select Parmesan Garlic	28 (1 oz)	140	1	9	15
Snack Stacks Original	1 pkg	140	1	10	12
Revolution Foods					
Organic Popalongs Whole Grains Cheesy Cheese	16 (0.7 oz)	90	2	3	14
Organic Popalongs Whole Grains Original	16 (0.7 oz)	100	2	3	15
Organic Popalongs Whole Grains Simply Cinnamon	16 (0.7 oz)	100	1	3	16
Robert's American Gourmet					
Soy Crisps Country Barbecue	1 oz	130	7	4	15
Salba Smart					
Organic Blue Corn Omega-3 Enriched	1 oz	104	2	6	19
Snyder's Of Hanover					
Kosher Dill	1 oz	140	2	6	20
MultiGrain Sunflower	1 oz	140	2	6	20
MultiGrain Sunflower Southwestern Cheddar	1 oz	140	2	6	20
MultiGrain Tortilla Lightly Salted	1 oz	130	2	5	20
MultiGrain Tortilla Strips Flaxseed Gold	1 oz	140	2	6	18
Organic Veggie Crisps	1 oz	140	1	7	18
Potato Original	1 oz	150	2	7	19
Sweet Potato Baked	1 oz	110	1	2	23
Tortilla Pounder Multi-Grain	1 oz	130	2	5	20
Tortilla White Corn	1 oz	140	2	5	23
Stacy's					
Pita Chips Multigrain	1 pkg	140	3	6	17
Pita Chips Parmesan Garlic & Herb	1 oz	140	4	5	19
Pita Chips Texarkana Hot	1 oz	130	3	5	19
Soy Thin Chips Sticky Bun	18 (1 oz)	130	6	5	15
Soy Thin Crisps Simply Cheese	18 (1 oz)	130	7	6	13

FOOD	PORTION	CALS	PROT	FAT	CARB
SunChips					
Original	16 (1 oz)	140	2	6	18
T.G.I. Friday's					
Potato Cheese Pizza	16 (1 oz)	160	2	9	17
Tater Skins					
Cheddar Bacon	16 (1 oz)	150	1	8	19
Original	16 (1 oz)	150	1	8	19
Terra					
Exotic Vegetable Original	14 (1 oz)	150	7	9	16
Exotic Vegetable Zesty Tomato	14 (1 oz)	150	1	9	16
Kettles Potato Sea Salt & Pepper	15 (1 oz)	140	2	6	18
Parsnip Chips	12 (1 oz)	150	2	10	13
Potato Au Natural	18 (1 oz)	150	2	9	15
Potato Blues	1 oz	130	2	6	19
Potato Frites Sea Salt & Vinegar	1 oz	150	2	8	18
Potato Golds Original	1 oz	130	2	5	19
Potato Potpourri	1 oz	140	2	7	17
Potato Red Bliss	1 oz	140	1	7	18
Stix Original Exotic Vegetable	1 oz	150	1	9	16
Sweet Potato	17 (1 oz)	160	1	11	15
Sweets & Beets	16 (1 oz)	150	2	9	15
Taro	1 oz	140	1	6	19
Thunder					
Potato Buffalo Wing w/ Blue Cheese	22 (1 oz)	150	1	8	16
Sour Cream & Onion	22 (1 oz)	150	2	9	15
Utz					
Pita Natural w/ Sea Salt	1 oz	120	3	5	18
Potato	20 (1 oz)	150	2	9	14
Potato Baked	1 oz	110	2	2	23
Potato BBQ	20 (1 oz)	150	2	10	14
Potato Grandma Kettle	1 oz	140	2	8	14
Potato Homestyle Kettle	1 oz	140	2	8	14
Potato Kettle Classics	20 (1 oz)	150	2	9	15
Potato Mystic Kettle	1 oz	150	2	9	15
Potato Mystic Kettle Reduced Fat	1 oz	130	2	6	18
Potato Natural Lightly Salted Kettle	1 oz	140	2	8	15
Potato No Salt Added	20 (1 oz)	150	2	9	14

FOOD	PORTION	CALS	PROT	FAT	CARB
Potato Onion & Garlic	1 oz	150	2	9	14
Potato Ripple	20 (1 oz)	150	2	10	14
Sweet Potato Kettle Classics	20 (1 oz)	150	1	9	16
Tortilla Baked	10	120	2	2	23
Tortilla Organic Yellow Corn	1 oz	140	2	6	19
Vegetable Natural Exotic Medley	1 oz	160	2	10	15
Zapp's					
Potato Cajun Dill	1 oz	150	2	8	17
Potato No Salt	1 oz	150	2	9	18
Potato Original	1 oz	150	2	8	17
Potato Sizzlin Steak	1 oz	150	2	8	17
Sweet Potato Lightly Salted	1 oz	150	1	8	17

CHITTERLINGS

pork cooked	3 oz	258	9	24	0

CHIVES

freeze-dried	1 tbsp	1	tr	tr	tr
fresh chopped	1 tbsp	1	tr	tr	tr
fresh chopped	1 tsp	0	tr	tr	tr

CHOCOLATE (*see also* CANDY, CHOCOLATE SPREAD, CHOCOLATE SYRUP, COCOA, HOT CHOCOLATE, ICE CREAM TOPPINGS, MILK DRINKS)

BAKING

baking	1 oz	145	3	15	8
grated unsweetened	¼ cup	165	4	17	10
liquid unsweetened	1 oz	134	3	14	10
mexican baking	1 sq (0.7 oz)	85	1	3	15
squares unsweetened	1 sq (1 oz)	145	4	15	9
Hershey's					
Unsweetened Block	1 (0.5 oz)	70	2	7	4
CHIPS					
milk chocolate	1 cup (6 oz)	862	12	52	100
semisweet	60 pieces (1 oz)	136	1	9	18
semisweet	1 cup (6 oz)	804	7	50	106
E. Guittard					
Cappuccino	30 (0.5 oz)	80	tr	5	9
Milk Chocolate	12 (0.5 oz)	80	1	5	9
Semisweet	30 (0.5 oz)	70	tr	4	10

FOOD	PORTION	CALS	PROT	FAT	CARB
Hershey's					
Milk Chocolate	1 tbsp (0.5 oz)	70	1	5	9
Premier White	1 tbsp (0.5 oz)	80	1	4	9
Semi-Sweet	1 tbsp (0.5 oz)	70	tr	4	10
Special Dark	1 tbsp (0.5 oz)	70	tr	5	9
Sugar Free	1 tbsp (0.5 oz)	70	tr	5	9
MIX					
drink mix powder	2–3 heaping tsp	75	1	1	20
drink mix powder as prep w/ whole milk	9 oz	226	9	9	31
Nesquik					
Chocolate Powder	2 tbsp (0.6 oz)	60	tr	1	14
Chocolate Powder No Sugar Added	2 tbsp (0.4 oz)	35	1	1	7
Sunfood					
Organic Powder	2 tbsp (1 oz)	120	6	4	15

CHOCOLATE MILK (*see* MILK DRINKS)

CHOCOLATE SPREAD
Love'n Bake

Chocolate Schmear	2 tbsp	140	4	8	14

CHOCOLATE SYRUP

chocolate fudge	1 tbsp (0.7 oz)	73	1	3	12
chocolate fudge	1 cup (11.9 oz)	1176	15	46	200
syrup	1 cup	653	6	3	177
syrup	2 tbsp	82	1	tr	22
syrup as prep w/ whole milk	1 cup (9.9 oz)	254	9	8	36
Hershey's					
Lite	2 tbsp (1.2 oz)	45	0	0	11
Sugar Free	2 tbsp (1.1 oz)	15	tr	0	5
Sundae Syrup Double Chocolate	2 tbsp (1.3 oz)	100	tr	0	24
Syrup	2 tbsp (1.4 oz)	100	tr	0	24
Nesquik					
Calcium Fortified	2 tbsp (1.3 oz)	100	0	0	25
Santa Cruz					
Organic	2 tbsp	110	1	0	27

FOOD	PORTION	CALS	PROT	FAT	CARB
U-Bet					
Original	2 tbsp (1.4 oz)	128	1	0	29
CHUTNEY					
apple	1.2 oz	68	tr	0	18
coconut	2 oz	87	1	9	1
fresh mint	2 oz	18	1	0	3
mango	¼ cup (2 oz)	227	2	5	43
tomato	1 oz	90	1	7	6
Chukar Cherries					
Curried Cherry	1 tbsp	30	0	0	8
Patak's					
Major Grey	1 tbsp	60	0	0	14
Mango Hot	1 tbsp	60	0	0	14
Mango Sweet	1 tbsp	60	0	1	14
Robert Rothchild Farm					
Hot Peach & Apple	2 tbsp	45	0	0	12
School House Kitchen					
Bardshar	1 oz	80	0	0	20
The Gracious Gourmet					
Mango Pineapple	2 tbsp (1 oz)	45	0	1	9
Wild Thymes Farm					
Apricot Cranberry Walnut	1 tbsp	16	tr	0	4
Plum Currant Ginger	1 tsp	20	tr	0	5
CILANTRO					
fresh	¼ cup	1	tr	tr	tr
fresh sprigs	5 (5 g)	1	tr	tr	tr
CINNAMON					
cinnamon sugar	1 tsp	16	tr	tr	4
ground	1 tsp	6	tr	tr	2
sticks	0.5 oz	39	1	tr	8
CISCO					
raw	3 oz	84	16	2	0
smoked	1 oz	50	5	3	0
CLAMS					
CANNED					
liquid only	3 oz	2	tr	tr	tr
liquid only	1 cup	6	1	tr	tr
meat only	3 oz	126	22	2	4
meat only	1 cup	236	41	3	8

FOOD	PORTION	CALS	PROT	FAT	CARB
Polar					
Baby	¼ cup	30	5	0	3
FRESH					
cooked	20 sm	133	23	2	5
cooked	3 oz	126	22	2	4
raw	3 oz	63	11	1	2
raw	9 lg (6.3 oz)	133	23	2	5
raw	20 sm (6.3 oz)	133	23	2	5
FROZEN					
Mrs. Paul's					
Fried	18 (3 oz)	270	9	13	29
TAKE-OUT					
breaded & fried	20 sm	379	27	21	19
CLEMENTINE JUICE					
Izze					
Sparkling Clementine	1 bottle (12 oz)	120	0	0	30
CLEMENTINES					
Cuties					
Fresh	2 (6 oz)	80	1	1	17
Disney Garden					
Clementines	1	35	1	0	9
CLOVES					
ground	1 tsp	7	tr	tr	1
COCOA (*see also* HOT CHOCOLATE)					
cocoa butter	1 tbsp	120	0	14	0
powder unsweetened	1 tbsp	12	1	1	3
Hershey's					
Cocoa	1 tbsp (5 g)	10	tr	1	3
COCONUT					
dried sweetened shredded	¼ cup	116	1	8	11
dried toasted	1 oz	168	2	13	13
dried unsweetened	1 oz	187	2	18	7
fresh from 1 coconut	14 oz	1405	13	133	60
fresh shredded	¼ cup	71	1	7	3
Bob's Red Mill					
Shredded	3 tbsp	120	1	11	4
Let's Do Organic					
Organic Reduced Fat Shredded	1 can (0.5 oz)	70	1	6	4
Shredded	3 tbsp (0.5 oz)	110	1	10	4

FOOD	PORTION	CALS	PROT	FAT	CARB
Mounds					
Sweetened Flakes	2 tbsp (0.5 oz)	70	tr	5	6
Prosperity					
Organic Coconut Flax Butter Garlic & Onion	1 tbsp	140	0	15	0
COCONUT JUICE					
coconut water fresh	½ cup	23	1	tr	4
creamed sweetened canned	½ cup	264	1	12	39
milk canned	½ cup	276	3	29	7
Goya					
Coconut Water	1 can (11.8 oz)	120	0	1	29
Let's Do Organic					
Creamed	1 oz	220	4	19	8
Milk	¼ cup	100	1	11	2
O.N.E.					
Natural Coconut Water	1 box (11 oz)	60	1	0	15
Thai Kitchen					
Lite Coconut Milk	2 oz	45	0	4	1
Zico					
Coconut Water All Flavors	1 pkg (11 oz)	60	1	0	15
COD					
atlantic canned	3 oz	89	19	1	0
atlantic canned	1 can (11 oz)	327	71	3	0
atlantic dried	3 oz	246	53	2	0
atlantic fresh cooked	1 fillet (6.3 oz)	189	41	2	0
atlantic fresh cooked	3 oz	89	19	1	0
atlantic fresh raw	3 oz	70	15	1	0
pacific fresh baked	3 oz	95	21	1	0
roe canned	1 oz	34	6	1	tr
roe tarama	3.5 oz	547	8	55	6
Mrs. Paul's					
Filets Lightly Breaded	1 (4 oz)	220	12	11	17
TAKE-OUT					
roe baked w/ butter & lemon juice	1 oz	36	6	1	tr
COFFEE (*see also* COFFEE BEVERAGES, COFFEE SUBSTITUTES)					
INSTANT					
decaffeinated as prep	8 oz	2	tr	0	0
decaffeinated powder	1 rounded tsp	4	tr	0	1
regular powder	1 rounded tsp	4	tr	tr	1

FOOD	PORTION	CALS	PROT	FAT	CARB
REGULAR					
brewed	8 oz	2	tr	tr	0
roasted beans	1 oz	64	4	4	18
Spava					
Calm	1 cup	0	0	0	0
Decaffeinated					
COFFEE BEVERAGES					
Click					
Espresso Protein Drink as prep	2 scoops (1.1 oz)	120	15	2	12
Iced 'Spresso					
Ultra Light American Vanilla	1 bottle (9.5 oz)	90	6	3	11
Ultra Light Espresso Latte	1 bottle (9.5 oz)	70	6	0	11
N.O. Brew					
Iced Coffee not prep	1 serv (2.6 oz)	10	0	0	1
O.N.E.					
Coffee Fruit	1 bottle (11 oz)	107	tr	1	26
Wolfgang Puck					
Culinary Iced All Flavors	1 bottle (8.5 oz)	120	3	3	23
TAKE-OUT					
cafe amaretto w/ alcohol	1 serv	192	1	9	15
cafe au lait	1 cup (8 oz)	77	4	4	6
cafe brulot	1 cup	48	tr	0	3
cafe brulot w/ alcohol	1 serv	130	1	tr	16
cappuccino	1 cup (8 oz)	77	4	4	6
coffee con leche	1 cup (6 oz)	104	3	4	16
cuban coffee w/ rum & creme de cacao	1 (9 oz)	112	3	2	6
dutch coffee w/ gin	1 (7 oz)	181	1	10	6
espresso	1 cup (4 oz)	2	tr	tr	0
french coffee w/ orange liqueur & kahlua	1 (8 oz)	232	1	10	24
irish coffee	1 serv (8 oz)	209	1	11	5
italian coffee w/ strega	1 (7 oz)	163	1	10	12
latte w/ skim milk	1 serv (13 oz)	88	8	tr	12
latte w/ whole milk	1 serv (14 oz)	143	9	6	15
mocha	1 serv (17 oz)	403	11	9	69

FOOD	PORTION	CALS	PROT	FAT	CARB
puerto rican coffee w/ rum & kahlua	1 (8 oz)	166	1	10	9
turkish	1 cup (4 oz)	50	tr	1	12

COFFEE SUBSTITUTES
Pixie
Mate Latte Chai	½ cup (4 oz)	80	0	0	18
Mate Latte Dark Roast	½ cup (4 oz)	70	0	0	16
Mate Latte Mocha	½ cup (4 oz)	70	0	0	18
Mate Latte Original	½ cup (4 oz)	70	0	0	17

COFFEE WHITENERS
Farmland
Nondairy Creamer	2 tbsp	40	1	3	2

International Delight
Amaretto	1 tbsp	40	0	2	7
Fat Free Amaretto	1 tbsp	30	0	0	7
Fat Free French Vanilla	1 tbsp	30	0	0	7
Fat Free Irish Creme	1 tbsp	30	0	0	7
French Vanilla	1 tbsp	45	0	2	7
Sugar Free French Vanilla	1 tbsp	20	0	2	1

Silk
French Vanilla	1 tbsp (0.5 oz)	20	0	1	3
Original	1 tbsp (0.5 oz)	15	0	1	1

WildWood
Soymilk Creamer Plain	1 tbsp	15	0	2	1

COLESLAW
Fresh Express
3 Color Deli	1½ cups	20	1	0	5
Kit w/ Sweet & Creamy Dressing	3 cups	120	1	8	12
Old Fashioned	2 cups	25	1	0	5

Mann's
Broccoli Cole Slaw w/o Dressing	1 serv (3 oz)	25	2	0	5

TAKE-OUT
coleslaw w/ dressing	¾ cup	147	1	11	13
vinegar & oil coleslaw	3.5 oz	150	1	9	16

COLLARDS
fresh cooked	½ cup	17	1	tr	4
frzn chopped cooked	½ cup	31	3	tr	6
raw chopped	½ cup	6	tr	tr	1

FOOD	PORTION	CALS	PROT	FAT	CARB
Allens					
Seasoned Southern Style	½ cup (4.1 oz)	35	2	0	6
Glory					
Green Fresh	2 cups	25	2	0	5
Seasoned canned	½ cup	35	2	0	5
Sensibly Seasoned canned	½ cup	20	2	0	4
COOKIES					
MIX					
chocolate chip	1 (0.56 oz)	79	1	4	10
oatmeal	1 (0.6 oz)	74	1	3	10
oatmeal raisin	1 (0.6 oz)	74	1	3	10
Betty Crocker					
Caramelita Bars as prep	1	190	2	8	28
Chocolate Chip as prep	2	170	1	8	21
Oatmeal as prep	2	160	2	7	22
Peanut Butter as prep	2	150	2	7	20
Reese's Dessert Bar Mix No Bake as prep	1	180	2	10	20
Sugar as prep	2	160	1	8	21
Sunkist Lemon Bars as prep	1	140	tr	4	24
Turtle Cookie Bars as prep	1	180	2	8	27
Duncan Hines					
Chocolate Chip as prep	2 (1.1 oz)	180	1	9	23
READY-TO-EAT					
animal crackers	1 (2.5 g)	11	tr	tr	2
animal crackers	11 (1 oz)	126	2	4	21
animal crackers	1 box (2.4 oz)	299	4	9	51
australian anzac biscuit	1	98	1	3	17
butter	1 (5 g)	23	tr	1	3
chocolate chip	1 (0.4 oz)	48	1	2	7
chocolate chip	1 box (1.9 oz)	233	3	12	36
chocolate chip low sugar low sodium	1 (0.24 oz)	31	tr	1	5
chocolate chip lowfat	1 (0.25 oz)	45	1	2	7
chocolate chip soft-type	1 (0.5 oz)	69	1	4	9
chocolate w/ creme filling	1 (0.35 oz)	47	1	2	7
chocolate w/ creme filling chocolate coated	1 (0.60 oz)	82	1	5	11
chocolate w/ creme filling sugar free low sodium	1 (0.35 oz)	46	1	2	7

FOOD	PORTION	CALS	PROT	FAT	CARB
chocolate w/ extra creme filling	1 (0.46 oz)	65	1	3	9
chocolate wafer	1 (0.2 oz)	26	tr	1	4
cream cheese	1 (1.1 oz)	141	2	9	14
digestive biscuits plain	2	141	2	7	21
fig bars	1 (0.56 oz)	56	1	1	11
fortune	1 (0.28 oz)	30	tr	tr	7
fudge	1 (0.73 oz)	73	1	1	17
gingersnaps	1 (0.24 oz)	29	tr	1	5
graham	1 sq (0.24 oz)	30	1	1	5
graham chocolate covered	1 (0.49 oz)	68	1	3	9
graham honey	1 (0.24 oz)	30	1	1	5
hermits	1 (1 oz)	117	2	5	18
jumbles coconut	1 (1 oz)	121	1	7	13
ladyfingers	1 (0.38 oz)	40	1	1	7
macaroons	1 (0.8 oz)	97	1	3	17
madeleines	1 (0.8 oz)	86	2	5	10
marshmallow chocolate coated	1 (0.46 oz)	55	1	2	9
marshmallow pie chocolate coated	1 (1.4 oz)	165	2	7	26
molasses	1 (0.5 oz)	65	1	2	11
neapolitan tri-color cookie	1 (0.6 oz)	79	1	5	8
oatmeal	1 (0.6 oz)	81	1	3	12
oatmeal soft-type	1 (0.5 oz)	61	1	2	10
oatmeal raisin	1 (0.6 oz)	81	1	3	12
oatmeal raisin low sugar no sodium	1 (0.24 oz)	31	tr	1	5
oatmeal raisin soft-type	1 (0.5 oz)	61	1	2	10
peanut butter sandwich	1 (0.5 oz)	67	1	3	9
peanut butter sandwich sugar free low sodium	1 (0.35 oz)	54	1	3	5
peanut butter soft-type	1 (0.5 oz)	69	1	4	9
pinenut cookies	1 (1.1 oz)	134	4	9	11
raisin soft-type	1 (0.5 oz)	60	1	2	10
reginette queen's biscuit	1 (0.8 oz)	86	2	3	13
shortbread	1 (0.28 oz)	40	1	2	5
shortbread pecan	1 (0.49 oz)	79	1	5	8
spritz	1 (0.4 oz)	42	1	2	6
sugar	1 (0.52 oz)	72	1	3	10
sugar low sugar sodium free	1 (0.24 oz)	30	1	1	5
sugar wafers w/ creme filling	1 (0.12 oz)	18	tr	1	3

FOOD	PORTION	CALS	PROT	FAT	CARB
sugar wafers w/ creme filling sugar free sodium free	1 (0.14 oz)	20	tr	1	3
toll house original	1 (0.8 oz)	105	2	6	13
vanilla sandwich	1 (0.35 oz)	48	tr	2	7
vanilla wafers	1 (0.21 oz)	28	tr	1	4
zeppole	1 (0.8 oz)	78	1	6	6
ABC					
Vegan Colossal Chocolate Chip	1 (2.1 oz)	240	3	7	41
Vegan Double Chocolate Decadence	1 (2.1 oz)	240	3	8	39
Vegan Luscious Lemon Poppyseed	1 (2.1 oz)	240	3	7	40
Vegan Mac The Chip	1 (2.1 oz)	250	4	10	35
Vegan Peanut Butter Chocolate Chip	1 (2.1 oz)	240	4	8	39
Vegan Phenomenal Pumpkin Spice	1 (2.1 oz)	220	4	7	39
Almond Joy					
Cookies	2 (1 oz)	140	2	8	17
Anna's Swedish Thins					
Almond Cinnamon	6 (1 oz)	140	2	7	18
Cappuccino	6 (1 oz)	140	2	7	18
Chocolate Mint	6 (1 oz)	150	2	8	17
Orange	6 (1 oz)	140	2	7	19
Archway					
Coconut Macaroon	2 (1.3 oz)	160	1	8	22
Frosty Lemon	1 (0.9 oz)	110	1	5	18
Fruit Filled Raspberry	1 (0.8 oz)	90	1	3	15
Arico					
Gluten Free Casein Free Almond Cranberry	1 bar (1.4 oz)	140	3	6	22
Gluten Free Casein Free Double Chocolate	1 (0.9 oz)	100	2	5	15
Gluten Free Casein Free Lemon Ginger	1 (0.9 oz)	90	2	4	15
Gluten Free Casein Free Peanut Butter	1 bar (1.4 oz)	160	5	7	19
Arrowroot					
Biscuit	1 (5 g)	20	0	1	4

FOOD	PORTION	CALS	PROT	FAT	CARB
Aunt Gussie's					
Biscotti Almond	1 (0.8 oz)	110	2	6	13
Biscotti Almond Sugar Free	2 (1 oz)	150	2	10	14
Biscotti Cinnamon Raisin No Sugar Added	1 (0.8 oz)	110	2	6	14
Biscotti Italian w/ Olive Oil	2 (1.2 oz)	160	3	5	25
Coconut Crisp	2 (1.1 oz)	170	2	9	18
Latte Sugar Free	1 (0.9 oz)	110	2	6	18
Lemon Sugar Free	3 (1.2 oz)	160	2	9	22
Mexican Wedding Cakes	3 (1.2 oz)	160	2	10	19
Snickerdoodle	2 (1.1 oz)	180	2	12	16
Vanilla Spritz Sugar Free Gluten Free	2 (0.9 oz)	110	0	5	17
Back To Nature					
Granola Cranberry Pecan	1 (1.1 oz)	130	2	6	20
Granola Honey Nut	1 (1.1 oz)	140	3	7	18
Bahlsen					
Delice	6 (1.1 oz)	150	2	8	19
Hannover Waffeln	6 (1.1 oz)	180	1	11	19
Hit Minis Chocolate Filled	5 (1.2 oz)	170	2	8	23
Waffeletten	4 (1 oz)	160	2	9	18
Barbara's Bakery					
Fig Bars Traditional	1	60	0	1	14
Fig Bars Wheat Free	1	60	0	0	13
Organic 100 Calorie Mini Ginger	1 pkg (0.9 oz)	100	1	2	19
Snackimals Chocolate Chip	10	120	1	4	19
Snackimals Wheat Free Oatmeal	10	120	1	5	17
Barnum's					
Animal Crackers	10 (1 oz)	120	2	4	22
Barry's Bakery					
French Twists Wild Raspberry	2 (0.5 oz)	60	0	2	9
Breaktime					
Ginger	4 (1 oz)	130	2	4	23
Oatmeal	4 (1 oz)	130	2	4	22
Brown & Haley					
Almond Roca	6 (1 oz)	110	1	4	19
Buzz Strong's					
Real Coffee	1 (1.2 oz)	150	2	7	22
Cameo					
Sandwich Creme	2 (1 oz)	130	1	5	21

FOOD	PORTION	CALS	PROT	FAT	CARB
Chips Ahoy!					
Chocolate Chip	1 pkg (1.4 oz)	190	2	9	27
Mini	1 pkg (1.2 oz)	170	2	8	24
Reduced Fat	1 pkg (1.1 oz)	140	2	5	23
Comfort Care					
Cabin Hearth Chocolate Chip	1 (2 oz)	250	3	11	38
Cabin Hearth Oatmeal Peach	1 (2 oz)	200	3	7	31
Cabin Hearth Oatmeal Raisin	1 (2 oz)	200	3	7	31
Country Choice Organic					
Fit Kids Snackin' Grahams Chocolate	18 (1 oz)	110	2	3	20
Oatmeal Chocolate Chip	1 (0.8 oz)	100	1	4	15
Oatmeal Raisin	1 (0.8 oz)	100	1	3	16
Dare					
Lemon Creme	1 (0.7 oz)	100	tr	4	14
Maple Leaf Creme	1 (0.6 oz)	80	tr	4	12
DiCamillo					
Biscotti DiPrato	5 (1 oz)	130	3	4	21
Divvies					
Chocolate Chip Vegan	1	130	1	7	17
Oatmeal Raisin Vegan	1	120	1	5	17
Earthbound Farms					
Organic Ginger Snaps	2	120	2	6	18
Emily's					
Fortune Dark Chocolate Covered	2 (1.4 oz)	140	2	6	23
Graham Cracker Milk Chocolate Covered	1 (1 oz)	150	2	9	17
Enjoy Life					
Allergen Gluten Free Gingerbread Spice	2 (1 oz)	100	1	4	19
Allergen Gluten Free No Oats Oatmeal	2 (1 oz)	120	1	4	21
Allergen Gluten Free Snickerdoodle	2 (1 oz)	130	1	5	21
Snack Bar Sunbutter Crunch	1 (1 oz)	140	3	5	20
Erin Baker's					
Breakfast Banana Toasted Flax	1 (3 oz)	300	6	5	55

FOOD	PORTION	CALS	PROT	FAT	CARB
Breakfast Caramel Apple	1 (3 oz)	290	5	4	57
Breakfast Mocha Cappuccino	1 (3 oz)	300	6	6	54
Breakfast Morning Glory	1 (3 oz)	310	6	8	54
Breakfast Peanut Butter & Jelly	1 (3 oz)	320	7	9	52
Breakfast Vegan Chocolate Chip	1 (3 oz)	310	6	6	57
Organic Breakfast Mini Oatmeal Raisin	1 (1 oz)	100	2	2	18
Organic Breakfast Mini Peanut Butter	1 (1 oz)	110	3	3	16
Fauchon					
Assorted Chocolate	4 (2 oz)	330	4	15	34
French Meadow Bakery					
Coconutty Macaroons	2 (1.1 oz)	150	2	8	17
Gluten Free Chocolate Chip	1 (2.1 oz)	320	1	16	43
Rhubarb Bar	1 (2.7 oz)	250	3	11	34
Vegan Peanut Butter Bliss	2 (1.2 oz)	150	2	7	19
Gak's Snacks					
Organic Brownie Chip	1 (1 oz)	130	2	5	20
Organic Chocolate Chip	1 (1 oz)	140	1	6	21
Organic Oatmeal	1 (1 oz)	120	2	4	19
Ginger Snaps					
Cookies	4 (1 oz)	120	1	3	23
Girl Scout					
Lemon Chalet Cremes	3 (1.3 oz)	170	1	7	26
Gluten-Free Pantry					
Gluten Free Buckwheat Raisin	1 (1 oz)	140	1	6	21
Gluten Free Chocolate Chunk	1 (1 oz)	140	1	8	19
Glutino					
Gluten Free Wafers Chocolate	4	160	1	8	19
Gluten Free Wafers Lemon	3	150	0	6	24
Gottena					
Exquisit	5	170	2	10	19
Gourmet Pastries					
Kourabiethes Butter Almond	1 (1.1 oz)	150	2	9	15
Phoenicia Honey & Spice	1 (1.3 oz)	140	2	5	20
Health Valley					
Mini Mint Chocolate Chip	4 (1 oz)	120	1	6	16
Oatmeal Raisin	1 (0.8 oz)	90	2	4	14
Raisin Oatmeal Low Fat	3	110	2	2	23
White Chocolate Chunk	1 (1 oz)	140	1	7	17

FOOD	PORTION	CALS	PROT	FAT	CARB
Home Free					
Organic Chocolate Chip	1 (1 oz)	140	1	6	21
Organic Oatmeal	1 (1 oz)	120	2	4	19
Honey Maid					
Grahams Honey	1 (1.1 oz)	130	2	4	24
Grahams Honey Low Fat	1 (1.1 oz)	120	2	2	25
Kashi					
TLC Happy Trail Mix	1 (1 oz)	130	2	5	21
TLC Oatmeal Raisin Flax	1 (1 oz)	130	2	5	20
TLC Oatmeal Dark Chocolate	1 (1 oz)	130	2	5	21
Kedem					
Tea Biscuits Chocolate	2 (0.3 oz)	32	1	1	6
Tea Biscuits Vanilla	2 (0.3 oz)	32	1	1	6
Keebler					
100 Calorie Right Bites Fudge Shoppe Fudge Grahams	1 pkg (0.7 oz)	100	1	4	15
100 Calorie Pack RightBites Sandies Shortbread	1 pkg (0.7 oz)	100	1	3	17
Animal Crackers Frosted	8	150	1	7	22
Chips Deluxe Chocolate Lovers	1	90	tr	5	10
Chips Deluxe Coconut	2	150	2	9	18
Chips Deluxe Fudge Stripes	1	100	1	6	13
Chips Deluxe Original	1 pkg (2 oz)	300	3	16	37
Chocolate Dip & Cookie Sticks	1 pkg (1 oz)	130	1	6	18
Danish Wedding	4	130	1	6	18
Dipping Delights Cheesecake	1	90	<2	4	13
E.L. Fudge Original	1	90	1	4	13
Fudge Shoppe Fudge Stripes	3	150	1	7	21
Fudge Shoppe Grasshoppers	4	140	1	7	19
Fudge Shoppe Mint Creme Filled	2	160	tr	9	20
Graham Honey	8 (1 oz)	110	2	2	22
Graham Original	8 (1 oz)	130	2	4	22
Oatmeal Country Style	2	130	2	6	18
Sandies Drops Butter Pecan	4	140	1	7	18
Sandies Fudge Drops	4 (1 oz)	140	1	7	18
Sandies Pecan Shortbread Reduced Fat	1	80	tr	4	11
Scooby-Doo Graham Sticks	9	130	2	4	21
S'mores Snack	1 pkg (0.8 oz)	110	1	6	14

FOOD	PORTION	CALS	PROT	FAT	CARB
Soft Batch Chocolate Chip	1	80	tr	4	11
Vanilla Wafers	8	140	1	6	21
Vienna Fingers	2 (1.1 oz)	150	1	6	23
Vienna Fingers Reduced Fat	2	140	1	5	24
Khaya					
Krunchi Orange & Chocolate	5 (1.53 oz)	240	3	12	29
Shortbread Grapeseed	13 (1.15 oz)	193	tr	10	27
Shortbread Orange Rooibos	13 (1.15)	259	tr	14	36
La Choy					
Fortune	4 (1 oz)	110	2	0	25
Lance					
Oatmeal Creme	1 (2.5 oz)	300	3	12	45
Van-O-Lunch	1 pkg (1.6 oz)	230	3	10	34
Late July					
Organic Sandwich Dark Chocolate	3 (1.2 oz)	150	2	6	21
Organic Sandwich Vanilla Bean w/ Green Tea	2 (0.8 oz)	110	1	5	16
Lean Body					
Cookie Bar Hi-Protein S'Mores	1 (3.2 oz)	360	30	13	30
Liz Lovely					
Vegan Cowboy	½ cookie (1.3 oz)	190	3	9	24
Vegan Cowgirl	½ cookie (1.5 oz)	210	2	9	30
Vegan Ginger Snapdragons	½ cookie (1.5 oz)	190	2	7	29
Loacker					
Quadratini Dark Chocolate	9 (1.1 oz)	160	2	8	20
Lorna Doone					
Shortbread	4 (1 oz)	140	1	7	20
LU					
Le Fondant	4 (1.1 oz)	170	2	10	19
Le Petit Beurre	4 (1.2 oz)	140	3	4	28
Petit Ecolier Dark Chocolate	2 (0.9 oz)	130	1	6	17
Petit Ecolier Milk Chocolate	2 (0.9 oz)	130	2	6	17
Shortbread	2 (1 oz)	140	1	8	16
Luna					
Berry Pomegranate	1 (1.4 oz)	140	3	3	27
Peanut Butter Chocolate	1 (1.4 oz)	150	4	6	23

FOOD	PORTION	CALS	PROT	FAT	CARB
M&M's					
Milk Chocolate	1 pkg (1.15 oz)	150	2	5	22
Mallomars					
Cookies	2	120	1	5	18
Mauna Loa					
Macadamia Nut Chocolate Chip	4 (1 oz)	150	1	9	17
Montana Monster Munchies					
Original	½ (1.4 oz)	177	4	9	21
Raisin	½ (1.4 oz)	172	3	9	22
MoonPie					
Mini All Flavors	1 pkg (1.2 oz)	130	2	4	23
Mrs. Fields					
Cookie Dough Snacks Brownie Chocolate Chip	7 (1 oz)	120	tr	3	18
Cookie Dough Snacks Chocolate Chip	7 (1 oz)	120	1	4	19
Murray's					
Sugar Free Chocolate Chip	3 (1.1 oz)	160	2	9	20
Sugar Free Chocolate Sandwich	3 (1 oz)	130	1	7	19
Sugar Free Fudge Dipped Grahams	4 (1 oz)	150	2	8	19
Sugar Free Ginger Snap	7 (1.1 oz)	130	2	5	23
Sugar Free Oatmeal	3 (1.1 oz)	140	2	7	21
Sugar Free Shortbread	8 (1 oz)	130	2	5	21
Nabisco					
100 Calorie Pack Alpha-Bits Mini	1 pkg	100	1	3	16
100 Calorie Pack Barnum's Animal Choco	1 pkg	100	1	3	17
100 Calorie Pack Lorna Doone	1 pkg	100	1	3	16
100 Calorie Pack Teddy Grahams Mini Cinnamon	1 pkg	100	1	3	16
Nana's					
No Gluten Berry Vanilla	1 bar (1.2 oz)	130	1	4	22
No Gluten Chocolate	1 (3.5 oz)	360	4	12	62
No Gluten Ginger	1 (3.5 oz)	360	4	10	64
No Gluten Nana Banana	1 bar (1.2 oz)	130	1	5	23
No Wheat Oatmeal Raisin	1 (3.5 oz)	280	6	10	46
Vegan Chocolate Chip	1 (4 oz)	320	6	14	48
Vegan Peanut Butter	1 (4 oz)	360	8	16	46
Vegan Sunflower	1 (3.5 oz)	380	8	14	60

FOOD	PORTION	CALS	PROT	FAT	CARB
Natural Ovens					
Oatmeal Raisin	1 (1.3 oz)	120	2	4	20
New York Style					
Biscotti Almond	3 (1 oz)	130	3	5	20
Newtons					
Fig	2 (1.1 oz)	110	1	2	22
Fig 100% Whole Grain	2 (1.3 oz)	130	1	3	26
Fig Fat Free	2 (1 oz)	90	1	0	22
Raspberry	2 (1 oz)	100	1	2	21
Nilla Wafers					
Cookies	1 oz	140	1	6	21
Reduced Fat	1 oz	110	1	2	24
Nonni's					
Biscotti Cioccolati	1 (0.8 oz)	110	2	5	17
Biscotti Limone	1 (0.8 oz)	110	2	5	17
Biscotti Original	1 (0.7 oz)	90	2	3	14
NutraBalance					
High Fibre	1 (0.7 oz)	90	1	4	13
Nutter Butter					
Bites	1 pkg (1.2 oz)	170	3	7	24
Sandwich Cookie	1 (1 oz)	130	2	6	19
Oreo					
Cakesters	2 (2 oz)	250	2	12	36
Cakesters Mini Golden 100 Calorie Pack	1 pkg (0.8 oz)	100	1	5	15
Double Stuff	1 (1 oz)	140	1	7	21
Sandwich Cookie	2 (1.2 oz)	160	2	7	25
Orion					
Choco Pie	1 (1 oz)	120	1	5	19
Pepperidge Farm					
Bordeaux	4 (1 oz)	130	2	5	19
Chantilly Raspberry	2	120	1	3	23
Chessmen	3 (0.9 oz)	120	2	5	18
Dark Chocolate Mint Chocolate Chunk	1	140	2	7	16
Gingerman	4	130	2	4	21
Medallion Milk Chocolate	5	160	2	8	20
Milano	3	180	2	10	21
Milano French Vanilla	2	130	1	5	18
Milano Mint Chocolate Covered	4	130	2	6	18

FOOD	PORTION	CALS	PROT	FAT	CARB
Milano Sugar Free	3	170	2	9	21
Nantucket Chocolate Dipped	1	150	2	8	20
Nantucket Dark Chocolate Chunk	1	140	2	7	16
Pirouettes Cappuccino	2	120	1	5	18
Pirouettes Chocolate Mint	2	120	1	5	18
Sausalito Milk Chocolate Macadamia Nut	1	140	2	8	16
Shortbread	2	140	2	7	16
Soft Baked Milk Chocolate	1	150	1	7	21
Soft Baked Oatmeal Cranberry	1	130	2	4	22
Soft Baked Sugar	1	140	2	5	22
Tahiti	2	170	2	10	17
Verona Apricot Raspberry	3	140	2	5	22
Pirouette					
Sandwich Vanilla Creamed	3 (1.1 oz)	133	1	4	22
Polar					
Fortune	2	56	2	0	12
Q.bel					
Wafer Rolls Dark Chocolate	1 pkg (0.9 oz)	120	1	6	18
Wafer Rolls Milk Chocolate	1 pkg (0.9 oz)	130	2	6	18
Quaker					
Breakfast Cookie Oatmeal Raisin	1	180	3	5	33
Ruger					
Wafers Vanilla	3 (1 oz)	160	1	9	20
SnackWell's					
Cookie Cakes Chocolate Mint	1 (0.6 oz)	50	1	1	12
Devil's Food Fat Free	1 (0.5 oz)	50	1	0	12
Sugar Free Lemon Creme	2 (1.1 oz)	130	1	6	23
Sugar Free Shortbread	2 (1 oz)	130	2	6	21
Snikiddy					
Cherry Oaties	1 pkg (0.8 oz)	110	2	4	17
South Beach					
Fiber Fit Double Chocolate Chunk	1 pkg (0.8 oz)	100	1	5	17
Fiber Fit Oatmeal Chocolate Chunk	1 pkg (0.8 oz)	100	1	5	17
Wafer Sticke Dark Chocolate Hazelnut Creme	1 pkg	100	5	6	10

FOOD	PORTION	CALS	PROT	FAT	CARB
Wafer Sticke Dark Chocolate Peanut Butter	1 pkg	100	5	6	10
Starbucks					
Almond Roca Buttercrunch Toffee	6 (1 oz)	110	1	4	19
Biscotti Chocolate Hazelnut	1 (0.9 oz)	100	2	5	14
White Chocolate & Raspberry	2 (0.9 oz)	120	1	6	15
Stella D'Oro					
100 Calorie Pack Breakfast Treats Original	1 pkg (0.8 oz)	100	2	2	19
Almond Delight	1 (1 oz)	150	2	8	18
Angelica Goodies	1 (0.7 oz)	90	1	3	15
Anginetti	4 (1.1 oz)	130	1	3	25
Biscotti Almond	1 (0.7 oz)	90	2	4	15
Biscotti French Vanilla	1 (0.7 oz)	90	1	3	15
Breakfast Treats Chocolate	1 (0.9 oz)	110	1	4	19
Breakfast Treats Original	1 (0.7 oz)	90	1	3	14
Coffee Treats Almond Toast	2 (0.9 oz)	100	2	2	20
Coffee Treats Angel Wings	3 (1 oz)	160	2	10	16
Coffee Treats Anisette Sponge	2 (0.9 oz)	90	2	1	18
Coffee Treats Anisette Toast	3 (1.2 oz)	130	2	1	27
Coffee Treats Roman Egg Biscuits	1 (1.1 oz)	130	3	5	19
Egg Jumbo	3 (1.2 oz)	120	2	2	25
Lady Stella	3 (1 oz)	130	1	5	19
Margherite	2 (1 oz)	130	2	5	20
Swiss Fudge	3 (1.2 oz)	170	2	9	22
Teddy Grahams					
Chocolate	24 (1.1 oz)	130	2	5	22
Honey	24 (1 oz)	130	2	4	23
Temptations					
Chocolate Alps	1 bar (1.6 oz)	170	2	7	28
Chocolate Mocha	1 bar (1.6 oz)	170	2	6	27
No Gluten Chocolate Rush	1 bar (1.6 oz)	170	1	9	25
Voortman					
Chinese Almond	1 (0.9 oz)	130	1	7	16
Coconut Delight	1 (0.6 oz)	90	1	6	10
Dutch Creme	1 (0.8 oz)	110	1	4	16
Fudge Swirl	1 (0.6 oz)	80	1	4	10
Gingerboy	1 (0.7 oz)	100	1	4	15

FOOD	PORTION	CALS	PROT	FAT	CARB
Maple Leaf	1 (0.6 oz)	90	1	4	13
Molasses	1 (1 oz)	110	2	3	20
Oatmeal Apple	1 (0.7 oz)	90	2	4	13
Peanut Delight	1 (0.9 oz)	130	2	7	15
Shortbread	1 (0.6 oz)	90	1	5	11
Sugar Free Chocolate Chip	1 (0.7 oz)	80	1	5	13
Sugar Free Vanilla Creme	2 (0.7 oz)	100	1	6	13
Sugar Free Wafers Lemon	3 (1 oz)	130	0	8	17
Sugar Free Wafers Peanut Butter	4 (1 oz)	150	2	8	17
Sugar Free Wafers Vanilla	3 (1 oz)	130	0	8	17
Turnover Blueberry	1 (0.9 oz)	110	1	4	18
Turnover Cherry	1 (0.9 oz)	110	1	4	18
Turnover Strawberry	1 (0.9 oz)	110	1	4	18
Wafers Chocolate Covered	1 (0.7 oz)	100	tr	5	13
Wafers Mini Chocolate	5 (1 oz)	130	tr	6	19
Wafers Vanilla	3 (1 oz)	140	1	7	20
Walkers					
Shortbread	1	100	1	6	11
Shortbread Chocolate Chip	2 (1 oz)	140	1	8	17
Whippet					
Original	2 (1.2 oz)	150	1	5	24
World Of Grains					
Apple Cinnamon	1 pkg	130	3	4	21
Cranberry	1 pkg	130	3	4	21
Multigrain	1 pkg	130	3	5	21
Zwieback					
Toast	1 (8 g)	35	1	1	6
REFRIGERATED					
chocolate chip	1 (0.42 oz)	59	1	3	8
chocolate chip unbaked	1 oz	126	1	6	17
oatmeal	1 (0.4 oz)	56	1	3	8
oatmeal raisin	1 (0.4 oz)	56	1	3	8
peanut butter	1 (0.4 oz)	60	1	3	7
peanut butter dough	1 oz	130	2	7	15
sugar	1 (0.42 oz)	58	1	3	8
sugar dough	1 oz	124	1	6	17
Pillsbury					
Chocolate Chip	2 (1.3 oz)	170	2	9	22
Gingerbread	2 (1.1 oz)	170	1	7	18

FOOD	PORTION	CALS	PROT	FAT	CARB
Oatmeal Chocolate Chip	2 (1.3 oz)	170	2	8	23
Peanut Butter	2 (1 oz)	130	2	6	16
S'Mores	2 (1.3 oz)	160	1	7	23
Sugar	2 (1.3 oz)	170	2	9	22
TAKE-OUT					
biscotti w/ nuts chocolate dipped	1 (1.3 oz)	117	2	6	16
black & white	1 lg (3 oz)	302	4	9	52
finikia	1 (1.2 oz)	171	2	5	16
koulourakia butter cookie twist	1 (0.9 oz)	113	2	6	14
linzer tart	1 (2.4 oz)	280	2	14	34
CORIANDER					
cilantro fresh	1 tsp (2 g)	tr	tr	tr	tr
leaf dried	1 tsp	2	tr	tr	tr
leaf fresh	¼ cup	1	tr	tr	tr
seed	1 tsp	5	tr	tr	1
CORN					
CANNED					
cream style	½ cup	93	2	1	23
w/ red & green peppers	½ cup	86	3	1	21
white	½ cup	66	2	1	15
yellow	½ cup	66	2	1	15
Del Monte					
Savory Sides In Butter Sauce	½ cup	90	2	3	14
Savory Sides Santa Fe	½ cup	70	3	1	16
Green Giant					
Mexicorn	⅓ cup	70	2	1	14
Super Sweet Yellow & White	⅓ cup	60	2	1	12
Orchids					
Whole Young Spears	½ cup (4.6 oz)	25	2	0	4
FRESH					
white cooked	½ cup	89	3	1	21
white raw	½ cup	66	2	1	15
yellow cooked	1 ear (2.7 oz)	83	3	1	19
yellow cooked	½ cup	89	3	1	21
yellow raw	1 ear (3 oz)	77	3	1	17
yellow raw	½ cup	66	2	1	15

FOOD	PORTION	CALS	PROT	FAT	CARB
FROZEN					
cooked	½ cup	67	2	tr	17
on the cob cooked	1 ear (2.2 oz)	59	2	tr	14
Birds Eye					
Steamfresh Singles Super Sweet	1 pkg (3.2 oz)	80	3	1	14
Steamfresh Southwestern	⅔ cup (2.9 oz)	90	2	2	16
Steamfresh Sweet Mini Corn On The Cob	1 (3 oz)	90	3	1	19
C&W					
Cheddar Bacon	½ cup	130	4	5	18
Early Harvest Supersweet Petite	⅔ cup	70	3	1	14
Salsa Corn	1 cup	90	3	1	17
Glory					
Savory Accents Fried Corn	½ cup	110	3	2	24
Green Giant					
Cream Style	½ cup	110	2	1	24
Nibblers On-The-Cob	1 (2.1 oz)	70	2	1	14
Health Is Wealth					
Creamed	½ pkg (4.5 oz)	110	4	2	23
Stouffer's					
Souffle	½ pkg (6 oz)	150	5	5	22
TAKE-OUT					
fritters	1 (1 oz)	62	2	2	9
on the cob w/ butter cooked	1 ear	155	4	3	32
scalloped	1 cup	257	10	11	34

CORN CHIPS (see CHIPS)

CORNISH HEN (see CHICKEN)

CORNMEAL

FOOD	PORTION	CALS	PROT	FAT	CARB
cornmeal mush as prep w/ water	1 cup	223	5	1	47
cornmeal yellow	½ cup (2.2 oz)	236	4	1	52
whole grain blue	½ cup (1.9 oz)	201	5	3	41
yellow self-rising	½ cup (3 oz)	296	7	2	62
Indian Head					
Stone Ground	¼ cup	100	3	1	20
Martha White					
White Enriched	3 tbsp (1.2 oz)	120	3	1	24
White Self Rising	3 tbsp (1.1 oz)	100	2	1	22
Yellow	3 tbsp (1.1 oz)	110	2	1	22

FOOD	PORTION	CALS	PROT	FAT	CARB
Quaker					
Quick Grits not prep	¼ cup	130	3	1	29
TAKE-OUT					
corn pone	1 piece (2.1 oz)	128	2	3	23
fritter puerto rican style	1 (1.4 oz)	109	3	7	8
harina de maize con coco	½ cup	383	4	27	36
harina de maize con leche	1 cup	295	8	7	51
hush puppies	1 (0.8 oz)	74	2	3	10
johnnycake	1 piece (1.7 oz)	134	4	4	21
CORNSTARCH					
cornstarch	1 tbsp (0.3 oz)	34	tr	0	8
cornstarch	¼ cup (1.1 oz)	122	tr	tr	29
Argo					
Cornstarch	1 tbsp (0.3 oz)	30	0	0	7
Bob's Red Mill					
Cornstarch	1 tbsp	30	0	0	7
COTTAGE CHEESE					
creamed large curd	½ cup (4 oz)	110	13	5	4
creamed small curd	½ cup (3.7 oz)	103	12	5	4
dry curd	½ cup (2.5 oz)	52	8	tr	5
lowfat 1%	½ cup (4 oz)	81	14	1	3
lowfat 1% lactose reduced	½ cup (4 oz)	84	14	1	4
Axelrod					
Lowfat 1%	½ cup (4 oz)	90	14	2	6
Breakstone's					
LiveActive	1 pkg (4 oz)	90	10	2	8
LiveActive Mixed Berries	1 pkg (4 oz)	120	8	2	18
Cabot					
Cottage Cheese	½ cup	100	13	5	4
No Fat	½ cup	70	13	0	5
Friendship					
1% Lowfat	½ cup	90	16	1	3
1% Lowfat No Salt Added	½ cup	90	16	1	4
1% Lowfat Whipped	½ cup	90	16	1	3
2% Digestive Health	½ cup	90	14	3	5
2% Pot Style	½ cup	90	15	3	3
4% California Style	½ cup	110	15	5	3
Nonfat	½ cup	80	15	0	4

FOOD	PORTION	CALS	PROT	FAT	CARB
Horizon Organic					
Lowfat	½ cup	100	13	3	4
Regular	½ cup	120	13	5	4
Knudsen					
LiveActive Pineapple	1 pkg (4 oz)	110	8	2	17
Land O' Lakes					
1% Lowfat	½ cup (4 oz)	90	13	2	5
2% Lowfat	½ cup (3.7 oz)	100	13	3	5
Cottage Cheese	½ cup (3.7 oz)	110	11	5	5
Fat Free	½ cup (4 oz)	80	14	0	6
Nancy's					
Organic Lowfat	½ cup	80	14	1	3
Organic Valley					
Low Fat	½ cup	100	15	2	4
COTTONSEED					
kernels roasted	1 tbsp	51	3	4	2
COUSCOUS					
cooked	1 cup (5.5 oz)	176	6	tr	36
dry	1 cup (6.1 oz)	650	22	1	134
Marrakesh Express					
Mango Salsa as prep	1 cup	190	7	0	38
Mushroom as prep	1 cup	190	8	1	39
Plain as prep	1 cup	270	10	0	57
Near East					
Mediterranean Curry as prep	1 cup	220	8	4	40
Original Plain as prep	1 cup	190	7	2	37
Parmesan as prep	1 cup	220	8	4	39
Toasted Pine Nut as prep	1 cup	230	8	5	39
Wild Mushroom & Herb as prep	1 cup	230	8	4	40
CRAB					
CANNED					
blue	½ cup	67	14	1	0
blue drained	1 can (6.5 oz)	124	26	2	0
Ace Of Diamonds					
Fancy w/ Leg Meat	¼ cup (2 oz)	40	7	0	2
Polar					
Claw Meat	¼ cup (2 oz)	37	10	0	1
Jumbo Lump Meat	¼ cup (2 oz)	39	8	1	0

FOOD	PORTION	CALS	PROT	FAT	CARB
FRESH					
alaska king meat only steamed	3 oz	82	16	1	0
blue cooked flaked	1 cup (4 oz)	120	24	2	0
dungeness steamed	3 oz	94	19	1	1
queen steamed	3 oz	98	20	1	0
FROZEN					
Mama Belle's					
Crab Cakes Maryland Style	1 (2 oz)	100	9	5	4
Mrs. Paul's					
Deviled Crab Cakes	1 (3 oz)	220	20	12	12
TAKE-OUT					
alaska king leg steamed	1 leg (4.7 oz)	130	26	2	0
baked	1 (3.8 oz)	160	29	2	4
cakes	2 (4.2 oz)	186	24	9	1
crab imperial	1 crab (6.8 oz)	289	30	15	6
crab salad	1 serv (5.5 oz)	285	21	21	3
crab thermidor	1 serv (6.4 oz)	456	22	37	8
deviled	1 serv (4.5 oz)	254	17	13	17
dungeness steamed	1 crab (4.5 oz)	140	28	2	1
empanada de jueyes	1 (4.4 oz)	341	12	16	38
fried crab puffs	4 (3.2 oz)	323	10	18	30
kenagi korean crab cooked	1 serv (3 oz)	71	16	tr	0
salmorejo de jueyes (in tomato sauce)	1 serv (4.5 oz)	215	20	14	3
soft-shell breaded & fried	1 med (2.3 oz)	216	13	13	11
taco de jueyes	1 (4.2 oz)	266	16	14	18
CRACKER CRUMBS					
cracker meal	1 cup	440	11	2	93
graham cracker crumbs	1 cup	355	6	8	65
Honey Maid					
Graham Cracker Crumbs	2½ tbsp (0.6 oz)	70	1	2	13
Keebler					
Graham	¼ cup	93	1	2	17
CRACKERS					
melba toast round	1	12	tr	tr	2
oyster cracker	¼ cup	48	1	1	8
saltines	1	13	tr	tr	2
water biscuits	3	92	2	3	16
zwieback	1 oz	107	3	1	21

FOOD	PORTION	CALS	PROT	FAT	CARB
34 Degrees					
Crispbread Sesame	19 (1.1 oz)	140	5	3	26
Athenos					
Pita Chips Whole Wheat	11 (1 oz)	120	4	4	18
Aunt Gussie's					
Cracker Flats Spelt Cinnamon Raisin	1 (1 oz)	100	3	2	19
Cracker Flats Spelt Everything	1 (0.8 oz)	60	2	2	12
Back To Nature					
Poppy Thyme	17 (1 oz)	130	2	4	21
Rice Thin Sesame Ginger	16	120	2	3	23
Sesame Tarragon	17 (1 oz)	130	2	5	21
Barbara's Bakery					
Rite Rounds Lite Original	5 (0.5 oz)	60	1	2	11
Wheatines Original	4	60	1	1	11
Better Cheddars					
Original	1.1 oz	160	3	8	18
Bremner Wafers					
Cracked Wheat	7 (0.5 oz)	70	2	2	11
Original	7 (0.5 oz)	70	2	2	11
Soup & Chili Crackers	50 (0.5 oz)	60	2	2	11
Breton					
Garden Vegetable	4 (0.7 oz)	100	1	4	13
Minis Cheddar Cheese	20 (0.7 oz)	100	3	5	13
Brown Rice Snaps					
Cheddar	6	60	1	1	12
Original Tamari Seaweed	9	60	1	0	12
Unsalted Plain	8	60	1	0	13
Cheese Nips					
Cheddar	1 pkg (1.2 oz)	170	3	7	22
Chicken Biskit					
Original	1.1 oz	160	2	8	19
Dare					
Crackers	3 (0.5 oz)	70	1	4	9
Original	4 (0.7 oz)	90	2	4	13
Reduced Fat & Salt	5 (0.7 oz)	80	3	2	16
Dr. Kracker					
Flatbread Klassic Seed	1 (1 oz)	120	6	5	13
Flatbread Pumpkin Seed Cheddar	1 (1 oz)	120	5	5	12

FOOD	PORTION	CALS	PROT	FAT	CARB
Flatbread Seeded Spelt	1 (1 oz)	120	5	6	12
Flatbread Seedlander	1 (1 oz)	120	5	5	15
Flatbread Spelt Sunflower Cheddar	1 (1 oz)	120	5	6	12
Krispy Grahams	5 (1 oz)	110	2	3	17
Glutino					
Gluten Free	4 (0.5 oz)	70	tr	2	12
Gluten Free Rusks	2 (0.7 oz)	80	0	2	15
GrainsFirst					
Autumn Harvest	7 (1.1 oz)	140	3	7	16
Grissol					
Crispy Baguettes Garden Herb	8 (1 oz)	110	3	2	19
Health Valley					
Organic Bruschetta Vegetable	4	70	1	3	10
Organic Cracked Pepper	4	70	1	3	10
Organic Cracker Stix Garlic Herb	8	70	1	3	9
Organic Whole Wheat	4	70	2	3	9
Kashi					
Heart To Heart Whole Grain	7 (1 oz)	120	3	4	22
TLC Natural Ranch	15 (1 oz)	130	4	3	22
TLC Original 7 Grain	15 (1 oz)	130	3	3	22
TLC Party Mediterranean Bruschetta	4	120	3	4	18
TLC Snack Fire Roasted Vegetable	5	130	3	4	21
TLC Toasted Asiago	15 (1.1 oz)	130	3	4	21
Keebler					
Club Multi-Grain	4	70	1	3	10
Club Original	4	70	1	3	9
Club Reduced Fat	5	70	1	3	12
Club Snack Sticks	12	130	1	6	19
Puffed Original	24	140	2	6	20
Sandwich Cheese & Peanut Butter	1 pkg (1.4 oz)	200	4	10	23
Sandwich Toast & Peanut Butter	1 pkg (1.4 oz)	200	4	10	23
Sandwich Wheat & Cheddar	1 pkg (1.3 oz)	190	2	10	23
Toasteds Harvest Wheat	16	130	2	6	20
Toasteds Sesame	5	80	1	4	10
Toasteds Wheat	5	80	1	4	10

FOOD	PORTION	CALS	PROT	FAT	CARB
Town House Bistro	2	80	1	3	11
Town House FlipSides Original	5	70	1	4	10
Town House Original	5	80	tr	5	10
Town House Reduced Fat	6	60	tr	2	11
Town House Reduced Sodium	5	80	tr	5	10
Town House Toppers	3	70	1	3	9
Wheatables 33% Less Fat	19	140	2	4	22
Wheatables Original	17	140	2	6	20
Zesta Saltine Fat Free	5	60	1	0	13
Zesta Saltine Original	5	60	1	2	11
Kellogg's					
All Bran Garlic Herb	18 (1 oz)	120	3	6	19
Kitchen Table Bakers					
Aged Parmesan	3	80	7	6	tr
Everything	3	80	7	6	tr
Garlic	3	80	6	6	tr
Jalapeno	3	80	6	6	2
Lance					
Captain Wafers	4	70	1	3	9
Nekot	1 pkg (1.7 oz)	240	7	11	30
Nipchee	1 pkg (1.4 oz)	190	4	11	22
Peanut Butter On Wheat	1 pkg (1.4 oz)	200	4	9	21
Toastchee	1 pkg (1.5 oz)	220	5	11	23
Toastchee Reduced Fat	1 pkg (1.4 oz)	180	6	7	23
Larzaroni					
Bruschette w/ Olives	9 (1.1 oz)	140	4	5	21
Late July					
Organic Classic Rich	4 (0.5 oz)	70	1	2	11
Organic Classic Saltine	4 (0.5 oz)	60	1	3	10
Mary's Gone Crackers					
Wheat Free Gluten Free Black Pepper	13 (1 oz)	140	3	5	21
Wheat Free Gluten Free Onion	13 (1 oz)	140	3	5	21
Wheat Free Gluten Free Original Seed	13 (1 oz)	140	3	5	21
Nabisco					
Garden Harvest Apple Cinnamon	16 (1 oz)	120	2	3	22
Garden Harvest Banana	16 (1 oz)	120	2	3	22
Garden Harvest Tomato Basil	16 (1 oz)	120	2	4	20

FOOD	PORTION	CALS	PROT	FAT	CARB
Garden Harvest Vegetable Medley	16 (1 oz)	120	2	4	20
Vegetable Thins	21 (1 oz)	150	2	7	20
New York Style					
Crispini Seeds & Spice	6	120	4	4	19
Panetini Original	2	80	2	4	10
Panetini Three Cheese	2	80	2	5	9
Pita Chips Garlic	7	130	3	5	17
Pita Chips Natural Whole Wheat	7	120	3	5	17
Nonni's					
Panetini Roasted Garlic	5 (1 oz)	120	4	4	19
Panetini Sun Dried Tomato Basil	5 (1 oz)	120	4	4	17
Orkney					
Oatcakes Thin	4 (1.8 oz)	227	6	12	25
Pepperidge Farm					
100 Calorie Pack Goldfish Cheddar	1 pkg	100	3	4	14
100 Calorie Pack Goldfish Pretzel	1 pkg	100	2	2	18
Goldfish Cinnamon Graham	1 pkg	210	3	8	32
Goldfish Pizza	55	140	3	5	20
Goldfish Reduced Sodium Cheddar	60	140	4	5	20
Goldfish w/ Whole Grain	55	140	4	5	19
Snack Sticks Pumpernickel	15	120	3	2	24
Water Crackers	4	60	0	1	12
Wheat Crisps Spicy Salsa	16	140	2	6	21
Premium					
Saltines Fat Free	5 (0.5 oz)	60	1	0	12
Saltines Low Sodium	5 (0.5 oz)	80	1	2	11
Saltines Multigrain	5 (0.5 oz)	60	1	2	10
Saltines Original	5 (0.5 oz)	60	1	2	11
Ritz					
Crackerfuls Classic Cheddar	1 (1 oz)	130	2	7	17
Hint Of Salt	0.5 oz	80	1	4	10
Original	0.5 oz	80	1	5	10
Reduced Fat	5 (0.5 oz)	70	1	2	11
Whole Wheat	0.5 oz	70	1	3	11

FOOD	PORTION	CALS	PROT	FAT	CARB
Sociables					
Original	0.5 oz	70	1	4	9
Triscuit					
Cracked Pepper & Olive Oil	6 (1 oz)	120	3	4	20
Deli-Style Rye	1 oz	120	3	5	19
Original	1 oz	120	3	5	19
Reduced Fat	1 oz	120	3	3	21
True North					
Peanut Crunches	¼ cup (1 oz)	150	5	8	13
Pistachio Crisps	12 (1 oz)	140	5	7	15
Utz					
Cheese Peanut Butter	6	200	4	10	21
Vegetable Thins					
Original	21 (1.1 oz)	150	2	7	19
Vinta					
Original	3 (0.7 oz)	100	2	5	12
Wasa					
Hearty	1 (0.5 oz)	45	1	0	11
Light Rye	2 (0.6 oz)	60	2	0	14
Multi Grain	1 (0.5 oz)	45	2	0	10
Sourdough	1 (0.4 oz)	35	1	0	9
Whole Grain	1 (0.4 oz)	40	1	0	10
Whole Wheat	1 (0.5 oz)	50	2	1	10
Water Crackers					
Original	6 (0.5 oz)	60	2	2	11
Westminster					
Oyster	1 pkg (0.5 oz)	66	1	2	11
Wheat Thins					
100% Whole Grain	1 oz	140	2	6	21
Low Sodium	1.1 oz	150	2	6	22
Original	1.1 oz	150	2	6	21
Reduced Fat	1 oz	130	3	4	21
Wheatsworth					
Crackers	5 (0.5 oz)	80	2	4	10
CRANBERRIES					
cranberry orange relish	¼ cup	118	tr	tr	31
dried	½ cup	85	tr	tr	23
fresh chopped	1 cup	13	tr	tr	3
fresh whole	1 cup	11	tr	tr	3
sauce	1 slice (2 oz)	86	tr	tr	22
sauce	¼ cup	109	tr	tr	27

FOOD	PORTION	CALS	PROT	FAT	CARB
Chukar Cherries					
North Cove Dried	¼ cup	100	0	0	24
De-Lite					
Dried Sweetened	1 oz	92	tr	tr	23
Earthbound Farms					
Organic Dried	⅓ cup	130	0	0	34
Emily's					
Milk Chocolate Covered	¼ cup (1.4 oz)	180	tr	10	24
Fool					
Cranberry Spread	1 tbsp	30	0	0	7
Fruitaceuticals					
OmegaCrans Dried	¼ cup	91	0	1	22
Mariani					
Dried Sweetened	⅓ cup	130	0	0	35
Ocean Spray					
Whole Berry Sauce	¼ cup (2.5 oz)	110	0	0	25
S&W					
Sauce Jellied	¼ cup (2.5 oz)	100	0	0	26
Sauce Whole Berry	¼ cup (2.5 oz)	100	0	0	26
Stoneridge Orchards					
Dried	⅓ cup (¼ oz)	140	0	0	33
Sun-Maid					
Dried Cape Cod	⅓ cup (1.4 oz)	130	0	0	33
Sunsweet					
Dried	⅓ cup (1.5 oz)	140	0	0	35
Tree Of Life					
Organic Jellied	¼ cup (2.5 oz)	100	0	0	26
Wild Thymes Farm					
Cranberry Fig Sauce	1 tsp	19	tr	0	5
Original Cranberry Sauce	1 tbsp	21	0	0	5
CRANBERRY BEANS					
canned	½ cup	108	7	tr	20
dried cooked w/o salt	½ cup	120	8	tr	22
Goya					
Roman Beans Dried not prep	¼ cup (1.4 oz)	80	8	0	24
CRANBERRY JUICE					
cranberry juice cocktail low calorie w/ vitamin C	8 oz	46	tr	tr	11

FOOD	PORTION	CALS	PROT	FAT	CARB
cranberry juice cocktail w/ vitamin C	8 oz	137	0	tr	34
unsweetened	8 oz	116	1	tr	31
Apple & Eve					
100% Juice	8 oz	130	0	0	32
Lakewood					
Organic	6 oz	50	1	0	12
Organic Light	6 oz	45	1	0	18
Nantucket Nectars					
Cranberry Cocktail	8 oz	130	0	0	33
Northland					
100% Juice No Sugar Added	8 oz	130	0	0	33
Ocean Spray					
Cran.Grape	8 oz	120	0	0	31
Cran.Pomegranate	8 oz	120	0	0	30
Cranberry Juice Cocktail	8 oz	120	0	0	30
White Cran Peach	8 oz	120	0	0	31
Old Orchard					
Cocktail	8 oz	140	0	0	34
Santa Cruz					
Organic Nectar	8 oz	110	tr	0	27
SSips					
Cocktail	1 box (7 oz)	110	0	0	28
CRAYFISH					
cooked	3 oz	97	20	1	0
raw	3 oz	76	16	1	0
raw	8	24	5	tr	0
CREAM (*see also* WHIPPED TOPPINGS)					
clotted cream	2 tbsp (1 oz)	164	tr	18	1
creme fraiche	2 tbsp (1 oz)	100	1	11	1
half & half	1 tbsp (0.5 oz)	20	tr	2	1
half & half	1 cup (8.5 oz)	315	7	28	10
heavy whipping	1 tbsp (0.5 oz)	52	tr	6	tr
heavy whipping whipped	1 cup (4.1 oz)	411	5	44	7
light coffee	1 tbsp (0.5 oz)	29	tr	3	1
light coffee	1 cup (8.4 oz)	496	6	46	9
light whipping	1 tbsp (0.5 oz)	44	tr	5	tr
light whipping whipped	1 cup (4.2 oz)	345	5	37	7
Cabot					
Whipped	2 tbsp	15	0	2	1

FOOD	PORTION	CALS	PROT	FAT	CARB
Horizon Organic					
Half & Half	2 tbsp	35	1	3	1
Heavy Whipping	1 tbsp	50	0	5	0
Land O' Lakes					
Aerosol Whipped Light Cream	2 tbsp (0.2 oz)	20	0	2	1
Half & Half	2 tbsp (1.1 oz)	35	tr	4	1
Half & Half Fat Free	2 tbsp (1.1 oz)	20	tr	0	3
Heavy Whipping	1 tbsp (0.5 oz)	50	0	5	0
Organic Valley					
Half & Half	2 tbsp (1 oz)	40	tr	4	1
Straus					
Organic Whipping Cream	1 tbsp (0.5 oz)	52	0	6	0
CREAM CHEESE					
cream cheese	1 oz	99	2	10	1
cream cheese	1 pkg (3 oz)	297	6	30	2
Connoisseur					
Wheel Mango Peach	2 tbsp	110	1	7	10
Wheel Wild Blueberry	2 tbsp	100	1	7	9
Earth Balance					
Brick	2 tbsp	80	3	6	2
Tub	2 tbsp	80	3	6	2
Horizon Organic					
Reduced Fat	2 tbsp	70	2	7	2
Spreadable	2 tbsp	110	2	10	tr
Lifeway					
Lox & Onion	2 tbsp	80	2	8	1
Vegetable	2 tbsp	80	2	7	1
Whipped	2 tbsp	80	2	8	1
Nancy's					
Organic	2 tbsp	95	1	9	2
Organic Valley					
Cream Cheese	1 oz	100	2	10	1
Soft	2 tbsp	90	1	9	2
Philadelphia					
⅓ Less Fat	1 oz	70	2	6	tr
Original	1 oz	100	2	9	1
Whipped	2 tbsp	60	1	6	1

FOOD	PORTION	CALS	PROT	FAT	CARB
CREAM CHEESE SUBSTITUTES					
Vegan Gourmet					
Alternative Cream Cheese	2 tbsp (1 oz)	90	2	8	3
CREAM OF TARTAR					
cream of tartar	1 tsp	8	0	0	2
CREPES					
basic crepe unfilled	1 (7 in)	112	4	6	11
Ekizian					
Chickpea Crepe	1 (7-in) (1.5 oz)	212	7	13	16
CROAKER					
atlantic breaded & fried	3 oz	188	15	11	6
atlantic raw	3 oz	89	15	3	0
CROCODILE					
cooked	3 oz	78	17	1	0
CROISSANT					
apple	1 (2 oz)	145	4	5	21
butter	1 lg (2.4 oz)	272	5	14	31
butter mini	1 (1 oz)	114	2	6	13
cheese	1 (1.5 oz)	174	4	9	20
chocolate	1 (2 oz)	237	5	14	25
TAKE-OUT					
w/ egg & cheese	1 (4.5 oz)	368	13	25	24
w/ egg & sausage	1 (5 oz)	497	16	34	31
w/ egg cheese & bacon	1 (4.1 oz)	385	16	24	25
w/ egg cheese & ham	1 (5.1 oz)	402	21	24	25
w/ egg cheese & sausage	1 (5.6 oz)	539	20	39	26
w/ ham & cheese	1 (4 oz)	338	15	20	25
CROUTONS					
plain	1 cup (1 oz)	122	4	2	22
seasoned	1 cup (1.4 oz)	186	4	7	25
Edward & Sons					
Organic Lightly Salted	2 tbsp	30	tr	1	5
Fresh Gourmet					
Butter & Garlic	7 (7 g)	35	1	2	4
Cheese & Garlic	12 (0.5 oz)	70	1	3	9
Classic Caesar	6 (7 g)	35	1	2	4

FOOD	PORTION	CALS	PROT	FAT	CARB
Cornbread Sweet Butter	½ cup (1 oz)	110	3	1	22
Country Ranch	6 (7 g)	35	1	2	4
Fat Free Garlic Caesar	12 (7 g)	30	1	0	5
Italian Seasoned	6 (7 g)	35	1	2	4
Organic Seasoned	5 (7 g)	30	1	2	4
Pepperidge Farm					
Whole Grain Seasoned	6	30	1	1	5
Zesty Italian	6	30	tr	1	5
CUCUMBER					
fresh peeled	1 med (7 oz)	24	1	tr	4
fresh sliced	1 cup	14	1	tr	3
fresh w/ peel sliced	½ cup	34	tr	tr	2
TAKE-OUT					
cucumber & onion salad w/ vinegar	1 cup	52	1	tr	12
cucumber raita	1 serv (3.3 oz)	40	2	3	3
cucumber salad w/ oil & vinegar	1 cup	183	1	15	11
cucumber salad w/ sour cream dressing	1 cup	68	1	6	3
kimchee	½ cup (1.8 oz)	36	tr	2	4
tzatziki	½ cup (3.4 oz)	72	2	6	4
CUMIN					
seed	1 tsp (2 g)	8	tr	tr	1
seed	1 tbsp (6 g)	22	1	1	3
CURRANT JUICE					
black currant nectar	7 oz	110	tr	0	26
red currant nectar	7 oz	108	tr	tr	26
CURRANTS					
black fresh	½ cup	36	1	tr	9
zante dried	½ cup	204	3	tr	53
Sun-Maid					
Zante	¼ cup (1.4 oz)	120	1	0	30
CURRY					
curry powder	1 tsp	7	tr	tr	1
paste	1 tube (6 oz)	465	7	36	30
Ethnic Gourmet					
Gujarati Vegetable Curry	1 pkg (10 oz)	380	8	11	63
Malay Chicken Curry	1 pkg (10 oz)	410	18	11	59
Simmer Sauce Bombay Curry	4 oz	70	2	3	10

FOOD	PORTION	CALS	PROT	FAT	CARB
Fortun's					
Finishing Sauce Mulligatawny Curry	¼ cup (2 oz)	60	1	2	10
French Meadow Bakery					
Fragrant Chicken Curry	1 pkg (12 oz)	280	28	5	36
Helen's Kitchen					
Indian Curry w/ Tofu Steaks & Rice	1 pkg (9 oz)	300	14	8	63
Patak's					
Curry Paste Biryani	2 tbsp	180	1	16	6
Garam Masala Paste	2 tsp	130	1	12	4
Tandoori Paste	2 tbsp	30	1	1	5
Vegetable Curry w/ Rice Rich Creamy Coconut	1 pkg	400	6	18	54
Vegetable Curry w/ Rice Rich Tomato & Onion	1 pkg (10.5 oz)	290	6	6	53
Vegetable Curry w/ Rice Tangy Lemon & Cilantro	1 pkg	300	5	7	54
Vindaloo Paste	2 tbsp	160	1	16	4
Spice Hunter					
Curry Seasoning Salt Free	¼ tsp	0	0	0	0
TastyBite					
Green Curry Vegetables & Jasmine Rice	1 pkg (12 oz)	320	6	10	52
Yellow Curry Vegetables & Jasmine Rice	1 pkg (12 oz)	380	7	13	61
Thai Kitchen					
Green Curry Paste	1 tbsp (0.5 oz)	15	0	0	3
TAKE-OUT					
beef curry	1 cup	432	27	31	14
beef kurma	1 serv (10 oz)	611	41	47	6
chicken curry ½ breast	1 serv	160	15	9	6
chicken curry boneless	1 serv (6.2 oz)	219	20	12	8
chicken curry leg & thigh	1 serv	180	17	10	7
chickpea curry	1 serv (8.3 oz)	305	18	15	23
eggplant curry	1 serv (8 oz)	241	4	19	12
lamb curry	1 cup	257	28	14	4
mixed vegetable curry	1 serv (7.7 oz)	398	4	33	22
pea & potato curry	1 serv (7 oz)	284	5	22	19
potato curry	1 serv (5.5 oz)	791	29	60	35
sambhar dhal curry	1 serv (10 oz)	177	8	7	21

FOOD	PORTION	CALS	PROT	FAT	CARB
CUSK					
fillet baked	3 oz	106	23	1	0
CUSTARD					
MIX					
as prep w/ 2% milk	½ cup (4.7 oz)	148	7	4	24
as prep w/ whole milk	½ cup (4.7 oz)	163	6	5	23
flan as prep w/ 2% milk	½ cup (4.7 oz)	135	4	2	26
flan as prep w/ whole milk	½ cup (4.7 oz)	150	4	4	25
TAKE-OUT					
baked	½ cup (5 oz)	148	7	7	15
flan	½ cup (5.4 oz)	220	7	6	35
flan de calabaza	1 piece (3.5 oz)	225	5	10	30
flan de coco	1 piece (4.2 oz)	340	10	13	48
tocino del cielo heaven's delight	1 cup	856	14	21	156
zabaione	½ cup (57.2 g)	135	3	5	13
CUTTLEFISH					
steamed	3 oz	134	28	1	1
DANDELION GREENS					
fresh cooked	½ cup	17	1	tr	3
raw chopped	½ cup	13	1	tr	3
DANISH PASTRY					
TAKE-OUT					
cheese	1 (2.5 oz)	266	6	16	26
cinnamon	1 (5 oz)	572	10	32	63
fruit	1 (5 oz)	527	8	27	68
lemon	1 (2.5 oz)	263	4	13	34
raisin nut	1 (2.3 oz)	280	5	16	30
DATES					
deglet noor chopped	¼ cup (1.3 oz)	104	1	tr	28
deglet noor dried	1 (7 g)	20	tr	tr	5
jujube dried	1 oz	75	1	tr	19
jujube fresh	1 oz	30	tr	tr	7
jujube preserved in sugar	1 oz	91	tr	tr	22
medjool	1 (0.8 oz)	66	tr	tr	18
Bob's Red Mill					
Dried Crumbles	⅓ cup	130	1	0	33

FOOD	PORTION	CALS	PROT	FAT	CARB
Earthbound Farms					
Organic Dried	6 (1.4 oz)	120	1	0	31
SunDate					
Fancy Medjool	3 (1.4 oz)	120	1	0	31
Sun-Maid					
Pitted	¼ cup (1.4 oz)	110	1	0	30
Sunsweet					
California Pitted	5 to 6 (1.4 oz)	120	1	0	30
Tree Of Life					
Deglet Noor Pitted	5 (1.5 oz)	120	1	0	31
Organic Medjool	5 (1.5 oz)	120	1	0	31

DEER (see JERKY, VENISON)

DELI MEATS/COLD CUTS (see also BEEF, CHICKEN, HAM, MEAT SUBSTITUTES, TURKEY)

FOOD	PORTION	CALS	PROT	FAT	CARB
barbecue loaf pork & beef	1 slice (0.8 oz)	40	4	2	1
beerwurst beef	2 oz	155	8	13	2
berliner pork & beef	1 slice (0.8 oz)	53	4	4	1
blood sausage	1 slice (0.9 oz)	95	4	9	tr
bologna beef	1 slice (1 oz)	88	3	8	1
bologna beef & pork	1 slice (1 oz)	87	4	7	2
bologna beef & pork low fat	1 slice (1 oz)	64	3	5	1
bologna beef lowfat	1 slice (1 oz)	57	3	4	1
bologna beef reduced sodium	1 slice (1 oz)	88	3	8	1
braunschweiger pork	1 slice (1 oz)	92	4	8	1
corned beef brisket	2 oz	90	11	5	0
dutch brand loaf pork & beef	1 slice (1.3 oz)	104	5	9	1
headcheese pork	1 slice (1.6 oz)	71	6	5	0
honey loaf pork & beef	1 slice (1 oz)	35	4	1	1
lebanon bologna beef	2 slices (1 oz)	105	11	6	tr
mortadella beef & pork	1 slice (0.5 oz)	47	2	4	tr
olive loaf pork	2 slices (2 oz)	134	7	9	5
pastrami beef	1 slice (1 oz)	41	6	2	tr
peppered loaf pork & beef	1 slice (1 oz)	41	5	2	1
pepperoni pork & beef	15 slices (1 oz)	135	6	12	1
picnic loaf pork & beef	1 slice (1 oz)	65	4	5	1
salami cooked beef & pork	1 slice (0.8 oz)	58	3	5	1
salami hard pork	3 slices (0.9 oz)	14	6	8	1
salami hard pork & beef less sodium	1 slice (1 oz)	113	4	9	2
sandwich spread pork & beef	¼ cup	141	5	10	7

FOOD	PORTION	CALS	PROT	FAT	CARB
summer sausage thuringer cervelat	2 oz	203	10	17	2
Applegate Farms					
Organic Genoa Salami Sliced	1 oz	100	7	7	0
Butterball					
Turkey Bologna	1 slice (1 oz)	60	3	5	3
Turkey Ham	1 slice (1 oz)	35	4	2	1
Carl Buddig					
Beef	2 oz	90	10	5	1
Corned Beef	2 oz	90	10	5	1
Healthy Ones					
Pastrami 97% Fat Free	4 slices (2 oz)	60	10	2	3
Oscar Mayer					
Salami Beef	3 slices (1.8 oz)	150	8	13	1
DILL					
seed	1 tsp	6	tr	tr	1
sprigs fresh	5 (0.3 oz)	0	tr	tr	tr
weed dry	1 tbsp	8	1	tr	2
DINNER (see also ASIAN FOOD, CURRY, PASTA DINNERS, POT PIE, SPANISH FOOD)					
A La Carte					
Stuffed Zucchini w/ Barley Risotto Chicken Stuffing in Tomato Sauce	1 serv (5 oz)	140	6	7	14
Amy's					
Country Dinner Vegetable Salisbury Steak	1 pkg (10.9 oz)	380	12	16	50
Banquet					
Boneless Pork Ribs	1 pkg	370	6	17	47
Chicken Fingers	1 pkg	460	13	15	69
Corn Dog Meal	1 pkg	470	11	18	68
Crock Pot Classics Chicken & Dumplings	⅔ cup	200	10	8	21
Crock Pot Classics Hearty Beef & Vegetables	⅔ cup	140	12	6	15
Crock Pot Classics Meatballs In Stroganoff Sauce	⅔ cup	300	14	14	29
Fish Sticks	1 pkg	360	13	13	46
Fried Beef Steak	1 pkg	390	14	19	41
Meatloaf	1 pkg	300	14	15	28

FOOD	PORTION	CALS	PROT	FAT	CARB
Original Fried Chicken	1 pkg	380	14	20	35
Salisbury Steak	1 pkg	300	14	16	25
Swedish Meatballs	1 pkg	430	20	23	35
Turkey	1 pkg	200	14	8	27
Betty Crocker					
Complete Meals Chicken & Buttermilk Biscuits	⅕ pkg (5.4 oz)	280	9	11	37
Complete Meals Stroganoff	⅕ pkg (5 oz)	200	10	5	30
Birds Eye					
Steamfresh Meals For Two Asian Chicken Vegetable Medley	½ pkg (11.9 oz)	290	20	6	36
Steamfresh Meals For Two Grilled Chicken Marinara	½ pkg (11.9 oz)	360	21	10	45
Steamfresh Meals For Two Sweet & Spicy Chicken	½ pkg (11.9 oz)	370	20	10	53
Voila! Pasta Primavera w/ Chicken	1⅔ cups	250	14	3	42
Voila! Shrimp Scampi	1¾ cups	190	11	3	31
Voila! Southwestern Chicken	2 cups	250	14	6	32
C&W					
Stir Fry Feast Pot Sticker + Sauce	2 cups	200	10	4	30
Stir Fry Feast Ultimate + Sauce	1½ cups	190	11	5	25
Campbell's					
Supper Bakes Cheesy Chicken w/ Pasta	⅙ pkg	170	6	4	28
Supper Bakes Garlic Chicken w/ Pasta	⅙ pkg	220	9	2	42
Supper Bakes Savory Pork Chops w/ Herb Stuffing	⅙ box	160	5	2	30
Supper Bakes Traditional Roast Chicken w/ Stuffing	⅙ pkg	160	5	3	29
Contessa					
Beef Goulash not prep	1¾ cups	210	12	5	32
Chicken Cacciatore not prep	1¾ cups	230	14	7	24
Chicken Alfredo not prep	1¾ cups	330	15	18	28
Fillo Factory					
Organic Fillo Pie Eggplant & Red Pepper	1 serv (5 oz)	230	4	9	35

FOOD	PORTION	CALS	PROT	FAT	CARB
French Meadow Bakery					
Garlic Ginger Chicken	1 pkg (12 oz)	310	24	5	42
Glory					
Savory Singles Chicken & Dumplings	1 pkg	290	16	8	40
Savory Singles Chicken Smoked Sausage & Rice Casserole	1 pkg	440	18	18	49
Savory Singles Ham & Sausage Jambalaya	1 pkg	400	17	18	42
Savory Singles Turkey & Gravy w/ Cornbread Stuffing	1 pkg	440	18	18	49
Gluten Free Cafe					
Lemon Basil Chicken	1 pkg (9.2 oz)	340	18	11	42
Glutino					
Gluten Free Chicken Pomodoro w/ Brown Rice & Vegetables	1 pkg (9.1 oz)	190	11	3	33
Gluten Free Chicken Ranchero w/ Brown Rice	1 pkg (9.1 oz)	180	14	2	30
Green Giant					
Create A Meal Stir Fry Sweet & Sour as prep	1 cup	280	2	7	36
Skillet Meal Chicken Teriyaki as prep	1½ cups	240	13	1	46
Healthy Choice					
Beef Pot Roast w/ Gravy	1 pkg (11 oz)	310	15	7	45
Beef Tips Portabello	1 pkg	300	20	8	33
Cafe Steamers Beef Merlot	1 pkg (10 oz)	220	17	6	22
Cafe Steamers Cajun Style Chicken & Shrimp	1 pkg (10.4 oz)	250	18	3	36
Cafe Steamers Chicken Margherita	1 pkg (10 oz)	340	23	8	43
Cafe Steamers Creamy Dill Salmon	1 pkg (9.8 oz)	240	19	6	26
Cafe Steamers Grilled Basil Chicken	1 (10.6 oz)	290	20	6	37
Cafe Steamers Grilled Whiskey Steak	1 pkg (9.4 oz)	250	18	4	34
Chicken Parmigiana	1 pkg (11.6 oz)	350	17	9	48
Country Herb Chicken	1 pkg (11.35 oz)	240	15	5	34

FOOD	PORTION	CALS	PROT	FAT	CARB
Fresh Mixers Southwestern Chicken	1 pkg (7.9 oz)	310	13	3	60
Lemon Pepper Fish	1 pkg (10.7 oz)	310	13	5	53
Mandarin Chicken	1 pkg (9.1 oz)	240	13	3	39
Salisbury Steak	1 pkg (12.5 oz)	360	20	9	46
Slow Roasted Turkey Medallions	1 pkg (8.5 oz)	220	14	5	28
Sweet & Sour Chicken	1 pkg (12 oz)	430	16	9	69
Traditional Turkey Breast	1 pkg	300	21	4	42
Hormel					
Compleats Microwave Meals Beef Steak & Peppers w/ Noodles	1 pkg (9.9 oz)	210	20	5	22
Compleats Microwave Meals Chicken Breast & Dressing	1 pkg (9.9 oz)	270	23	7	29
Compleats Microwave Meals Chicken Breast & Gravy w/ Mashed Potatoes	1 pkg (9.9 oz)	200	19	3	24
Compleats Microwave Meals Homestyle Beef w/ Potatoes & Gravy	1 pkg (9.9 oz)	220	11	6	30
Compleats Microwave Meals Meatloaf w/ Potatoes & Gravy	1 pkg (9.9 oz)	310	18	11	34
Compleats Microwave Meals Salisbury Steak w/ Slice Potato & Gravy	1 pkg (9.9 oz)	280	16	11	30
Compleats Microwave Meals Santa Fe Chicken w/ Rice & Beans	1 pkg (9.9 oz)	280	20	4	41
Compleats Microwave Meals Swedish Meatballs	1 pkg (9.9 oz)	350	15	18	32
Compleats Microwave Meals Sweet & Sour Chicken w/ Rice	1 pkg (9.9 oz)	290	13	2	54
Compleats Microwave Meals Teriyaki Chicken w/ Rice	1 pkg (9.9 oz)	270	13	2	50
Compleats Microwave Meals Tuna Casserole	1 pkg (9.9 oz)	240	17	7	26
Compleats Microwave Meals Turkey & Dressing w/ Gravy	1 pkg (9.9 oz)	290	20	9	31

FOOD	PORTION	CALS	PROT	FAT	CARB
Compleats Microwave Meals Turkey & Hearty Vegetables	1 pkg (9.9 oz)	180	14	4	24
Joy Of Cooking					
Braised Beef Tips & Egg Noodles	1 cup (7.7 oz)	220	17	7	24
Roasted Herb Chicken	1 cup (7.7 oz)	170	11	3	27
Kashi					
Black Bean Mango	1 pkg (10 oz)	340	8	8	58
Lemon Rosemary Chicken	1 pkg (10 oz)	330	17	9	45
Lime Cilantro Shrimp	1 pkg (10 oz)	250	12	8	33
Southwest Style Chicken	1 pkg (10 oz)	240	16	5	32
Sweet & Sour Chicken	1 pkg (10 oz)	320	18	4	55
Lean Cuisine					
Cafe Classics Sweet & Sour Chicken	1 pkg (10 oz)	300	18	3	51
Dinnertime Selects Lemon Garlic Shrimp	1 pkg (12 oz)	350	18	7	54
Marie Callender's					
Chicken Fried Beef	1 meal	540	19	28	51
Chicken Teriyaki	1 meal	430	19	4	78
Golden Battered Filet Dinner	1 meal	450	22	16	53
Herb Roasted Chicken	1 meal	460	30	25	26
Meat Loaf w/ Gravy	1 meal	480	31	22	39
Old Fashioned Beef Pot Roast	1 meal	330	27	10	32
Salisbury Steak	1 meal	400	27	16	38
Slow Roasted Beef	1 meal	370	25	13	37
Sweet & Sour Chicken	1 meal	600	22	20	88
Turkey w/ Stuffing	1 meal	400	32	9	45
Mon Cuisine					
Vegan Moroccan Couscous	1 pkg (10 oz)	280	20	4	46
Vegan Veal Schnitzel In Sauce	1 pkg (10 oz)	300	24	8	38
Vegetarian Stuffed Cabbage In Tomato Sauce	1 pkg (10 oz)	220	13	5	36
Moosewood					
Organic Vegetarian Moroccan Stew	1 pkg (10 oz)	150	5	3	29
Organic Bistro					
Chicken Citron	1 pkg (13.5 oz)	490	31	17	53
Ginger Chicken	1 pkg (13.25 oz)	490	31	17	53

FOOD	PORTION	CALS	PROT	FAT	CARB
Jamaican Shrimp Cakes	1 pkg (12 oz)	380	23	8	55
Savory Turkey	1 pkg (12 oz)	430	35	14	43
Sockeye Salmon Cakes	1 pkg (12.2 oz)	600	34	36	36
Spiced Chicken Morocco	1 pkg (12.2 oz)	390	26	11	46
Wild Salmon	1 pkg (13.1 oz)	500	35	23	41
Organic Classics					
Chicken Marsala w/ Mashed Potatoes	1 pkg (9.5 oz)	330	14	16	31
Jamaican Style Jerk Chicken w/ Wehani Rice	1 pkg (9.5 oz)	270	16	7	37
Lemon Chicken w/ Wehani Rice	1 pkg (9.5 oz)	320	14	8	49
South Beach					
Chicken Santa Fe Style Rice & Beans	1 pkg (8.9 oz)	340	22	12	35
Meatloaf w/ Gravy	1 pkg (8.9 oz)	210	16	9	17
Roasted Turkey	1 pkg (9.4 oz)	240	17	9	27
Stouffer's					
Beef Stew	1 pkg (11 oz)	280	21	9	28
Beef Stroganoff	1 pkg (9.75 oz)	380	22	17	34
Chicken A La King	1 pkg (11.5 oz)	360	18	12	44
Corner Bistro Bourbon Steak Tips	1 pkg (12 oz)	520	25	22	56
Corner Bistro Sesame Chicken	1 pkg (12.63 oz)	510	22	15	72
Country Fried Beef Steak	1 pkg (16 oz)	610	22	33	55
Creamed Chipped Beef	½ pkg (5.5 oz)	140	9	7	9
Fish Filet	1 pkg (9 oz)	400	27	16	36
Fried Chicken Breast	1 pkg (8.88 oz)	360	20	18	30
Green Pepper Steak	1 pkg (10.5 oz)	240	18	4	32
Grilled Chicken Teriyaki	1 pkg (9.38 oz)	300	21	4	45
Grilled Lemon Pepper Chicken	1 pkg (9 oz)	240	19	8	24
Meatloaf	1 pkg (6 oz)	560	34	29	40

FOOD	PORTION	CALS	PROT	FAT	CARB
Pork Cutlet	1 pkg (10 oz)	370	13	21	31
Roast Pork	1 pkg (9.5 oz)	320	17	11	39
Roast Turkey Breast	1 pkg (16 oz)	390	21	13	48
Salisbury Steak	1 pkg (16 oz)	470	29	24	34
Stuffed Pepper	1 pkg (10 oz)	220	11	10	22
Swedish Meatballs	1 pkg (11.5 oz)	560	32	27	47
Sukhis					
Tikka Masala Chicken	1 serv (5 oz)	170	25	6	46
Swanson					
Chicken & Dumplings	1 cup	230	11	10	24
Chicken A La King	1 can	270	14	18	12
Taste Above					
Meatless Zesty BBQ w/ Veggie Beef & Rice	1 pkg (10 oz)	280	16	6	48
TastyBite					
Beans Marsala & Basmati Rice	1 pkg (12 oz)	426	14	8	75
Spinach Dal & Basmati Rice	1 pkg (12 oz)	372	12	9	62
Stir Fry Vegetables & Jasmine Rice	1 pkg (12 oz)	450	7	16	67
Vegetable Supreme & Basmati Rice	1 pkg (12 oz)	317	11	6	55
Yves					
Meatless Santa Fe Beef	1 pkg (10.5 oz)	360	15	9	57

DIP

FOOD	PORTION	CALS	PROT	FAT	CARB
spinach sour cream	¼ cup	155	2	15	4
Cabot					
French Onion	2 tbsp	50	1	5	1
Ranch	2 tbsp	50	1	5	1
Cedarlane					
Organic Five Layer Mexican	2 tbsp	60	3	3	4
Emerald Valley					
Organic Black Bean	1 tbsp (1 oz)	45	2	2	6
Guiltless Gourmet					
Black Bean Mild	2 tbsp (1.1 oz)	40	2	0	7
Health Is Wealth					
Vegetarian Spinach & Artichoke	3 tbsp (1 oz)	30	1	2	3
Kraft					
Green Onion	2 tbsp	60	tr	5	3
LiteHouse					
Avocado	2 tbsp	140	1	15	2

FOOD	PORTION	CALS	PROT	FAT	CARB
Caramel Low Fat	1 tbsp	110	1	0	27
Caramel Original	2 tbsp	110	1	2	25
Dilly	2 tbsp	150	1	16	1
Fruit Dip Chocolate Yogurt	2 tbsp	110	1	6	14
Fruit Dip Vanilla Yogurt	2 tbsp	60	1	2	10
Lite Ranch Veggie	2 tbsp	70	1	7	3
Organic Ranch	2 tbsp	130	1	13	2
Marie's					
French Onion Roasted	2 tbsp	100	1	10	2
Guacamole	2 tbsp	40	1	3	3
Honey Vanilla Cream Fruit Dip	2 tbsp	60	1	5	5
Spinach Parmesan	2 tbsp	90	2	9	2
Naturally Fresh					
Caramel	2 tbsp	100	0	4	15
Chocolate	2 tbsp	70	1	0	17
Cream Cheese Strawberry	2 tbsp	90	1	4	14
Ranch Lite	2 tbsp	80	1	8	2
Ranch Vegetable	2 tbsp	120	1	12	2
Road's End Organics					
Nacho Cheese Gluten Free	2 tbsp	20	2	0	3
Robert Rothchild Farm					
Artichoke	2 tbsp	60	2	5	2
Snyder's Of Hanover					
Three Bean	2 tbsp	25	1	0	5
Utz					
Jalapeno Cheddar	2 tbsp	260	0	4	2
Sour Cream & Onion	2 tbsp	60	1	5	2
Wild Thymes Farm					
Indian Vindaloo Curry	1 tbsp	12	tr	1	1
Indonesian Peanut Sauce	1 tbsp	32	1	2	2
DOCK					
fresh cooked	3½ oz	20	2	1	3
raw chopped	½ cup	15	1	tr	2
DOUGHNUTS					
chocolate glazed	1 med (1.5 oz)	175	2	8	24
chocolate w/ chocolate icing	1 med (2 oz)	218	3	12	26
creme filled	1 (3 oz)	307	5	21	26
custard filled	1 (2.3 oz)	235	4	16	20
french cruller glazed	1 med (1.4 oz)	169	1	8	24

FOOD	PORTION	CALS	PROT	FAT	CARB
jelly filled	1 (3 oz)	289	5	16	33
old fashioned plain	1 med (2 oz)	226	3	13	25
oriental okinawan	1 (0.6 oz)	75	1	4	10
plain chocolate frosted	1 med (1.5 oz)	194	2	11	22
plain glazed	1 med (1.6 oz)	192	2	10	23
whole wheat sugared	1 med (1.6 oz)	162	3	9	19
Entenmann's					
PoP'ettes Chocolate Frosted	3 (2.2 oz)	330	2	24	28

DRINK MIXERS

FOOD	PORTION	CALS	PROT	FAT	CARB
whiskey sour mix not prep	1 pkg (0.6 oz)	64	tr	0	16
whiskey sour mix	2 oz	55	0	0	14
Angostura					
Bloody Mary	4 oz	20	0	0	4
Daiquiri	2 oz	72	0	0	18
Grenadine	1 tsp	10	0	0	3
Margarita	4 oz	80	0	0	30
Pina Colada	4 oz	60	0	0	16
Strawberry Daiquita	8 oz	120	0	0	31
Dave's Gourmet					
Bloody Mary Original	2 oz	25	1	0	5
McIlhenny					
Bloody Mary Mix as prep	1 cup	70	2	0	15

DRUM

FOOD	PORTION	CALS	PROT	FAT	CARB
freshwater fillet baked	5.4 oz	236	35	10	0
freshwater baked	3 oz	130	19	5	0

DUCK

FOOD	PORTION	CALS	PROT	FAT	CARB
boneless roasted	½ duck (7.8 oz)	444	52	25	0
boneless w/o skin roasted	3.5 oz	201	23	11	0
boneless w/o skin roasted diced	1 cup (4.9 oz)	281	33	16	0
chinese pressed	1 cup (4.9 oz)	267	10	14	26
chinese pressed	3 oz	162	6	8	16
pekin breast boneless w/ skin roasted	1 (4.2 oz)	242	29	13	0
pekin breast w/o skin broiled	3 oz	133	26	2	0
pekin leg w/ skin w/o bone roasted	1 (3.2 oz)	200	25	10	0
pekin leg w/o skin & bone roasted	1 (2.6 oz)	134	22	5	0

FOOD	PORTION	CALS	PROT	FAT	CARB
w/ skin & bone roasted	½ duck (13 oz)	1287	73	108	0
w/ skin & bone roasted	1 serv (6 oz)	583	33	49	0
wing roasted bone removed	1 (1.1 oz)	101	6	8	0
Grimaud Farms					
Muscovy Duck Confit	1 serv (3 oz)	170	20	10	tr
Muscovy Duck Whole	1 serv (3.7 oz)	200	19	14	tr
TAKE-OUT					
breast battered & fried bone removed	½ (3.2 oz)	199	20	10	6
leg battered & fried bone removed	1 (2.5 oz)	155	16	8	5

DUMPLING
Health Is Wealth

FOOD	PORTION	CALS	PROT	FAT	CARB
Potstickers Vegan	2 (1.6 oz)	90	6	3	13
Joyce Chen					
Chinese Style Potstickers Chicken & Vegetable	6	170	8	2	30
Chinese Style Potstickers Pork & Vegetable	6	170	8	3	30
Kahiki					
Potstickers Chicken	5 (3.3 oz)	230	7	11	24
Samosas Coconut Curry Chicken	4 (2.8 oz)	170	8	3	26
Pepperidge Farm					
Apple	1	250	3	11	32
Peach	1	320	3	11	50
Traveling Chef					
Potstickers Chicken + Dipping Sauce 42	5 pieces + 1 tbsp sauce	285	13	7	
TAKE-OUT					
apple	1 (6.7 oz)	661	7	34	83
cherry	1 (2.7 oz)	238	3	12	31
cornmeal	1 (2.8 oz)	134	5	4	20
fried pork	1 (3.5 oz)	338	13	21	25
fried puerto rican style	1 med (1.1 oz)	117	2	7	11
gyoza potstickers vegetable	8 (4.9 oz)	210	8	4	34
peach	1 (2.7 oz)	253	3	12	33
piroshki meat filled	1 (3.4 oz)	348	12	22	25
steamed meat	1 (1.3 oz)	41	4	1	4

FOOD	PORTION	CALS	PROT	FAT	CARB
DURIAN					
fresh	3.5 oz	141	3	2	29
EDAMAME (see SOYBEANS)					
EEL					
fresh cooked	3 oz	200	20	13	0
fresh cooked	1 fillet (5.6 oz)	375	38	24	0
raw	3 oz	156	16	10	0
smoked	3.5 oz	330	19	28	0
EGG (see also EGG DISHES, EGG SUBSTITUTES)					
CHICKEN					
hard or soft cooked	1	77	6	5	1
pickled	1	72	6	5	1
poached	1	73	6	5	tr
scrambled plain	2	199	13	15	2
sunny side up	2	155	11	12	1
white cooked	1	17	4	tr	tr
yolk cooked	1	55	3	4	1
Davidson's					
Pasteurized Shell Eggs	1 lg	75	6	5	0
Egg Innovations					
100% Organic Cage Free Large	1 (1.8 oz)	70	6	5	1
Egg-Land's Best					
Extra Large	1 (2 oz)	80	7	5	0
Large	1	70	6	4	0
Good Earth Organics					
Organic Instant Whites	1 pkg (0.5 oz)	50	12	0	1
Horizon Organic					
Jumbo	1 (2.2 oz)	90	8	5	1
Land O' Lakes					
Farm Fresh Brown Extra Large	1 (1.8 oz)	70	6	5	1
Organic Valley					
Egg Whites Pasteurized	¼ cup	25	5	0	1
Large Omega-3	1	70	7	5	tr
Pete & Gerry's					
Organic Large	1 (1.8 oz)	70	6	5	1
Tree Of Life					
White Large Natural Omega-3	1 (1.8 oz)	70	<6	5	tr
OTHER POULTRY					
duck 100 year old	1 (1 oz)	49	4	3	1

FOOD	PORTION	CALS	PROT	FAT	CARB
duck cooked	1 (2.5 oz)	129	9	10	1
duck preserved hard core	1 (1.8 oz)	80	6	6	1
duck preserved soft core	1 (1.8 oz)	80	7	6	1
duck salted	1 (1 oz)	54	4	4	2
goose cooked	1 (5 oz)	265	20	19	2
quail canned	1 (0.3 oz)	14	1	1	tr
quail cooked	1 (0.5 oz)	24	2	2	0
turkey raw	1 (2.8 oz)	135	11	9	1

EGG DISHES
Aunt Jemima
Eggs & Sausage	1 pkg (6.2 oz)	370	14	27	16
Omelet Ham & Cheese	1 pkg (5.2 oz)	250	13	15	17

Cedarlane
Zone Omelette Cheese	1 pkg (10.4 oz)	350	25	14	31

Jimmy Dean
Breakfast Bowls D-Lights Sausage	1 pkg	230	23	7	19
Breakfast Bowls Eggs Potato & Ham	1 pkg	390	24	23	23
Breakfast Bowls Eggs Potatoes Sausage & Cheddar Cheese	1 pkg	490	23	34	20
Breakfast Skillets Bacon as prep	1 serv (4.5 oz)	370	10	24	14
Breakfast Skillets Ham as prep	1 serv (4.5 oz)	270	8	15	16
Breakfast Skillets Smoked Sausage as prep	1 serv (4.5 oz)	380	8	25	20
Omelets Ham & Cheese	1 (4.2 oz)	280	16	19	4
Omelets Sausage & Cheese	1 (4.3 oz)	270	15	22	5

TAKE-OUT
deviled	1 half	62	4	5	tr
eggs benedict	2	825	35	64	26
omelet cheese	3 eggs	387	25	29	6
omelet mushroom	3 eggs	251	18	17	6
omelet mushroom & onion	3 eggs	294	20	20	7
omelet plain	3 eggs	338	24	25	4
omelet spanish	3 eggs	496	23	38	17
omelet spinach	3 eggs	279	20	19	6
omelet western	3 eggs	355	24	23	6
salad	½ cup	353	10	34	2
scotch egg	1 (4.2 oz)	301	14	21	16

FOOD	PORTION	CALS	PROT	FAT	CARB
tortilla de amarillo omelet w/ plantain	3 eggs	536	16	35	43

EGG ROLLS

FOOD	PORTION	CALS	PROT	FAT	CARB
egg roll wrapper fresh	1 (1.1 oz)	93	3	tr	19
spring roll deep fried	1 (0.8 oz)	70	1	4	7
Blue Horizon Organic					
Spring Rolls Chinese Shrimp	3 (2.1 oz)	130	3	4	16
Spring Rolls Indian	3 (2.1 oz)	110	3	4	15
Spring Rolls Thai	3 (2.1 oz)	110	3	4	16
Spring Rolls Thai Shrimp	3 (2.1 oz)	130	3	4	15
Health Is Wealth					
Spinach	1 (3 oz)	170	8	8	18
Thai Spring Roll	2 (1.6 oz)	90	3	3	13
Kahiki					
Chicken	1 (3 oz)	160	7	6	19
Chipotle Lime Chicken	1 (3 oz)	170	8	4	26
Lemongrass Chicken Stix	3 (2.6 oz)	100	7	2	13
Pork & Shrimp	1 (3 oz)	140	8	4	20
Vegetable	1 (3 oz)	90	2	4	12
TAKE-OUT					
chicken	1 (3 oz)	140	7	4	20
lobster	1 (4.8 oz)	270	8	7	43
lumpia vegetable & shrimp	2 (3 oz)	120	4	0	26
meat & shrimp	1 (4.8 oz)	320	10	12	41
pork & shrimp	1 (5 oz)	300	13	10	41
shrimp	1 (3 oz)	170	6	5	24
spicy pork	1 (3 oz)	200	6	9	23
vegetable	1 (3 oz)	170	5	4	28

EGG SUBSTITUTES

FOOD	PORTION	CALS	PROT	FAT	CARB
Bob's Red Mill					
Egg White Dried	2 tsp	15	3	0	0
Vegetarian Egg Replacer	1 tbsp	30	3	1	2
Egg Beaters					
Original	¼ cup (2.1 oz)	30	6	0	1
EggPro					
Powder	1 tbsp	15	4	0	tr
Horizon Organic					
Liquid Egg	¼ cup	35	6	0	1

FOOD	PORTION	CALS	PROT	FAT	CARB
Quick Eggs					
Fat Free Cholesterol Free	¼ cup	30	6	0	1
EGGNOG					
eggnog	1 cup	342	10	19	34
eggnog	1 qt	1368	39	76	138
eggnog flavor mix as prep w/ milk	9 oz	260	8	8	39
Farmland					
Egg Nog	½ cup	180	4	8	23
Horizon Organic					
Lowfat	½ cup	140	6	3	22
Organic Valley					
Ultra Pasteurized	½ cup	180	5	10	18
Straus					
Organic Cream Top	4 oz	160	5	10	13
TAKE-OUT					
eggnog	1 cup	306	5	22	16
EGGNOG SUBSTITUTES					
Silk					
Nog	½ cup (4 oz)	90	3	2	15
EGGPLANT					
cubed cooked w/ oil	1 cup	133	2	8	17
pickled	½ cup	33	1	tr	7
slices grilled	1 (2 oz)	36	tr	2	5
Cedarlane					
Eggplant Mediterranean	1 pkg (10 oz)	230	13	10	22
Celentano					
Eggplant Parmigiana	1 serv (7 oz)	330	9	22	26
Peloponnese					
Baba Ganoush	2 tbsp	40	1	3	2
Stonewall Kitchen					
Eggplant Spread	1 tbsp	25	0	1	4
TastyBite					
Punjab Eggplant	½ pkg (5 oz)	144	4	9	13
The Gracious Gourmet					
Tapenade Roasted Eggplant	2 tbsp (1 oz)	35	1	4	3
TAKE-OUT					
baba ghannouj	¼ cup	55	2	4	5
caponata	2 tbsp (1 oz)	30	1	2	3

FOOD	PORTION	CALS	PROT	FAT	CARB
iman bayildi eggplant w/ onion & tomato	1 serv (15.6 oz)	345	3	28	25
indian eggplant runi	1 serv	180	2	14	13
moussaka	1 serv (9 oz)	372	20	24	18
papoutsaki little shoes	1 serv (15.5 oz)	245	12	16	15
tempura	1 serv (1.5 oz)	118	1	10	5
ELDERBERRIES					
fresh	1 cup	105	1	1	27
ELDERBERRY JUICE					
elderberry	7 oz	76	4	0	16
ELK					
eye of round roasted	3.5 oz	151	31	3	1
ground cooked	3.5 oz	143	29	3	0
Natural Frontier Foods					
Filet	1 (4 oz)	140	26	3	0
ENERGY BARS (see also CEREAL BARS, NUTRITION SUPPLEMENTS)					
Activex					
Organic All Flavors	1 (1.6 oz)	200	8	12	17
Attune					
Wellness Chocolate Crisp	1 (0.7 oz)	100	2	6	11
Wellness Cool Mint Chocolate	1 (0.7 oz)	100	2	6	11
Balance					
100 Calories Peanut Butter Crisp	1 (1 oz)	100	6	5	14
100 Calories Vanilla Crisp	1 (1 oz)	100	5	4	15
Carbwell Chocolate Fudge	1 (1.8 oz)	190	14	6	23
Gold Chocolate Peanut Butter	1 (1.8 oz)	210	14	6	23
Gold S'mores Crunch	1 (1.8 oz)	210	15	6	23
Organic Apricot Mango Crisp	1 (1.6 oz)	180	10	7	23
Organic Cranberry Pomegranate Crisp	1 (1.6 oz)	180	10	7	23
Original Almond Brownie	1 (1.8 oz)	200	14	6	22
Original Mocha Crisp	1 (1.8 oz)	200	15	6	21
Pure Banana Cashew	1 (1.6 oz)	180	9	6	23
Pure Cherry Pecan	1 (1.6 oz)	190	9	7	22
Boomi Bar					
Almond Protein Plus	1	270	12	18	20

FOOD	PORTION	CALS	PROT	FAT	CARB
Cashew Almond Delicacy	1	260	8	17	23
Cranberry Apple	1	210	4	9	28
Merry Macadamia	1	220	3	14	26
Pistachio Pineapple	1	200	5	9	28
Bora Bora					
Organic Cranberry Crunch	1 (1.4 oz)	170	5	10	18
Organic Peanut Peanut	1 (1.4 oz)	230	6	17	10
Organic Sesame Raisin	1 (1.4 oz)	170	5	11	17
Clif					
Apricot	1 (2.4 oz)	230	10	3	45
Black Cherry Almond	1 (2.4 oz)	250	10	5	44
Builders Chocolate	1 (2.4 oz)	270	20	8	30
Builders Lemon	1 (2.4 oz)	270	20	8	31
Chocolate Almond Fudge	1 (2.4 oz)	250	10	5	44
Chocolate Chip Peanut Crunch	1 (2.4 oz)	260	11	6	42
Crunchy Peanut Butter	1 (2.4 oz)	250	11	6	42
Mojo Chocolate Peanut	1 (1.6 oz)	210	9	10	22
Mojo Honey Roasted Peanuts	1 (1.6 oz)	200	10	10	20
Mojo Mountain Mix	1 (1.6 oz)	180	9	8	21
Mojo Peanut Butter & Jelly	1 (1.6 oz)	220	9	11	21
Nectar Cherry Pomegranate	1 (1.6 oz)	150	3	5	29
Nectar Dark Chocolate Walnut	1 (1.6 oz)	160	3	6	27
Oatmeal Raisin Walnut	1 (2.4 oz)	240	10	5	43
Spiced Pumpkin Pie	1 (2.4 oz)	240	10	5	45
Vanilla Almond	1 (2.4 oz)	270	20	8	30
ZBar Blueberry	1 (1.3 oz)	120	3	3	23
ZBar Honey Graham	1 (1.3 oz)	130	3	3	26
ZBar Spooky S'mores	1 (1.3 oz)	130	2	4	23
Glucerna					
All Flavors	1 (0.7 oz)	80	4	3	12
Gnu					
Flavor & Fiber Banana Walnut	1 (1.4 oz)	130	3	3	30
Flavor & Fiber Chocolate Brownie Bar	1 (1.4 oz)	140	3	3	32
Green SuperFood					
Whole Food	1 (2.1 oz)	220	5	8	36
Whole Food Chocolate	1 (2.1 oz)	230	5	9	37
JojoBar					
Chocolate Cashew	1 (1.8 oz)	220	11	14	18
Peanut Butter & Jelly	1 (1.8 oz)	220	13	13	17

FOOD	PORTION	CALS	PROT	FAT	CARB
Kashi					
GoLean Chocolate Almond Toffee	1 (2.7 oz)	290	13	6	45
GoLean Cookies 'N Cream	1 (2.7 oz)	290	13	6	50
GoLean Malted Chocolate Chip	1 (2.7 oz)	290	13	6	49
GoLean Oatmeal Raisin Cookie	1 (2.7 oz)	280	13	5	49
GoLean Peanut Butter & Chocolate	1 (2.7 oz)	290	13	6	48
GoLean Crunchy Chocolate Peanut	1 (1.8 oz)	180	9	5	30
GoLean Roll Caramel Peanut	1 (1.9 oz)	200	12	5	29
GoLean Roll Fudge Sundae	1 (1.9 oz)	190	12	5	27
TLC Chewy Granola Cherry Dark Chocolate	1 (1.2 oz)	120	5	2	24
TLC Crunchy Granola Honey Toasted 7 Grain	1 (1.4 oz)	180	7	6	26
TLC Crunchy Granola Pumpkin Spice	1 (1.4 oz)	180	6	6	26
TLC Crunchy Granola Roasted Almond	1 (1.4 oz)	180	7	6	26
LaraBar					
Jocalat Chocolate	1 (1.7 oz)	190	5	10	24
Lean Body					
Gold Caramel Cookie Twist	1 (2.9 oz)	330	30	7	36
Living Harvest					
Organic Hemp Protein Forbidden Fruit	1 (1.6 oz)	170	6	6	25
Luna					
Berry Almond	1 (1.7 oz)	170	9	4	29
Chai Tea	1 (1.7 oz)	190	9	5	26
Dulce De Leche	1 (1.7 oz)	170	9	4	28
Mini Caramel Nut Brownie	1 (0.7 oz)	70	3	3	11
Mini S'mores	1 (0.7 oz)	80	4	2	11
Sunrise Apple Cinnamon	1 (1.7 oz)	180	8	5	27
Sunrise Strawberry Crunch	1 (1.7 oz)	170	8	5	26
Toasted Nuts 'N Cranberry	1 (1.7 oz)	170	9	5	26
Mrs. May's					
Trio Blueberry	1 (1.2 oz)	170	5	12	15
Trio Tropical	1 (1.2 oz)	170	5	12	14

FOOD	PORTION	CALS	PROT	FAT	CARB
Nature's Path					
Optimum Pomegran Cherry	1 (2 oz)	230	4	5	39
Nutiva					
Organic Flax & Raisin	1 (1.4 oz)	200	7	15	15
Organic Flaxseed Flax Chocolate	1 (1.4 oz)	200	6	12	19
Organic Original Hempseed	1 (1.4 oz)	210	9	14	11
Odwalla					
Berries GoMega	1	220	5	5	41
Carrot	1	220	4	4	43
Choco-walla	1	240	5	6	42
Cranberry C Monster	1	220	4	3	44
Super Protein	1	230	16	5	31
Superfood	1	230	4	4	43
Prana Bar					
Apricot Goji	1 (1.7 oz)	220	4	13	26
Coconut Acai	1 (1.7 oz)	220	4	13	26
Pear Ginseng	1 (1.7 oz)	220	5	15	21
PureFit					
Almond Crunch	1 (2 oz)	230	18	6	25
Peanut Butter Crunch	1 (2 oz)	240	18	7	26
Sencha Naturals					
Green Tea Bar Lively Lemongrass	1 (2 oz)	220	9	8	29
Green Tea Bar Original	1 (2 oz)	220	9	9	29
Simply Nutrilite					
Sweet & Salty	1 (1.6 oz)	170	4	6	27
South Beach					
Energy Mix	1 pkg (1 oz)	160	6	13	8
SoyJoy					
Fruit & Soy Bar Berry	1 (1.1 oz)	130	4	5	17
Fruit & Soy Bar Mango Coconut	1 (1.1 oz)	140	4	6	16
Fruit & Soy Bar Raisin Almond	1 (1.1 oz)	130	4	6	16
Think5					
Red Berry	1 (2.5 oz)	240	4	4	48
Red Berry Chocolate Covered	1 (2.8 oz)	290	4	8	52
ThinkPink					
Blueberry Dark Chocolate	1 (2.1 oz)	240	20	8	26
Lemon Burst	1 (2.1 oz)	230	20	7	27
Peanut Butter Caramel	1 (2.1 oz)	230	20	8	26
White Chocolate Raspberry	1 (2.1 oz)	240	20	8	28

FOOD	PORTION	CALS	PROT	FAT	CARB
ENERGY DRINKS					
180					
Blue w/ Acai	1 can (8.2 oz)	120	0	0	31
Blue w/ Acai Low Calorie	1 can (8.2 oz)	15	0	0	4
Orange Citrus Blast	1 can (8.2 oz)	120	0	0	33
Orange Citrus Blast Sugar Free	1 can (8.2 oz)	5	0	0	1
Red w/ Gogi	1 can (8.2 oz)	130	0	0	31
1In3Trinity					
Energy Drink	1 can (8.4 oz)	10	0	0	3
B52					
Zero Sugar Citrus Berry	8 oz	10	0	0	1
Bai					
Antioxidant Infusion Jamaica Blueberry	8 oz	70	0	0	18
Antioxidant Infusion Kenya Peach	8 oz	70	0	0	17
Antioxidant Infusion Mango Kauai	8 oz	70	0	0	18
Bawls					
Guarana	8 oz	90	0	0	25
Guaranexx Sugar Free	1 bottle (10 oz)	0	0	0	0
Bloom					
All Flavors	1 can (10.5 oz)	100	tr	0	24
Boost					
Beauty	1 bottle (12 oz)	220	2	0	52
Youth	1 bottle (12 oz)	200	2	0	48
Boozer					
Hangover Remedy	1 can (8.4 oz)	110	0	0	28
Brain Toniq					
Functional Drink	1 can (8.4 oz)	80	0	0	20
C1.5					
Extreme	1 can (8.4 oz)	120	0	0	30
Cintron					
Citrus Mango	8 oz	110	tr	0	27
Citrus Mango Sugar Free	8 oz	0	tr	0	0
Clif					
Quench Fruit Punch	8 oz	45	0	0	11
Quench Orange	8 oz	45	0	0	11

FOOD	PORTION	CALS	PROT	FAT	CARB
Coca-Cola					
Zero	8 oz	1	0	0	tr
Coolah					
Original	8 oz	120	0	0	31
DNA Energy					
Low Carb Citrus	8 oz	0	0	0	0
Dr. Tim's					
ISO-5	1 bottle (11.2 oz)	60	0	0	15
Jungle Juice	1 bottle (4 oz)	20	2	0	8
Emu					
Energy Drink	1 bottle (8.4 oz)	170	tr	0	41
EQ Thirst Equalizer					
All Flavors	8 oz	60	0	0	15
Function					
Alternative Energy	8 oz	60	0	0	15
Brainiac Carambola Punch	8 oz	60	0	0	15
Urban Detox Citrus Prickly Pear	8 oz	60	0	0	17
Youth Trip Acai Grape	8 oz	60	0	0	15
Fuze					
Refresh Banana Coconut	8 oz	90	0	0	25
Refresh Peach Mango	8 oz	90	0	0	23
Refresh Strawberry Banana	8 oz	100	0	0	25
Slenderize Cranberry Raspberry	8 oz	5	0	0	2
Slenderize Low Carb Tropical Punch	8 oz	5	0	0	tr
Slenderize Tangerine Grapefruit	8 oz	10	0	0	2
Vitalize Blackberry Grape	8 oz	100	0	0	26
Vitalize Orange Mango	8 oz	100	0	0	25
Gatorade					
All Flavors	8 oz	50	0	0	14
Ginger Boost					
Ginger Orange	8 oz	110	1	0	24
Gleukos					
Performance All Flavors	8 oz	70	0	0	17
Go Girl					
Bliss	1 can (11.5 oz)	35	0	0	8

FOOD	PORTION	CALS	PROT	FAT	CARB
Glo	1 can (12 oz)	35	0	0	9
Sugar Free	1 can (12 oz)	<5	0	0	tr
Guayaki					
Organic Empower Mint	8 oz	38	0	0	9
Organic Raspberry Revolution	8 oz	50	0	0	12
Organic Unsweetened	8 oz	15	0	0	3
Hiro					
Thermo	1 can (8.33 oz)	10	0	0	2
Vitality	1 can (8.33 oz)	10	0	0	2
IChill					
Relaxation Shot Blissful Berry	1 bottle (2 oz)	0	0	0	0
Kidstrong					
All Flavors	8 oz	30	0	0	7
King 888					
Original	8 oz	110	0	0	28
Sugar Free	8 oz	0	0	0	0
Liv Naturals					
All Flavors	8 oz	70	0	0	16
Marquis Platinum					
Vitality Drink	1 can	30	0	0	16
Me					
Curious Blueberry Lime	1 can	70	0	0	17
Vivacious Tangerine Pineapple	1 can	70	0	0	17
Mix1					
All Flavors	1 bottle (11 oz)	200	15	3	29
Mr. Re					
Restorative	1 can (11 oz)	80	0	0	22
Neuro					
Bliss	1 bottle (14.5 oz)	35	0	0	9
Gasm	1 bottle (14.5 oz)	35	0	0	9
Sleep	1 bottle (14.5 oz)	35	0	0	9
Sonic	1 bottle (14.5 oz)	35	0	0	9
Sport	1 bottle (14.5 oz)	35	0	0	9

FOOD	PORTION	CALS	PROT	FAT	CARB
Trim	1 bottle (14.5 oz)	35	0	0	9
NOS					
High Performance	1 bottle (11 oz)	150	2	0	38
Ocean Spray					
Cranergy Cranberry Life	1 bottle (12 oz)	50	0	0	12
Cranergy Raspberry Cranberry Lift	1 bottle (12 oz)	50	0	0	13
Odwalla					
Berries GoMega	8 oz	160	3	2	34
Mo' Beta	8 oz	150	1	0	37
Super Protein Original	8 oz	190	10	1	35
Superfood	8 oz	130	1	1	30
Wellness	8 oz	150	2	1	33
OOBA					
All Flavors	8 oz	90	0	0	22
Pimpjuice					
Energy Drink	1 can (8 oz)	140	0	0	35
PJ Tight	1 can (8 oz)	20	0	0	3
Purity Organic					
Acerola Cherry	1 bottle	60	0	0	15
Pomegranate Blueberry	1 bottle	60	0	0	15
Pomegranate Raspberry	1 bottle	60	0	0	15
Quench Aid					
Berry	1 pkg	10	0	0	2
Dragonfruit	1 pkg	10	0	0	2
Rehab					
Recovery Supplement	1 can (12 oz)	150	0	0	38
Rockstar					
Energy Drink	8 oz	140	0	0	31
Simply Nutrilite					
Berry Antioxidant	1 can (8.4 oz)	120	1	0	29
Source Burn					
2	8 oz	130	1	0	31
Energy Drink	8 oz	140	0	0	36
Sugar Free	8 oz	10	1	0	0
Steaz					
Organic Fuel	8 oz	90	0	0	23
T-Fusion					
Energy Tea	8 oz	0	0	0	1

FOOD	PORTION	CALS	PROT	FAT	CARB
Therafizz					
Vitamin C	1 pkg	5	0	0	tr
UnderWay					
Appetite Suppressing All Flavors	8 oz	10	0	0	2
Venga					
Brainstorm	8 oz	130	0	0	31
Calorie Burn	8 oz	10	0	0	2
Energize	8 oz	100	0	0	24
Health&Zen	8 oz	80	0	0	20
VIB					
Chill-N	1 can (8 oz)	40	0	0	10
XOOD					
Endurance Drink All Flavors as prep	1 serv	135	3	0	30
Youth Juice					
Drink	2 oz	10	tr	0	3
Zenergize					
Chill	1 tablet	2	0	0	1
Energy+	1 tablet	2	0	0	1
Hydrate	1 tablet	2	0	0	1
ENGLISH MUFFIN					
READY-TO-EAT					
apple cinnamon	1	138	4	2	28
crumpets	1 (1.5 oz)	80	3	0	16
granola	1	155	6	1	31
mixed grain	1	155	6	1	31
plain	1	134	4	1	26
plain toasted	1	133	4	1	26
raisin cinnamon	1	138	4	2	28
sourdough	1	134	4	1	26
wheat	1	127	5	1	26
whole wheat	1	134	6	1	27
Aunt Gussie's					
Gluten Free Cinnamon Raisin	1 (3 oz)	200	3	3	41
Gluten Free Original	1 (3 oz)	200	3	3	41
Fiber One					
100% Whole Wheat	1 (2 oz)	100	5	0	22

FOOD	PORTION	CALS	PROT	FAT	CARB
Milton's					
Healthy Multi-Grain	1 (2 oz)	150	4	1	33
Pepperidge Farm					
100% Whole Wheat	1	140	6	2	26
Original	1	130	5	2	25
Roman Meal					
English Muffin	1 (2.3 oz)	140	6	1	29
Rudi's Organic Bakery					
MultiGrain w/ Flax	1 (2 oz)	130	5	1	25
Whole Grain Wheat	1 (2 oz)	120	5	1	23
Sun-Maid					
Raisin	1 (2.5 oz)	170	5	1	36
Thomas'					
100 Calories	1	100	4	1	24
Griller Multi Grain	1 (3.2 oz)	210	7	2	41
Griller Onion	1 (3.2 oz)	200	7	1	40
Light Multi-Grain	1	100	6	2	24
Oatmeal & Honey	1	130	5	1	25
Original Whole Grain	1	130	5	1	26
Sandwich Size Original	1	190	7	2	38
TAKE-OUT					
w/ butter	1 (2.2 oz)	189	5	6	30
w/ cheese & sausage	1 (4 oz)	393	15	24	29
w/ egg cheese & canadian bacon	1 (4.8 oz)	289	17	13	28
w/ egg cheese & sausage	1 (5.8 oz)	487	22	31	31
EPAZOTE					
fresh	1 tbsp (1 g)	tr	0	0	tr
fresh sprig	1 (2 g)	1	tr	tr	tr
EPPAW					
raw	½ cup	75	2	1	16
FALAFEL					
Near East					
Falafel Patties Vegetarian as prep	2.5	220	10	13	18
TAKE-OUT					
falafel	1 (1.2 oz)	57	2	3	5

FOOD	PORTION	CALS	PROT	FAT	CARB
FAT (*see also* BUTTER, BUTTER SUBSTITUTES, MARGARINE, OIL)					
bacon grease	1 tbsp	116	0	13	0
beef shortening	1 tbsp	115	0	13	0
beef suet	1 oz	242	tr	27	0
chicken	1 tbsp (0.4 oz)	115	0	13	0
duck	1 tbsp (0.4 oz)	113	0	13	0
goose	1 oz	257	0	29	0
goose	1 tbsp	115	0	13	0
lamb new zealand	1 oz	182	2	19	0
lard	1 tbsp (0.5 oz)	115	0	13	0
lard	1 cup (7.2 oz)	1849	0	205	0
meat pan drippings	½ tbsp	124	0	14	0
pork raw	1 oz	230	1	25	0
salt pork	1 cube (1 oz)	215	2	23	0
shortening	1 cup	1812	0	205	0
shortening	1 tbsp	113	0	13	0
turkey	1 tbsp	116	0	13	0
ucuhuba butter	1 tbsp	120	0	14	0
whale blubber	1 oz	248	tr	28	0
Crisco					
Butter Flavor	1 tbsp	110	0	12	0
Shortening	1 tbsp	110	0	12	0
Earth Balance					
Natural Shortening	1 tbsp	130	0	14	0
Nebraska Land					
Pork Fatback	½ oz	110	1	11	0
FAVA BEANS					
canned	½ cup	91	7	tr	16
fava fresh cooked	½ cup	94	6	tr	17
Progresso					
Fava Beans	½ cup (4.6 oz)	100	6	1	17
FEIJOA					
fresh	1 (1.75 oz)	25	1	tr	5
puree	1 cup	119	3	2	26
FENNEL					
fresh bulb	1 (8.2 oz)	73	3	tr	17
fresh sliced	1 cup	27	1	tr	6
leaves	1 oz	7	tr	tr	1
seed	1 tsp	7	tr	tr	1
stir fried	1 cup	85	2	6	9

FOOD	PORTION	CALS	PROT	FAT	CARB
Ocean Mist					
Fennel Sweet Anise Sliced Fresh	1 cup	27	1	1	6
FENUGREEK					
seed	1 tsp	12	1	tr	2
FIBER					
Benefiber					
Supplement	1 pkg (4 g)	20	0	0	4
Fiber Supreme					
Fiber	1 round tbsp (0.5 oz)	36	1	tr	12
ND Labs					
Apple Fiber	1 round tbsp (7 g)	15	0	tr	7
Liquid Fiber Flow	1 tbsp (0.5 oz)	42	0	0	11
UniFiber					
Natural Fiber	1 pkg (4 g)	4	0	0	tr
Wellements					
Fiber-Psyll	1 scoop (0.5 oz)	55	0	0	14
FIDDLEHEAD FERNS					
fresh	3.5 oz	34	5	tr	6
FIG JUICE					
Smart Juice					
Organic 100% Juice	8 oz	131	1	0	35
FIGS					
calimyrna	3 (5.4 oz)	120	1	0	28
canned in heavy syrup	½ cup	114	tr	tr	30
canned in light syrup	½ cup	87	tr	tr	23
canned water pack	½ cup	66	1	tr	17
dried california	½ cup (3.5 oz)	200	4	1	58
dried cooked	½ cup	139	2	1	36
dried small	1 (1.4 oz)	30	tr	tr	8
dried whole	1 (8 g)	21	tr	tr	5
fresh large	1 (2.2 oz)	47	tr	tr	12
California Fresh					
Fresh	3 (5.4 oz)	120	1	0	31
Hermes					
Organic Adriatic Fig Spread	1 tbsp	60	0	0	15

FOOD	PORTION	CALS	PROT	FAT	CARB
Nuta Figs					
Mission	¼ cup (1.4 oz)	110	1	0	26
Orchard Choice					
Mission	4-5 (1.4 oz)	110	1	0	26
Sun-Maid					
California Mission	4 (1.5 oz)	120	1	0	28
Calimyrna	3 (1.5 oz)	120	1	0	28
FIREWEED					
leaves chopped	1 cup (0.8 oz)	24	1	1	4
FISH (see also individual names, SUSHI)					
FROZEN					
breaded fillet	1 (2 oz)	155	9	7	14
sticks	1 stick (1 oz)	76	4	3	7
Dr. Praeger's					
Breaded Fillets	1 (2.1 oz)	100	5	4	12
Fishies	3 (1.5 oz)	90	4	4	9
Gorton's					
Classic Crispy Battered Fillets	2	230	6	10	22
Classic Crunchy Golden Fillets	2	140	9	12	23
Fillets Beer Battered	2 (3.6 oz)	250	8	17	17
Fillets Breaded Lemon Herb	2 (3.6 oz)	240	9	13	21
Fillets Potato Crunch	2 (3.6 oz)	240	9	14	20
Fish Sticks Classic Breaded	6	290	10	18	19
Grilled Fillets Cajun Blackened	1 (3.8 oz)	100	17	3	1
Grilled Fillets Lemon Pepper	1 (3.7 oz)	100	17	3	1
Tenders Original Batter	3 pieces (3.6 oz)	230	8	12	23
Van de Kamp's					
Battered Tenders	4 (4 oz)	210	9	10	22
Crisp & Healthy Breaded Fish Sticks	6 (3.6 oz)	140	9	1	24
Crunchy Fillets	2 (3.5 oz)	230	8	13	21
Sticks	6 (4 oz)	260	11	13	26
TAKE-OUT					
fish cake	1 (4.7 oz)	166	18	7	6
jamaican brown fish stew	1 serv	426	48	22	9
kedgeree	5.6 oz	242	21	11	15
mousse	1 serv (3.5 oz)	185	13	14	3
stew	1 cup (7.9 oz)	157	19	4	10
taramasalata	2 tbsp	124	1	14	1

FOOD	PORTION	CALS	PROT	FAT	CARB
FISH OIL					
cod liver	1 tbsp	123	0	14	0
herring	1 tbsp	123	0	14	0
menhaden	1 tbsp	123	0	14	0
salmon	1 tbsp	123	0	14	0
sardine	1 tbsp	123	0	14	0
shark	1 oz	270	0	29	0
whale beluga	1 oz	256	0	29	0
whale bowhead	1 oz	252	0	28	0
Nordic Naturals					
Omega-3 Effervescent as prep	1 pkg (9.7 g)	39	0	2	3
FISH PASTE					
fish paste	2 tsp	15	1	1	tr
FLAXSEED					
Arrowhead Mills					
Organic	3 tbsp (1 oz)	140	6	9	9
Bob's Red Mill					
Flaxseed Meal	2 tbsp	60	3	5	4
Carrington Farms					
Organic Flax Paks	1 pkg (0.4 oz)	50	2	5	3
Flax USA					
Flax Sprinkles	2 tbsp (0.5 oz)	70	2	5	4
Natural Ovens					
Flax Complete Supplement	1 tbsp (0.4 oz)	60	2	4	4
Tree Of Life					
Flax Seed	3 tbsp (1 oz)	140	5	10	11
FLOUNDER					
FRESH					
cooked	3 oz	99	21	1	0
cooked	1 fillet (4.5 oz)	148	31	2	0
FROZEN					
Mrs. Paul's					
Filets Lightly Breaded	1 (2.7 oz)	150	8	7	12
TAKE-OUT					
breaded & fried	3.2 oz	211	13	11	15
stuffed w/ crab	1 piece (7.6 oz)	332	43	11	14

FOOD	PORTION	CALS	PROT	FAT	CARB
FLOUR					
all-purpose self-rising	½ cup (2.2 oz)	221	6	1	46
all-purpose unbleached	½ cup (2.2 oz)	228	6	1	48
arrowroot	½ cup (2.2 oz)	228	tr	tr	56
bread flour	½ cup (2.4 oz)	247	8	1	50
buckwheat whole groat	½ cup (2.1 oz)	201	8	2	42
cake	½ cup (2.4 oz)	248	6	1	53
carob	½ cup (1.8 oz)	114	2	tr	46
carob	1 tbsp (0.2 oz)	13	tr	tr	5
chickpea besan	½ cup (1.6 oz)	178	10	3	27
peanut low fat	½ cup (1.1 oz)	128	10	7	9
potato	½ cup (2.8 oz)	286	6	tr	66
rice brown	½ cup (2.8 oz)	287	6	2	60
rice white	½ cup (2.8 oz)	289	5	1	63
rye dark	½ cup (2.2 oz)	207	9	2	44
rye light	½ cup (1.8 oz)	187	4	1	41
soy lowfat	½ cup (1.5 oz)	165	20	4	15
triticale whole grain	½ cup (2.3 oz)	220	9	1	48
white all-purpose enriched bleached	½ cup (2.2 oz)	228	6	1	48
whole wheat	½ cup (2.1 oz)	203	8	1	44
Arrowhead Mills					
Organic Barley	⅓ cup	95	3	1	19
Organic Brown Rice	⅓ cup	130	3	1	27
Organic Kamut	⅓ cup	130	5	1	25
Organic Oat	⅓ cup	120	4	3	21
Organic Rye	¼ cup	110	3	1	24
Organic Spelt	⅓ cup	130	4	1	25
Organic Unbleached White	¼ cup	120	3	1	26
Organic White Rice	⅓ cup	120	2	0	28
Bob's Red Mill					
Brown Rice	¼ cup	140	3	1	31
Corn	¼ cup	160	2	1	22
Graham	¼ cup	120	5	1	21
Kamut Organic	¼ cup	94	3	1	21
Sorghum Sweet White Gluten Free	¼ cup	120	4	1	25
Spelt	¼ cup	120	4	1	22
Whole Wheat	¼ cup	110	4	1	23

FOOD	PORTION	CALS	PROT	FAT	CARB
Whole Wheat Hard White Organic	¼ cup	120	4	1	24
Domata Living Flour					
Gluten Free Casein Free	¼ cup	110	tr	0	26
Gold Medal					
All Purpose	¼ cup (1 oz)	100	3	0	22
Self Rising	¼ cup (1 oz)	100	3	0	23
Whole Wheat	¼ cup (1 oz)	100	4	1	21
Wondra	¼ cup (1 oz)	100	3	0	23
Lundberg					
Brown Rice	¼ cup	110	2	2	26
Manitoba Harvest					
Hemp Seed Flour	¼ cup	120	10	4	14

FOOD COLORS

blue	1 tsp	0	0	0	0
orange	1 tsp	0	0	0	0
yellow	1 tsp	tr	tr	0	0

FRENCH BEANS

dried cooked	1 cup	228	12	1	43

FRENCH FRIES (see POTATO)

FRENCH TOAST

french toast frzn	1 slice (2 oz)	126	4	4	19
Aunt Jemima					
Cinnamon	2 slices (4 oz)	240	8	6	39
Whole Grain	2 slices (4 oz)	240	8	6	39
Farm Rich					
Original Sticks	5 (4.2 oz)	330	6	15	42
TAKE-OUT					
plain	1 slice	151	7	7	16
sticks	5 (4.9 oz)	513	8	29	58
w/ butter	2 slices	356	10	19	36

FROG LEGS

frog legs	3 oz	175	15	–	–
TAKE-OUT					
as prep w/ seasoned flour & fried	1 (0.8)	70	4	5	15

FOOD	PORTION	CALS	PROT	FAT	CARB
FRUCTOSE					
liquid	1 oz	84	0	0	23
powder	¼ cup (1.7 oz)	180	0	0	49
powder	1 tsp (4.2 g)	15	0	0	4
Bob's Red Mill					
Fructose	1 tsp	15	0	0	4
Tree Of Life					
Fructose	1 tsp (4 g)	15	0	0	4
FRUIT DRINKS (see also individual names, SMOOTHIES, YOGURT DRINKS)					
FROZEN					
Chiquita					
Banana Colada as prep	8 oz	125	0	2	25
Mixed Berry as prep	8 oz	120	0	0	28
Peach Mango as prep	8 oz	120	1	0	28
MIX					
Crystal Light					
LiveActive On The Go	1 pkg	10	0	0	3
South Beach					
Tide Me Over Strawberry Banana	1 pkg	30	3	0	6
Tide Me Over Tropical Breeze	1 pkg	30	3	0	6
READY-TO-DRINK					
fruit punch	6 oz	87	tr	tr	22
Apple & Eve					
100% Cranberry Apple Juice	8 oz	100	1	0	24
Mango Mangosteen	8 oz	120	0	0	30
Back To Nature					
100% Juice Berry	1 pkg (6 oz)	90	0	0	21
Brazsoy					
Fruit Juice w/ Soy	8 oz	94	1	1	21
Crayons					
Kiwi Strawberry	1 bottle (12 oz)	130	0	0	45
Outrageous Orange Mango	1 bottle (12 oz)	140	0	0	45
Redder Than Ever Fruitpunch	1 bottle (12 oz)	130	0	0	45
Drenchers					
Super Fruit Endurance Grape Apple	8 oz	120	1	0	29
Super Juice Fit N' Lean Heart Healthy Tropical Passion	8 oz	10	0	0	2

FOOD	PORTION	CALS	PROT	FAT	CARB
Super Juice Fit N' Lean Power Protein Orange Cream	8 oz	20	2	0	2
Super Juice Immunity Fruit & Veggie Berry	8 oz	110	1	0	26
Essn					
Sparkling Blood Orange & Cranberry	1 can (8.4 oz)	160	1	0	38
Fizz Ed.					
Pomegranate Cherry	1 can (8.4 oz)	90	0	0	22
Frutzzo					
Organic 100% Juice Pomegranate Passionfruit	1 bottle (12 oz)	140	0	0	34
Organic 100% Juice Pomegranate Acai	1 bottle (12 oz)	140	0	0	35
GoodBelly					
Black Currant Probiotic Drink	8 oz	120	tr	0	31
Blueberry Acai Probiotic Drink	1 bottle (2.7 oz)	50	tr	0	12
Cranberry Watermelon Probiotic Drink	8 oz	100	tr	0	24
Peach Mango Probiotic Drink	1 bottle (2.7 oz)	50	tr	0	13
Strawberry Rosehips Probiotic Drink	1 bottle (2.7 oz)	50	tr	0	12
Juicy Juice					
Harvest Surprise Orange Mango	8 oz	130	1	0	31
Lakewood					
Lean Green	6 oz	90	1	0	26
Organic Acai Amazon Berry	6 oz	95	2	3	21
Land O' Lakes					
Juice Cranberry Apple	1 cup (8 oz)	120	0	0	30
Minute Maid					
Pomegranate Blueberry 100% Juice	8 oz	120	0	1	31
Mott's					
Apple Blueberry	8 oz	130	0	0	15
Fruit Medley	1 bottle (14 oz)	230	1	0	54
Nantucket Nectars					
100% Juice Peach Orange	8 oz	130	0	0	32

FOOD	PORTION	CALS	PROT	FAT	CARB
100% Juice Pomegranate Cherry	8 oz	120	0	0	29
Kiwi Berry	8 oz	120	0	0	29
Organic Banana Mango Carrot	8 oz	140	0	0	32
Pineapple Orange Guava	8 oz	120	0	0	29
Noble					
Organic 100% Juice Orange Tangerine	8 oz	120	1	0	29
Northland					
100% Juice Cranberry Pomegranate	8 oz	140	0	0	34
NutraShake					
Fruit Punch Plus Fiber	1 pkg (8 oz)	120	0	0	29
Ocean Spray					
100% Juice Cranberry & Concord Grape	8 oz	150	0	0	37
Cran.Apple	8 oz	130	0	0	32
Cran.Raspberry	8 oz	110	0	0	28
Ruby Tangerine	8 oz	120	0	0	31
Odwalla					
Quenchers AntioxiDance	8 oz	90	0	0	23
Quenchers B Berrier	8 oz	120	0	0	30
Old Orchard					
100% Juice Pomegranate Black Currant	8 oz	130	0	0	30
100% Juice Pomegranate Cherry	8 oz	140	0	0	34
Cocktail Apple Passion Mango	8 oz	120	0	0	29
Healthy Balance Apple Kiwi Strawberry	8 oz	31	0	0	6
Sabor Latino					
Guava Mango Drink	1 box (7 oz)	110	0	0	29
Nectar Strawberry Banana + Calcium	8 oz	150	0	0	37
Pina Colada	8 oz	130	0	0	32
Santa Cruz					
Organic Cranberry Goji	8 oz	120	0	0	30
Snapple					
100% Juiced Fruit Punch	8 oz	170	0	0	42
Juice Drink Acai Blackberry	8 oz	110	0	0	27

FOOD	PORTION	CALS	PROT	FAT	CARB
Juice Drink Cranberry Raspberry	8 oz	100	0	0	26
SSips					
Cherry Berry	1 box (7 oz)	110	0	0	26
Sun Shower					
100% Juice Nectarine Mango	8 oz	93	1	0	21
Sundia					
Tropical Medley	½ cup	70	1	0	18
Tree Ripe					
Organic Fruit Punch	8 oz	150	1	0	36
Tropical Grove					
Fruit Punch	8 oz	110	0	0	26
Tropicana					
Fruit Punch	1 cup	130	0	0	32
Light Fruit Punch	8 oz	10	0	0	3
Orange Tangerine Juice	8 oz	110	2	0	25
Orchard Berry	8 oz	110	1	0	27
Organic Orchard Medley	8 oz	120	0	0	29
Twister Berry Blast	8 oz	120	tr	0	29
Twister Citrus Spark	8 oz	120	0	0	30
Twister Fruit Fury	8 oz	120	tr	0	30
Twister Light Strawberry Spiral	8 oz	40	0	0	10
V8					
Light Peach Mango	8 oz	50	0	0	13
Splash Diet Berry Blend	8 oz	10	0	0	3
Splash Mango Peach	8 oz	80	0	0	20
V-Fusion Acai Mixed Berry	8 oz	110	0	0	27
V-Fusion Pomegranate Blueberry	8 oz	100	0	0	25
V-Fusion Light Peach Mango	8 oz	50	0	0	13
Vruit					
Apple Carrot	1 box (8.45 oz)	120	1	0	29
Berry Veggie	1 box (8.45 oz)	110	1	0	27
Orange Veggie	1 box (8.45 oz)	110	1	1	26
Tropical Blend	1 box (8.45 oz)	110	1	0	27
Wadda Juice					
All Flavors	1 bottle (4 oz)	25	0	0	7
Walnut Acres					
Organic Orange Carrot	8 oz	110	0	0	27

FOOD	PORTION	CALS	PROT	FAT	CARB
Welch's					
Light Strawberry Mango	8 oz	50	0	0	13
FRUIT MIXED (see also individual names)					
CANNED					
fruit cocktail in heavy syrup	½ cup	93	1	tr	24
fruit cocktail juice pack	½ cup	56	1	tr	15
fruit cocktail water pack	½ cup	40	1	tr	10
fruit salad in heavy syrup	½ cup	94	tr	tr	24
fruit salad in light syrup	½ cup	73	tr	tr	19
fruit salad juice pack	½ cup	62	1	tr	16
fruit salad water pack	½ cup	37	tr	tr	10
mixed fruit in heavy syrup	½ cup	92	tr	tr	24
tropical fruit salad in heavy syrup	½ cup	110	1	tr	29
Del Monte					
Carb Clever Fruit Cocktail	½ cup	40	0	0	11
Dole					
Mixed Fruit Light Syrup	½ cup (4.3 oz)	80	0	0	21
Homemade Harvey's					
Crushed Fruit Apple Pear & Spices	1 pkg (4.5 oz)	60	0	0	17
Crushed Fruit Mango Pineapple Banana & Passion Fruit	1 pkg (4.5 oz)	90	1	0	22
Crushed Fruit Strawberries Bananas & Kiwis	1 pkg (4.5 oz)	100	1	1	23
Mott's					
Healthy Harvest Pomegranate	1 pkg (3.9 oz)	50	0	0	13
Polar					
Mixed Fruit Light Syrup	½ cup (4.9 oz)	50	0	0	12
S&W					
Chunky Mixed In Sweetened Juice	½ cup (4.3 oz)	80	tr	0	19
Fruit Cocktail	½ cup (4.4 oz)	80	0	0	20
DRIED					
mixed	11 oz pkg	712	7	1	188
Brothers-All-Natural					
Crisps Strawberry Banana	1 pkg (0.42 oz)	45	1	0	10
Elizabeth's Natural					
Fancy Mixed	5 pieces	80	1	0	20

FOOD	PORTION	CALS	PROT	FAT	CARB
Fruitaceuticals					
PomaCrans	¼ cup	100	0	0	24
Mariani					
Berries 'N Cherries	¼ cup	140	tr	0	38
Sun-Maid					
Fruit Bits	¼ cup (1.4 oz)	120	1	0	29
Mixed	¼ cup (1.4 oz)	100	1	0	26
Sunsweet					
Berry Blend	¼ cup (1.4 oz)	120	1	0	32
Orchard Mix	¼ cup (1.4 oz)	100	1	0	25
Tropical Mix	⅓ cup	150	0	0	33
FRESH					
Chiquita					
Apple & Grape Bites	1 pkg (2.5 oz)	40	0	0	10
FROZEN					
mixed fruit sweetened	1 cup	245	4	tr	61
FRUIT SNACKS					
fruit leather	1 bar (0.8 oz)	81	tr	1	18
fruit leather pieces	1 pkg (0.9 oz)	92	tr	2	21
fruit leather pieces	1 oz	97	tr	2	22
fruit leather rolls	1 sm (0.5 oz)	49	tr	tr	12
fruit leather rolls	1 lg (0.7 oz)	73	tr	1	18
Bare Fruit					
Bananas & Cherries	1 pkg (0.6 oz)	55	2	1	12
Clif					
Twisted Fruit Grape	1 piece (0.7 oz)	70	0	0	16
Twisted Fruit Pineapple	1 piece (0.7 oz)	70	0	0	16
Twisted Fruit Tropical Twist	1 piece (0.7 oz)	70	0	0	16
Funky Monkey					
Bananamon	1 pkg (1 oz)	110	1	0	27
Carnaval Mix	1 pkg (1 oz)	110	1	0	26
Jivealime	1 pkg (1 oz)	110	1	0	27
Purple Funk	1 pkg (1 oz)	120	1	1	26
Jelly Belly					
Fruit Snacks	1 pkg (2.5 oz)	220	0	0	58
Peeled Snacks					
Fruit & Nuts FigSated	⅓ cup	150	3	6	20
Fruit & Nuts Plu-what?	⅓ cup	150	3	6	22
Revolution Foods					
Organic Mashups Berry	1 pkg (3.2 oz)	40	0	0	10
Organic Mashups Tropical	1 pkg (3.2 oz)	60	1	0	13

FOOD	PORTION	CALS	PROT	FAT	CARB
Stretch Island					
Fruit Leather Bountiful Blueberry	1 pkg (0.5 oz)	45	0	0	12
Fruit Leather Harvest Grape	1 pkg (0.5 oz)	45	0	0	12
Fruit Leather Mango Sunrise	1 pkg (0.5 oz)	45	0	0	11
Fruit Leather Truly Tropical	1 pkg (0.5 oz)	45	0	0	11
Organic Smooshed Fruit Apple	1 piece (0.4 oz)	40	0	0	10
Organic Smooshed Fruit Strawberry	1 piece (0.4 oz)	40	0	0	10
Tahitian Noni					
Soft Chews Raspberry	1 pkg (2 oz)	240	2	3	50
Tropicana					
Fruit Wise Bars All Flavors	1 bar (1.4 oz)	140	0	0	36
Fruit Wise Strips All Flavors	1 strip (0.7 oz)	70	0	0	17
Welch's					
Fruit'N Yogurt Strawberry	1 pkg (0.9 oz)	90	1	2	17
Mixed Fruit	1 pkg (0.9 oz)	80	1	0	19
GARLIC					
clove	1	4	tr	tr	1
fresh chopped	1 tbsp	18	1	tr	4
powder	1 tsp	9	tr	tr	2
McSweet					
Pickled	8 pieces (1 oz)	40	0	0	5
Spice World					
Ajo Garlic Clove	1 (3 g)	5	0	0	1
GEFILTE FISH					
sweet	1 piece (1.5 oz)	35	4	1	3
Mrs. Adler's					
Gefilte Fish	1 piece (1.8 oz)	50	5	2	3
Ungar's					
Gefilte Fish	2 slices (1.8 oz)	83	6	5	5
Lite	2 slices (2.4 oz)	80	7	3	5
No Sugar	2 slices (1.8 oz)	70	6	4	3
GELATIN					
READY-TO-EAT					
Jell-O					
Sugar Free Lemon Lime	1 serv (3.2 oz)	10	1	0	0

FOOD	PORTION	CALS	PROT	FAT	CARB
GIBLETS					
capon simmered	1 cup (5 oz)	238	38	8	0
chicken fried	1 cup (5 oz)	402	47	20	6
chicken simmered	1 cup (5 oz)	289	30	17	1
turkey simmered	1 cup (5 oz)	243	39	7	3
GINGER					
ground	1 tsp	6	tr	tr	1
pickled	0.5 oz	5	tr	0	1
preserved	1.5 oz	34	0	0	8
root fresh	5 slices	9	tr	tr	2
root fresh sliced	¼ cup	19	tr	tr	4
Tree Of Life					
Crystallized Pieces	7 (1.4 oz)	150	0	0	37
GINKGO NUTS					
canned	1 oz	32	1	tr	6
dried	1 oz	99	3	tr	21
raw	1 oz	52	1	tr	11
GINSENG					
dried	1 oz	90	5	tr	20
fresh	1 oz	28	1	tr	6
GIZZARDS					
chicken simmered	1 cup (5 oz)	212	44	4	0
turkey simmered	1 (3 oz)	103	18	3	tr
Perdue					
Fresh Chicken	3 oz	130	23	3	1
GNOCCHI					
Racconto					
Potato Whole Wheat as prep w/o salt	1 cup (5.8 oz)	248	1	0	60
Vantia					
Gnocchi Whole Wheat	¾ cup	210	5	1	46
GOAT					
roasted	3 oz	122	23	3	0
GOJI BERRIES					
dried	1 oz	106	2	3	19

FOOD	PORTION	CALS	PROT	FAT	CARB
Kopali					
Organic Dark Chocolate Covered	½ pkg (1 oz)	120	2	6	18
Navitas Naturals					
Dried	1 oz	90	4	0	18
Sunfood					
Organic	1 oz	90	4	0	18
Superfood Snacks					
Organic Chocolate Goji Treats	3 pieces (1.4 oz)	150	4	4	24
Tree Of Life					
Organic	1 oz	110	<4	0	25

GOJI JUICE

Arthur's					
Goji Plus	1 bottle (11 oz)	210	3	tr	49
Gojilania					
Organic	8 oz	110	5	0	23

GOOSE

boneless roasted	2.7 oz	231	19	17	0
meat only raw	6.5 oz	298	42	13	0
w/ skin & bone roasted	1 serv (6.6 oz)	573	47	41	0
wild boneless roasted diced	1 cup (4.9 oz)	426	35	31	0

GOOSEBERRIES

canned in light syrup	1 cup	184	2	1	47
fresh	1 cup	66	1	1	15
Kopali					
Organic Goldenberry	1 pkg (1.8 oz)	150	4	0	31
Navitas Naturals					
Cape Gooseberry Dried	1 oz	80	2	0	17

GRAINS

Kashi					
7 Whole Grain Pilaf Fiery Fiesta	1 cup (4.9 oz)	210	8	5	40
7 Whole Grain Pilaf Moroccan Curry	1 cup (4.9 oz)	220	8	5	42
7 Whole Grain Pilaf Original	1 cup (4.9 oz)	220	8	4	45

GRAPE JUICE

bottled unsweetened	1 cup	154	1	tr	38

FOOD	PORTION	CALS	PROT	FAT	CARB
Apple & Eve					
Vintage Concord	8 oz	150	0	0	40
Cascadian Farm					
Organic frzn as prep	8 oz	150	0	0	38
First Blush					
All Flavors	8 oz	154	1	0	38
Juicy Juice					
Harvest Surprise	8 oz	120	1	0	28
Kedem					
100% Juice	8 oz	150	tr	0	37
Lakewood					
Organic Concord	6 oz	105	1	0	25
Mott's					
100% Juice Grape Medley	1 bottle (14 oz)	230	1	0	55
Nantucket Nectars					
Grapeade	8 oz	140	0	0	33
Organic Concord Grape	8 oz	130	0	0	31
Old Orchard					
100% Juice White	8 oz	160	0	0	38
Santa Cruz					
Organic Concord Grape	8 oz	160	tr	0	40
Snapple					
100% Juiced Grape	8 oz	170	0	0	43
Grapeade	8 oz	100	0	0	26
Tree Ripe					
Organic 100% Juice	6 oz	120	1	0	28
Tropicana					
Grape	1 bottle (14 oz)	270	tr	0	67
Walnut Acres					
Organic	8 oz	120	0	0	31
GRAPE LEAVES					
canned	1 (4 g)	3	tr	tr	tr
fresh raw	1 (3 g)	3	tr	tr	1
TAKE-OUT					
dolmas w/ beef & rice	1 (0.7 oz)	50	2	4	2
dolmas w/ lamb & rice	1 (0.7 oz)	56	2	4	3
dolmas w/ rice	1 (2 oz)	92	1	6	8

FOOD	PORTION	CALS	PROT	FAT	CARB
GRAPEFRUIT					
CANNED					
sections juice pack	½ cup (4.4 oz)	46	1	tr	11
sections light syrup	½ cup (4.5 oz)	76	1	tr	20
sections water pack	½ cup (4.3 oz)	44	1	tr	11
FRESH					
pink or red	½ (4.6 oz)	52	1	tr	13
sections pink or red	1 cup (8.1 oz)	97	2	tr	25
sections white	1 cup (8.1 oz)	76	2	tr	19
white	½ (4.1 oz)	39	1	tr	10
Ocean Spray					
Sweet Ruby Red	½ med (5.4 oz)	60	1	0	16
GRAPEFRUIT JUICE					
canned sweetened	1 cup (8.8 oz)	115	1	tr	28
canned unsweetened	1 cup (8.7 oz)	94	1	tr	22
fresh white	1 cup (8.7 oz)	96	1	tr	23
pink fresh	1 cup (8.7 oz)	96	1	tr	23
Apple & Eve					
Ruby Red	8 oz	130	0	0	32
Izze					
Sparkling Fortified Grapefruit	1 can (8.4 oz)	90	0	0	23
Odwalla					
100% Juice	8 oz	90	2	0	20
Sundia					
Ruby	½ cup	70	1	0	18
Tropicana					
Sweet	8 oz	130	1	0	31
GRAPES					
muscadine	10–12 (3.5 oz)	76	5	0	14
scuppernongs	10–12 (3.5 oz)	68	5	0	12
seedless red or green	20	69	1	tr	18
seedless red or green	1 cup	110	1	tr	29
thompson seedless in heavy syrup	½ cup	93	1	tr	25
thompson seedless water pack	½ cup	49	1	tr	13
with seeds red or green	20	80	1	tr	21
with seeds red or green	1 cup	106	1	tr	28
Chiquita					
Grapes	1 cup (3.2 oz)	62	1	0	16

FOOD	PORTION	CALS	PROT	FAT	CARB
Earthbound Farms					
Organic Black	1½ cups	190	1	1	24
Revolution Foods					
Organic Mashups Grape	1 pkg (3.2 oz)	60	0	0	14
GRAVY					
CANNED					
beef	1 cup	124	9	6	11
beef	1 can (10 oz)	155	11	7	14
chicken	1 cup	189	5	14	13
mushroom	1 cup	120	3	6	13
turkey	1 cup	122	6	5	12
Campbell's					
Au Jus	¼ cup	5	1	0	0
Chicken	¼ cup	40	0	3	3
Fat Free Beef	¼ cup	15	1	0	3
Fat Free Turkey	¼ cup	20	1	0	4
Mushroom	¼ cup	20	0	1	3
Franco-American					
Fat Free Slow Roast Chicken	¼ cup	20	tr	0	4
Slow Roast Chicken	¼ cup	20	1	1	3
Heinz					
Classic Chicken Fat Free	¼ cup	15	0	0	3
HomeStyle Classic Chicken	¼ cup	25	0	1	4
Roasted Turkey Fat Free	¼ cup (2.1 oz)	20	1	0	3
MIX					
au jus as prep w/ water	1 cup	32	1	1	4
brown as prep w/ water	1 cup	75	2	2	13
chicken as prep	1 cup	83	3	2	14
mushroom as prep	1 cup	70	2	1	14
onion as prep w/ water	1 cup	77	2	1	16
pork as prep	1 cup	76	2	2	13
turkey as prep	1 cup	87	3	2	15
Bournvita					
Extract	2 heaping tsp	34	1	1	7
Bovril					
Extract	1 heaping tsp	9	2	0	tr
Butterball					
Turkey	¼ cup (2 oz)	30	0	0	6

FOOD	PORTION	CALS	PROT	FAT	CARB
Knorr					
Au Jus Instant as prep	2 oz	10	tr	0	2
Beef Instant as prep	2 oz	20	1	1	3
Brown Instant as prep	2 oz	25	1	0	6
Brown Low Sodium Instant as prep	2 oz	25	1	tr	5
Chicken Instant as prep	2 oz	25	tr	tr	5
Chicken Low Sodium Instant as prep	2 oz	25	1	1	4
Leahey Gardens					
No Beef Brown Gluten Free	¼ cup	9	tr	tr	3
No Chicken Golden	¼ cup	18	tr	2	3
Marmite					
Extract	1 heaping tsp	9	2	0	tr
Road's End Organics					
Savory Herb Cholesterol Free Gluten Free	¼ cup	25	tr	0	5
TAKE-OUT					
au jus	1 cup	62	1	6	1
giblet gravy	¼ cup	45	3	3	3
GREAT NORTHERN BEANS					
canned	1 cup	299	19	1	55
dried cooked	1 cup	209	15	1	37
HamBeens					
Great Northerns as prep	½ cup	120	7	1	22
GREEN BEANS					
CANNED					
drained	1 cup	27	2	tr	6
Allens					
No Salt	½ cup	15	0	0	3
Del Monte					
Fresh Cut Italian	½ cup	30	1	0	6
Gertie's Finest					
Pickled	1 oz	15	1	0	3
Green Giant					
50% Less Sodium Cut	½ cup	20	1	0	4
McSweet					
Dilly Beans Whole	5 (1 oz)	30	0	0	7

FOOD	PORTION	CALS	PROT	FAT	CARB
S&W					
Cut	½ cup (4.2 oz)	20	1	0	4
Dilled	1 oz	20	0	0	5
FRESH					
cooked w/o salt	1 cup	44	2	tr	10
raw	1 cup	34	2	tr	8
raw whole beans	10	17	1	tr	4
FROZEN					
cooked	1 cup	38	2	tr	9
Birds Eye					
Steamfresh Whole	1 cup (2.9 oz)	35	1	0	5
C&W					
French Cut	1 cup	30	1	0	5
Cascadian Farm					
Organic Petite Whole	1 cup	25	1	0	5
Green Giant					
Green Bean Casserole	⅔ cup	110	2	8	8
TAKE-OUT					
casserole w/ mushroom sauce	1 cup	108	3	6	11
pickled	½ cup	19	1	tr	4
GREENS					
Allens					
Seasoned Mixed	½ cup	45	4	1	6
GROUNDCHERRIES					
fresh	½ cup	37	1	tr	8
GROUPER					
cooked	1 fillet (7.1 oz)	238	50	3	0
cooked	3 oz	100	21	1	0
raw	3 oz	78	16	1	0
GUAR GUM					
Bob's Red Mill					
Guar Gum	1 tbsp	20	0	0	6
GUAVA					
fresh	1	45	1	1	11
guava sauce	½ cup	43	tr	tr	11

FOOD	PORTION	CALS	PROT	FAT	CARB
GUAVA JUICE					
Apple & Eve					
Nectar	5 oz	130	0	0	32
OKF					
Sparkling Fresh Guava	1 bottle (8.3 oz)	20	0	0	13
Sabor Latino					
Nectar + Calcium	8 oz	160	0	0	39
GUINEA HEN					
boneless w/o skin raw	½ hen (9.3 oz)	290	54	7	0
w/ skin raw	½ hen (12 oz)	545	81	22	0
Grimaud Farms					
Guinea Fowl	1 serv (3.7 oz)	130	25	4	tr
HADDOCK					
fresh broiled	4 oz	127	27	1	0
roe raw	1 oz	37	7	tr	tr
smoked	1 oz	33	7	tr	0
Van de Kamp's					
Battered Fillets	2 (3.6 oz)	210	9	11	21
TAKE-OUT					
breaded & fried	4 oz	229	23	10	10
HAGGIS					
scottish haggis	1 serv (6.4 oz)	473	16	32	31
Caledonian Kitchen					
Highland Beef	3 oz	173	8	10	12
Vegetarian	3 oz	190	7	13	12
House of Kenton					
Vegetarian	1 serv (3.5 oz)	249	3	20	14
MacSween					
Traditional	1 (8 oz)	260	12	16	18
Vegetarian	1 (8 oz)	238	7	12	22
HALIBUT					
atlantic & pacific cooked	3 oz	119	23	2	0
atlantic & pacific cooked	½ fillet (5.6 oz)	223	42	5	0
atlantic & pacific raw	3 oz	93	18	2	0
greenland baked	3 oz	203	16	15	0
greenland baked	5.6 oz	380	29	28	0

FOOD	PORTION	CALS	PROT	FAT	CARB
FROZEN					
Van de Kamp's					
Battered Fillets	3 (4 oz)	230	10	11	22
HAM					
boneless extra lean roasted	3 oz	123	18	5	1
boneless roasted	3 oz	151	19	8	0
canned extra lean roasted	3 oz	116	18	4	tr
canned lean roasted	3 oz	142	18	7	tr
center slice lean & fat roasted	3 oz	173	17	11	tr
deviled	¼ cup	188	7	17	1
ham salad spread	2 tbsp	65	3	5	3
patty grilled	1 patty (2 oz)	205	8	19	1
prosciutto	4 slices (1.3 oz)	72	10	3	tr
sliced	3 slices (2.9 oz)	137	14	7	3
sliced extra lean	3 slices (2.2 oz)	69	11	2	2
westphalian smoked	1 oz	105	5	10	0
whole roasted	3 oz	207	18	14	0
Applegate Farms					
Organic Uncured	2 oz	70	10	2	1
Carl Buddig					
Ham Sliced	2 oz	85	10	5	1
Honey Ham Sliced	2 oz	90	10	5	2
Healthy Ones					
Honey 97% Fat Free	7 slices (2 oz)	90	9	2	2
Hormel					
Chunk Ham canned	2 oz	90	9	6	0
Deli Cooked	4 slices (2 oz)	70	10	2	1
Deli Honey	4 slices (2 oz)	70	9	2	3
Deli Smoked	4 slices (2 oz)	60	9	2	1
Dinner	2 oz	70	10	2	2
Organic Prairie					
Hardwood Smoked Bone In Spiral Sliced	3 oz	110	19	3	tr
Oscar Mayer					
Ham Brown Sugar Thin Sliced	⅓ pkg (2 oz)	70	10	2	4
Virginia Shaved	2 oz	50	9	1	1
Sara Lee					
Virginia Baked	4 slices (1.8 oz)	60	10	2	2

FOOD	PORTION	CALS	PROT	FAT	CARB
Tyson					
Glazed Ham Maple & Brown Sugar	1 serv (5 oz)	180	17	5	18
Honey Ham	2 slices (1.6 oz)	50	9	2	1
TAKE-OUT					
croquette	1 (2.2 oz)	149	9	9	8
salad	½ cup	287	16	23	5
spam musubi	1 serv (6 oz)	253	6	6	42
thick slice fried	1 (2.2 oz)	140	13	9	tr
HAMBURGER					
Applegate Farms					
Organic Beef Cooked	1 (3 oz)	195	21	12	0
Organic Turkey Burger	1 (4 oz)	190	22	11	0
Hot Pockets					
Cheeseburger	1 (4.5 oz)	310	11	13	37
Lean Pockets					
Cheeseburger	1 (4.5 oz)	280	12	7	40
Oscar Mayer					
Lunchables All-Star Burgers	1 pkg	420	14	14	60
Quaker Maid					
Pure Beef Patties	1 (4 oz)	240	19	18	0
TAKE-OUT					
cheeseburger + condiments	1 reg (4.5 oz)	347	17	17	28
double hamburger + condiments	1 reg (5.8 oz)	384	23	19	30
single patty + condiments	1 reg (4 oz)	299	15	11	35
HAMBURGER SUBSTITUTES (*see also* MEAT SUBSTITUTES)					
Amy's					
All American Burger	1 (2.5 oz)	120	10	3	15
Cheddar Veggie Burger	1 (2.5 oz)	160	8	5	20
Texas Burger	1 (2.5 oz)	120	12	3	14
Dr. Praeger's					
Veggie Burger Bombay	1 (2.78 oz)	110	6	5	13
Veggie Burger California	1 (2.75 oz)	110	5	5	13
Veggie Burger California Gluten Free	1 (2.75 oz)	120	5	6	13
Gardenburger					
Black Bean Chipotle	1 (2.5 oz)	80	5	3	13
Flamed Grilled	1 (2.5 oz)	90	11	4	5

FOOD	PORTION	CALS	PROT	FAT	CARB
GardenVegan	1 (2.5 oz)	100	10	1	12
Original	1 (2.5 oz)	100	5	4	14
Portabella	1 (2.5 oz)	90	5	3	15
Morningstar Farms					
Classic Burger	1 (2.2 oz)	150	14	7	10
Okara Pattie	1 (2.2 oz)	120	12	5	6
Vegan Burger	1 (2.5 oz)	100	13	2	8
Sunshine Burgers					
Garden	1 (2.6 oz)	190	8	13	14
Original	1 (2.6 oz)	190	8	13	14
WildWood					
Organic Original Burgers Tofu-Veggie	1 (3.2 oz)	180	12	13	8
HAZELNUTS					
chocolate hazelnut spread	2 tbsp (1.3 oz)	200	2	11	23
chopped	¼ cup (1 oz)	181	4	17	5
ground	¼ cup (0.7 oz)	118	3	11	3
whole	¼ cup (1.2 oz)	212	5	21	6
whole nuts	21 (1 oz)	178	4	17	5
Chukar Cherries					
Chocolate Covered Spiced	3 tbsp (1.4 oz)	228	4	17	21
Fisher					
Chopped	¼ cup (1 oz)	180	4	17	5
Love'n Bake					
Hazelnut Praline	2 tbsp	170	3	12	13
HEART					
beef simmered	3 oz	140	24	4	tr
chicken cooked	1 (3 g)	5	1	tr	0
chicken diced simmered	½ cup	134	19	6	tr
lamb braised	3 oz	157	21	7	2
pork braised	1 (4.5 oz)	191	30	7	1
turkey simmered	½ cup	94	16	3	tr
veal braised	3 oz	158	25	6	tr
Rumba					
Beef	4 oz	130	19	4	3
HEARTS OF PALM					
canned	½ cup	20	2	tr	3
canned	1 (1.2 oz)	9	1	tr	2

FOOD	PORTION	CALS	PROT	FAT	CARB
Native Forest					
Organic	1 oz	15	1	0	2
HEMP					
Living Harvest					
Organic Hemp Nuts	2 tbsp (1 oz)	170	10	12	5
Organic Protein Powder	2 scoops (1 oz)	110	14	3	9
Manitoba Harvest					
Hemp Seed Butter	2 tbsp	160	11	10	7
Protein Powder	2 scoops (1 oz)	134	15	6	5
Shelled Seed	2 tbsp	160	11	10	7
Nutiva					
Organic Protein Powder	2 scoops (1 oz)	120	11	3	14
Shelled Hempseed	2 tbsp	110	6	8	2
HERBAL TEA (see TEA/HERBAL TEA)					
HERBS/SPICES (see also individual names)					
cajun seasoning	1 tbsp	19	1	1	3
chinese five spice	1 tsp	7	0	tr	2
garam masala	1 tsp	8	tr	tr	1
poultry seasoning	1 tsp	5	tr	tr	1
pumpkin pie spice	1 tsp	6	tr	tr	1
Bragg					
Herb & Spice Seasoning	¼ tsp	0	0	0	0
Dave's Gourmet					
Insanity Spice	¼ tsp (1 g)	5	0	0	0
Ribber City					
Rib-A-Dub-Rub Dry Rub Seasoning	¼ tsp (0.8 oz)	3	0	0	1
Spice Hunter					
All Purpose Blend	¼ tsp	0	0	0	0
Greek Seasoning Salt Free	¼ tsp	0	0	0	0
HERRING					
atlantic baked	4 oz	230	26	13	0
dried salted	1 fillet (1.4 oz)	161	18	9	0
pickled	1 oz	74	4	5	3
pickled in cream sauce	1 oz	72	3	5	2
roe	1 tbsp	39	6	2	tr
smoked kippered	1 oz	62	7	4	0

FOOD	PORTION	CALS	PROT	FAT	CARB
TAKE-OUT					
breaded fried	1 serv (4 oz)	225	15	14	9
HIBISCUS					
flowers dried sweetened	⅓ cup	100	0	0	23
Santa Cruz					
Organic Hibiscus Cooler	8 oz	100	tr	0	24
HICKORY NUTS					
dried	1 oz	187	4	18	5
HOMINY					
white canned	1 cup	119	2	1	24
yellow canned	½ cup	115	2	1	23
Allens					
White	½ cup	100	2	1	22
Bush's					
Golden	½ cup	60	1	0	13
HONEY					
honey	¼ cup (3 oz)	258	tr	0	70
honey	1 tbsp (0.7 oz)	64	tr	0	17
orange blossom	1 tbsp	60	0	0	17
wild honey	1 tbsp	60	0	0	17
Comfort Care					
Raw Clover	1 tbsp (0.7 oz)	60	0	0	17
Dutch Gold					
Clover	1 tbsp	60	0	0	17
Tree Of Life					
Alfalfa Honey Raw Unfiltered	1 tbsp	60	0	0	17
Avocado Honey Raw Unfiltered	1 tbsp (0.7 oz)	60	0	0	17
Buckwheat Honey Raw Unfiltered	1 tbsp	60	0	0	17
Tupelo Honey Raw Unfiltered	1 tbsp	60	0	0	17
Wholesome Sweeteners					
Organic Fair Trade Amber	1 tbsp	60	0	0	17
Organic Fair Trade Raw	1 tbsp	60	0	0	17
HONEYDEW					
balls frzn	1 cup (8 oz)	83	1	tr	21
fresh cut up	1 cup	61	1	tr	15
fresh wedge	⅛ melon (4.5 oz)	45	1	tr	11
whole fresh	1 (35 oz)	360	5	1	91

FOOD	PORTION	CALS	PROT	FAT	CARB
Chiquita					
Fresh Cut Up	1 cup (6.2 oz)	64	1	0	16
HORSE					
roasted	3 oz	149	24	5	0
HORSERADISH					
sauce	1 tbsp	7	tr	tr	2
wasabi root raw	1 (5.9 oz)	184	8	1	40
wasabi root raw sliced	½ cup (2.3 oz)	71	3	tr	15
Gold's					
Horse Radish	1 tsp (5 g)	0	0	0	0
Robert Rothchild Farm					
Sauce	1 tsp	20	0	2	1
Zatarain's					
Prepared	1 tbsp	15	0	0	2
HOT CHOCOLATE					
mix not prep	1 pkg (1 oz)	111	2	1	23
mix w/ no calorie sweetener as prep w/ water	8 oz	72	3	1	14
mix w/ sugar as prep w/ nonfat milk	8 oz	209	9	1	30
mix w/ sugar as prep w/ water	8 oz	138	2	1	29
Hershey's					
Goodnight Hugs	1 pkg (1.2 oz)	140	3	3	27
Nestle					
Hot Cocoa Carb Select Fat Free	1 pkg	25	1	0	5
Hot Cocoa Milk Chocolate	1 pkg (1 oz)	80	tr	3	15
Hot Cocoa Rich Chocolate as prep w/ water	1 pkg	80	tr	3	15
Silhouette Solution					
Down East not prep	1 pkg (0.88 oz)	90	15	2	5
Starbucks					
Hot Cocoa Mix	1 pkg	130	4	2	28
Swiss Miss					
Cocoa Caramel as prep	1 pkg	120	1	3	22
Cocoa No Sugar Added as prep	1 pkg	60	2	1	10
Cocoa Rich Creamy as prep	1 pkg	110	2	2	22
Cocoa w/ Marshmallows as prep	1 pkg	120	1	2	24

FOOD	PORTION	CALS	PROT	FAT	CARB
Cocoa w/ Marshmallows Fat Free as prep	1 pkg	140	1	3	29
French Vanilla as prep	1 pkg	110	2	2	24
Milk Chocolate as prep	1 pkg	120	1	3	23
TAKE-OUT					
chocolate caliente w/ lowfat milk	1 serv (8.4 oz)	221	11	9	27
chocolate caliente w/ whole milk	1 serv (8.4 oz)	276	10	17	25
hot chocolate	1 cup (8.7 oz)	192	9	6	30
mexican hot chocolate	1 cup	173	10	6	20
HOT DOG (see also HOT DOG SUBSTITUTES)					
beef	1 (1.5 oz)	149	5	13	2
beef & pork	1 (1.5 oz)	137	5	12	1
beef low fat	1 (2 oz)	133	7	11	1
chicken	1 (1.5 oz)	116	6	9	3
fat free	1 (2 oz)	62	7	1	6
low fat	1 (2 oz)	88	6	6	3
low sodium	1 (2 oz)	180	7	16	1
pork and beef cheese smokie	1 (1.5 oz)	141	6	12	1
turkey	1 (1.5 oz)	102	6	8	1
Applegate Farms					
Natural Beef	1 (1.5 oz)	80	5	6	0
Organic Chicken	1 (1.5 oz)	70	7	5	0
Dietz & Watson					
New York Style Beef	1 (2.3 oz)	130	8	15	2
Healthy Ones					
Beef	1 (1.8 oz)	70	6	3	7
Franks	1 (1.8 oz)	70	6	3	6
Johnsonville					
Stadium Beef	1 (2.7 oz)	240	9	22	2
Organic Prairie					
Beef Uncured	1 (1.5 oz)	120	5	11	0
Chicken Uncured	1 (1.5 oz)	100	7	6	1
Pork Uncured	1 (1.5 oz)	130	5	12	0
Turkey Uncured	1 (1.5 oz)	80	8	6	1
Oscar Mayer					
Beef	1 (1.6 oz)	140	5	13	1
Beef Light	1 (1.6 oz)	90	5	6	2
Cheese Dogs	1 (1.6 oz)	140	5	13	1

FOOD	PORTION	CALS	PROT	FAT	CARB
Corn Dogs	1	210	6	12	21
Smokies	1 (1.8 oz)	150	6	13	1
TAKE-OUT					
corndog	1	460	17	19	56
w/ bun chili	1	297	14	13	31
w/ bun plain	1	242	10	15	18

HOT DOG SUBSTITUTES
Health Is Wealth

FOOD	PORTION	CALS	PROT	FAT	CARB
Vegetarian Cocktail Franks	3 (2.4 oz)	220	8	16	16
Loma Linda					
Big Franks	1 (1.8 oz)	110	11	6	3
Big Franks Low Fat Vegan	1 (1.8 oz)	80	12	3	3
Morningstar Farms					
Corn Dog Veggie	1 (2.5 oz)	170	8	6	22
Yves					
Meatless Hot Dog	1	50	10	1	2
Tofu Dogs	1	45	8	1	2

HUMMUS
Athenos

FOOD	PORTION	CALS	PROT	FAT	CARB
Original	2 tbsp	80	2	5	5
Roasted Garlic	2 tbsp	80	2	5	5
Roasted Red Pepper	2 tbsp	80	2	6	5
Emerald Valley					
Organic Greek Olive & Roasted Garlic	2 tbsp (1 oz)	60	2	3	6
Organic Original	2 tbsp (1 oz)	50	2	2	7
Organic Spinach Feta	2 tbsp (1 oz)	50	2	2	6
Guiltless Gourmet					
Original	2 tbsp (1.1 oz)	50	2	2	8
Tribe					
40 Spices	2 tbsp	50	1	4	3
French Onion	2 tbsp	50	1	4	4
Organic Classic	2 tbsp	50	2	4	4
Organic Roasted Red Peppers	2 tbsp	40	1	3	3
Roasted Eggplant	2 tbsp	35	1	3	3
Scallion	2 tbsp	50	1	4	4
Zesty Lemon	2 tbsp	50	1	3	4
Wholesome Valley					
Organic Classic	2 tbsp (1 oz)	60	2	4	5

FOOD	PORTION	CALS	PROT	FAT	CARB
Wild Garden					
Hummus Dip	2 tbsp	35	2	2	4
WildWood					
Organic Low Fat	2 tbsp	50	2	2	6
Organic Mid-Eastern	2 tbsp	65	2	4	6
TAKE-OUT					
hummus	¼ cup (2.2 oz)	109	3	5	12
HYACINTH BEANS					
dried cooked	1 cup	228	16	1	40

ICE CREAM AND FROZEN DESSERTS (*see also* ICES AND ICE POPS, SHERBET, YOGURT FROZEN)

FOOD	PORTION	CALS	PROT	FAT	CARB
chocolate	½ cup (4 fl oz)	143	3	7	19
dixie cup chocolate	1 (3.5 fl oz)	125	2	6	16
dixie cup strawberry	1 (3.5 fl oz)	112	2	5	16
dixie cup vanilla	1 (3.5 fl oz)	116	2	6	14
freeze dried ice cream chocolate strawberry & vanilla	1 pkg (0.75 oz)	158	2	5	24
strawberry	½ cup (4 fl oz)	127	2	6	18
vanilla	½ cup (4 fl oz)	132	2	7	16
vanilla soft serve	½ cup	111	4	2	19
Breyers					
Butter Pecan	½ cup	150	2	10	14
Carb Smart Chocolate	½ cup	90	2	6	13
Carb Smart Fudge Bar	1 (3.5 oz)	100	3	7	9
Carb Smart Vanilla	½ cup	90	2	6	13
Carb Smart Vanilla Bar Chocolate Coated	1 (3 oz)	170	2	15	9
Cherry Vanilla	½ cup	130	2	6	18
Chocolate Crackle	½ cup	160	2	10	15
Chocolate Extra Creamy	½ cup	140	2	7	17
Coffee	½ cup	130	2	7	15
Cookies & Cream	½ cup	150	2	7	19
Double Churn ½ Fat Chocolate Mocha Silk	½ cup	130	3	5	19
Double Churn ½ Fat Creamy Vanilla	½ cup	100	2	3	17
Double Churn ½ Fat Mint Chocolate Chip	½ cup	130	2	5	19

FOOD	PORTION	CALS	PROT	FAT	CARB
Double Churn ½ Fat Rocky Road	½ cup	130	3	5	22
Double Churn Fat Free Chocolate Fudge Brownie	½ cup	110	3	0	25
Double Churn Fat Free Creamy Vanilla	½ cup	90	3	0	21
Double Churn Fat Free French Chocolate	½ cup	90	3	0	22
Double Churn No Sugar Added Vanilla	½ cup	80	2	4	14
Dulce De Leche	½ cup	150	2	6	21
French Vanilla	½ cup	140	3	7	14
Heath English Toffee	½ cup	160	2	6	25
Overload Very Chocolate Cherry	½ cup	120	2	3	21
Overload Waffle Cone	½ cup	130	2	3	22
Peach	½ cup	120	2	5	17
Sandwich Mrs. Fields Brownie	1 (6 oz)	450	5	19	64
Sandwich Mrs. Fields Cookie	1 (3 oz)	190	2	8	29
Sandwich Oreo	1 (3 oz)	170	2	6	26
Snicker	½ cup	170	3	8	20
Strawberry	½ cup	120	2	5	15
Strawberry Cheesecake Sara Lee	½ cup	150	2	6	20
Vanilla Fudge Brownie	½ cup	150	2	7	20
Vanilla Lactose Free	½ cup	130	2	7	14
Celestial Seasonings					
Tea Dreams Cinnamon Apple Spice	½ cup	140	0	6	24
Tea Dreams Vanilla Ginger Spice Chai	½ cup	140	0	6	24
Tea Dreams Bars Chocolate Caramel Chai	1 (2.7 oz)	240	tr	15	28
Ciao Bella					
Gelato Chocolate	1 pkg (3.5 oz)	210	4	13	22
Gelato Hazelnut	1 pkg (3.5 oz)	210	3	13	21
Gelato Vanilla	1 pkg (3.5 oz)	184	3	11	19
Dippin' Dots					
Banana Split	½ cup	170	3	10	16
Chocolate	½ cup	165	3	10	15

FOOD	PORTION	CALS	PROT	FAT	CARB
Fudge Fat Free No Sugar Added	½ cup	92	4	0	18
Horchata	½ cup	170	3	10	16
Java Delight	½ cup	170	3	10	16
Root Beer Float	½ cup	111	1	3	20
Vanilla	½ cup	170	3	10	16
Fat Boy					
Casco Nut Sundae On A Stick	1 (3 oz)	310	7	24	21
Casco Nut Sundae On A Stick Cherry Cordial	1 (3 oz)	300	3	22	26
Sandwich Chocolate	1 (3 oz)	210	4	9	31
Sandwich Egg Nog	1 (3 oz)	220	4	10	31
Sandwich Jr. Vanilla	1 (1.6 oz)	120	2	5	17
Sandwich Vanilla	1 (3 oz)	220	4	10	30
Glace De Vino					
Chocolate Amarreto Cream Sherry	½ cup	180	2	7	21
Raspberry Merlot Cheesecake	½ cup	180	2	7	22
Good Humor					
Bar Chocolate Eclair	1 (3 oz)	160	2	8	21
Bar Cookies & Cream	1 (3 oz)	190	2	11	21
Bar Vanilla Chocolate Coated	1 (4 oz)	260	3	17	24
Cone King Giant	1 (8 oz)	390	7	21	44
Cone Sundae	1 (4.3 oz)	260	4	15	29
King Bar Heath	1 (4 oz)	310	3	20	31
King Cone Vanilla	1 (4.6 oz)	250	4	13	30
Sandwich Giant Vanilla	1 (6 oz)	220	4	4	43
Sandwich Oreo	1 (4.5 oz)	240	4	10	36
Sandwich Vanilla	1 (3 oz)	130	2	2	26
Swirlwind	1 (6 oz)	160	4	3	31
Haagen-Dazs					
Bailey's Irish Cream	½ cup (3.6 oz)	260	5	17	21
Bar Chocolate & Dark Chocolate	1 (3 oz)	290	4	20	24
Bar Vanilla & Almonds	1 (3 oz)	310	5	22	22
Bar Vanilla & Milk Chocolate	1 (3 oz)	290	4	21	22
Butter Pecan	½ cup (3.7 oz)	310	5	23	21
Caramel Cone	½ cup (4 oz)	320	4	19	32
Cherry Vanilla	½ cup (3.5 oz)	240	4	15	23
Chocolate Chip Cookie Dough	½ cup (3.6 oz)	310	4	20	29
Chocolate Peanut Butter	½ cup (3.8 oz)	360	8	24	27
Cookies & Cream	½ cup (3.6 oz)	270	5	17	23

FOOD	PORTION	CALS	PROT	FAT	CARB
Dulce De Leche	½ cup (3.7 oz)	290	5	17	28
Five Coffee	½ cup (3.6 oz)	220	5	12	23
Five Milk Chocolate	½ cup (3.6 oz)	220	6	12	22
Five Passion Fruit	½ cup (3.6 oz)	220	4	11	25
Five Vanilla	½ cup (3.7 oz)	270	5	18	21
Green Tea	½ cup (3.6 oz)	250	5	17	20
Mango	½ cup (3.7 oz)	250	4	14	28
Reserve Amazon Valley Chocolate	½ cup (3.7 oz)	290	5	19	25
Reserve Caramelized Hazelnut Gianduja	½ cup (3.5 oz)	290	4	18	27
Reserve Fleur De Sel Caramel	½ cup (3.7 oz)	280	4	17	28
Reserve Hawaiian Lehua Honey & Sweet Cream	½ cup (3.8 oz)	270	4	17	26
Rocky Road	½ cup (3.6 oz)	300	5	18	29
Strawberry	½ cup (3.7 oz)	250	4	16	23
Vanilla Honey Bee	½ cup (3.6 oz)	270	5	17	23
Hershey's					
Banana Split	½ cup (2.5 oz)	160	2	9	18
Chocolate	½ cup (2.5 oz)	140	3	8	15
Cookies And Cream	½ cup (2.5 oz)	160	2	9	16
Fudge Royale	½ cup (2.5 oz)	180	2	9	19
Mint Moose Tracks	½ cup (2.5 oz)	200	3	14	21
Raspberry	½ cup (2.5 oz)	170	2	9	21
Tally-Ho Low Fat Butter Pecan	½ cup (2.5 oz)	90	3	2	14
Vanilla	½ cup (2.5 oz)	150	3	9	14
Klondike					
Bar Caramel Pretzel	1 (4 oz)	260	3	14	30
Bar Original Vanilla	1 (4.5 oz)	250	3	17	22
Bar Reese's	1 (4 oz)	260	4	16	26
Bar Whitehouse Cherry	1 (4.5 oz)	250	2	17	24
Cone Crunchy Vanilla	1 (4.3 oz)	280	5	16	30
Slim A Bear 100 Calorie Sandwich Vanilla	1 (3 oz)	100	2	2	21
Slim A Bear Bar Vanilla	1 (4 oz)	170	6	9	21
Land O' Lakes					
Vanilla	½ cup (2.4 oz)	150	2	8	17
Vanilla Light	½ cup (2.3 oz)	100	3	3	17
Molli Coolz					
Cup Banana Cream Pie	1	120	2	9	9

FOOD	PORTION	CALS	PROT	FAT	CARB
Cup Chocolate Fusion	1	140	2	10	10
Cup Chocolate Peanut Butter	1	160	2	12	12
Ionz Cotton Candy	1 cup	100	2	7	8
Ionz S'mores	1 cup	110	2	9	7
Rocks Cherry Blue Raz & Lemon	1 cup	80	tr	2	15
Rocks Lemon Lime	1 cup	80	tr	2	15
Shakers Chocolate	1 (10.2 oz)	250	3	11	35
Natural Choice					
Organic Double Chocolate	½ cup	230	3	14	25
Organic Strawberry	½ cup	210	2	13	22
Organic Vanilla	½ cup	220	2	14	22
Popsicle					
Creamsicle	1 (2.5 oz)	100	1	2	20
Purely Decadent					
Dairy Free Bar Chocolate Coated Vanilla	1 (2.7 oz)	200	2	9	26
Dairy Free Bar Chocolate Coated Vanilla Almond	1 (2.7 oz)	210	2	10	28
Organic Coconut Milk Chocolate	½ cup	150	1	9	20
Organic Coconut Milk Vanilla Bean	½ cup	150	1	8	19
Organic Dairy Free Belgian Chocolate	½ cup	180	1	7	30
Organic Dairy Free Chocolate Obsession	½ cup	210	2	9	36
Organic Dairy Free Gluten Free Cookie Dough	½ cup	230	1	8	36
Organic Dairy Free Mocha Almond Fudge	½ cup	200	3	9	32
Organic Dairy Free Snickerdoodle	½ cup	190	1	6	34
Organic Dairy Free Vanilla	½ cup	170	1	8	29
Rice Dream					
Bar Vanilla Chocolate Coating	1 (3 oz)	230	1	15	24
Bar Vanilla Nutty	1 (3.3 oz)	320	5	24	27
Carob Almond	½ cup	180	0	10	26
Frozen Pie Chocolate	1 (3.4 oz)	330	3	19	40
Mint Carob Chip	½ cup	170	1	8	25
Strawberry	½ cup	160	0	8	25

FOOD	PORTION	CALS	PROT	FAT	CARB
Sheer Bliss					
Bar Pomegranate	1 (3.1 oz)	260	3	16	24
Blissbites	2 (1.1 oz)	100	1	7	9
Blisswich	1 (3.3 oz)	270	3	10	39
Freedom	½ cup (4 oz)	290	3	16	32
Mediterranean Coffee	½ cup (4 oz)	260	3	18	25
Pomegranate	½ cup (4 oz)	290	3	16	32
Vanilla	½ cup (4 oz)	300	6	19	29
Skinny Cow					
Bar Dippers Vanilla & Caramel	1	80	2	3	11
Bar Truffle Caramel	1	100	3	2	19
Bar Truffle French Vanilla	1	100	3	2	18
Cone Chocolate w/ Fudge	1	150	4	3	29
Cone Vanilla w/ Caramel	1	150	4	3	29
Fudge Bar	1	100	4	1	22
Sandwich Chocolate Peanut Butter	1	150	4	2	30
Sandwich Cookies 'N Cream	1	150	4	2	31
Sandwich Vanilla	1	140	4	2	30
Sandwich Vanilla No Sugar Added	1	140	4	2	30
SoDelicious					
Dairy Free Sandwich Minis Pomegranate	1 (1.4 oz)	90	2	2	18
Dairy Free Sandwich Mint	1 (2.2 oz)	150	3	3	28
Dairy Free Sandwich Vanilla	1 (2 oz)	150	3	3	28
Dairy Free Sugar Free Chocolate Coated Vanilla Bar	1 (2.2 oz)	150	2	14	15
Dairy Free Sugar Free Fudge Bar	1 (2 oz)	80	2	5	12
Organic Dairy Free Sandwich Neapolitan	1 (2.2 oz)	150	3	3	28
Soy Dream					
Butter Pecan	½ cup	140	1	9	17
Sandwich Lil' Dreamers Chocolate	1 (1.4 oz)	100	1	5	15
Vanilla	½ cup	140	1	7	18
Starbucks					
Caramel Macchiato	½ cup (3.6 oz)	240	3	13	27
Coffee	½ cup (3.5 oz)	210	3	13	21
Java Chip Frappuccino	½ cup (3.5 oz)	250	3	15	25

FOOD	PORTION	CALS	PROT	FAT	CARB
Mocha Frappuccino	½ cup (3.5 oz)	220	3	13	23
Mocha Bar	1	280	4	19	26
Straus					
Organic Coffee	4 oz	240	4	15	19
Organic Vanilla Bean	4 oz	240	4	15	19
The Greek Gods					
Pagoto Ice Krema Baklava	½ cup (4 oz)	240	5	12	29
Pagoto Ice Krema Chocolate Fig	½ cup (4 oz)	240	4	11	32
Pagoto Ice Krema Honey Pomegranate	½ cup (4 oz)	230	4	11	31
Turkey Hill					
Banana Split	½ cup	150	2	7	19
Choco Mint Chip	½ cup	160	2	9	17
Chocolate All Natural	½ cup	150	3	8	18
Chocolate Marshmallow	½ cup	160	2	6	24
Coconut Cream Pie	½ cup	170	2	9	20
Cookies 'N Cream	½ cup	150	2	8	19
Duetto Cherry	½ cup	120	1	3	21
Duetto Lemon	½ cup	120	1	4	21
Duetto Root Beer	½ cup	120	0	3	21
French Vanilla	½ cup	140	2	7	16
Light Banana Split	½ cup	110	2	3	19
Light Dulce De Chocolate	½ cup	120	2	3	22
Light Moose Tracks	½ cup	140	3	6	20
Light Vanilla Bean	½ cup	100	2	2	17
No Sugar Added Cherry Fudge Ripple	½ cup	80	3	0	22
No Sugar Added Vanilla Bean	½ cup	70	3	0	19
Original Vanilla	½ cup	140	2	7	16
Peanut Butter Ripple	½ cup	170	3	11	16
Rocky Road	½ cup	170	3	8	23
Sandwich Chocolate Chunk	1 (3.2 oz)	320	3	15	44
Sandwich Vanilla Bean	1 (2.5 oz)	190	3	7	29
Sandwich Light Vanilla Bean	1 (2.5 oz)	160	3	3	32
Sundae Cone Vanilla Fudge	1 (3.3 oz)	320	6	18	35
Tin Roof Sundae	½ cup	150	2	8	19
TAKE-OUT					
cone vanilla light soft serve	1 (4.6 oz)	164	4	6	24
gelato chocolate hazelnut	½ cup (5.3 oz)	370	9	29	26
gelato vanilla	½ cup (3 oz)	211	3	15	18

FOOD	PORTION	CALS	PROT	FAT	CARB
ice cream pie no crust	1 slice (3.4 oz)	218	3	14	21
mud pie	⅛ pie (8 oz)	698	9	32	96
sundae caramel	1 (5.4 oz)	303	7	9	49
sundae hot fudge	1 (5.4 oz)	284	6	9	48
sundae strawberry	1 (5.4 oz)	269	6	8	45

ICE CREAM CONES AND CUPS

FOOD	PORTION	CALS	PROT	FAT	CARB
brown sugar cone	1 (10 g)	40	1	tr	8
wafer cone	1	17	tr	tr	3
waffle cone	1 lg	121	2	2	23
Keebler					
Cone Sugar	1	50	1	1	10
Ice Creme Cone	1	15	0	0	4
Waffle Bowl	1	50	tr	1	10
Waffle Cone	1	50	tr	1	10

ICE CREAM TOPPINGS

FOOD	PORTION	CALS	PROT	FAT	CARB
butterscotch	2 tbsp (1.4 oz)	103	1	tr	27
caramel	2 tbsp (1.4 oz)	103	1	tr	27
marshmallow cream	1 oz	88	1	tr	23
marshmallow cream	1 jar (7 oz)	615	3	tr	157
nuts in syrup	2 tbsp	184	2	9	24
pineapple	2 tbsp (1.5 oz)	106	tr	0	28
pineapple	1 cup (11.5 oz)	861	1	–	226
strawberry	2 tbsp (1.5 oz)	107	tr	tr	28
strawberry	1 cup (11.5 oz)	863	1	1	225

ICED TEA
MIX
Nestea

FOOD	PORTION	CALS	PROT	FAT	CARB
Lemon Liquid Concentrate as prep	8 oz	80	0	0	19
Peach Liquid Concentrate as prep	8 oz	90	0	0	21
Sugar Free w/ Lemon	2 tsp	5	0	0	2
Sweetened w/ Lemon	1⅓ tbsp	60	0	0	15
Unsweetened w/ Lemon	2 tsp	5	0	0	1
READY-TO-DRINK					
Bina					
Lemon	8 oz	70	0	0	17
Peach	8 oz	114	0	0	29

FOOD	PORTION	CALS	PROT	FAT	CARB
Bolthouse Farms					
Perfectly Protein Vanilla Chai Tea w/ Soy	8 oz	160	10	3	25
Bombilla & Gourd					
Organic Eco Teas All Flavors	8 oz	40	0	0	11
Cafe Sepia					
Matcha Latte	1 can (8.6 oz)	130	3	3	23
Delta Blues					
Tea Punch Black Tea Sumptuous Spearmint	8 oz	90	0	0	21
Tea Punch Green Tea Peach & Delectable Lemongrass	8 oz	90	0	0	22
Tea Punch Green Tea Peach Apricot Pineapple Quince	8 oz	100	0	0	24
Fuze					
Antioxidant Tea	8 oz	60	0	0	15
Green Tea	8 oz	60	0	0	16
White Tea	8 oz	60	0	0	15
Gold Peak Tea					
Green Tea Sweetened	1 bottle (16.9 oz)	170	0	0	45
Hawaiian					
Iced Tea	1 can (11.5 oz)	120	0	0	35
Ito En					
Apricot	8 oz	60	0	0	15
Green Tea Apple	8 oz	70	0	0	18
Mango	8 oz	50	0	0	15
Sencho Shot	1 can (6.4 oz)	0	0	0	0
White Tea Grape	8 oz	60	0	0	15
Kombucha					
Wonder Drink Asian Pear Ginger	1 bottle (8.5 oz)	65	0	0	16
Wonder Drink Rooibus Red Peach	1 bottle (8.5 oz)	60	0	0	15
Nantucket Nectars					
Half & Half	8 oz	90	0	0	22
Original Lemon	8 oz	80	0	0	22
Nestea					
Green Tea Diet Peach	8 oz	0	0	0	0

FOOD	PORTION	CALS	PROT	FAT	CARB
Green Tea Peach	1 bottle (20 oz)	220	0	0	57
Lemon	1 bottle (20 oz)	210	0	0	56
Lemon Diet	8 oz	0	0	0	0
Sweetened	8 oz	60	0	0	17
Sweetened Diet Green Tea	8 oz	0	0	0	0
Sweetened Green Tea	8 oz	80	0	0	20
Old Orchard					
Green Tea w/ Lemon & Honey	8 oz	45	0	0	12
Green Tea w/ Pomegranate	8 oz	45	0	0	12
Osteo					
Fruit Tea All Flavors	1 can (12 oz)	120	0	0	32
Pixie					
Black Tea Mate Lemon Ginger	8 oz	35	0	0	8
Yerba Mate Authentic	8 oz	30	0	0	7
POM					
Light Tea Pomegranate Hibiscus Green	8 oz	35	0	0	16
Light Tea Pomegranate Orange Blossom	8 oz	35	0	0	14
Light Tea Pomegranate Wildberry White	8 oz	35	0	0	16
Santa Cruz					
Organic Lemon	8 oz	60	0	0	15
Organic Peppermint	8 oz	60	0	0	15
Organic TeaZer Passionfruit	(12 oz) 1 bottle	90	0	0	22
Organic TeaZer Pear	(12 oz) 1 bottle	90	0	0	21
Snapple					
Black Tea Lemon	8 oz	80	0	0	21
Diet Lemon Tea	8 oz	10	0	0	0
Diet Lemonade Iced Tea	8 oz	10	0	0	2
Diet Peach	8 oz	0	0	0	0
Diet Plum-A-Granate	8 oz	5	0	0	0
Green Tea Mango Metabolism	8 oz	60	0	0	15
Peach	8 oz	90	0	0	23
Red Tea Pomegranate Raspberry	8 oz	80	0	0	21
White Tea Apple Plum	8 oz	80	0	0	21

FOOD	PORTION	CALS	PROT	FAT	CARB
SSips					
Diet Green Tea w/ Honey & Ginseng	1 box (7 oz)	0	0	0	0
Green Tea w/ Honey & Ginseng	1 box (7 oz)	60	0	0	15
Lemon	8 oz	100	0	0	24
Sweet Leaf					
Diet Mint & Honey Green Tea	8 oz	0	tr	0	tr
Lemon & Lime Unsweet	8 oz	0	0	0	0
Original Sweet	8 oz	70	0	0	18
Pomegranate Green Tea	8 oz	60	tr	0	16
Swiss Tea					
Diet	8 oz	0	0	0	1
Diet Decafe	8 oz	0	0	0	0
Green Tea w/ Ginseng & Honey	8 oz	80	0	0	20
Sweet Tea Southern Style	8 oz	90	0	0	23
W/ Lemon	8 oz	100	0	0	24
White Tea Sweetened w/ Raspberry	8 oz	90	0	0	24
True Brew					
Cranberry Orange	8 oz	72	0	0	18
Green Tea	8 oz	64	0	0	16
Sweet Tea	8 oz	76	0	0	19
Turkey Hill					
Decaffeinated	8 oz	80	0	0	20
Diet Decaffeinated	8 oz	0	0	0	0
Nature's Accents Blueberry Oolong	8 oz	100	0	0	24
Nature's Accents Chai Spiced Zero Calorie	8 oz	0	0	0	1
Nature's Accents Green Tea	8 oz	70	0	0	17
Southern Brew Extra Sweet	8 oz	90	0	0	21
VidaTea					
All Flavors	1 can	90	0	0	24
VitaZest					
Green Tea Vitamin Enriched	8 oz	0	0	0	0
Weil For Tea					
Gyokuro	1 can (8.6 oz)	0	0	0	0
Turmeric	1 can (8.6 oz)	0	0	0	0

FOOD	PORTION	CALS	PROT	FAT	CARB
ICES AND ICE POPS					
Breeze Freeze					
100% Fruit Juice	1 (8 oz)	54	0	0	13
Fruit Granita	1 (8 oz)	120	1	0	28
Breyers					
Pure Fruit Pop Lemon Lime	1 (1.75 oz)	40	0	0	10
Pure Fruit Pop Pomegranate Blends	1 (1.75 oz)	40	0	0	10
Dippin' Dots					
Cherry Berry	½ cup	90	0	0	23
Watermelon	½ cup	90	0	0	23
Haagen-Dazs					
Fat Free Sorbet Mango	½ cup (4 oz)	120	0	0	37
Fat Free Sorbet Raspberry	½ cup (3.7 oz)	120	0	0	30
Fat Free Sorbet Zesty Lemon	½ cup (4 oz)	110	0	0	29
Lowfat Sorbet Chocolate	½ cup (3.7 oz)	130	2	1	28
Luigi's					
Italian Ice Cherry	1 (6 oz)	130	0	0	32
Italian Ice Lemon Strawberry	1 (6 oz)	120	0	0	31
Italian Ice No Sugar Added Lemon	1 (6 oz)	60	0	0	20
Italian Ice Pina Colada	1 (6 oz)	130	0	0	33
Swirl Blue Ribbon Lemonade	1 (6 oz)	150	0	0	39
Mr. J					
All Flavors	1 bar (2.25 oz)	50	tr	tr	12
Natural Choice					
Organic Vegan Fruit Bars Coconut	1 (2.75 oz)	90	0	4	16
Organic Vegan Fruit Bars Pink Lemonade	1 (2.75 oz)	50	0	0	13
Organic Vegan Grape	1 (2.75 oz)	50	0	0	13
Organic Vegan Sorbet Blueberry	½ cup	110	0	0	29
Organic Vegan Sorbet Lemon	½ cup	110	0	0	30
Organic Vegan Sorbet Mango	½ cup	110	0	0	29
PickleSickle					
Pop	1 (2 oz)	3	0	0	1
Popsicle					
Creamsicle Pop No Sugar Added	2 (1.65 oz)	45	1	1	10

FOOD	PORTION	CALS	PROT	FAT	CARB
Creamsicle Pop Sugar Free	2 (1.65 oz)	40	1	2	10
Diet Soda Pops	1 (1.6 oz)	15	0	0	3
Firecracker	1 (1.6 oz)	35	0	0	9
Fudgsicle Bar	1 (2.5 oz)	100	2	2	17
Fudgsicle Pops No Sugar Added	1 (1.65 oz)	40	2	1	10
Lifesavers Pop	1 (3.5 oz)	90	0	0	22
Pop Ups Orange Burst	1 (2.75 oz)	90	1	1	18
Rainbow Pops	1 (1.65 oz)	40	0	0	10
Snow Cone	1 (7 oz)	30	0	0	7
SoDelicious					
Dairy Free Creamy Orange Bar	1 (2.2 oz)	80	1	2	18
Sweet Nothings					
Bar Mango Raspberry	1 (2.6 oz)	100	1	0	23
The Power Of Fruit					
Original Fruit Bar	1 (1.75 oz)	28	tr	tr	7
Turkey Hill					
Venice Mango	½ cup	100	0	0	23
Venice Pomegranate Blueberry w/ Acai	½ cup	100	0	0	25

JACKFRUIT

fresh	3.5 oz	70	1	tr	4

JALAPENO (*see* PEPPERS)

JAM/JELLY/PRESERVES

apple butter	1 tbsp (0.6 oz)	31	tr	tr	8
jam all flavors	1 pkg (0.5 oz)	39	tr	tr	10
jam all flavors	1 tbsp (0.7 oz)	56	tr	tr	14
jam apricot	1 tbsp (0.7 oz)	48	tr	tr	13
jam diet all flavors	1 tbsp (0.5 oz)	18	tr	tr	8
jelly all flavors	1 tbsp (0.7 oz)	51	tr	0	13
jelly reduced sugar all flavors	1 tbsp (0.7 oz)	34	tr	tr	9
jelly diet all flavors	1 tbsp (0.7 oz)	25	tr	tr	10
orange marmalade	1 tbsp (0.7 oz)	49	tr	0	13
preserves all flavors	1 tbsp (0.7 oz)	56	tr	tr	14
Cascadian Farm					
Organic Fruit Spread Blackberry	1 tbsp	45	0	0	11
Organic Fruit Spread Raspberry	1 tbsp	45	0	0	11
Organic Sweet Orange Marmalade	1 tbsp	45	0	0	11

FOOD	PORTION	CALS	PROT	FAT	CARB
Chukar Cherries					
Preserves No Sugar Added Cherry Amaretto	1 tbsp	24	0	0	18
Preserves Red Sour Cherry	1 tbsp	40	0	0	10
Preserves Vanilla Peach	1 tbsp	28	0	0	19
Columia Empire Farms					
Marionberry Seedless Perserves	1 tbsp	60	0	0	14
Comfort Care					
Country Apple Butter	1 tbsp (1 oz)	40	0	0	11
Delicia					
Fruit Spread Black Cherry	1 tbsp (0.7 oz)	40	0	0	10
Gedney					
State Fair Preserves Strawberry Rhubarb	1 tbsp	50	0	0	12
Hero					
Swiss Preserves Black Cherry	1 tbsp (0.7 oz)	50	tr	0	13
Revolution Foods					
Organic Jelly Grape	1 tbsp (0.7 oz)	60	0	0	14
Organic Preserves Strawberry	1 tbsp (0.7 oz)	60	0	0	14
Robert Rothchild Farm					
Preserves Cherry Acai	1 tbsp	35	0	0	9
Trappist					
Jelly Pomegranate	1 tbsp (0.7 oz)	50	0	0	14
Tree Of Life					
Organic Fruit Spread Grape	1 tbsp (0.6 oz)	30	8	0	8
Organic Fruit Spread Peach	1 tbsp (0.6 oz)	30	0	0	8
Welch's					
Grape Jelly	1 tbsp	50	0	0	13

JAPANESE FOOD (see ASIAN FOOD, SUSHI)

JELLY (see JAM/JELLY/PRESERVES)

FOOD	PORTION	CALS	PROT	FAT	CARB
JELLYFISH					
pickled	½ cup (1 oz)	10	2	tr	0
JERKY					
beef	1 piece (0.7 oz)	82	7	5	2
pork	1 strip (0.5 oz)	62	5	4	2
venison	1 strip (0.5 oz)	55	5	3	2
Applegate Farms					
Natural Joy Stick	1 (1 oz)	100	9	7	0

FOOD	PORTION	CALS	PROT	FAT	CARB
Dakota Gourmet					
Fruit Jerky Strawberry Kiwi	1	70	tr	0	16
Frank's RedHot					
Chile'N Lime Steak Strips	1 oz	80	10	4	2
Original Beef	1 oz	80	11	1	5
Gary West					
Beef Strips Hickory Smoked	1 oz	70	12	1	5
Buffalo Strips	½ pkg (1 oz)	60	11	0	3
Elk Strips	½ pkg (1 oz)	70	13	1	4
Organic Prairie					
Beef	1 oz	75	9	2	5
Outpost					
Beef	1 oz	70	13	1	4
Beef Steak	1 pkg (0.9 oz)	60	8	3	2
Beef Stick	1 (0.4 oz)	60	2	5	2
Primal					
Mealtless Vegan Hickory Smoke	1 pkg (1 oz)	99	10	3	8
Meatless Vegan Mesquite Lime	1 pkg (1 oz)	74	10	2	7
Meatless Vegan Texas BBQ	1 pkg (1 oz)	81	10	1	11
Meatless Vegan Thai Peanut	1 pkg (1 oz)	74	10	2	8
Slim Jim					
Beef	7 pieces	130	11	8	3
Beef Jerky Hickory Smoked	1 oz	80	12	2	4
Classic Handipack	1 box	210	8	19	3
Giant Caddy Pepperoni	1 pkg	150	6	13	3
Twin Pack Cheese & Pepperoni	1 pkg	150	9	12	2
Tanka					
Natural Buffalo Cranberry Bar	1 (1 oz)	70	7	2	7
Natural Buffalo Cranberry Bite	1 (0.5 oz)	35	4	1	3
Tony's Smokehouse					
Salmon	1 pkg (0.5 oz)	40	7	1	2
JICAMA					
fresh	1 sm (12.8 oz)	139	3	tr	32
raw sliced	1 cup	46	1	tr	11
JUJUBE					
dried	1 oz	82	1	tr	21
JUTE					
cooked	1 cup	32	3	tr	6

FOOD	PORTION	CALS	PROT	FAT	CARB
KALE					
chopped cooked w/o salt	1 cup	36	2	1	7
fresh cooked w/ fat	1 cup	69	2	4	7
scotch chopped cooked w/o salt	1 cup	36	2	1	7
Allens					
Seasoned	½ cup	35	3	1	5
Glory					
Fresh Greens	1 serv (2.8 oz)	40	3	1	8
Seasoned canned	½ cup	35	2	1	5
KANGAROO					
kangaroo	3 oz	120	24	2	–
KEFIR					
kefir	8 oz	98	8	2	12
Evolve					
Plain	8 oz	120	11	3	15
Strawberry	8 oz	180	10	2	31
Helios					
Organic All Fruit Flavors	8 oz	160	8	4	26
Organic Plain	8 oz	120	8	4	12
Lifeway					
Greek Style	8 oz	202	7	14	12
Nonfat All Fruit Flavors	8 oz	188	14	0	33
Nonfat Plain	8 oz	116	14	0	15
Organic Lowfat All Fruit Flavors	8 oz	160	14	2	25
Organic Lowfat Plain	8 oz	110	14	2	12
Original	8 oz	162	8	8	15
Probugs All Flavors	1 bottle	130	9	5	15
Slim6 All Flavors	8 oz	110	14	2	8
Nancy's					
Organic Lowfat Blackberry	1 cup	180	7	3	34
Organic Lowfat Plain	1 cup	110	8	3	14
Organic Lowfat Raspberry	1 cup	180	7	3	35
KETCHUP					
banana	1 tsp	10	0	0	2
ketchup	1 pkg (0.2 oz)	6	tr	tr	2
ketchup	1 tbsp	15	tr	tr	4
low sodium	1 tbsp	15	tr	tr	4
Heinz					
Ketchup	1 tbsp	15	0	0	4
Organic	1 tbsp	20	0	0	5

FOOD	PORTION	CALS	PROT	FAT	CARB
Muir Glen					
Organic	1 tbsp	20	0	0	4
OrganicVille					
No Added Sugar	1 tbsp (0.6 oz)	20	0	0	4
Texas Sassy					
Tequila Ketchup	1 tbsp (0.5 oz)	20	0	0	5
Tree Of Life					
Organic	1 tbsp (0.6 oz)	20	0	0	4
Wholemato					
Organic Agave	1 tbsp	15	0	0	3
KIDNEY					
beef simmered	3 oz	134	23	4	0
lamb braised	3 oz	116	20	3	1
pork braised	3 oz	128	22	4	0
veal braised	3 oz	139	22	5	0
Rumba					
Beef	4 oz	120	19	4	2
KIDNEY BEANS					
canned	½ cup	108	7	1	19
dried cooked w/o salt	½ cup	112	8	tr	20
B&M					
Red Kidney Baked Beans	½ cup (4.6 oz)	200	8	3	36
Progresso					
Cannellini	½ cup (4.6 oz)	110	8	0	20
Van Camp's					
New Orleans	½ cup	90	6	0	19
KIWI					
fresh	1 med (2.6 oz)	46	1	tr	11
fresh	1 lg (3.2 oz)	56	1	tr	13
Chiquita					
Fresh	1 (2.7 oz)	46	1	0	11
KIWI JUICE					
Auna					
Kiwifruit Juice	1 bottle (12 oz)	120	0	0	33
KNISH					
TAKE-OUT					
cheese	1 (2.1 oz)	205	6	12	19
meat	1 (1.8 oz)	174	7	11	13

FOOD	PORTION	CALS	PROT	FAT	CARB
potato	1 lg (7 oz)	332	8	12	49
potato	1 (2.1 oz)	212	5	12	21

KOHLRABI
raw sliced	1 cup	36	2	tr	8
sliced cooked w/o salt	1 cup	48	3	tr	11

TAKE-OUT
creamed	1 cup	150	5	9	14

KRILL
fresh	1 oz	22	3	1	tr

KUMQUATS
canned in syrup	1	13	tr	tr	3
fresh	1	13	tr	tr	3

LAMB
cubed lean & fat braised	4 oz	253	38	10	0
cubed lean broiled	4 oz	211	32	8	0
ground broiled	4 oz	321	28	22	0
leg roasted	4 oz	213	19	15	0
loin chop lean & fat broiled	1 chop (4 oz)	222	17	16	0
rib chop lean & fat broiled	1 chop (1.6 oz)	165	10	14	0
rib roast baked	4 oz	386	25	31	0
shank lean & fat braised	4 oz	360	42	20	0
shoulder chop lean & fat cooked	1 chop (5.5 oz)	274	22	20	0
shoulder w/ bone braised	4 oz	231	19	17	0

LAMB DISHES
TAKE-OUT
keema w/ coconut milk	1 serv (8 oz)	380	13	28	18
moussaka	4 in sq (16 oz)	659	35	43	32
shepherd's pie	1 (21.3 oz)	742	42	31	76
stew w/ potatoes & vegetables	1 cup	260	22	6	29

LAMBSQUARTERS
chopped cooked w/ salt	1 cup	58	6	1	9

LECITHIN
lecithin	1 tbsp	104	0	14	0
Bob's Red Mill					
Lecithin Granules	1 tbsp	60	0	4	1
Tree Of Life					
Granules	1 tbsp (0.3 oz)	55	0	4	1

FOOD	PORTION	CALS	PROT	FAT	CARB
LEEKS					
chopped cooked w/o salt	¼ cup	8	tr	tr	2
cooked	1 (4.4 oz)	38	1	tr	9
freeze dried	1 tbsp	1	tr	0	tr
LEMON					
fresh	1 med (4 oz)	22	1	tr	12
peel	1 tsp	1	tr	0	tr
peel	1 tbsp	3	tr	tr	1
wedge	1 (7 g)	2	tr	tr	1
True Lemon					
Crystallized Lemon	1 pkg (1 g)	0	0	0	tr
LEMON CURD					
lemon curd made w/ egg	2 tsp	29	tr	1	4
Robert Rothchild Farm					
Lemon Curd & Tart Filling	1 tbsp	50	0	2	8
LEMON GRASS					
fresh	1 tbsp	5	tr	tr	1
LEMON JUICE					
bottled	1 tbsp	3	tr	tr	1
bottled	1 oz	6	1	tr	2
fresh	1 oz	8	tr	0	3
from 1 lemon	1.6 oz	12	tr	0	4
from wedge	6 g	1	tr	0	1
Canarino					
Italian Hot Lemon Beverage as prep	1 cup	0	0	0	0
Essn					
Sparkling Meyer Lemon Juice	1 can (8.4 oz)	170	1	0	41
Natalie's Orchid Island Juice					
100% Juice	1 tsp	1	0	0	0
Santa Cruz					
Organic 100% Juice	1 tsp	0	0	0	0
LEMONADE					
READY-TO-DRINK					
Apple & Eve					
Organic	8 oz	130	0	0	32
Minute Maid					
Lemonade	1 can (12 oz)	150	0	0	42

FOOD	PORTION	CALS	PROT	FAT	CARB
Nantucket Nectars					
Lemondade	8 oz	110	0	0	28
Natalie's Orchid Island Juice					
Lemonade	8 oz	130	0	0	33
Odwalla					
PomaGrand	8 oz	110	0	0	28
Pure Squeezed	8 oz	120	0	0	30
Santa Cruz					
Organic Sparkling	8 oz	110	0	0	27
Simply					
Lemonade	8 oz	120	0	0	30
SSips					
Lemonade	8 oz	110	0	0	27
Sweet Leaf					
Half & Half Lemonade Tea	8 oz	85	0	0	20
Original	8 oz	90	tr	0	24
Tropicana					
Light	1 cup	10	0	0	2
Orchard Style	8 oz	120	0	0	31
Twister Light	8 oz	50	0	0	12
Twister Strawberry	8 oz	140	tr	0	35
Turkey Hill					
Lemonade	8 oz	120	0	0	29
Uncle Matt's					
Organic	8 oz	120	tr	0	30
LENTILS					
dried cooked	1 cup	230	18	1	40
Near East					
Lentil Pilaf as prep	1 cup	200	11	3	36
TastyBite					
Jodhpur Lentils	½ pkg (5 oz)	106	6	4	12
Madras Lentils	½ pkg (5 oz)	120	6	5	14
TruRoots					
Organic Sprouted Green not prep	¼ cup (1.4 oz)	140	10	1	25
TAKE-OUT					
lentil loaf	1 slice (1.6 oz)	83	4	4	10
yemiser selatta ethiopian lentil salad	1 serv (3 oz)	115	4	7	11

FOOD	PORTION	CALS	PROT	FAT	CARB
LETTUCE (*see also* SALAD)					
arugula	6 leaves (0.4 oz)	3	tr	tr	tr
arugula shredded	1 cup	5	1	tr	1
boston	1 head (5.7 oz)	21	2	tr	4
boston chopped	6 leaves	7	1	tr	1
cornsalad field salad	1 cup (1.9 oz)	7	1	tr	1
iceberg	6 med leaves	7	tr	tr	1
iceberg	1 lg head (26.5 oz)	106	7	1	22
iceberg shredded	1 cup	10	1	tr	2
looseleaf outer leaves	6 (5 oz)	22	2	tr	4
looseleaf shredded	1 cup	5	tr	tr	1
red leaf	6 leaves (3.6 oz)	16	1	tr	2
red leaf shredded	1 cup	4	tr	tr	1
romaine	3 leaves (3 oz)	14	1	tr	3
romaine heart	6 leaves (1.3 oz)	6	tr	tr	1
romaine shredded	1 cup	8	1	tr	2
Dole					
Classic Romaine	1½ cups (3 oz)	15	1	0	4
Earthbound Farms					
Organic Baby Romaine Salad	2 cups	15	1	0	2
Fresh Express					
5 Lettuce Mix	3 cups	15	1	0	1
Lettuce Trio	2½ cups	15	1	0	3
Organic Baby Arugula	3 cups	20	2	1	3
Organic Hearts Of Romaine	1½ cups	15	1	0	2
Premium Romaine	2 cups	15	1	0	3
Shreds Iceberg	1½ cups	15	1	0	3
Sweet Butter	2½ cups	10	1	0	2
Mann's					
Romaine Hearts	6 leaves (3 oz)	15	1	1	3
Ocean Mist					
Butter Leaf Shredded	1 cup (2 oz)	7	1	0	1
Green Or Green Leaf Shredded	1 cup (1.3 oz)	5	0	0	1
Iceberg	⅙ head (3 oz)	15	1	0	3
LILY ROOT					
dried	1 oz	89	2	1	21
fresh	1 oz	32	1	tr	8

FOOD	PORTION	CALS	PROT	FAT	CARB
LIMA BEANS					
CANNED					
lima beans	½ cup	95	6	tr	18
Allens					
Baby Butter Beans	½ cup	120	7	1	22
Medium Green	½ cup	140	9	1	26
East Texas Fair					
Green	½ cup	120	7	0	23
Hanover					
Butter Beans In Sauce	½ cup	100	7	0	18
DRIED					
cooked	½ cup	150	6	tr	20
FROZEN					
C&W					
Baby	½ cup	110	6	0	20
Green Giant					
Baby & Butter Sauce as prep	⅔ cup	100	5	2	18
LIME					
fresh	1 (2.4 oz)	20	tr	tr	7
wedge	1 (8 g)	2	tr	tr	1
True Lime					
Crystallized Lime	1 pkg	0	0	0	0
LIME JUICE					
bottled	1 oz	6	tr	tr	2
fresh	1 oz	8	tr	tr	3
from 1 lime	1.1 oz	11	tr	tr	4
Angostura					
Lime Mixer	1 tsp	5	0	0	2
Natalie's Orchid Island Juice					
100% Juice	1 tsp	0	0	0	0
Sabor Latino					
Limeade	8 oz	160	0	0	39
Santa Cruz					
Organic 100% Juice	1 tsp	0	0	0	0
Simply					
Limeade	8 oz	120	0	0	31
Sweet Leaf					
Limeade Cherry	8 oz	90	tr	0	24

FOOD	PORTION	CALS	PROT	FAT	CARB
Turkey Hill					
Limonade	8 oz	120	0	0	29
LING					
blue raw	3.5 oz	83	17	1	0
fresh baked	3 oz	95	21	1	0
fresh fillet baked	5.3 oz	168	37	1	0
LINGCOD					
baked	3 oz	93	19	1	0
fillet baked	5.3 oz	164	34	2	0
LIQUOR/LIQUEUR (*see also* BEER AND ALE, CHAMPAGNE, MALT, WINE)					
7&7	1 serv	178	0	0	19
alabama slammer	1 serv	103	tr	tr	7
amaretto sour	1 serv	295	2	tr	57
angel's kiss	1 serv	85	tr	1	5
antifreeze	1 serv	177	1	tr	31
apricot sour	1 serv	164	tr	tr	8
aquavit	1 oz	65	0	0	0
b 52	1 serv	247	1	4	25
b&b	1 serv	75	0	0	0
bahama breeze	1 serv	70	tr	tr	9
bahama mama	1 serv	153	1	tr	23
bailey's & amaretto	1 serv	184	1	5	16
banana colada	1 serv	376	2	1	64
bay breeze	1 serv	173	1	tr	18
bend me over	1 serv	242	1	tr	32
betsy ross	1 serv	206	tr	0	5
black devil	1 serv	220	tr	tr	1
black russian	1 serv	184	0	tr	12
bloody mary	1 serv	150	1	tr	5
blue whale	1 serv	222	tr	tr	23
bourbon & soda	1 serv (4 oz)	105	0	0	0
bourbon sour	1 serv	166	tr	tr	8
brandy alexander	1 serv	266	1	6	12
brandy sour	1 serv	164	tr	tr	8
bushwacker	1 serv	286	tr	5	27
coffee liqueur	1 serv (1.5 oz)	175	tr	tr	24
cognac	1 oz	67	0	0	tr
cosmopolitan martini	1 serv	126	tr	tr	7
creme de menthe	1 serv (1.5 oz)	186	0	tr	21

FOOD	PORTION	CALS	PROT	FAT	CARB
daiquiri	1 serv (2 oz)	112	tr	tr	4
daiquiri banana	1 serv	277	1	tr	32
dark & stormy	1 serv	64	0	0	0
doctor pepper	1 serv	95	0	0	12
frozen daiquiri pineapple	1 serv	186	1	tr	28
frozen tequila screwdriver	1 serv	159	1	tr	17
fuzzy navel	1 serv	247	1	tr	10
gin	1 serv (1.5 oz)	110	0	0	0
gin & tonic	1 serv (7.5 oz)	171	0	0	16
gin ricky	1 serv	114	tr	tr	1
grasshopper	1 serv	275	1	5	26
happy hawaiian	1 serv	434	2	8	60
harvey wallbanger	1 serv	198	1	tr	16
head banger	1 serv	165	0	0	4
hot buttered rum	1 serv (8.8 oz)	316	tr	12	4
hot toddy	1 serv	188	tr	1	13
hurricane	1 serv	205	tr	tr	19
kamikaze	1 serv	136	0	0	2
long island iced tea	1 serv	292	tr	tr	7
lynchburg lemonade	1 serv	465	tr	tr	85
mai tai	1 serv	165	tr	tr	17
manhattan	1 serv	171	tr	tr	3
margarita	1 serv	173	0	0	11
margarita strawberry	1 serv	106	tr	tr	11
martini	1 serv (3 oz)	206	tr	0	2
martini apple	1 serv	147	tr	tr	4
martini rum	1 serv	131	tr	0	tr
mellow yellow	1 serv	95	0	0	4
mexican grasshopper	1 serv	638	1	19	52
mint julep	1 serv	136	tr	tr	17
mississippi mud	1 serv	496	3	12	46
mudslide	1 serv	566	2	10	46
narragansett	1 serv	168	0	0	2
nutcracker	1 serv	730	2	10	64
old fashioned	1 serv	223	tr	tr	4
orange crush	1 serv	461	0	0	65
pain killer	1 serv	277	1	tr	20
peppermint pattie	1 serv	344	tr	tr	37
pina colada	1 serv (4.5 oz)	245	1	3	32
planter's cocktail	1 serv	105	tr	0	3

FOOD	PORTION	CALS	PROT	FAT	CARB
planter's punch	1 serv	233	2	tr	34
presbyterian	1 serv	170	tr	0	8
purple passion	1 serv	215	tr	tr	22
rob roy	1 serv	171	tr	0	3
rum	1 serv (1.5 oz)	97	0	0	0
rum boogie	1 serv	134	tr	tr	12
rum cola	1 serv	209	tr	tr	21
rum highball	1 serv	170	0	0	11
rum punch	1 serv	448	1	1	88
rum screwdriver	1 serv	166	1	tr	16
rum sour	1 serv	156	tr	tr	8
rum swizzle	1 serv	187	0	0	15
rusty nail	1 serv	159	0	0	6
sake	1 serv (1 oz)	39	tr	0	1
salty dog	1 serv	210	1	tr	19
scotch & soda	1 serv	104	tr	0	tr
sea breeze	1 serv	207	tr	tr	19
sex on the beach	1 serv	190	tr	tr	18
slippery nipple	1 serv	142	tr	2	11
sloe gin fizz	1 serv (2.5 oz)	132	0	0	4
snake bite	1 serv	362	0	0	22
tequila gimlet	1 serv	150	tr	tr	6
tequila sour	1 serv	156	tr	tr	8
tequila stinger	1 serv	221	0	tr	14
tequila sunrise	1 serv (6.8 oz)	232	1	tr	24
tom collins	1 serv (7.5 oz)	121	tr	0	3
vermouth cassis	1 serv	97	tr	tr	5
vodka	1 serv (1.5 oz)	97	0	0	0
vodka gimlet	1 serv	150	tr	tr	6
vodka sour	1 serv	138	tr	tr	3
vodka stinger	1 serv	378	0	tr	28
whiskey	1 serv (1.5 oz)	105	0	0	tr
whiskey sour	1 serv (3.5 oz)	162	tr	tr	14
white russian	1 serv	290	tr	8	17
zombie	1 serv	235	tr	tr	10

LIVER (see also PATE)

FOOD	PORTION	CALS	PROT	FAT	CARB
beef braised	1 slice (2.4 oz)	130	20	4	3
beef pan-fried	1 slice (2.8 oz)	142	21	4	4
chicken fried	3 oz	146	22	5	1
chicken simmered	3 oz	142	21	6	1

FOOD	PORTION	CALS	PROT	FAT	CARB
duck raw	1 (1.5 oz)	60	8	2	2
goose raw	1 (3.3 oz)	125	15	4	6
lamb braised	3 oz	187	26	7	2
lamb fried	3 oz	202	22	11	3
moose braised	3 oz	132	21	4	3
pork braised	3 oz	140	22	4	3
turkey simmered	1 liver (2.9 oz)	227	17	17	1
veal braised	1 slice (2.8 oz)	154	23	5	3
veal pan fried	1 slice (2.4 oz)	129	18	4	3
Organic Prairie					
Beef	2 oz	80	11	2	2
Perdue					
Chicken Fresh	4 oz	130	19	6	0
Rumba					
Beef	4 oz	160	22	5	7
TAKE-OUT					
calves liver w/ onions	1 serv (5 oz)	177	24	4	10
LLAMA					
llama	3 oz	120	22	3	–
LOBSTER					
northern cooked	3 oz	83	17	1	1
northern cooked	1 cup	142	30	1	2
northern raw	3 oz	77	77	1	tr
northern raw	1 lobster (5.3 oz)	136	28	1	1
spiny steamed	3 oz	122	22	2	3
spiny steamed	1 (5.7 oz)	233	43	3	5
TAKE-OUT					
newburg	1 cup	485	46	27	13
LOGANBERRIES					
fresh	½ cup (2.5 oz)	40	1	tr	9
frzn thawed	½ cup (2.6 oz)	40	1	tr	10
LONGANS					
fresh	1	2	tr	0	tr
LOQUATS					
fresh	1 sm (0.5 oz)	6	tr	tr	2
fresh	1 lg (0.7 oz)	9	tr	tr	2
fresh cubed	½ cup (2.6 oz)	35	tr	tr	9

FOOD	PORTION	CALS	PROT	FAT	CARB
LOTUS					
root raw sliced	10 slices	45	2	tr	14
root sliced cooked	10 slices	59	1	tr	14
seeds dried	1 oz	94	4	1	18
LOX (see SALMON)					
LUPINES					
dried cooked	1 cup	197	26	5	16
LYCHEES					
canned in syrup	½ cup (4.4 oz)	114	1	tr	29
canned in syrup	1 (0.7 oz)	19	tr	tr	5
dried	1 (2.5 g)	7	tr	tr	2
fresh	1 (0.3 oz)	6	tr	tr	2
fresh cut up	½ cup (3.3 oz)	63	1	tr	16
Polar					
Lychee	1	110	tr	0	27
MACA ROOT					
Navitas Naturals					
Powder Gelatanized	1 tsp (5 g)	20	1	0	3
Raw Powder	1 tsp (5 g)	20	1	0	4
MACADAMIA NUTS					
dry roasted w/ salt	11 nuts (1 oz)	200	2	22	4
oil roasted	1 oz	204	2	22	4
Chukar Cherries					
Extra Dark Chocolate Covered	3 tbsp (1.4 oz)	216	2	20	14
Emily's					
Milk Chocolate Covered	4 (1.5 oz)	260	3	19	21
Fisher					
Macadamia Nuts	¼ cup (1 oz)	200	2	21	4
Hawaiian Host					
White Choco	3 pieces (1.4 oz)	230	1	15	22
Mauna Loa					
Dry Roasted Salted	¼ cup (1 oz)	230	2	24	4
Dry Roasted Unsalted	¼ cup (1 oz)	230	2	24	4
Honey Roasted	¼ cup (1 oz)	200	2	19	9
Kona Coffee	¼ cup (1 oz)	180	1	15	12
Maui Onion & Garlic	1 pkg (1.2 oz)	230	2	23	5

FOOD	PORTION	CALS	PROT	FAT	CARB
MACE					
ground	1 tsp	8	tr	1	1
MACKEREL					
CANNED					
jack	1 can (12.7 oz)	563	84	23	0
jack	1 cup	296	44	12	0
Polar					
Jack	1/3 cup	90	13	4	0
FRESH					
atlantic cooked	3 oz	223	20	15	0
atlantic raw	3 oz	174	16	12	0
jack baked	3 oz	171	22	9	0
jack fillet baked	6.2 oz	354	45	18	0
king baked	3 oz	114	22	2	0
king fillet baked	5.4 oz	207	40	4	0
pacific baked	3 oz	171	22	9	0
pacific fillet baked	6.2 oz	354	45	18	0
spanish cooked	3 oz	134	20	5	0
spanish cooked	1 fillet (5.1 oz)	230	34	9	0
spanish raw	3 oz	118	16	5	0
SMOKED					
atlantic	3.5 oz	296	19	24	0
MAHI MAHI					
fresh baked	4 oz	192	18	13	1
MALANGA					
dasheen mashed	1 cup	226	3	tr	53
dasheen pieces boiled	1 cup	212	3	tr	50
pieces fried	1 cup	304	1	11	52
root raw	1 (10.7 oz)	299	5	1	72
MALT					
malt liquor	1 bottle (12 oz)	148	1	0	13
nonalcoholic	1 bottle (12 oz)	133	1	tr	29
MALTED MILK					
chocolate as prep w/ milk	1 cup	179	8	5	27
chocolate flavor powder	3 heaping tsp (0.7 oz)	79	1	1	18
natural flavor as prep w/ milk	1 cup	186	9	6	24

FOOD	PORTION	CALS	PROT	FAT	CARB
natural flavor powder	3 heaping tsp (0.7 oz)	87	2	2	16

MAMMY-APPLE
fresh	1	431	4	4	106

MANGO
dried	1 slice (5 g)	16	tr	tr	4
dried	½ cup (1.8 oz)	74	1	tr	41
fresh	1 (7.3 oz)	135	1	1	35
fresh sliced	½ cup (3 oz)	54	tr	tr	14
pickled	1 slice (1 oz)	38	tr	tr	10
C&W					
Chunks	¾ cup	90	tr	0	24
Kopali					
Organic Dried	1 pkg (1.8 oz)	140	0	0	38
Peeled Snacks					
Fruit Picks Go-Mango-Man-Go	1 pkg (1.4 oz)	120	2	0	28
Polar					
Sliced	3 pieces (5 oz)	100	0	0	24
Sunsweet					
Philippine dried	6 pieces (1.5 oz)	130	1	0	30
Thailand dried	⅓ cup (1.4 oz)	140	0	0	34

MANGO JUICE
nectar canned	1 cup (8.8 oz)	128	tr	tr	33
GoodBelly					
Mango Probiotic Drink	8 oz	100	tr	0	25
Old Orchard					
Nectar Cocktail	8 oz	120	0	0	30
Snapple					
Juice Drinks Mango Madness	8 oz	100	0	0	26

MANGOSTEEN
canned in syrup	½ cup (3.4 oz)	72	tr	1	18

MARGARINE
margarine butter blend	1 tbsp (0.5 oz)	101	tr	11	tr
squeeze	1 pkg (0.2 oz)	36	tr	4	0
squeeze liquid	1 tbsp (0.5 oz)	102	tr	11	0
stick	1 tbsp (0.5 oz)	100	tr	11	tr
stick	1 stick (4 oz)	810	tr	91	1

FOOD	PORTION	CALS	PROT	FAT	CARB
tub diet	1 tbsp (0.5 oz)	26	0	3	tr
tub fat free	1 tbsp (0.5 oz)	27	tr	tr	1
tub light	1 tbsp (0.5 oz)	59	tr	7	tr
tub salted	1 tbsp (0.5 oz)	101	tr	11	tr
whipped salted	1 tbsp (0.3 oz)	67	tr	8	tr
Benecol					
Spread Light	1 tbsp	50	0	5	0
Spread Regular	1 tbsp	70	0	8	0
Brummel & Brown					
Creamy Fruit Spread Strawberry	1 tbsp	50	0	4	3
Spread w/ Natural Yogurt	1 tbsp (0.5 oz)	45	0	5	0
Country Crock					
Light	1 tbsp (0.5 oz)	50	0	5	0
Regular	1 tbsp (0.5 oz)	90	0	7	0
Spread w/ Calcium + Vitamin D	1 tbsp (0.5 oz)	50	0	5	0
Earth Balance					
Butter Blend Salted	1 tbsp	100	0	11	0
Buttery Spread Original	1 tbsp	100	0	11	0
Buttery Spread Soy Garden	1 tbsp	100	0	11	0
Buttery Sticks Vegan	1 tbsp	100	0	11	0
Land O' Lakes					
Soft	1 tbsp (0.5 oz)	100	0	11	0
Stick	1 tbsp (0.5 oz)	100	0	11	0
Move Over Butter					
Spread	1 tbsp	50	0	6	0
Promise					
Buttery Spread	1 tbsp	80	0	8	0
Buttery Spread Activ	1 tbsp	70	0	8	0
Fat Free	1 tbsp	5	0	0	0
Light	1 tbsp	45	0	5	0
Light Activ	1 tbsp	45	0	5	0
Smart Balance					
Omega Plus w/ Flax Oil	1 tbsp	80	0	9	0

MARINADE (see SAUCE)

MARJORAM

dried	1 tsp	2	tr	tr	tr

MARLIN

raw	3 oz	110	20	3	0

FOOD	PORTION	CALS	PROT	FAT	CARB
MARSHMALLOW					
chocolate coated	1 (0.4 oz)	41	tr	1	8
coconut coated	1 (0.4 oz)	33	tr	1	7
marshmallow regular	1 (0.3 oz)	23	tr	tr	6
miniatures	1 cup (1.8 oz)	159	1	tr	41
miniatures	10 (0.3 oz)	22	tr	tr	6
MATZO					
brie	1 piece (0.5 oz)	54	1	3	5
egg	1 (1 oz)	109	3	1	22
matzo ball	1 med (1.2 oz)	48	2	2	6
plain	1 (1 oz)	111	3	tr	23
whole wheat	1 (1 oz)	98	4	tr	22
Holiday Candies					
Dark Chocolate Coated	1 oz	130	2	5	20
Manischewitz					
Egg & Onion	1 (1 oz)	100	3	1	23
Matzo Ball Mix	2 tbsp	50	1	0	11
Yehuda					
Organic	1 (1 oz)	110	4	1	23
MAYONNAISE					
diet	1 tbsp	36	tr	3	3
imitation	1 tbsp	35	tr	3	2
mayonnaise	1 tbsp	99	tr	11	1
Cains					
All Natural	1 tbsp	100	0	11	0
Light	1 tbsp	50	0	5	2
Hellman's					
Light	1 tbsp	45	0	5	tr
Real	1 tbsp	90	0	10	0
Real Canola No Cholesterol	1 tbsp	90	0	10	0
Reduced Fat	1 tbsp	20	0	2	2
W/ Extra Virgin Olive Oil	1 tbsp	50	0	5	tr
Hollywood					
Canola	1 tbsp	100	0	11	0
Safflower	1 tbsp	100	0	11	0
Kraft					
Mayo	1 tbsp	90	0	10	0
Mayo W/ Olive Oil	1 tbsp	45	0	4	2

FOOD	PORTION	CALS	PROT	FAT	CARB
Miracle Whip					
Free	1 tbsp	15	0	0	3
Light	1 tbsp	25	0	2	3
Original	1 tbsp	40	0	3	2
NatureNaise					
Organic Spread	1 tbsp (0.5 oz)	40	1	3	2
Smart Balance					
Omega	1 tbsp	120	0	14	0
Omega Plus	1 tbsp	50	0	5	2
Vegenaise					
Grapeseed Oil	1 tbsp (0.5 oz)	90	0	9	0
Organic	1 tbsp (0.5 oz)	90	0	9	0
Original	1 tbsp (0.5 oz)	90	0	9	0

MEAT SUBSTITUTES (*see also* BACON SUBSTITUTES, CANADIAN BACON SUBSTITUTES, CHICKEN SUBSTITUTES, HAMBURGER SUBSTITUTES, MEATBALL SUBSTITUTES, SAUSAGE SUBSTITUTES, TURKEY SUBSTITUTES)

FOOD	PORTION	CALS	PROT	FAT	CARB
Amy's					
Veggie Loaf w/ Mashed Potatoes & Vegetables	1 pkg (10 oz)	290	9	8	47
Gardenburger					
BBQ Riblets w/ Sauce	1 serv (5 oz)	240	17	5	33
Helen's Kitchen					
GardenSteak Tofu Steak	1 (3 oz)	150	12	2	14
Loma Linda					
Dinner Cuts	2 slices (3.2 oz)	90	18	1	4
Swiss Stake	1 piece (3.2 oz)	130	9	6	9
Morningstar Farms					
Meal Starters Steak Strips	12 pieces (3 oz)	140	23	3	5
Veat					
Gourmet Bites	1 serv (2.5 oz)	90	8	3	8
Vegetarian Fillet	1 (1.8 oz)	170	15	5	19
Worthington					
Bolono	3 slices (2 oz)	80	11	3	3
Choplets	2 slices (3.2 oz)	90	18	1	4
Corned Beef Vegetarian	3 slices (2 oz)	140	10	9	5
Dinner Roast	1 slice (3 oz)	180	14	11	6
Multigrain Cutlets	2 slices (3.2 oz)	100	17	1	5

FOOD	PORTION	CALS	PROT	FAT	CARB
Prime Stakes	1 piece (3.2 oz)	120	9	6	7
Vegetable Skallops	½ cup (3 oz)	90	17	1	4
Wham	2 slices (2 oz)	110	10	7	3
Yves					
Meatless Beef Skewers	1 (2.8 oz)	100	14	1	10
Meatless Bologna	4 slices	60	14	3	2
Meatless Ground Round Original	⅓ cup	60	10	1	5
Meatless Pepperoni	6 slices	90	14	1	4

MEATBALL SUBSTITUTES

FOOD	PORTION	CALS	PROT	FAT	CARB
meatless	2 (1.3 oz)	71	8	3	3
Gardenburger					
Mama Mia Meatballs	6 (3 oz)	110	12	5	7
Loma Linda					
Tender Rounds	6 (2.8 oz)	120	13	5	6

MEATBALLS

FOOD	PORTION	CALS	PROT	FAT	CARB
beef cocktail	1 (0.2 oz)	18	2	1	0
beef lg	1 (1.5 oz)	111	11	7	0
beef med	1 (1 oz)	74	7	5	0
chicken cocktail	1 (0.2 oz)	12	1	tr	1
chicken lg	1 (1.5 oz)	71	8	3	3
chicken med	1 (1 oz)	47	6	2	2
turkey med	1 (1 oz)	47	6	2	2
Butterball					
Seasoned Italian frzn	6 (3 oz)	170	21	6	6
DelGrosso					
Italian Style	3 (3 oz)	180	13	12	5
Honeysuckle White					
Turkey Italian Style frzn	3 (3 oz)	190	17	10	6
Mama Lucia					
Homestyle	4	207	14	20	8
Italian Style	4	280	11	23	8
Sausage Beef	8	220	14	17	3
Organic Classics					
Italian Beef	3 (3 oz)	180	17	11	5
Perdue					
Turkey Italian Style	4 (3 oz)	180	15	10	5

FOOD	PORTION	CALS	PROT	FAT	CARB
Shady Brook					
Turkey Meatballs Appetizer Size + Sweet & Sour Sauce	6 + 2 tbsp sauce	235	17	10	17
Tyson					
Italian Style Chicken	6 (3 oz)	180	13	11	6
TAKE-OUT					
albondigas w/ sauce	3 + sauce (5.3 oz)	372	21	27	11
porcupine + tomato sauce	3 + sauce	160	11	7	14
swedish w/ cream sauce	3 + sauce (4.7 oz)	215	17	12	9
sweet & sour	3 + sauce (4.5 oz)	188	15	11	8

MELON

FOOD	PORTION	CALS	PROT	FAT	CARB
sprite	1 (10.6 oz)	110	1	0	29

MEXICAN FOOD (see SALSA, SPANISH FOOD, TORTILLA)

MILK
CANNED

FOOD	PORTION	CALS	PROT	FAT	CARB
condensed sweetened	1 tbsp (0.7 oz)	61	2	2	10
condensed sweetened	1 cup (10.7 oz)	982	24	27	166
evaporated nonfat	1 cup (9 oz)	200	19	1	29
evaporated nonfat	1 tbsp (0.5 oz)	12	1	tr	2
Borden					
Sweetened Condensed Low Fat	2 tbsp	120	3	2	23
Carnation					
Evaporated	2 tbsp	40	2	2	3
Evaporated Fat Free	2 tbsp (1 oz)	25	2	0	4
Evaporated Lowfat 2%	2 tbsp (1 oz)	25	2	1	3
DRIED					
buttermilk	1 tbsp (0.2 oz)	25	2	tr	3
buttermilk	¼ cup (1 oz)	111	10	2	14
nonfat instant	1 pkg (3.2 oz)	326	32	1	47
nonfat instant	1 tbsp (0.6 oz)	61	6	tr	9
whole milk	¼ cup (1.1 oz)	159	8	9	12
Alba					
Instant Non-Fat as prep	1 cup	80	8	0	11
Bob's Red Mill					
Buttermilk Sweet Cream as prep	8 oz	60	5	1	7
Non Fat as prep	8 oz	80	7	0	11

FOOD	PORTION	CALS	PROT	FAT	CARB
Carnation					
Instant Nonfat as prep	1 cup	80	8	0	12
Organic Valley					
Buttermilk	3 tbsp	110	10	1	16
Nonfat	3 tbsp	90	9	0	13
Sanalac					
Powder	¼ cup (0.8 oz)	80	8	0	13
REFRIGERATED					
1%	1 cup (8.6 oz)	102	8	3	12
2%	1 cup (8.6 oz)	122	8	5	11
buffalo	7 oz	224	8	16	10
buttermilk lowfat	1 cup (8.6 oz)	98	8	2	12
camel	7 oz	160	10	8	10
donkey	7 oz	86	4	2	12
fat free	1 cup (8.6 oz)	83	8	tr	12
goat	1 cup (8.6 oz)	168	9	10	11
human	1 cup (8.6 oz)	172	3	11	17
indian buffalo	1 cup (8.6 oz)	237	9	17	13
mare	7 oz	98	4	4	12
sheep	1 cup (8.6 oz)	265	15	17	13
whole	1 cup (8.6 oz)	146	8	8	11
Active Lifestyle					
Fat Free w/ Plant Sterols	8 oz	90	8	0	13
Dairy Ease					
Fat Free Lactose Free	1 cup (8 oz)	90	8	0	12
Reduced Fat 2% Lactose Free	1 cup (8 oz)	130	9	5	12
Whole Lactose Free	1 cup (8 oz)	160	8	9	11
Farmland					
Buttermilk	8 oz	160	12	4	19
Fat Free	8 oz	80	8	0	12
Special Request 1% Plus Omega-3	8 oz	130	11	3	17
Special Request Skim Plus	8 oz	110	11	0	17
Special Request Skim Plus 100% Lactose Free	8 oz	110	11	0	17
Whole	8 oz	160	12	4	19
Friendship					
Buttermilk Lowfat	1 cup	120	9	4	12
Horizon Organic					
Fat Free	8 oz	90	9	0	12

FOOD	PORTION	CALS	PROT	FAT	CARB
Land O' Lakes					
1%	1 cup (8 oz)	100	8	3	13
2%	1 cup (8 oz)	120	8	5	12
Skim	1 cup (8 oz)	90	8	0	13
Whole	1 cup (8 oz)	150	8	8	12
Organic Valley					
Fat Free	1 cup	90	8	0	13
Lactose Free Fat Free	1 cup	90	8	0	14
Whole Nonhomogenized	1 cup	150	8	8	12
Straus					
Organic Reduced Fat 2% Cream Top	8 oz	130	10	5	13
SunMilk					
Heart Healthy 1% Sunflower Oil	8 oz	120	11	2	15
Heart Healthy 2% Sunflower Oil	8 oz	120	10	3	15
Turkey Hill					
Cool Moos Whole Milk	8 oz	160	8	3	27
Tuscan					
Whole	8 oz	150	8	8	12
Valio					
100% Lactose Free 0% Fat	8 oz	80	11	0	7
100% Lactose Free 2% Fat	8 oz	120	11	5	7
Welsh Farms					
Fat Free	8 oz	80	8	0	12
SHELF-STABLE					
Parmalat					
2% Reduced Fat	8 oz	130	8	5	12
Fat Free	8 oz	80	8	0	12
Lactose Free 2% Reduced Fat	8 oz	130	8	5	12
MILK DRINKS					
chocolate milk	1 cup (8.8 oz)	208	8	8	26
chocolate milk lowfat	1 cup (8.8 oz)	158	8	3	26
Bravo!					
Blenders Creamy Double Chocolate	1 bottle (11 oz)	180	17	4	19
Blenders Creamy French Vanilla	1 bottle (11 oz)	160	17	4	20
Cocio					
Chocolate Milk	8 oz	140	6	4	20

FOOD	PORTION	CALS	PROT	FAT	CARB
CocoaVia					
Indulgence Rich Chocolate	1 bottle (5.65 oz)	150	6	3	28
Dove					
Bravo! Dark Chocolate	1 bottle	310	8	16	37
Bravo! Milk Chocolate	1 bottle	310	8	16	36
Farmland					
Really Really Good! Chocolate Milk	8 oz	160	8	3	25
Horizon Organic					
Lowfat Chocolate Milk	8 oz	170	8	3	27
Strawberry	8 oz	200	8	5	31
Land O' Lakes					
2% Swiss Chocolate	1 cup (8.4 oz)	190	8	5	26
Chocolate Skim	1 cup (8 oz)	160	8	0	31
Strawberry	1 cup (8 oz)	190	7	8	22
Lifeway					
La Fruta All Flavors	8 oz	180	8	2	33
Nesquik					
Chocolate Powder No Sugar Added as prep w/ lowfat milk	1 cup (8 oz)	160	1	5	18
Chocolate Powder as prep w/ lowfat milk	1 cup (8 oz)	180	tr	5	27
Ready-To-Drink Banana	1 cup (8 oz)	200	7	5	30
Ready-To-Drink Chocolate	1 cup (8 oz)	200	8	5	32
Ready-To-Drink Strawberry	1 cup (8 oz)	200	8	5	33
Ready-To-Drink Vanilla	1 cup (8 oz)	200	8	5	30
Strawberry Powder as prep w/ lowfat milk	1 cup (8 oz)	190	0	4	27
Strawberry Powder not prep	2 tbsp (0.6 oz)	60	0	0	15
Organic Valley					
Buttermilk Lowfat 1%	1 cup	100	8	3	12
Parmalat					
Chocolate Milk 2% Reduced Fat	1 cup	190	8	5	28
Sipahh					
Straw Banana	1 straw	15	0	0	3
Straw Cookies and Cream	1 straw	15	0	0	3
Turkey Hill					
Cool Moos 2% Reduced Fat	8 oz	120	8	5	12
Cool Moos Chocolate	8 oz	180	8	3	32

FOOD	PORTION	CALS	PROT	FAT	CARB
MILK SUBSTITUTES					
soy milk	1 cup	79	7	5	4
Brazsoy					
Condensed Soy Milk	1 serv (0.7 oz)	54	1	1	10
Soy Cream	1 tbsp (0.5 oz)	27	0	3	0
Lifeway					
SoyTreat All Flavors	8 oz	160	7	4	23
Living Harvest					
Hempmilk Original	1 cup	130	4	3	20
Hempmilk Vanilla	1 cup	130	4	3	20
Lundberg					
Organic Drink Rice Original	8 oz	120	1	3	22
Manitoba Harvest					
Hemp Bliss Chocolate	8 oz	160	5	7	17
Hemp Bliss Original	1 cup	110	5	7	7
Hemp Bliss Vanilla	8 oz	150	5	7	14
Odwalla					
Soy Smart Chai	8 oz	150	6	4	22
Soy Smart Vanilla	8 oz	120	6	4	15
Soymilk Plain	8 oz	110	7	4	12
Soymilk Vanilla Being	8 oz	100	4	3	13
Organic Valley					
Soy Original	1 cup	100	7	3	11
Soy Unsweetened	1 cup	80	7	4	3
Rice Dream					
Carob	8 oz	150	1	3	30
Heartwise Vanilla	8 oz	140	1	2	30
Horchata	8 oz	130	7	4	16
Original	8 oz	120	1	3	24
Original Enriched	8 oz	120	1	3	23
Vanilla Enriched	8 oz	130	1	3	26
Silk					
Chocolate	1 cup (8 oz)	140	5	4	23
Plain	8 oz	100	7	4	8
Soy Heart Health	1 cup	80	6	2	10
Soy Plain Light	1 cup	70	6	2	8
Soy Plus DHA Omega-3	1 cup	110	7	5	8
Soy Pumpkin Spice	1 cup	170	6	4	28
Soy Unsweetened	1 cup	80	7	4	4
Vanilla	1 cup (8 oz)	100	6	4	10

FOOD	PORTION	CALS	PROT	FAT	CARB
Soy Dream					
Classic Vanilla	8 oz	140	7	4	18
Original Enriched	8 oz	100	7	4	8
SoyZen					
Soy Milk Cappuccino	8 oz	150	7	4	22
WildWood					
Organic Probiotic Soymilk Blueberry	8 oz	190	7	3	33
Organic Probiotic Soymilk Pomegranate	8 oz	180	7	3	31
Organic Soymilk Plain	8 oz	100	7	4	8
Organic Soymilk Unsweetened	8 oz	72	7	4	3
ZenSoy					
Soy Milk Chocolate	8 oz	170	7	4	27
Soy Milk Plain	8 oz	90	7	4	9
Soy Milk Vanilla	8 oz	110	7	4	14
Soy On The Go Vanilla w/ Omega 3	1 pkg (8.25 oz)	110	7	4	14
MILKFISH (AWA)					
baked	4 oz	215	30	10	0
MILKSHAKE					
chocolate	1 serv (10.6 oz)	357	9	8	63
malted milkshake	1 serv (10 oz)	402	9	14	62
vanilla	1 (11 oz)	351	12	9	56
Buffy's Cool Cow					
Chocolate	1 pkg (8 oz)	150	9	3	23
Vanilla	1 pkg (8 oz)	150	9	3	24
Lean Body					
Hi-Protein Chocolate Ice Cream	1 (17 oz)	260	40	9	9
Molli Coolz					
Shakers Vanilla as prep w/ skim milk	1 (10.2 oz)	240	3	10	30
Nesquik					
Ready-To-Drink Chocolate	1 cup (8 oz)	170	8	5	26
Silhouette Solution					
Colossal Chocolate not prep	1 pkg (1.05 oz)	110	15	3	8
Vanilla Creme not prep	1 pkg (1.02 oz)	100	15	2	8

FOOD	PORTION	CALS	PROT	FAT	CARB
MILLET					
cooked	1 cup (6.1 oz)	207	6	2	41
Arrowhead Mills					
Organic Hulled not prep	¼ cup	150	4	2	33
MINERAL WATER (*see* WATER)					
MISO					
dried	1 oz	86	7	3	10
miso	½ cup	284	16	8	39
MOLASSES					
blackstrap	1 tbsp (0.7 oz)	47	0	0	12
molasses	¼ cup (3 oz)	244	0	tr	63
molasses	1 tbsp (0.7 oz)	58	0	tr	15
Tree Of Life					
Blackstrap Unsulphured	1 tbsp	45	0	0	11
MONKFISH					
baked	3 oz	82	16	2	0
MOOSE					
roasted	4 oz	142	31	1	0
MOTH BEANS					
dried cooked	1 cup	207	14	1	37
MOUSSE					
TAKE-OUT					
chocolate	½ cup	454	8	32	32
fish timbale	1 cup	329	22	25	3
MUFFIN					
MIX					
blueberry as prep	1 (1.75 oz)	149	3	4	24
corn as prep	1 (1.75 oz)	160	4	5	25
wheat bran as prep	1 (1.75 oz)	138	5	5	23
Betty Crocker					
Banana Nut as prep	1	120	2	3	22
Blueberry as prep	1	120	2	3	23
Cornbread Muffin as prep	1	160	2	6	24
Fiber One Banana Nut as prep	1	170	2	7	27
Fiber One Blueberry as prep	1	160	2	6	30
Lemon Poppyseed as prep	1	200	2	8	29

FOOD	PORTION	CALS	PROT	FAT	CARB
Duncan Hines					
Blueberry Streusel as prep	1	210	3	8	32
Cinnamon Swirl 100% Whole Grain as prep	1	220	3	8	34
Triple Chocolate Chunk 100% Whole Grain as prep	1	240	4	11	35
Glory					
Golden Sweet Corn as prep	1	170	2	5	27
Martha White					
Whole Grain Apple Cinnamon not prep	¼ cup (1.2 oz)	140	2	4	24
Whole Grain Blueberry not prep	¼ cup (1.2 oz)	140	2	4	24
Yellow Corn not prep	¼ cup (1.2 oz)	140	2	3	26
Miracle Muffins					
Banana w/ Splenda as prep	1	86	9	3	12
READY-TO-EAT					
blueberry	1 (2 oz)	158	3	4	27
oat bran wheat free	1 (2 oz)	154	4	4	28
toaster type blueberry	1	103	2	3	18
toaster type corn	1	114	2	4	19
toaster type wheat bran w/ raisins	1 (1.3 oz)	106	2	3	19
Hostess					
100 Calorie Pack Mini Banana Streusel	1 pkg (1.2 oz)	100	2	4	19
100 Calorie Pack Mini Blueberry Streusel	1 pkg (1.2 oz)	100	2	3	20
VitaMuffin					
AppleBerryBran	1 (2 oz)	100	3	0	25
BlueBran	1 (2 oz)	100	3	0	24
CranBran	1 (2 oz)	100	3	0	24
Sugar Free Low Carb Banana Nut	1 (2 oz)	90	5	2	24
VitaTops Banana Nut	1 (2 oz)	100	5	2	19
VitaTops Dark Chocolate Pomegranate	1 (2 oz)	100	3	2	21
VitaTops Deep Chocolate	1 (2 oz)	100	4	2	25
VitaTops Golden Corn	1 (2 oz)	100	4	1	25
VitaTops MultiBran	1 (2 oz)	100	4	1	22

FOOD	PORTION	CALS	PROT	FAT	CARB
TAKE-OUT					
corn	1 lg (2.5 oz)	214	5	7	32
raisin bran lowfat	1 (4 oz)	270	5	1	61
MULBERRIES					
fresh	20 (1 oz)	13	tr	tr	3
fresh	½ cup (2.5 oz)	30	1	tr	7
Kopali					
Organic Dark Chocolate Covered	½ pkg (1 oz)	140	2	6	20
Organic Dried	1 pkg (1.7 oz)	240	5	1	38
Navitas Naturals					
Dried	1 oz	91	3	0	21
MULLET					
striped cooked	3 oz	127	21	4	0
striped raw	3 oz	99	16	3	0
MUNG BEANS					
dried cooked	1 cup	213	14	1	39
TruRoots					
Organic Sprouted not prep	¼ cup (1.4 oz)	140	10	1	30
MUNGO BEANS					
dried cooked	1 cup	190	14	1	33
MUSHROOMS					
CANNED					
caps	8 (1.6 oz)	12	1	tr	2
caps pickled	6 (0.8 oz)	5	1	tr	1
chanterelle	3.5 oz	12	1	1	tr
pickled	1 cup	33	4	tr	5
pieces	½ cup	20	1	tr	2
straw	1 cup	58	7	1	8
Green Giant					
Pieces & Stems	½ cup	25	2	0	4
Polar					
Straw	½ cup	20	3	0	4
Whole Button	½ cup	30	3	0	4
Whole Shiitake	½ cup	30	1	1	4
DRIED					
chanterelle	1 oz	25	5	tr	tr
shiitake	1 (3.6 g)	11	tr	tr	3

FOOD	PORTION	CALS	PROT	FAT	CARB
tree ear	½ cup (0.4 oz)	36	1	tr	10
wood ear mok yee	½ cup (0.4 oz)	25	2	tr	8
FRESH					
brown italian or crimini sliced	1 cup	19	2	tr	3
brown italian or crimini whole	1 (0.7 oz)	5	1	tr	1
chanterelle	3.5 oz	11	2	tr	tr
enoki raw	1 lg (5 g)	2	tr	tr	tr
enoki sliced	1 cup	29	2	tr	5
enoki whole	1 cup	28	2	tr	5
maitake diced	1 cup	26	1	tr	5
maitake whole	1 (6.6 g)	2	tr	tr	tr
morel	3.5 oz	9	2	tr	0
oyster	1 sm (0.5 oz)	5	1	tr	1
oyster sliced	1 cup	30	3	tr	6
portabella raw	1 cap (3 oz)	22	2	tr	4
portabella sliced grilled	1 cup (4.2 oz)	42	5	1	6
shiitake cooked	4 (2.5 oz)	40	1	tr	10
shiitake pieces cooked	1 cup	81	2	tr	21
white	1 (0.6 oz)	4	1	tr	1
white sliced cooked	1 cup	28	4	tr	4
white sliced raw	½ cup	8	1	tr	1
Giorgio					
Mushrooms	3 oz	20	2	0	3
Golden Gourmet					
Beech Brown	4 oz	20	3	1	7
Beech White	4 oz	13	3	1	6
King Trumpet	4 oz	20	3	0	7
Maitake	4 oz	20	3	1	8
Hokto					
Organic Bunashimeji Beech Mushrooms	1 pkg (3.5 oz)	30	3	1	3
Organic Maitake Hen Of The Wood	1 pkg (3.5 oz)	30	2	1	4
FROZEN					
Farm Rich					
Breaded	5 (3 oz)	120	3	2	23
TAKE-OUT					
battered fried	1 lg (0.6 oz)	39	1	3	3
creamed	1 cup	171	6	11	15
stuffed	1 (0.8 oz)	67	3	4	6

FOOD	PORTION	CALS	PROT	FAT	CARB
MUSKRAT					
roasted	3 oz	199	26	10	0
MUSSELS					
blue raw	1 cup	129	18	3	6
blue raw	3 oz	73	10	2	3
fresh blue cooked	3 oz	147	20	4	6
Polar					
Mussels	2 oz	60	10	3	tr
MUSTARD					
dry mustard	1 tsp	15	1	1	1
hot chinese	1 tsp	3	tr	tr	tr
organic yellow	1 tsp	5	0	0	0
seed	1 tsp	15	1	1	1
yellow prepared	1 tbsp	3	tr	tr	tr
Bone Suckin'					
Fat Free Gluten Free	1 tbsp	25	0	0	5
Dave's Gourmet					
Insanity	1 tsp (5 g)	5	0	0	1
D'Oni					
Bold As Love Honey Habanero	1 tsp	5	0	0	2
French's					
Classic Yellow	1 tsp	0	0	0	0
Honey	1 tsp	10	0	0	1
Honey Dijon	1 tsp	10	0	0	1
Horseradish	1 tsp	5	0	0	0
Spicy Brown	1 tsp	5	0	0	0
Hellman's					
Deli	1 tsp	5	0	0	tr
Dijonnaise	1 tsp	5	0	0	1
Honey Mustard	1 tsp	10	0	0	2
Robert Rothchild Farm					
Champagne Garlic	1 tsp	6	0	0	1
School House Kitchen					
Sweet Smooth Hot	1 tsp	15	0	1	1,
Texas Sassy					
Mustard Sauce	2 tbsp (1 oz)	15	0	0	3
Vivi's					
Classic	1 tbsp (0.5 oz)	15	0	0	4
Sizzlin' Chipotle	1 tbsp (0.5 oz)	15	0	0	4

FOOD	PORTION	CALS	PROT	FAT	CARB
MUSTARD GREENS					
canned	1 cup	23	3	tr	3
fresh as prep w/ fat	1 cup	50	3	3	3
fresh chopped boiled w/o salt	1 cup	21	3	tr	3
fresh raw chopped	1 cup	15	2	tr	3
frozen chopped boiled w/o salt	1 cup	28	3	tr	5
Allen's					
Seasoned	½ cup	45	4	1	6
Glory					
Seasoned canned	½ cup	35	2	0	3
Sylvia's					
Specially Seasoned	½ cup	30	2	0	5
NATTO					
natto	½ cup	187	16	10	13
House					
Natto	2 oz	120	10	6	5
NAVY BEANS					
canned	1 cup	296	20	1	54
dried cooked	1 cup	259	16	1	48
NECTARINE					
fresh	1 sm (4.5 oz)	57	1	tr	14
fresh	1 lg (5.5 oz)	69	2	1	16
fresh sliced	1 cup (5 oz)	63	2	tr	15
Chiquita					
Fresh	1 (5 oz)	63	2	0	15
Sunsweet					
Dried	3 pieces (1.4 oz)	100	1	0	25
NECTARINE JUICE					
Sun Shower					
100% Juice	8 oz	93	1	0	21
NEUFCHATEL					
neufchatel	1 oz	74	3	7	1
neufchatel	1 pkg (3 oz)	221	8	20	3
Organic Valley					
Soft	2 tbsp	70	2	6	2

FOOD	PORTION	CALS	PROT	FAT	CARB
NONI JUICE					
Lakewood					
Noni Pure Juice	2 oz	8	0	0	2
Snapple					
Juice Drink Low Calorie Metabolism Noni Berry	8 oz	15	0	0	2
Tree Of Life					
100% Juice Concentrate	2 tbsp	15	0	0	4
NOODLES					
cellophane	1 cup	492	tr	tr	121
chow mein	1 cup (1.6 oz)	237	4	14	25
egg	1 cup (38 g)	145	5	2	27
egg cooked	1 cup (5.6 oz)	213	8	2	40
japanese soba cooked	1 cup (4 oz)	113	6	tr	24
japanese somen cooked	1 cup (6.2 oz)	231	7	tr	48
korean acorn noodles not prep	2 oz	195	7	tr	41
rice cooked	1 cup (6.2 oz)	192	2	tr	44
spinach/egg cooked	1 cup (5.6 oz)	211	8	3	39
House					
Shirataki Tofu Noodles	2 oz	20	1	1	3
Shirataki Yam Noodles	2 oz	5	0	0	1
Krasdale					
Egg Wide not prep	1 cup (2 oz)	210	8	2	41
La Choy					
Chow Mein Noodles	½ cup (1 oz)	130	3	5	19
Rice	½ cup	130	2	4	21
Light 'N Fluffy					
Egg Extra Wide cooked	1½ cups	210	8	3	40
No Yolks					
Dumplings	2 oz	210	8	1	41
Ronzoni					
Healthy Harvest Whole Grain Extra Wide not prep	2 oz	180	8	1	41
Thai Kitchen					
Stir-Fry Rice Linguini not prep	2 oz	210	4	1	46
NUTMEG					
ground	1 tsp	12	tr	1	1
nutmeg butter	1 tbsp	120	0	14	0

FOOD	PORTION	CALS	PROT	FAT	CARB

NUTRITION SUPPLEMENTS (see also CEREAL BARS, ENERGY BARS, ENERGY DRINKS)

Clif

FOOD	PORTION	CALS	PROT	FAT	CARB
Shot Bloks Black Cherry	3 (1 oz)	100	0	0	24
Shot Bloks Cola	3 (1 oz)	100	0	0	24
Shot Bloks Margarita	3 (1 oz)	90	0	0	24
Shot Bloks Orange	3 (1 oz)	100	0	0	24
Ensure					
Shake Creamy Milk Chocolate	1 bottle (8 oz)	250	9	6	40
Shake Strawberries & Cream	1 bottle (8 oz)	250	9	6	40
Glowelle					
Beauty Drink All Flavors	1 bottle	100	0	0	24
Glucerna					
Shake Creamy Chocolate Delight	1 bottle (8 oz)	200	10	7	27
Shake Homemade Vanilla	1 bottle (8 oz)	200	10	7	26
Jelly Belly					
Sport Beans Lemon Lime	1 pkg (1 oz)	100	0	0	25
Joint Juice					
Tropical Fruit	1 can (8 oz)	25	0	0	6
Luna					
Electrolyte Splash	1 pkg	80	0	0	20
Moons Energy Chews Watermelon	6 (1 oz)	100	0	0	24
Recovery Smoothie	1 pkg	120	0	0	21
Oxylent					
Oxygenating Multivitamin Drink	1 pkg	10	0	0	2
S/7					
Prenatal Vitamin Drink Berry	1 pkg (0.5 oz)	45	0	1	9
Slim-Fast					
Optima Ready-To-Drink Creamy Milk Chocolate	1 can (11 oz)	190	10	6	25

NUTS MIXED (see also individual names)

FOOD	PORTION	CALS	PROT	FAT	CARB
dry roasted w/ peanuts salted	¼ cup	203	6	18	9
dry roasted w/ peanuts w/o salt	¼ cup	203	6	18	9
mixed nuts chocolate covered	¼ cup (1.5 oz)	240	4	17	20
oil roasted w/o peanuts salted	¼ cup	221	6	20	8
oil roasted w/o peanuts w/o salt	¼ cup	221	6	20	8

FOOD	PORTION	CALS	PROT	FAT	CARB
Back To Nature					
Tuscan Herb Roast	1 oz	170	5	15	7
Dave's Gourmet					
Burning Nuts	1 oz	200	9	17	7
Emily's					
Roasted Mixed Nuts	¼ cup (1.3 oz)	230	6	20	8
Mauna Loa					
Mixed Nuts	¼ cup (1 oz)	180	5	16	6
NuttZo					
Multi-Nut Butter Organic	2 tbsp (1.1 oz)	180	7	16	7
Planters					
Mixed	30 nuts (1 oz)	170	6	15	6
NUT-rition Energy Mix	¼ cup	180	5	14	10
True North					
Clusters Pecan Almond Peanut	8 (1 oz)	170	5	13	13
OCTOPUS					
dried boiled	3 oz	144	26	2	4
fresh steamed	3 oz	139	25	2	4
smoked	1 oz	40	7	1	1
TAKE-OUT					
ensalada de pulpo	1 cup	299	17	21	10
OHELOBERRIES					
fresh	1 cup	39	1	tr	10
OIL					
almond	1 tbsp	120	0	14	0
almond	1 cup	1927	0	218	0
apricot kernel	1 tbsp	120	0	14	0
apricot kernel	1 cup	1927	0	218	0
avocado	1 cup	1927	0	218	0
avocado	1 tbsp	124	0	14	0
babassu palm	1 tbsp	120	0	14	0
butter oil	1 cup	1795	1	204	0
butter oil	1 tbsp	112	tr	13	0
canola	1 cup	1927	0	218	0
canola	1 tbsp	124	0	14	0
coconut	1 tbsp	117	0	14	0
corn	1 tbsp	120	0	14	0
corn	1 cup	1927	0	218	0
cottonseed	1 tbsp	120	0	14	0

FOOD	PORTION	CALS	PROT	FAT	CARB
cottonseed	1 cup	1927	0	218	0
cupu assu	1 tbsp	120	0	14	0
garlic oil	1 tbsp	150	0	17	0
grapeseed	1 tbsp	120	0	14	0
hazelnut	1 cup	1927	0	218	0
hazelnut	1 tbsp	120	0	14	0
mustard	1 tbsp	124	0	14	0
mustard	1 cup	1927	0	218	0
oat	1 tbsp	120	0	14	0
olive	1 tbsp	119	0	14	0
olive	1 cup	1909	0	216	0
palm	1 tbsp	120	0	14	0
palm	1 cup	1927	0	218	0
palm kernel	1 cup	1879	0	218	0
palm kernel	1 tbsp	117	0	14	0
peanut	1 cup	1909	0	216	0
peanut	1 tbsp	119	0	14	0
poppyseed	1 tbsp	120	0	14	0
pumpkin seed	1 oz	217	0	29	0
rice bran	1 tbsp	120	0	14	0
safflower	1 tbsp	120	0	14	0
safflower	1 cup	1927	0	218	0
sesame	1 tbsp	120	0	14	0
sheanut	1 tbsp	120	0	14	0
soybean	1 cup	1927	0	218	0
soybean	1 tbsp	120	0	14	0
sunflower	1 cup	1927	0	218	0
sunflower	1 tbsp	120	0	14	0
teaseed	1 tbsp	120	0	14	0
tomatoseed	1 tbsp	120	0	14	0
vegetable	1 tbsp	120	0	14	0
vegetable	1 cup	1927	0	218	0
walnut	1 cup	1927	0	218	0
walnut	1 tbsp	120	0	14	0
wheat germ	1 tbsp	120	0	14	0
Bell Plantation					
Extra Virgin Roasted Peanut	1 tbsp	120	0	14	0
Bragg					
Olive Extra Virgin	1 tbsp	120	0	14	2

FOOD	PORTION	CALS	PROT	FAT	CARB
Carapelli					
Grapeseed	1 tbsp	120	0	14	0
Olive Extra Virgin	1 tbsp	120	0	14	0
Colavita					
Olive Extra Virgin	1 tbsp (0.5 oz)	120	0	14	0
Crisco					
Cooking Spray	⅓ sec	0	0	0	0
Original	spray				
Frying Oil Blend	1 tbsp	130	0	14	0
Light Olive	1 tbsp	120	0	14	0
Peanut	1 tbsp	120	0	14	0
Pure Vegetable	1 tbsp	120	0	14	0
Gaea					
Olive Carbon Neutral	1 tbsp (0.5 oz)	130	0	14	0
Gourme Mist					
Extra Virgin Olive Cold Pressed	1 sec spray	4	0	tr	0
Hollywood					
Canola Enriched	1 tbsp	120	0	14	0
Peanut Enriched Gold	1 tbsp	120	0	14	0
Safflower Expeller Pressed	1 tbsp	120	0	14	0
House Of Tsang					
Mongolian Fire	1 tsp	45	0	5	0
Wok Oil	1 tbsp	130	0	14	0
Kinloch Plantation					
100% Virgin Pecan	1 tbsp	130	0	14	0
Living Harvest					
Organic Hemp Oil	2 tbsp	250	0	28	0
Lucini					
Extra Virgin Premium Select	1 tbsp (0.5 oz)	120	0	14	0
Manitoba Harvest					
Hemp Seed Oil	1 tbsp	126	0	14	0
Martinis					
Kalamata Olive Extra Virgin Cold Pressed	1 tbsp (0.5 oz)	120	0	15	0
Mazola					
Corn	1 tbsp	120	0	14	0
Monini					
Grapeseed	1 tbsp (0.5 oz)	120	0	14	0
Navitas Naturals					
Organic Virgin Coconut	1 tbsp (0.5 oz)	120	0	14	0

FOOD	PORTION	CALS	PROT	FAT	CARB
Nutiva					
Organic Coconut Extra Virgin	1 tbsp	120	0	14	0
Organic Hemp Cold Pressed	1 tbsp	120	0	14	0
Olivo					
Spray Olive Oil 100% Extra Virgin	⅓ sec spray	0	0	0	0
Pam					
Organic Canola spray	⅓ sec	0	0	0	0
Robert Rothchild Farm					
Basil Infused	1 tbsp	120	0	14	0
Smart Balance					
Omega Oil	1 tbsp	120	0	14	0
Tree Of Life					
Almond Expeller Pressed	1 tbsp (0.5 oz)	120	0	14	0
Avocado Expeller Pressed	1 tbsp (0.5 oz)	120	0	14	0
Macadamia Nut Expeller Pressed	1 tbsp (0.5 oz)	120	0	14	0
Organic Coconut Expeller Pressed	1 tbsp	120	0	14	0
Walnut Expeller Pressed	1 tbsp (0.5 oz)	120	0	14	0
Wesson					
Canola	1 tbsp	120	0	14	0
OKRA					
CANNED					
pickled	6 pods (2.3 oz)	18	1	tr	4
Allens					
Cut	½ cup	30	1	0	6
McIlhenny					
Spicy Pickled	1 oz	10	0	0	2
Trappey's					
Creole Gumbo	½ cup	35	2	0	6
FRESH					
cooked w/ salt	8 pods	19	2	tr	4
luffa chinese okra cooked	1 cup	39	3	tr	8
sliced cooked w/ salt	½ cup	18	2	tr	4
TAKE-OUT					
batter dipped fried	10 pieces (2.6 oz)	142	2	10	12

FOOD	PORTION	CALS	PROT	FAT	CARB
OLIVES					
black	2 med (0.3 oz)	8	tr	1	tr
greek	1 (0.5 oz)	16	tr	1	1
green	2 lg (0.3 oz)	11	tr	1	tr
green	2 med (0.2 oz)	10	tr	1	tr
green	1 sm (0.2 oz)	8	tr	1	tr
green	2 extra lg (0.5 oz)	19	tr	2	1
green chopped	¼ cup (1.2 oz)	48	tr	5	1
green olive tapenade	1 tbsp	25	0	3	1
green stuffed	2 sm (0.2 oz)	9	tr	1	tr
green stuffed	2 med (0.3 oz)	10	tr	1	tr
green stuffed	¼ cup (1.3 oz)	47	tr	5	1
green stuffed	2 lg (0.3 oz)	12	tr	1	tr
ripe	2 extra lg (0.4 oz)	12	tr	1	1
ripe	2 sm (0.2 oz)	7	tr	1	tr
ripe	2 lg (0.3 oz)	10	tr	1	1
ripe sliced	¼ cup (1.2 oz)	35	tr	3	2
spanish stuffed	5 (0.5 oz)	15	0	1	1
Dave's Gourmet					
Olives In Pain	⅛ jar (0.5 oz)	15	0	2	0
Peloponnese					
Amfissa	3	45	0	5	1
Ionian Green	3	25	0	3	1
Kalamata Pitted	5	45	0	5	1
Kalamata Spread	1 tsp	15	0	2	0
Stonewall Kitchen					
Mixed Olive Spread	1 tbsp	35	0	2	5
ONION					
CANNED					
cocktail	½ cup	41	2	tr	9
French's					
Original French Fried	2 tbsp	45	0	4	3
McSweet					
Pickled Onions	4 (1 oz)	10	0	0	2
The Gracious Gourmet					
Balsamic Four Onion Spread	1 tbsp (0.5 oz)	20	0	0	6
DRIED					
flakes	1 tbsp	17	tr	tr	4

FOOD	PORTION	CALS	PROT	FAT	CARB
powder	1 tsp	7	tr	tr	2
shallots	1 tbsp	3	tr	0	1
Bob's Red Mill					
Minced	1 tbsp	40	1	1	8
FRESH					
cooked w/o salt	1 sm (2 oz)	26	1	tr	6
cooked w/o salt	1 med (3.3 oz)	41	1	tr	10
cooked w/o salt	1 lg (4.5 oz)	56	2	tr	13
cooked w/o salt chopped	1 tbsp	7	tr	tr	2
raw chopped	1 tbsp	4	tr	tr	1
raw chopped	½ cup	32	1	tr	7
raw slice	1 (0.5 oz)	6	tr	tr	1
raw sliced	½ cup	23	1	tr	5
scallions raw	1 med (0.5 oz)	5	tr	tr	1
scallions raw chopped	¼ cup	8	tr	tr	2
shallots raw chopped	¼ cup	29	1	tr	7
sweet whole raw	1 (11.6 oz)	106	3	tr	25
whole raw	1 sm (2.5 oz)	28	1	tr	7
whole raw	1 med (4 oz)	44	1	tr	10
whole raw	1 lg (5.3 oz)	60	2	tr	14
Bland Farms					
Vidalia Sweet	1 (5 oz)	60	1	0	14
Blue Ribbon					
Yellow	1 med (5.2 oz)	60	2	0	14
Earthbound Farms					
Organic Green Onions	¼ cup	10	0	0	2
Organic Red	1 med (5.2 oz)	60	2	0	14
Ocean Mist					
Green Onions Chopped	¼ cup	10	0	0	2
OsoSweet					
Onion	1 med (5 oz)	60	2	0	14
FROZEN					
C&W					
Petite Whole	⅔ cup (3 oz)	30	0	0	6
Farm Rich					
Petals Breaded + Sauce	10 (3 oz)	200	2	12	22
TAKE-OUT					
creamed	1 cup	187	5	9	22
fried	½ cup	57	tr	5	3
rings breaded & fried	8 to 9 (3 oz)	276	4	16	31

FOOD	PORTION	CALS	PROT	FAT	CARB
OPOSSUM					
roasted	3 oz	188	26	9	0
ORANGE					
FRESH					
california valencia	½ cup (3.2 oz)	44	1	tr	11
california valencia	1 (4.2 oz)	59	1	tr	14
florida	1 (5.3 oz)	69	1	tr	17
florida sections	½ cup (3.2 oz)	43	1	tr	11
navel	1 (4.9 oz)	69	1	tr	18
navel sections	1 cup (5.8 oz)	81	2	tr	21
peel	1 tbsp (0.2 oz)	3	tr	tr	1
Darling					
Mandarine	1 med (3.8 oz)	50	1	0	13
ORANGE JUICE					
chilled	1 cup (8.7 oz)	112	2	1	26
fresh	1 cup (8.7 oz)	112	2	1	26
mandarin orange	7 oz	94	2	tr	20
Florida's Natural					
Calcium & Vitamin D	8 oz	110	2	0	26
Izze					
Sparkling Esque Mandarin Orange	1 bottle (12 oz)	50	0	0	12
Land O' Lakes					
Juice	1 cup (8 oz)	110	1	0	25
Juice w/ Calcium	1 cup (8 oz)	120	1	0	29
Mott's					
100% Juice Sunkist Orange Sensation	1 bottle (14 oz)	210	0	0	50
Mr. J					
100% Juice Calcium Fortified	1 pkg (4 oz)	60	0	0	19
NutraBalance					
Fortified	1 pkg (4 oz)	60	1	0	17
Odwalla					
100% Juice	8 oz	110	1	0	25
Organic Valley					
W/ Calcium	1 cup	110	2	0	26
Simply					
Orange Calcium Fortified	8 oz	110	2	0	26
Orange Original	8 oz	110	2	0	26

FOOD	PORTION	CALS	PROT	FAT	CARB
Snapple					
Orangeade	8 oz	100	0	0	26
SSips					
Orangeade	8 oz	120	0	0	31
Tree Ripe					
100% Juice + Calcium & Vitamins	8 oz	120	1	0	29
Organic 100% Juice	6 oz	90	0	0	22
Tropicana					
Antioxidant Advantage	8 oz	110	2	0	26
Calcium + Vitamin D	8 oz	110	2	0	26
Fiber	8 oz	120	2	0	29
Healthy Heart	8 oz	120	2	0	26
Healthy Kids	8 oz	110	2	0	26
Light'n Healthy w/ Calcium	8 oz	50	tr	0	13
No Pulp	8 oz	110	2	0	26
Orangeade	8 oz	111	0	0	33
Organic	8 oz	120	1	0	28
Trop50' Orange Juice Beverage	8 oz	50	tr	0	13
Uncle Matt's					
Organic 100% Juice Pulp Free	8 oz	110	2	0	26
Organic 100% Juice w/ Pulp	8 oz	110	2	0	26
Welsh Farms					
Juice	8 oz	110	0	0	27
TAKE-OUT					
orange julius	1 cup (9.2 oz)	212	14	tr	39
OREGANO					
crumbled	1 tsp	3	tr	tr	1
ground	1 tsp	6	tr	tr	1

ORGAN MEATS (see BRAINS, GIBLETS, GIZZARDS, HEART, KIDNEY, LIVER, SWEETBREAD)

FOOD	PORTION	CALS	PROT	FAT	CARB
OSTRICH					
cooked	4 oz	195	29	8	0
cooked diced	1 cup (4.7 oz)	215	35	9	0
Natural Frontier Foods					
Filets	1 (4 oz)	130	28	3	0
Ground Lean	4 oz	130	28	3	0
OYSTERS					
canned eastern	1 cup	112	11	4	6
eastern baked	6 med	47	4	1	4

FOOD	PORTION	CALS	PROT	FAT	CARB
eastern raw	6 med	50	4	1	5
eastern sauteed	6 med	76	5	5	3
smoked	6	33	3	1	2
Polar					
Whole	¼ cup	70	7	3	4
Whole Smoked	⅓ cup	95	8	5	4
TAKE-OUT					
breaded & fried	6	368	13	18	40
fritter	1 (1.4 oz)	121	4	6	12
oysters rockefeller	1 cup	302	18	17	22
stew	1 cup	208	11	13	11
PANCAKE/WAFFLE SYRUP					
lite	¼ cup	98	0	0	27
pancake syrup	¼ cup	209	0	tr	55
pancake syrup	1 pkg (2 oz)	156	0	tr	41
Aunt Jemima					
Butter Lite	¼ cup (2.1 oz)	100	0	0	26
Naturally Fresh					
Maple Mountain Sugar Free	2 tbsp	0	0	0	0
Wholesome Sweeteners					
Organic	¼ cup	240	0	0	60
PANCAKES					
FROZEN					
Aunt Jemima					
Buttermilk	3 (3 oz)	210	6	4	40
Buttermilk Low Fat	3 (3 oz)	210	6	4	40
Whole Grain	3 (3 oz)	230	7	6	38
Dr. Praeger's					
Broccoli	1 (2 oz)	80	2	4	9
Potato	1 (2.2 oz)	100	2	4	13
Golden					
Potato Latkes	1 (1.3 oz)	70	2	3	10
Zucchini	1 (1.3 oz)	70	2	3	8
Jimmy Dean					
Breakfast Bowls Pancake & Sausage Links	1 pkg	710	13	31	93
Griddle Cake Sandwich Sausage Egg & Cheese	1 (4 oz)	370	8	23	32
Original Pancakes & Sausage On A Stick	1 (2.5 oz)	110	6	13	21

FOOD	PORTION	CALS	PROT	FAT	CARB
Pillsbury					
Blueberry	3 (4 oz)	230	5	4	46
Buttermilk	3 (4 oz)	240	6	4	47
Original	3 (4 oz)	250	6	4	49
Ratner's					
Potato Latkes	1 (1.5 oz)	80	2	2	15
MIX					
Arrowhead Mills					
Gluten Free Pancake & Waffle as prep	2 (5 in)	240	11	6	42
Batter Blaster					
Organic Original Pancake & Waffle Batter not prep	¼ cup (2 oz)	112	3	1	23
Bisquick					
Shake 'N Pour Buttermilk as prep	3	220	6	3	42
TAKE-OUT					
buckwheat	1 (7 in)	142	5	5	19
norwegian lefse	1 (9 in) (2.7 oz)	163	3	5	27
plain	1 (7 in)	183	4	3	35
potato	1 (1.3 oz)	70	2	4	8
w/ butter & syrup	2 (8.1 oz)	520	8	14	91
whole wheat	1 (7 in)	183	6	8	23

PANCREAS (see SWEETBREAD)

PANINI (see SANDWICHES)

PAPAYA

canned in syrup	½ cup (2.3 oz)	50	tr	tr	13
dried	1 strip (0.8 oz)	59	1	tr	15
fresh	1 sm (5.3 oz)	59	1	tr	15
fresh	1 lg (13.3 oz)	148	2	1	37
fresh cubed	1 cup (4.9 oz)	55	1	tr	14
green cooked	½ cup (2.3 oz)	18	tr	tr	5

PAPAYA JUICE

nectar	1 cup (8.8 oz)	142	tr	tr	36
Lakewood					
Red	8 oz	80	1	0	20
Yellow	8 oz	105	2	0	26

FOOD	PORTION	CALS	PROT	FAT	CARB
Old Orchard					
Nectar Cocktail	8 oz	120	0	0	30
PAPRIKA					
dried	1 tsp	1	tr	tr	tr
Bob's Red Mill					
Hungarian	½ tsp	11	0	0	2
PARSLEY					
dried	1 tbsp	4	tr	tr	1
freeze dried	1 tbsp	1	tr	tr	tr
fresh chopped	1 tbsp	1	tr	tr	tr
fresh chopped	¼ cup	5	tr	tr	1
fresh sprigs	5 (1.8 oz)	18	1	tr	3
PARSNIPS					
fresh sliced cooked w/o salt	½ cup (2.7 oz)	55	1	tr	13
whole cooked	1 (5.6 oz)	114	2	tr	27
TAKE-OUT					
creamed	1 cup (8 oz)	237	6	11	31
PASSION FRUIT					
fresh	1 (0.6 oz)	17	tr	tr	4
fresh cut up	½ cup (4.1 oz)	114	3	1	28
PASSION FRUIT JUICE					
nectar	1 cup (8.8 oz)	168	tr	tr	44
yellow lilikoi	1 cup (8.7 oz)	138	1	tr	35
Santa Cruz					
Organic 100% Juice Nectar	8 oz	150	1	0	40
PASTA (*see also* NOODLES, PASTA DINNERS, PASTA SALAD)					
DRY					
corn cooked	1 cup (4.9 oz)	176	4	1	39
elbows not prep	1 cup	389	13	2	78
elbows cooked	1 cup (4.9 oz)	197	7	1	40
shells small cooked	1 cup (4 oz)	162	5	1	33
spaghetti cooked	1 cup (4.9 oz)	197	7	1	40
spinach spaghetti cooked	1 cup (4.9 oz)	182	6	1	37
spirals cooked	1 cup (4.7 oz)	189	6	tr	38
vegetable cooked	1 cup (4.7 oz)	172	6	tr	36
whole wheat all shapes cooked	1 cup	174	7	tr	37

FOOD	PORTION	CALS	PROT	FAT	CARB
Amish Natural					
Fettuccine Fiber Rich not prep	2 oz	200	6	1	42
Fettuccine not prep	2 oz	201	8	1	41
Fettuccine Whole Wheat not prep	2 oz	210	8	2	41
Barilla					
Plus Rotini not prep	2 oz	210	10	2	38
DeBoles					
Angel Hair Rice Pasta not prep	¼ pkg (2 oz)	210	4	1	46
Elbow Corn Pasta Wheat Free not prep	⅙ pkg (2 oz)	200	4	2	43
Fettuccine not prep	¼ pkg (2 oz)	210	7	1	41
Organic Angel Hair Whole Wheat not prep	¼ pkg (2 oz)	210	7	2	42
Organic Eggless Ribbon not prep	1 cup (2 oz)	210	7	1	43
Organic Fettucini Spinach not prep	¼ pkg (2 oz)	210	7	1	43
Organic Lasagna not prep	¼ pkg (2.5 oz)	260	9	1	54
Organic Rigatoni Whole Wheat not prep	1 cup (2 oz)	210	7	2	42
Rigatoni not prep	¼ pkg (2 oz)	210	7	1	41
Dreamfields					
Lasagna not prep	2 pieces (2 oz)	190	7	1	42
Rotini not prep	⅔ cup (2 oz)	190	7	1	42
Gillian's					
Penne Brown Rice Pasta Wheat Gluten Egg Free not prep	2 oz	200	4	2	43
Lundberg					
Organic Spaghetti Brown Rice not prep	2 oz	210	4	2	44
Maddy's					
Gluten Free not prep	4 oz	310	5	2	66
Mueller's					
Elbow Macaroni not prep	½ cup	210	7	1	41
Ronzoni					
Elbows not prep	½ cup (2 oz)	210	7	1	42
Garden Delight Radiatore not prep	2 oz	190	7	1	40

FOOD	PORTION	CALS	PROT	FAT	CARB
Garden Delight Spaghetti not prep	2 oz	190	7	1	40
Smart Pasta not prep	2 oz	180	6	1	43
Wacky Mac					
Veggie All Shapes not prep	2 oz	200	8	1	41
FRESH					
cooked	2 oz	75	3	1	14
spinach cooked	2 oz	74	3	1	14
Buitoni					
Ravioli Four Cheese 100% Whole Wheat	1¼ cups	320	16	10	42
Monterey Gourmet					
Whole Wheat Ravioli Vegetable & Cheese	1 cup (3.5 oz)	240	12	6	35
Whole Wheat Tortellini Italian Cheese	1 cup (3.5 oz)	290	13	6	48

PASTA DINNERS (see also PASTA SALAD)
CANNED

FOOD	PORTION	CALS	PROT	FAT	CARB
Chef Boyardee					
Beef Ravioli	1 cup	240	8	8	35
Mini Ravioli	1 cup	250	8	9	35
Mini-Bites Spaghetti & Meatballs	1 cup	250	10	10	30
Hormel					
Kid's Kitchen Microwave Meals Cheezy Mac 'N Beef	1 pkg (7.5 oz)	250	14	6	34
Kid's Kitchen Microwave Meals Cheezy Mac 'N Cheese	1 pkg (7.5 oz)	270	11	14	24
Kid's Kitchen Microwave Meals Mini Beef Ravioli	1 pkg (7.5 oz)	240	8	6	38
Kid's Kitchen Microwave Meals Spaghetti Rings & Franks	1 pkg (7.5 oz)	240	9	8	32
Lasagna w/ Meat Sauce	1 pkg (7.5 oz)	210	9	5	31
Spaghetti w/ Meat Sauce	1 pkg (7.5 oz)	210	10	5	31
SpaghettiOs					
A to Z's w/ Meatballs	1 cup	260	11	9	33
A to Z's w/ Sliced Franks	1 cup	230	9	6	32
Mini Beef Ravioli In Meat Sauce	1 cup	260	11	5	43
Pasta	1 cup	180	6	1	37
Plus Calcium	1 cup	170	6	1	35

FOOD	PORTION	CALS	PROT	FAT	CARB
FROZEN					
4Real					
Mac+Cheese	1 pkg (8 oz)	230	8	5	33
Meat Sauce w/ Beef Ravioli	1 pkg (8 oz)	190	8	4	32
Spaghetti Rings	1 pkg (8 oz)	180	6	1	37
Amy's					
Bowls Baked Ziti	1 pkg	390	9	12	62
Bowls Stuffed Pasta Shells	1 pkg	310	19	13	30
Lasagna Cheese	1 pkg (10.2 oz)	380	20	14	44
Lasagna Tofu Vegetable	1 pkg (9.4 oz)	310	13	11	41
Macaroni & Cheese	1 pkg (8.9 oz)	410	16	16	47
Macaroni & Cheese Light In Sodium	1 pkg (8.9 oz)	400	16	16	47
Macaroni & Soy Cheese	1 pkg (8.9 oz)	370	16	15	42
Rice Mac & Cheese	1 pkg (9 oz)	400	16	16	47
Banquet					
Lasagna Family Entree	1 cup	510	25	16	63
Macaroni & Cheese	1 cup	200	7	6	30
Noodles & Beef	1 cup	160	8	4	20
Birds Eye					
Steamfresh Meals For Two Shrimp Alfredo	½ pkg (11.9 oz)	420	21	12	55
Steamfresh Meals For Two Shrimp Pasta Primavera	½ pkg (11.9 oz)	450	15	24	39
Blue Horizon Organic					
Penne Alfredo w/ Shrimp	½ pkg (9.9 oz)	430	17	22	39
Penne Alla Vodka w/ Shrimp	½ pkg (9.9 oz)	270	17	6	38
Pesto Farfalle w/ Shrimp	½ pkg (9.9 oz)	280	17	6	38
Scampi Rotini w/ Shrimp	½ pkg (9.9 oz)	410	18	19	44
Cedarlane					
Zone Chicken & Vegetables Pasta & Ginger	1 pkg (10 oz)	340	24	12	35
Zone Lasagna Vegetable	1 pkg (10.9 oz)	310	24	12	33
Celentano					
Cheese Ravioli	4 (4.3 oz)	230	11	4	36
Contessa					
Ravioli Portobello	6 (6.7 oz)	360	14	17	39
Glory					
Macaroni & Cheese	1 pkg	480	21	23	47

FOOD	PORTION	CALS	PROT	FAT	CARB
Gluten Free Cafe					
Fettuccini Alfredo	1 pkg (9.2 oz)	400	4	16	55
Pasta Primavera	1 pkg (9.2 oz)	270	4	9	42
Glutino					
Gluten Free Duo Mushroom Penne	1 pgk (10.5 oz)	380	8	6	73
Gluten Free Macaroni & Cheese	1 pkg (8.8 oz)	430	19	20	44
Gluten Free Penne Alfredo	1 pkg (9.1 oz)	340	15	8	48
Green Giant					
Skillet Meal Chicken & Cheesy Pasta as prep	1¼ cups	270	15	6	42
Healthy Choice					
Creamy Garlic Shrimp w/ Bow Tie Pasta	1 pkg (11.5 oz)	280	13	5	44
Portabella Marsala Pasta	1 pkg (9 oz)	270	12	7	38
Tomato Basil Penne	1 pkg (10 oz)	280	13	6	39
Helen's Kitchen					
Farfalle & Basil Pasta w/ Tofu Steaks	1 pkg (9 oz)	320	20	11	70
Joy Of Cooking					
Al Dente Cavatappi Bolognese	1 cup (7.7 oz)	280	14	12	29
Best Loved Macaroni & Cheese	1 cup (5.4 oz)	280	10	18	36
Cheese Ravioli Pomodoro	1 cup (7.7 oz)	250	13	7	34
Creamy Fettuccine Carbonara	1 cup (7.5 oz)	330	15	16	31
Kashi					
Chicken Pasta Pomodoro	1 pkg (10 oz)	280	19	6	38
Marie Callender's					
Fettucine Chicken & Broccoli	1 meal	630	30	37	43
Meat Lasagna	1 cup	240	14	9	24
Milton's					
Lasagna Vegetable w/ Multi-Grain Pasta	1 cup (8 oz)	340	17	16	30
Mon Cuisine					
Vegetarian Spaghetti & Meatballs	1 pkg (10 oz)	360	29	4	54
Moosewood					
Organic Vegetarian Broccoli & Pasta Parmesan	1 pkg (10 oz)	380	14	13	52
Organic Vegetarian Farfalle & Spinach Pesto Sauce	1 pkg (10 oz)	370	14	11	56

FOOD	PORTION	CALS	PROT	FAT	CARB
Organic Vegetarian Spicy Penne Puttanesca	1 pkg (10 oz)	300	8	10	45
New York Ravioli					
Jolie Kid Shapes Ravioli Cheese	1 cup	330	15	9	47
Jolie Kid Shapes Ravioli Cheese & Broccoli	1 cup	340	15	8	53
Ravioli Four Cheese	1 cup	360	17	6	58
Ravioli Tomato Basil & Mozzarella	1 cup	340	12	5	64
Organic Bistro					
Pasta Puttanesca	1 pkg (12.15 oz)	330	12	6	57
Organic Classics					
Cajun Chicken Tetrazzine w/ Penne Pasta	1 pkg (10 oz)	370	25	10	43
Chicken Cacciatore w/ Penne Pasta	1 pkg (10 oz)	270	20	4	37
Macaroni & Meat Sauce	1 pkg (10 oz)	340	16	9	49
Plum Organics					
Bowtie Pasta	1 pkg (6.9 oz)	230	7	6	37
Cheese Filled Spinach Tortellini	1 pkg (6.9 oz)	190	8	2	37
Putney Pasta					
Ravioli Butternut Squash & Vermont Maple Syrup	1 cup	200	8	4	35
Ravioli Portobello & Grilled Onion	7 (5.2 oz)	240	11	5	39
Ravioli Whole Wheat Spinach & Cheese	9 (5 oz)	300	13	9	42
Skillet Meal Chicken Piccata	1 serv (9 oz)	300	14	11	35
Skillet Meal Shrimp Pesto	1 serv (9 oz)	540	18	38	32
Tortellini Spinach Mozzarella & Walnuts	1 cup	360	20	8	51
Tortellini Tri-Color Three Cheese	1 cup	340	16	8	51
Stouffer's					
Cheesy Spaghetti Bake	1 pkg (12 oz)	460	21	24	39
Chicken Parmigiana	1 pkg (13.13 oz)	460	18	18	56
Escalloped Chicken & Noodles	1 pkg (8 oz)	330	14	18	28
Homestyle Chicken & Noodles	1 pkg (12 oz)	340	25	12	33

FOOD	PORTION	CALS	PROT	FAT	CARB
Italian Sausage Stuffed Rigatoni	1 pkg (9.13 oz)	380	18	14	46
Lasagna Vegetable	1 pkg (10.5 oz)	390	17	18	40
Lasagna Bake w/ Meat Sauce	1 pkg (11.5 oz)	380	18	13	47
Macaroni & Beef	1 pkg (11.5 oz)	330	19	11	38
Macaroni & Cheese	1 cup (6 oz)	350	15	17	34
Manicotti Cheese	1 pkg (9 oz)	360	18	14	41
Shrimp Scampi	1 pkg (14 oz)	410	21	11	57
Tuna Noodle Casserole	1 pkg (10 oz)	350	18	15	35
Turkey Tettrazini	1 pkg (10 oz)	380	19	20	32
Taste Above					
Meatless Thai Peanut Coconut Sauce w/ Veggie Chicken & Vermicelli	1 pkg (10 oz)	320	26	19	22
Meatless Tuscan Marinara Sauce w/ Veggie Chicken & Penne Pasta	1 pkg (10 oz)	320	26	19	22
Weight Watchers					
Smart Ones Lasagna w/ Meat Sauce	1 pkg (10.5 oz)	300	17	6	43
Yves					
Meatless Lasagna	1 pkg (10.5 oz)	300	17	3	51
MIX					
Back To Nature					
Crazy Bugs Macaroni & Cheese as prep	1 cup	370	12	10	60
Harvest Wheat Elbows & Cheddar as prep	½ pkg	380	12	12	60
Organic Shells & Cheese as prep	½ pkg	380	12	12	60
Carapelli					
Penne Alfredo as prep	1 cup	240	9	1	47
Spirals Creamy Tomato as prep	1 cup	240	9	1	49
DeBoles					
Organic Macaroni & Cheese Whole Wheat as prep	1 cup	410	11	14	60

FOOD	PORTION	CALS	PROT	FAT	CARB
Pasta & Cheese as prep	1 cup	420	10	15	60
Rice Shells & Cheddar as prep	½ cup	260	3	8	57
Hamburger Helper					
Cheesy Jambalaya as prep	1 cup	330	4	13	30
Knorr					
Pasta & Sauce Jalapeno Jack as prep	1 cup	230	8	3	45
Pasta Sides w/ Whole Grains Alfredo as prep	⅔ cup	300	10	11	42
Kraft					
Bistro Deluxe Sundried Tomato Parmesan as prep	1 cup	300	12	10	40
La Bella Vita					
Chicken & Lemon Borsellini as prep	1 cup	270	14	6	39
Near East					
Basil & Herb as prep	1 cup	240	8	5	42
Spicy Tomato as prep	1 cup	230	7	5	38
Pasta Roni					
Angel Hair w/ Herbs as prep	1 cup	310	9	13	41
Chicken as prep	1 cup	300	9	12	39
Chicken Quesadilla as prep	1 cup	310	10	13	40
Fettuccine Alfredo as prep	1 cup	450	11	25	47
Nature's Way Mushrooms In Cream Sauce as prep	1 cup	280	9	10	39
Sour Cream & Chives as prep	1 cup	310	8	15	38
Stroganoff as prep	1 cup	350	12	14	47
Road's End Organics					
Mac & Cheese Dairy Free Gluten Free as prep	1 cup	310	8	1	63
Shells & Cheese as prep	1 cup	330	14	1	66
Thai Kitchen					
Stir-Fry Rice Noodles Thai Peanut as prep	½ pkg	310	9	6	54
REFRIGERATED					
Country Crock					
Elbow Macaroni & Cheese	1 cup (8 oz)	370	14	17	40
Four Cheese Pasta	1 cup (8 oz)	380	15	17	41

FOOD	PORTION	CALS	PROT	FAT	CARB
Rozzano					
Organic Ravioli Grilled Vegetable	1 cup (3.5 oz)	200	10	6	26
SHELF-STABLE					
Allergaroo					
Gluten Free Spaghetti	1 pkg (8 oz)	220	3	3	49
Gluten Free Spyglass Noodles	1 pkg (8 oz)	230	4	3	49
Betty Crocker					
Bowl Appetit! Cheddar Broccoli Pasta	1 bowl (2.8 oz)	330	11	11	49
Bowl Appetit! Garlic Parmesan Pasta	1 bowl (2.8 oz)	320	11	9	50
Healthy Choice					
Fresh Mixers Ziti & Meat Sauce	1 pkg (6.9 oz)	340	15	6	56
Hormel					
Compleats Microwave Meals Chicken & Noodles	1 pkg (9.9 oz)	240	15	8	27
TastyBite					
Peanut Sauce w/ Noodles	1 pkg (10 oz)	530	17	19	104
TAKE-OUT					
bami goreng indonesian noodle dish	1 cup	170	5	3	25
lasagna meatless	1 piece (9 oz)	356	19	11	46
lasagna w/ meat	1 piece (8 oz)	362	22	14	37
lasagna w/ vegetables	1 serv (9 oz)	315	17	10	41
macaroni & cheese w/ ham	1 cup	542	21	33	41
manicotti cheese filled w/ marinara sauce	1 (5 oz)	229	13	10	22
manicotti cheese filled w/ meat sauce	1 (5 oz)	239	14	11	20
pasta w/ pesto sauce	1 cup	370	10	25	27
ravioli cheese & spinach filled w/ cream sauce	1 cup	362	15	17	38
ravioli cheese w/ tomato sauce	1 cup	335	14	14	38
ravioli meat filled w/ marinara sauce	1 cup	372	22	16	36
rigatoni w/ sausage sauce	¾ cup	260	10	12	28
spaghetti w/ red clam sauce	1 cup	285	13	8	41
spaghetti w/ sauce & meatballs	2 cups	670	34	26	80
spaghetti w/ white clam sauce	1 cup	456	25	20	43

FOOD	PORTION	CALS	PROT	FAT	CARB
tortellini cheese w/ tomato sauce	1 cup	332	14	14	38
tortellini meat filled w/ marinara sauce	1 cup	281	14	10	33
tortellini spinach filled w/ marinara sauce	1 cup	238	10	8	32

PASTA SALAD
MIX
Suddenly Salad

Caesar as prep	1 cup (1.8 oz)	310	6	14	38
Classic as prep	¾ cup	250	6	8	39
Creamy Italian as prep	¾ cup	350	7	20	36
Creamy Parmesan as prep	¾ cup	370	5	22	33

TAKE-OUT

pasta salad w/ crab vegetables mayonnaise	1 cup	317	10	16	33
tortellini salad cheese filled w/ vinaigrette dressing	1 cup	333	12	18	30

PATE

chicken liver canned	1 tbsp	26	2	2	1
duck pate	1 oz	96	4	8	1
fish pate	1 oz	76	3	7	1
liver w/ truffle	1 serv (2 oz)	183	6	16	4
mushroom pate	1 can (2.25 oz)	130	2	11	7
pate de foie gras smoked canned	1 tbsp	60	1	6	1
pork pate	1 oz	107	3	10	1
pork pate en croute	1 oz	91	3	7	3
rabbit pate	1 oz	66	5	5	1
shrimp	1 can (2.25 oz)	140	6	10	7

Patchwork

All Flavors	2 oz	270	5	27	5

PEACH
CANNED

halves in light syrup	1 half (3.4 oz)	53	tr	tr	14
halves juice pack	1 half (3.4 oz)	43	1	tr	11
in heavy syrup	½ cup (2.6 oz)	85	1	tr	22
peach sauce	½ cup	120	tr	0	32
pickled	½ cup (4.2 oz)	143	1	tr	35

FOOD	PORTION	CALS	PROT	FAT	CARB
pickled whole	1 (3.1 oz)	104	1	tr	26
slices juice pack	½ cup (4.4 oz)	55	1	tr	14
slices light syrup	½ cup (4.4 oz)	68	1	tr	18
slices water pack	½ cup (4.3 oz)	29	1	tr	7
spiced in heavy syrup	½ cup (4.2 oz)	91	1	tr	24
Del Monte					
Carb Clever Sliced	½ cup	30	1	0	7
Sliced Light Syrup Raspberry Flavor	½ cup	80	tr	0	20
Polar					
White	½ cup	70	1	0	17
S&W					
Slices Natural Style	½ cup (4.4 oz)	80	1	0	19
DRIED					
halves	½ cup (2.8 oz)	191	3	1	49
halves	1 (0.5 oz)	31	tr	tr	8
halves cooked w/o sugar	½ cup (4.5 oz)	99	2	tr	25
Mrs. May's					
Fruit Chips	1 pkg	35	0	0	8
Stoneridge Orchards					
Whole	⅓ cup (1.4 oz)	140	0	0	31
FRESH					
peach	1 lg (6.1 oz)	68	2	tr	17
peach	1 med (5.3 oz)	58	1	tr	14
sliced	½ cup (2.7 oz)	30	1	tr	8
FROZEN					
C&W					
Ultimate Sliced	¾ cup	50	1	0	13
PEACH JUICE					
nectar	1 cup (8.7 oz)	134	1	tr	35
Froose					
Playful Peach	1 box (4.2 oz)	80	1	0	19
Izze					
Sparkling Peach	1 bottle (12 oz)	130	0	0	32
OKF					
Sparkling Fresh Peach	1 bottle (8.3 oz)	50	0	0	12
Santa Cruz					
Organic Nectar	8 oz	120	0	0	31

FOOD	PORTION	CALS	PROT	FAT	CARB
PEANUT BUTTER					
chunky	2 tbsp	188	8	16	7
chunky	1 cup	1520	62	129	56
chunky w/o salt	1 cup	1520	62	129	56
chunky w/o salt	2 tbsp	188	8	16	7
smooth	1 cup	1517	63	128	53
smooth	2 tbsp	188	8	16	7
smooth w/o salt	1 cup	1517	63	129	53
smooth w/o salt	2 tbsp	188	8	16	7
Arrowhead Mills					
Organic Creamy	2 tbsp	190	8	17	6
Organic Honey Sweetened Creamy	2 tbsp	190	7	16	7
Organic Natural Crunchy	2 tbsp	190	8	17	6
Barney Butter					
Crunchy	2 tbsp	180	6	16	7
Smooth	2 tbsp	180	6	15	8
Better'n Peanut Butter					
Creamy	2 tbsp (1.1 oz)	100	4	2	13
Low Sodium	2 tbsp (1.1 oz)	100	4	2	13
Chet's					
Chocolate	2 tbsp	180	7	14	10
Roasted Nut	2 tbsp	180	7	14	9
Earth Balance					
Creamy or Chunky	1 tbsp	190	7	17	7
Justin's					
Organic Cinnamon	2 tbsp (1.1 oz)	180	7	15	8
Organic Classic	2 tbsp (1.1 oz)	150	7	17	7
Naturally More					
Natural	2 tbsp	169	10	11	8
Organic	2 tbsp	170	10	11	8
PB2					
Powdered Chocolate	2 tbsp	52	4	13	6
Powdered Chocolate Chip	2 tbsp	53	6	2	3
Reese's					
Creamy	2 tbsp (1.1 oz)	190	8	16	7
Peanut Butter Chips	1 tbsp (0.5 oz)	80	2	5	8
Revolution Foods					
Organic Creamy & Crunchy	1 tbsp (1.1 oz)	200	10	16	5

FOOD	PORTION	CALS	PROT	FAT	CARB
Santa Cruz					
Organic Creamy	2 tbsp (1.1 oz)	210	8	16	6
Smart Balance					
Chunky Omega	2 tbsp	200	7	17	6
Wonder					
Peanut Spread	2 tbsp	100	4	3	13
Peanut Spread Low Sodium	2 tbsp	100	4	3	13
PEANUT BUTTER SUBSTITUTES					
NoNuts					
Golden Peabutter	1 tbsp	93	2	7	6
PEANUTS					
chocolate coated	¼ cup	193	5	12	18
chocolate coated	1	21	1	1	2
cooked w/ salt	½ cup	286	12	20	19
dry roasted w/ salt	1 oz	166	7	14	6
dry roasted w/ salt	28 (1 oz)	164	7	14	6
dry roasted w/o salt	28 (1 oz)	164	7	14	6
dry roasted w/o salt	¼ cup	214	9	18	8
honey roasted	¼ cup	191	8	16	8
sugar coated	¼ cup	203	6	13	18
yogurt coated	¼ cup	230	6	16	18
Fisher					
Butter Toffee	¼ cup (1 oz)	140	3	6	18
Honey Roasted	¼ cup (1 oz)	170	5	13	9
Lance					
Salted	1 pkg (1.1 oz)	200	9	15	6
Nuts Are Good					
Buffalo	1 oz	120	3	6	16
Pina Colada	1 oz	130	3	7	16
Raspberry	1 oz	130	3	7	16
Vanilla Rum	1 oz	130	3	7	17
Sunfood					
Organic Wild Jungle	1 oz	174	7	14	5
True North					
Clusters	6 (1 oz)	170	6	13	9
PEAR					
CANNED					
halves in heavy syrup	½ cup (3.5 oz)	74	tr	tr	19
halves in heavy syrup	1 (1.7 oz)	36	tr	tr	9

FOOD	PORTION	CALS	PROT	FAT	CARB
halves in light syrup	1 (2.7 oz)	43	tr	tr	12
halves juice pack	½ cup (4.4 oz)	62	tr	tr	16
halves juice pack	1 (2.7 oz)	38	tr	tr	10
halves light syrup	½ cup (4.4 oz)	72	tr	tr	19
halves water pack	1 (2.7 oz)	22	tr	tr	6
Del Monte					
Carb Clever Sliced	½ cup	40	0	0	10
Liberty Gold					
Bartlett In Heavy Syrup	½ cup (4.5 oz)	90	0	0	23
S&W					
Halves Light Syrup	½ cup (4.4 oz)	80	0	0	19
DRIED					
halves	5 (3 oz)	229	2	1	61
halves	½ cup (3.2 oz)	236	2	1	63
halves	1 (0.6 oz)	47	tr	tr	13
halves cooked w/o sugar	½ cup (4.5 oz)	162	1	tr	43
Bare Fruit					
Organic	1 pkg (0.6 oz)	46	1	0	12
Brothers-All-Natural					
Crisps Asian Pear	1 pkg (0.35 oz)	40	0	0	9
Crispy Green					
Pears	1 pkg (0.35 oz)	40	0	0	8
FRESH					
asian	1 lg (9.6 oz)	116	1	1	30
asian	1 med (4.3 oz)	51	1	tr	13
pear	1 sm (5.2 oz)	86	1	tr	23
pear	1 lg (8.1 oz)	133	1	tr	36
pear	1 med (6.2 oz)	103	1	tr	28
sliced w/ skin	1 cup (4.9 oz)	81	1	tr	22
Chiquita					
Pear	1 (6.2 oz)	103	1	0	28
PEAR JUICE					
nectar canned	1 cup (8.8 oz)	150	tr	tr	39
Froose					
Perfect Pear	1 box (4.2 oz)	80	0	0	18
Santa Cruz					
Organic Nectar	8 oz	120	0	0	30

FOOD	PORTION	CALS	PROT	FAT	CARB
PEAS					
CANNED					
green	½ cup	59	4	tr	11
green low sodium	½ cup	59	4	tr	11
Del Monte					
Sweet No Salt Added	½ cup	60	3	0	11
Green Giant					
50% Less Sodium Young Tender Sweet	½ cup	60	4	0	11
Young Tender Sweet	½ cup	60	4	0	12
Le Sueur					
50% Less Sodium Young Tender	½ cup	60	4	0	11
S&W					
Petit Pois	½ cup (4.4 oz)	60	3	0	10
DRIED					
split cooked	1 cup	231	16	1	41
Arrowhead Mills					
Organic Green Split not prep	¼ cup	160	12	1	24
HamPeas					
Green Split Peas as prep	½ cup	120	8	1	21
Jack Rabbit					
Green Split	¼ cup (1.6 oz)	110	11	0	27
Snapea Crisps					
Baked Original	22 (1 oz)	70	5	8	14
Tree Of Life					
Wasabi Peas	¼ cup (1.1 oz)	120	5	4	17
FRESH					
green cooked	½ cup	67	4	tr	13
green raw	½ cup	58	4	tr	11
snap peas cooked	½ cup	34	3	tr	6
snap peas raw	½ cup	30	2	tr	5
Mann's					
Snow Peas	1 serv (3 oz)	35	2	0	6
FROZEN					
green cooked	½ cup	63	4	tr	11
snap peas cooked	½ cup	42	3	tr	7
Birds Eye					
Steamfresh Garlic Baby Peas & Mushrooms	¾ cup	80	4	2	12
Steamfresh Singles Sweet Peas	1 pkg (3.2 oz)	70	5	0	13

FOOD	PORTION	CALS	PROT	FAT	CARB
C&W					
Alfredo	½ cup	110	6	5	11
Early Harvest Petite No Salt Added	⅔ cup	70	4	0	12
Sugar Snap	⅔ cup	40	2	0	7
Green Giant					
Early June No Sauce	⅔ cup	50	5	1	11
SHELF-STABLE					
TastyBite					
Agra Peas & Greens	½ pkg (5 oz)	138	4	10	9
PECANS					
candied	1 oz	190	tr	17	10
dry roasted	1 oz	187	2	18	6
dry roasted salted	1 oz	187	2	18	6
halves dry roasted w/ salt	20 (1 oz)	200	3	21	4
halves dried	1 cup	721	8	73	20
oil roasted	1 oz	195	2	20	5
oil roasted salted	1 oz	195	2	20	5
Emily's					
Roasted & Salted	¼ cup (1 oz)	210	3	22	4
Fisher					
Roasted & Salted	¼ cup (1 oz)	200	3	21	4
PECTIN					
liquid	1 oz	3	0	0	1
powder	1 pkg (1.75 oz)	162	0	tr	45
Sure Jell					
Fruit Pectin	1 pkg (1.75 oz)	0	0	0	0
PEPEAO					
dried	¼ cup	18	tr	tr	5
raw sliced	1 cup	25	tr	tr	7
PEPPER					
black	1 tsp	5	tr	tr	1
cayenne	1 tsp	6	tr	tr	1
white	1 tsp	7	tr	tr	2
PEPPERMINT					
fresh chopped	2 tbsp	2	tr	tr	tr

FOOD	PORTION	CALS	PROT	FAT	CARB
PEPPERS					
CANNED					
chili green	1 cup (5.5 oz)	29	1	tr	6
chili green hot chopped	½ cup	17	1	tr	4
chili pepper paste	1 tbsp	6	tr	1	1
chili red hot	1 (2.6 oz)	18	1	tr	4
chili red hot chopped	½ cup	17	1	tr	4
green halves	½ cup	13	1	tr	3
jalapeno chopped	½ cup	17	1	tr	3
red halves	½ cup	13	1	tr	3
Gedney					
Hot & Sweet Jalapeno Peppers	¼ cup	30	0	0	5
Hot Banana Pepper Rings	¼ cup	10	0	0	1
Gertie's Finest					
Piquillo	1 oz	10	1	0	2
Pace					
Green Chiles Diced	2 tbsp	10	0	0	2
DRIED					
ancho	1 tsp	3	tr	tr	1
ancho	1 (0.6 oz)	48	2	1	9
casabel	1 tsp	3	tr	tr	1
chipotle smoked	1 tsp	3	tr	tr	1
green	1 tbsp	1	tr	tr	tr
guajillo	1 tsp	3	tr	tr	1
mulato	1 tsp	3	tr	tr	1
pasilla	1 tsp	3	tr	tr	1
pasilla	1 (7 g)	24	1	1	4
red	1 tbsp	1	tr	tr	tr
FRESH					
banana	1 (4 in) (1.2 oz)	9	1	tr	2
banana	1 cup (4.4 oz)	33	2	1	7
chili green hot	1	18	1	tr	4
chili green hot chopped	½ cup	30	2	tr	7
chili red chopped	½ cup	30	2	tr	7
chili red hot	1 (1.6 oz)	18	1	tr	4
green	1 (2.6 oz)	20	1	tr	5
green chopped	½ cup	13	tr	tr	3
green chopped cooked	½ cup	19	1	tr	5
green cooked	1 (2.6 oz)	20	1	tr	5

FOOD	PORTION	CALS	PROT	FAT	CARB
habanero	1 tsp	9	1	tr	2
hungarian	1 (0.9 oz)	8	tr	tr	2
jalapeno	1 (0.5 oz)	4	tr	tr	1
jalapeno sliced	1 cup (3.2 oz)	27	1	1	5
red	1 (2.6 oz)	20	1	tr	5
red chopped	½ cup	13	tr	tr	3
red chopped cooked	½ cup	19	1	tr	5
red cooked	1 (2.6 oz)	20	1	tr	5
serrano	1 (6 g)	2	tr	tr	tr
serrano chopped	1 cup (3.7 oz)	34	2	tr	7
yellow	10 strips	14	1	tr	3
yellow	1 (6.5 oz)	50	2	tr	12
FROZEN					
green chopped	1 oz	6	tr	tr	1
red chopped	1 oz	6	tr	tr	1
C&W					
Strips	¾ cup	25	1	0	4

PERCH
FRESH

FOOD	PORTION	CALS	PROT	FAT	CARB
cooked	1 fillet (1.6 oz)	54	11	1	0
cooked	3 oz	99	21	1	0
ocean perch atlantic cooked	3 oz	103	20	2	0
ocean perch atlantic cooked	1 fillet (1.8 oz)	60	12	1	0
ocean perch atlantic raw	3 oz	80	16	1	0
raw	3 oz	77	16	1	0
red raw	3.5 oz	114	18	4	0
FROZEN					
Bell					
Cajun Nuggets	12 (4.5 oz)	170	21	3	16
Fillets Breaded	1 piece (4.5 oz)	170	21	3	16
Fillets Unbreaded	1 piece (3.5 oz)	80	18	1	0

PERSIMMONS

FOOD	PORTION	CALS	PROT	FAT	CARB
dried japanese	1 (1.2 oz)	93	tr	tr	25
fresh	1 (6 oz)	118	1	tr	31

PHEASANT

FOOD	PORTION	CALS	PROT	FAT	CARB
breast boneless cooked	½ (4.4 oz)	312	41	15	0
cooked diced	1 cup	332	44	16	0
drumstick & thigh cooked	1 (2.6 oz)	184	24	9	0

FOOD	PORTION	CALS	PROT	FAT	CARB
PHYLLO					
sheet	1 (0.7 oz)	57	1	1	10
Ekizian					
Sheets	2 (4 oz)	433	12	9	76
Fillo Factory					
Kataifi Shredded Fillo	1 (2 oz)	180	5	2	35
Organic	2 sheets (1.5 oz)	130	4	1	27
Organic Whole Wheat	2 sheets (1.8 oz)	140	4	1	30
Shells Large	1 (0.7 oz)	80	2	2	13
PICANTE (see SALSA)					
PICKLES					
bread & butter	6 slices	39	tr	tr	9
dill	1 lg (4.7 oz)	24	1	tr	6
dill low sodium	1 med (2.3 oz)	12	tr	tr	3
dill sliced	6 slices	7	tr	tr	2
sweet gherkin	1 (1.2 oz)	41	tr	tr	11
tsukemono japanese pickles	¼ cup	10	tr	tr	2
Claussen					
Bread 'N Butter sliced Chips	1 oz	20	0	0	4
Kosher Dills Halves	1 (1 oz)	5	0	0	1
Sweet Gerkins	1 (0.9 oz)	30	0	0	7
Gedney					
Baby Dills	3 (1 oz)	5	0	0	1
Organic Baby Dills	2 (1 oz)	5	0	0	1
Texas Sassy					
Pickle Chips	1 tbsp (0.5 oz)	30	0	0	7
Tree Of Life					
Organic Sweet Bread & Butter Chips	4 (1 oz)	30	0	0	8
PIE (see also PIE CRUST, PIE FILLING)					
FROZEN					
Mrs. Smith's					
Bake & Serve No Sugar Added Apple	1 slice (4.6 oz)	310	3	16	40
Blueberry Crumb	1 slice (4.2 oz)	320	3	14	48
Cherry	1 slice (4.6 oz)	330	3	16	44
Cinnabon Apple Crumb	1 slice (4.6 oz)	350	3	16	49

FOOD	PORTION	CALS	PROT	FAT	CARB
Classic Cream Key Lime	1 slice (4.2 oz)	410	5	19	56
Coconut Custard	1 slice (4.4 oz)	300	6	17	31
Deep Dish Berry Burst	1 slice (4.2 oz)	340	3	15	51
Dutch Apple Crumb	1 slice (4.6 oz)	370	3	17	52
Pumpkin Custard	1 slice (4.6 oz)	300	5	15	38
Soda Shoppe Boston Cream	1 slice (2.7 oz)	220	2	9	32
Soda Shoppe Chocolate Cream	1 slice (4.6 oz)	350	4	17	47
Soda Shoppe Lemon Meringue	1 slice (4.2 oz)	300	3	10	51
READY-TO-EAT					
Lance					
Pecan	1 (3 oz)	350	4	17	46
Lifestream					
Pie Oh-My Apple	1 (3.5 oz)	280	3	11	43
Pie Oh-My Pineapple	1 (3.5 oz)	280	3	11	45
TAKE-OUT					
apple one crust	1 slice (5.3 oz)	363	3	14	59
apple tart	1 (4.2 oz)	370	4	19	48
apple two crust	1 slice (5.3 oz)	356	3	17	51
apricot tart	1 (4.2 oz)	356	4	17	48
apricot two crust	1 slice (5.3 oz)	417	5	19	59
banana cream	1 slice (5.1 oz)	387	6	20	47
blackberry one crust	1 slice (4.4 oz)	341	4	17	44
blackberry two crust	1 slice (5.3 oz)	394	4	19	54
blueberry one crust	1 slice (4.8 oz)	292	3	12	45
blueberry tart	1 (4.2 oz)	346	3	17	47
blueberry two crust	1 slice (5.3 oz)	348	3	15	52
cherry one crust	1 slice (4.8 oz)	312	3	12	50
cherry two crust	1 slice (5.3 oz)	390	3	17	60
chess	1 slice (3 oz)	365	5	18	48
chocolate cream	1 slice (5 oz)	380	7	18	50
coconut creme	1 slice (5 oz)	429	3	24	54
custard	1 slice (4.8 oz)	286	7	16	28
grasshopper	1 slice (3.5 oz)	341	4	19	33
key lime	1 slice (5 oz)	420	4	14	71
lemon meringue	1 slice (4.8 oz)	367	2	12	65
lemon meringue tart	1 (4.1 oz)	298	4	14	41
mince two crust	1 slice (5.3 oz)	434	4	16	72
peach two crust	1 slice (5.3 oz)	334	3	15	49
pear two crust	1 slice (5.3 oz)	400	4	18	57
pecan	1 slice (4 oz)	456	5	21	65

FOOD	PORTION	CALS	PROT	FAT	CARB
pineapple two crust	1 slice (5.3 oz)	394	4	18	55
plum two crust	1 slice (5.3 oz)	441	4	21	61
prune one crust	1 slice (5.3 oz)	450	6	14	77
pumpkin	1 slice (5.4 oz)	323	6	15	42
raisin tart	1 (4.2 oz)	348	4	16	49
raisin two crust	1 slice (5.3 oz)	376	4	16	55
raspberry one crust	1 slice (4.8 oz)	330	3	13	52
raspberry two crust	1 slice (5.3 oz)	422	4	20	58
rhubarb two crust	1 slice (5.3 oz)	444	5	23	55
shoo-fly	1 slice (4 oz)	404	4	13	69
strawberry rhubarb two crust	1 slice (5.3 oz)	422	5	21	53
strawberry two crust	1 slice (6 oz)	386	4	16	58
sweet potato	1 piece (5.4 oz)	276	6	14	32

PIE CRUST

FOOD	PORTION	CALS	PROT	FAT	CARB
baked	⅙ crust (1 oz)	147	1	9	14
chocolate wafer	⅛ crust (1.2 oz)	177	2	11	19
chocolate wafer tart shell	1 (0.8 oz)	111	1	7	12
deep dish frzn	⅛ crust (1.8 oz)	266	3	16	27
graham cracker	⅙ crust (1.2 oz)	172	1	9	23
graham cracker tart shell	1 (0.8 oz)	109	1	5	14
puff pastry shell	1 (1.4 oz)	223	3	15	18
tart shell	1 (1 oz)	149	1	10	14
Honey Maid					
Graham Cracker Crumbs as prep	⅛ pie	160	1	9	18
Keebler					
Graham Reduced Fat	⅛ pie (0.7 oz)	100	1	4	15
Ready Crust Chocolate	⅛ pie (0.7 oz)	100	1	5	14
Ready Crust Graham	⅒ pie (0.9 oz)	130	1	6	18
Ready Crust Shortbread	⅛ pie (0.7 oz)	110	1	5	14
Mrs. Smith's					
Deep Dish Shell frzn	1 slice (1 oz)	130	2	7	14
Nilla Wafers					
Pie Crust	⅙ (1 oz)	140	1	8	18
Pepperidge Farm					
Puff Pastry Sheets frzn	⅙ sheet	170	3	11	14
Puff Pastry Shell frzn	1	190	4	13	16

FOOD	PORTION	CALS	PROT	FAT	CARB
Pillsbury					
Crusts Just Unroll	⅛ (1 oz)	110	tr	7	12
Deep Dish frzn	⅛ (0.7 oz)	90	1	5	11
Pet Ritz Deep Dish frzn	⅛ (0.6 oz)	90	1	5	11
PIE FILLING					
apple	1 cup	155	tr	tr	41
blueberry	1 cup	474	1	1	116
cherry	1 cup	317	2	2	76
lemon	1 cup	923	13	18	185
pumpkin pie mix canned	1 cup	281	3	tr	71
Chukar Cherries					
Triple Cherry	½ cup	190	tr	1	47
Comstock					
Country Cherry Original	⅓ cup (3.1 oz)	90	0	0	23
Farmer's Market					
Organic Pumpkin Pie Mix	½ cup	100	0	0	25
PIEROGI					
potato	1 (1.3 oz)	70	3	2	11
Mrs. T's					
Mini Potato & Cheddar	7 (3 oz)	130	4	2	25
Potato & Cheddar	4 (4 oz)	170	6	3	32
Potato & Onion	3 (4 oz)	160	5	2	32
Potato Broccoli & Cheddar	3 (4 oz)	190	6	5	31
Sauerkraut	3 (4 oz)	140	4	2	28
Sour Cream & Chive	3 (4 oz)	190	5	5	32
PIGEON PEAS					
dried cooked	1 cup	204	11	1	39
dried cooked	½ cup	102	6	tr	20
PIGNOLIA (see PINE NUTS)					
PIG'S FEET					
cooked	1	201	19	14	0
pickled	1	177	12	14	tr
Hormel					
Pigs Feet	2 oz	80	7	6	0
PIKE					
northern cooked	½ fillet (5.4 oz)	176	38	1	0
northern cooked	3 oz	96	21	1	0

FOOD	PORTION	CALS	PROT	FAT	CARB
northern raw	3 oz	75	16	1	0
roe raw	1 oz	37	7	tr	tr
walleye baked	3 oz	101	21	1	0
walleye fillet baked	4.4 oz	147	30	2	0

PILLNUTS

canarytree dried	1 oz	204	3	23	1

PIMIENTOS

canned	1 slice	0	tr	0	tr
canned	1 tbsp	3	tr	tr	1

PINE NUTS

pine nuts dried	¼ cup (1.2 oz)	277	5	23	4
pinyon dried	1 oz	178	3	17	5
pinyon dried	20 (2 g)	13	tr	1	tr
Fisher					
Pine Nuts	¼ cup (1 oz)	190	4	19	4

PINEAPPLE
CANNED

chunks in heavy syrup	1 cup	199	1	tr	52
chunks juice pack	1 cup	150	1	tr	39
crushed in heavy syrup	1 cup	199	1	tr	52
slices in heavy syrup	1 slice	45	tr	tr	12
slices in light syrup	1 slice	30	tr	tr	8
slices juice pack	1 slice	35	tr	tr	9
slices water pack	1 slice	19	tr	tr	5
tidbits in heavy syrup	1 cup	199	1	tr	52
tidbits in juice	1 cup	150	1	tr	19
tidbits in water	1 cup	79	1	tr	20
Gefen					
Chunks In Juice	½ cup (4.9 oz)	80	0	0	19
Liberty Gold					
Chunks In Natural Juice	½ cup (4.7 oz)	80	tr	0	21
Slices Natural Juice	½ cup	80	tr	0	21
DRIED					
Brothers-All-Natural					
Crisps	1 pkg (0.53 oz)	60	0	0	14
Crispy Green					
Freeze-Dried	1 pkg (0.35)	35	0	0	9

FOOD	PORTION	CALS	PROT	FAT	CARB
Kopali					
Organic	1 pkg (1.7 oz)	170	0	0	43
Mrs. May's					
Fruit Chips	1 pkg	35	0	0	8
Sunsweet					
Pineapples	⅓ cup (1.4 oz)	130	0	0	34
FRESH					
diced	1 cup	77	1	tr	19
slice	1 slice	42	tr	tr	10
Chiquita					
Bites	1 piece (2.8 oz)	40	1	0	9
Cut Up	1 cup (5.8 oz)	82	1	0	22
FROZEN					
chunks sweetened	½ cup	104	tr	tr	27
PINEAPPLE JUICE					
canned	1 cup	139	1	tr	34
frzn as prep	1 cup	129	1	tr	32
frzn not prep	6 oz	387	3	tr	96
Sundia					
Purely	½ cup	60	1	0	15
Walnut Acres					
Organic	8 oz	130	0	0	32
PINK BEANS					
dried cooked	1 cup	252	15	1	47
PINTO BEANS					
dried cooked	1 cup	245	15	1	45
Arrowhead Mills					
Organic Dried not prep	¼ cup	150	9	0	27
HamBeens					
Dried as prep	½ cup	120	7	1	22
Tree Of Life					
Organic	½ cup (4.6 oz)	120	8	0	23
TAKE-OUT					
stewed w/ viandas	1 cup	222	11	8	27
PISTACHIOS					
dry roasted w/ salt	49 nuts (1 oz)	161	6	13	8
dry roasted w/o salt	49 nuts (1 oz)	162	6	13	8
in shells	½ cup	165	6	13	8

FOOD	PORTION	CALS	PROT	FAT	CARB
Fisher					
Shelled	¼ cup (1 oz)	160	6	13	8
Love'n Bake					
Pistachio Paste	2 tbsp	160	4	11	14
True North					
Sea Salted In Shells	½ cup	170	6	14	7
Wonderful					
Roasted & Salted In Shells	½ cup	170	6	14	8
PITANGA					
fresh	1 cup	57	1	1	13
fresh	1	2	tr	tr	1
PIZZA (see also PIZZA CRUST)					
4Real					
Cheese	1 (4.2 oz)	220	11	4	38
Cheesy Pizza Quesadilla	1 (2.5 oz)	160	11	5	15
Turkey Pepperoni	1 (4.2 oz)	220	11	4	38
Amy's					
Cheese & Pesto Whole Wheat Crust	⅓ pie (4.6 oz)	360	13	18	37
Margherita	1 pie (6.2 oz)	360	16	17	47
Non Dairy Cheese Rice Crust	1 pie (6 oz)	460	10	28	46
Pocket Sandwich Spinach Feta	1 (4.5 oz)	260	11	9	34
Roasted Vegetable No Cheese	⅓ pie (4 oz)	270	6	9	42
Single Serve Spinach Light In Sodium	1 (7.2 oz)	440	19	18	54
Soy Cheese	⅓ pie (4.3 oz)	290	12	11	37
Toaster Pops Cheese Pizza	5–6 pieces (1.9 oz)	160	5	6	21
Cedarlane					
Zone Cheese	1 (6.5 oz)	380	27	14	39
Dayeinu					
Passover Pizza	1 slice (4 oz)	325	15	8	49
DiGiorno					
Crispy Flatbread Tuscan Chicken	⅓ pie (4.6 oz)	280	14	14	25
For One Thin Crust Grilled Chicken & Vegetable	1 (8.4 oz)	520	28	17	64
For One Traditional Crust Supreme	1 (9.9 oz)	790	31	36	85

FOOD	PORTION	CALS	PROT	FAT	CARB
Four Cheese	⅙ pie (4.7 oz)	310	15	11	40
Garlic Bread Pepperoni	⅙ pie (5 oz)	380	17	17	40
Rising Crust Four Cheese	⅓ pie (4 oz)	270	13	9	34
Rising Crust Italian Sausage	⅙ pie (5 oz)	350	15	14	40
Rising Crust Spinach Mushroom Garlic	⅙ pie (5 oz)	290	15	9	42
Rising Crust Three Meat	⅙ pie (5 oz)	350	16	15	41
Stuffed Crust Pepperoni	⅕ pie (5.3 oz)	380	19	16	40
Thin Crispy Crust Pepperoni	⅕ pie (4.4 oz)	320	16	15	31
Thin Crispy Crust Spinach Mushroom Garlic	⅕ pie (4.6 oz)	250	12	9	32
Ultimate Topping Four Meat	⅕ pie (5 oz)	380	19	19	34
Ultimate Topping Supreme	⅕ pie (5.3 oz)	360	16	18	35
Dr. Praeger's					
Bagel Pizza	1 (2 oz)	120	7	3	17
Farm Rich					
Slices Pepperoni	2 (3.5 oz)	280	14	14	22
Glutino					
Gluten Free Duo Cheese	1 (6.1 oz)	420	10	12	68
Gluten Free Spinach & Feta	1 (6.1 oz)	430	10	16	62
Health Is Wealth					
Vegetarian Mini Pizza Bagels	4 (3.1 oz)	150	8	0	28
Hot Pockets					
Croissant Five Cheese	1 (4.5 oz)	350	14	17	35
Croissant Pepperoni	1 (4.5 oz)	380	11	22	32
Sausage	1 (4.5 oz)	330	10	16	36
Jeno's					
Crisp 'N Tasty Cheese	1 pie (6.8 oz)	440	16	21	47
Crisp 'N Tasty Pepperoni	1 (6.7 oz)	490	16	26	50
Crisp 'N Tasty Supreme	1 (7.2 oz)	490	17	25	49
Kraft					
Rising Crust Three Meat	⅓ pie (4.4 oz)	320	15	14	25
Lean Pockets					
Pepperoni	1 (4.5 oz)	260	15	7	35
Sausage & Pepperoni	1 (4.5 oz)	280	12	7	39
Lunchables					
Pepperoni Sausage	1 pkg	440	16	12	68
Pizza Deep Dish Cheese	1 pkg	370	10	11	60
Red Baron					
Classic Crust 4 Cheese	1 pie (8.6 oz)	740	33	39	62

FOOD	PORTION	CALS	PROT	FAT	CARB
Stouffer's					
Corner Bistro Flatbread Chicken Bacon & Spinach	1 pkg (9.13 oz)	640	31	29	65
Corner Bistro Flatbread Margherita	1 pkg (9.13 oz)	540	22	22	65
Corner Bistro Flatbread Shrimp & Roasted Garlic	1 pkg (9.33 oz)	600	33	19	75
French Bread Grilled Vegetable	1 pkg (11.63 oz)	340	13	12	44
French Bread Sausage	1 pkg (4.2 oz)	420	15	21	43
French Bread Sausage & Pepperoni	1 pkg (4.2 oz)	460	17	24	42
French Bread White Pizza	1 pkg (10.13 oz)	470	22	23	44
Totino's					
Crisp Crust Canadian Bacon	½ pie (5.1 oz)	320	13	15	34
Crisp Crust Combination	½ pie (5.3 oz)	380	14	21	34
Crisp Crust Pepperoni Trio	½ pie (5 oz)	370	13	21	33
Crisp Crust Three Meat	½ pie (5.2 oz)	350	13	18	34
Pizza Rolls Combination	6 (3 oz)	220	8	11	24
Pizza Rolls Mega Ultimate Combination	3 (3.3 oz)	200	8	8	25
Pizza Rolls Supreme	6 (3 oz)	210	7	9	25
TAKE-OUT					
cheese	16 in pie	3384	151	144	372
cheese	⅛ of 16 in pie	423	19	18	46
cheese deep dish individual	1 (5.5 oz)	460	15	24	47
cheese & vegetables	⅛ of 16 in pie	428	17	16	55
ground beef	16 in pie	3753	151	172	392
ham & pineapple	⅛ of 16 in pie	439	19	16	55
no cheese	⅛ of 16 in pie	262	6	7	43
pepperoni	⅛ of 16 in pie	469	19	22	49
white pizza	⅛ of 16 in pie	484	20	17	61
PIZZA CRUST					
crust	1 slice (1.7 oz)	130	4	2	25
whole wheat	⅛ crust (2 oz)	120	4	2	24
Boboli					
100% Whole Wheat	⅕ crust (2 oz)	150	6	3	27
Original	⅛ crust (1.8 oz)	140	5	3	24

FOOD	PORTION	CALS	PROT	FAT	CARB
Original Mini	½ crust (2.5 oz)	190	6	3	35
Thin Crust	⅕ crust (2 oz)	170	6	4	28
French Meadow Bakery					
Gluten Free	¼ pie (1.9 oz)	160	2	4	29
Martha White					
Mix not prep	¼ pkg	160	5	1	32
Pillsbury					
Classic	⅙ crust (2.3 oz)	160	5	2	31
PLANTAINS					
cooked mashed	1 cup	232	2	tr	62
sliced cooked	1 cup	179	1	tr	48
Grab Em Snacks					
Chips Black Pepper	1 oz	150	tr	8	19
TAKE-OUT					
mofongo	1 serv	320	9	3	71
ripe fried	1 serv (2.8 oz)	214	1	7	38
sweet baked w/ ice cream	1 serv	285	2	8	57
PLUM JUICE					
Nantucket Nectars					
Red Plum	8 oz	120	0	0	30
Sunsweet					
PlumSmart Light	8 oz	60	0	0	15
PLUMS					
canned in heavy syrup	1 cup	163	1	tr	42
canned purple juice pack	1 cup	146	1	tr	38
canned purple water pack	1 cup	102	1	tr	27
dried japanese	1	9	tr	tr	2
fresh	1	30	tr	tr	8
pickled	1	34	tr	tr	9
Chiquita					
Fresh	1 (2.3 oz)	30	0	0	8
Oregon					
Whole In Heavy Syrup	½ cup (4.6 oz)	100	1	0	25
POI					
poi	1 cup	240	1	0	65

FOOD	PORTION	CALS	PROT	FAT	CARB
POKEBERRY SHOOTS					
cooked	½ cup	16	2	tr	3
fresh	½ cup	18	2	tr	3
POLENTA					
Bob's Red Mill					
Corn Grits Polenta not prep	¼ cup	130	3	1	27
POLLACK					
atlantic fillet baked	5.3 oz	178	38	2	0
atlantic baked	3 oz	100	21	1	0
POMEGRANATE					
fresh	1 (5.4 oz)	105	1	tr	26
Navitas Naturals					
Pomegranate Powder	1 tbsp (0.5 oz)	50	0	0	13
POMEGRANATE JUICE					
Apple & Eve					
Organic	8 oz	130	0	0	33
Arthur's					
Pom Plus	1 bottle (11 oz)	220	1	0	54
Frutzzo					
Organic 100% Juice	1 bottle (12 oz)	130	0	0	32
Langers					
100% Juice	8 oz	150	0	0	37
Odwalla					
PomaGrand 100% Juice	8 oz	160	0	0	40
Old Orchard					
100% Pure	8 oz	140	0	0	34
Smart Juice					
Organic 100% Juice	8 oz	149	1	0	37
Tart Is Smart					
Concentrate	0.5 oz	37	0	0	9
POMPANO					
smoked	2 oz	109	12	6	0
steamed or poached	4 oz	156	18	9	0
TAKE-OUT					
battered & fried	4 oz	304	20	21	8
breaded & fried	4 oz	242	16	15	10

FOOD	PORTION	CALS	PROT	FAT	CARB
POPCORN					
air popped	1 cup (0.3 oz)	31	1	tr	6
caramel coated	1 cup (1.2 oz)	152	1	5	28
caramel coated w/ peanuts	⅔ cup (1 oz)	114	2	2	23
cheese	1 cup (0.4 oz)	58	1	4	6
oil popped	1 cup (0.4 oz)	55	1	3	6
Divvies					
Caramel Corn Vegan	½ cup	80	tr	3	14
I.M. Healthy					
Roasted Sweet Corn Original Lightly Salted	1 oz	120	3	5	20
Jay's					
Caramel	¾ cup	110	tr	0	26
Ok-Ke-Doke Cheese	1 oz	160	2	11	13
Lance					
White Cheddar	1 pkg (0.7 oz)	100	1	11	8
Mrs. Fields					
Clusters Butter Toffee Crunch	⅔ cup	170	2	5	31
Poppycock					
Cashew Lovers	½ cup (1.1 oz)	148	2	6	21
Original	½ cup (1.1 oz)	160	2	8	20
Pecan Delight	½ cup (1.1 oz)	150	1	8	20
Smart Balance					
Low Fat Smart 'N Healthy as prep	5 cups	120	4	2	24
Snyder's Of Hanover					
Butter	0.6 oz	100	1	8	6
Tree Of Life					
Organic Lightly Salted	4 cups	100	3	2	21
Utz					
Butter	2 cups	170	2	12	13
Cheese	2 cups	160	2	11	14
Puff'n Corn Original Hulless	2 cups	150	1	17	11
POPOVER					
home recipe as prep w/ 2% milk	1 (1.4 oz)	87	4	3	11
home recipe as prep w/ whole milk	1 (1.4 oz)	90	4	3	11
mix as prep	1 (1.2 oz)	67	3	2	10

FOOD	PORTION	CALS	PROT	FAT	CARB
POPPY SEEDS					
poppy seeds	1 tbsp	47	2	4	2
Bob's Red Mill					
Poppy Seeds	3 tbsp	170	6	14	6
Love'n Bake					
Poppy Seed Filling	2 tbsp	120	2	5	18
PORGY					
fresh	3 oz	77	18	tr	0
PORK (see also HAM, JERKY, PORK DISHES)					
FRESH					
boneless loin lean & fat roasted	3.5 oz	195	26	9	0
center loin chop bone in broiled	1 (3 oz)	178	22	9	0
center rib chop lean & fat bone in broiled	1 (3 oz)	189	21	11	0
country style ribs bone in lean & fat braised	3.5 oz	288	28	19	0
dehydrated oriental style	1 cup (0.8 oz)	135	3	14	tr
fresh ham rump half lean & fat roasted	4 oz	278	32	16	0
fresh ham shank half lean & fat roasted	4 oz	319	28	22	0
fresh ham whole lean & fat roasted	4 oz	302	30	19	0
ground cooked	4 oz	328	28	23	0
ham hock cooked	1	167	14	12	0
shoulder chop bone in braised	1 (3 oz)	229	23	15	0
sirloin roast lean & fat bone in roasted	4 oz	231	27	13	0
spareribs bone in roasted	3 oz	304	18	26	0
tail simmered	3 oz	336	15	30	0
tenderloin roast boneless lean & fat roasted	4 oz	145	26	4	0
top loin chop boneless lean & fat broiled	1 (3.5 oz)	195	27	9	0
Organic Prairie					
Chop	1 (3.3 oz)	220	26	13	0
Ground	4 oz	300	19	24	0
Smithfield					
Boneless Smoked Pork Chop	3 oz	110	15	4	4
Smoked Pork Chop	3 oz	100	14	3	2

FOOD	PORTION	CALS	PROT	FAT	CARB
Tyson					
Baby Back Ribs Buffalo	4 oz	300	16	24	4
Ground Reduced Fat	4 oz	260	18	20	0
Half Loin Boneless	4 oz	190	20	12	0
Loin Chops Bone-In Center Cut	4 oz	190	20	13	0
Spareribs	4 oz	290	16	24	0
Stew Meat	4 oz	130	21	5	0
TAKE-OUT					
chicharrones pork cracklings fried	1 cup	492	34	38	1
chop breaded & fried	1 lg (5 oz)	441	30	26	19
chop breaded & fried	1 med (3.4 oz)	304	20	18	13
chop stewed	1 lg (4.6 oz)	315	36	18	0

PORK DISHES
A La Carte Gourmet

FOOD	PORTION	CALS	PROT	FAT	CARB
Pork Loin w/ Cream Spinach Feta Stuffing	1 serv (5 oz)	200	20	9	8
Hormel					
Always Tender Loin Filet Honey Mustard	1 serv (4 oz)	140	20	5	4
Always Tender Tenderloin Apple Burbon	1 serv (4 oz)	140	19	4	5
Pork Roast Au Jus	1 serv (2 oz)	90	8	3	10
Tyson					
Roast Pork w/ Vegetables	1 serv (4 oz)	190	21	4	18
Ventera					
Pork Carnitas	1 serv (5 oz)	190	23	8	6
TAKE-OUT					
kalua pork	1 cup (7 oz)	497	43	34	1
pork satay w/ peanut sauce	5 sticks (3.5 oz)	214	12	13	14
pulled pork w/ barbecue sauce	1 serv (5 oz)	240	14	14	15
spareribs barbecued w/ sauce	2 med (2.8 oz)	248	17	18	3
tourtiere	1 piece (4.9 oz)	451	15	34	21

PORK RINDS (*see also* SNACKS)

POT PIE
Amy's

FOOD	PORTION	CALS	PROT	FAT	CARB
Broccoli	1 (7.5 oz)	430	11	22	46

FOOD	PORTION	CALS	PROT	FAT	CARB
Shepherd's	1 (8 oz)	160	5	4	27
Shepherd's Pie Light In Sodium	1 (8 oz)	160	5	4	27
Vegetable	1 (7.5 oz)	360	10	13	50
Banquet					
Beef	1	450	14	27	36
Chicken	1	370	10	21	34
Chicken w/ Broccoli	1	350	10	20	32
Turkey	1	390	10	21	36
Hot Pockets					
Pot Pie Express Chicken	1 (4.5 oz)	330	8	18	34
Marie Callender's					
Beef	½ pie	540	16	32	46
Cheeesy Chicken	½ pie	600	17	37	46
Chicken	1	670	19	41	55
Creamy Mushroom & Chicken	½ pie	560	15	35	45
Turkey	1	670	19	41	56
Mon Cuisine					
Vegan	1 pkg (9 oz)	650	21	39	60
Pepperidge Farm					
Chili Beans & Cornbread	1 cup	360	11	17	40
Reduced Fat Roasted White Meat Chicken	1 cup	470	14	21	56
Roasted White Meat Chicken	1 cup	510	13	32	43
Stouffer's					
Chicken White Meat	1 pkg (10 oz)	660	19	37	62
TAKE-OUT					
beef	1 (14.6 oz)	938	34	57	72
chicken	1 (14.6 oz)	897	37	52	69
ham	1 serv (11 oz)	752	28	45	58
oyster	1 serv (11.5 oz)	817	19	53	67
puerto rican pastelon de carne	1 piece (5 oz)	666	22	48	35
st. stephen's day pie	1 serv (16.7 oz)	549	35	29	38
tuna	1 (27 oz)	1715	71	102	126
vegetarian w/ meat substitute	1 (8 oz)	511	17	32	39

POTATO (see also CHIPS, KNISH, PANCAKES)
CANNED

potatoes	½ cup	54	1	tr	12

FOOD	PORTION	CALS	PROT	FAT	CARB
Butterfield					
Whole White	3.5 pieces (5.8 oz)	90	2	0	20
Del Monte					
Savory Sides Au Gratin	½ cup	80	2	3	13
S&W					
New Whole	2 (5.5 oz)	60	1	0	13
Sunshine					
Whole White	3 pieces (5.9 oz)	90	2	0	20
FRESH					
baked skin only	1 skin (2 oz)	115	2	tr	27
baked w/ skin	1 (6.5 oz)	220	5	tr	51
baked w/o skin	1 (5 oz)	145	3	tr	34
baked w/o skin	½ cup	57	1	tr	13
boiled	½ cup	68	1	tr	16
microwaved	1 (7 oz)	212	5	tr	49
microwaved w/o skin	½ cup	78	2	tr	18
raw w/o skin	1 (3.9 oz)	88	2	tr	20
FROZEN					
french fries	10 strips	111	2	4	17
french fries thick cut	10 strips	109	2	4	17
hash browns	½ cup	170	2	9	22
potato puffs	½ cup	138	2	7	19
potato puffs	1	16	tr	1	2
Cascadian Farm					
Organic Country Style	¾ cup	50	1	0	12
Organic Hash Browns	1 cup	60	2	0	14
Funster					
BBQ Lite	14 pieces (3 oz)	140	2	3	25
Cheddar	14 pieces (3 oz)	135	2	3	25
Original	14 pieces (3 oz)	135	2	3	25
Green Giant					
Roasted Potatoes w/ Garlic & Herb Sauce as prep	½ cup	90	2	2	15
Health Is Wealth					
Twice Baked Cheddar Cheese	1 (5 oz)	200	4	10	25
Vegetarian Potato Skins	2 (2.7 oz)	110	5	7	8

FOOD	PORTION	CALS	PROT	FAT	CARB
Joy Of Cooking					
Elegant Scalloped	1 cup (8 oz)	300	9	17	21
Red Skin Mashed	1 cup (4.2 oz)	160	3	9	17
MIX					
au gratin as prep	½ cup	160	6	9	14
instant mashed flakes as prep w/ whole milk & butter	½ cup	118	2	6	16
instant mashed flakes not prep	½ cup	78	2	tr	18
instant mashed granules as prep w/ whole milk & butter	½ cup	114	2	5	15
instant mashed granules not prep	½ cup	372	8	1	86
scalloped	½ cup	105	4	5	13
Betty Crocker					
Au Gratin as prep	⅔ cup	150	2	5	24
Cheddar & Bacon as prep	⅔ cup	120	2	3	21
Cheesy Scalloped as prep	½ cup	120	2	3	21
Julienne as prep	⅔ cup	140	2	5	20
Mashed Four Cheese as prep	½ cup	170	2	7	21
Mashed Sour Cream & Chives as prep	½ cup	170	2	7	21
Scalloped as prep	½ cup	130	2	4	20
Seasoned Skillets Hash Browns as prep	½ cup	120	2	4	19
REFRIGERATED					
Bob Evans					
Mashed Potatoes Original	½ cup (4.4 oz)	150	3	7	20
Country Crock					
Garlic Mashed	⅔ cup (5 oz)	160	2	7	22
Homestyle Mashed	⅔ cup (5 oz)	180	2	9	23
Loaded Mashed	⅔ cup (5 oz)	200	4	11	22
Diner's Choice					
Mashed	⅔ cup	110	2	5	15
Reser's					
Potato Express Red Skinned Mashed	½ cup	140	3	5	22
Simply Potatoes					
Traditional Mashed	½ cup (4.4 oz)	120	2	6	15

FOOD	PORTION	CALS	PROT	FAT	CARB
SHELF-STABLE					
TastyBite					
Bombay Potatoes	½ pkg (5 oz)	105	5	4	13
TAKE-OUT					
au gratin w/ cheese	½ cup	178	7	10	17
baked topped w/ cheese sauce	1	475	15	29	47
baked topped w/ cheese sauce & bacon	1	451	18	26	44
baked topped w/ cheese sauce & broccoli	1	402	14	14	47
baked topped w/ cheese sauce & chili	1	481	23	22	56
baked topped w/ sour cream & chives	1	394	7	22	50
french fries	1 reg	235	3	12	29
hash browns	½ cup (2.5 oz)	151	2	9	16
indian yogurt potatoes	1 serv	315	7	9	52
mashed	½ cup	111	2	4	18
o'brien	1 cup	157	5	3	30
potato pancakes	1 (1.3 oz)	101	2	7	11
potato salad	½ cup	179	3	10	14
red new boiled	5 sm (5 oz)	120	3	0	27
scalloped	½ cup	127	4	5	18
twice baked w/ cheese	1 half (10 oz)	392	8	18	48
POTATO STARCH					
potato starch	1 oz	96	tr	tr	24
Bob's Red Mill					
Potato Starch	1 tbsp	40	0	0	10
POUT					
ocean baked	3 oz	86	18	1	0
ocean fillet baked	4.8 oz	139	29	2	0
PRETZELS					
chocolate covered	1 (0.4 oz)	47	1	1	8
soft	1 lg (5 oz)	483	12	4	99
twists salted	10 (2.1 oz)	229	6	2	48
twists w/o salt	10 (2.1 oz)	229	5	2	48
whole wheat	2 sm (1 oz)	103	3	1	23
yogurt covered	1 (4 g)	19	tr	1	3
yogurt covered	1 cup (3 oz)	391	7	13	61

FOOD	PORTION	CALS	PROT	FAT	CARB
Braids					
Honey Wheat	7 (1 oz)	110	3	2	23
Mini Knots	17 (1 oz)	110	3	1	23
Glenny's					
Organic Original Salted	8 (1 oz)	110	3	0	23
Organic Sourdough	6 (1 oz)	110	3	0	23
Glutino					
Gluten Free All Shapes	44 (1.4 oz)	190	1	8	28
New York Style					
Pretzel Flatz Original Salt	12	110	3	1	23
Rold Gold					
Braided Twists	1 oz	110	2	1	22
Braided Twists Honey Wheat	1 oz	110	2	1	23
Dipped Twists Fudge Coated	1 oz	140	2	6	18
Mini Sticks Honey Mustard & Onion	1 oz	140	2	6	19
Pretzel Waves Cheddar	1 oz	130	2	5	20
Pretzel Waves Dark Chocolate Drizzle	1 oz	130	2	4	20
Pretzel Waves Vanilla Yogurt Drizzle	1 oz	130	2	5	21
Sourdough Hard	1	100	2	1	21
Sticks Classic	1 oz	100	2	0	23
Tiny Twists	1 oz	100	3	0	23
Salba Smart					
Omega-3 Enriched	1 oz	110	2	2	21
Snyder's Of Hanover					
100 Calorie Pack Snaps	1 pkg (0.9 oz)	100	3	1	22
Dips Milk Chocolate	1 oz	140	2	6	19
Dips Special Dark Chocolate	1 oz	140	2	5	22
Mini Unsalted	1 oz	110	3	0	25
MultiGrain Sticks Lightly Salted	1 oz	120	3	2	23
MultiGrain Twists	1 oz	120	3	2	22
Nibblers Sourdough	1 oz	120	3	0	25
Old Tyme	1 oz	120	3	1	24
Organic Honey Wheat	1 oz	130	3	2	24
Organic Oat Bran	1 oz	120	3	0	25
Pieces Garlic Bread	1 oz	140	3	7	18
Pieces Honey Mustard & Onions	1 oz	140	2	7	18

FOOD	PORTION	CALS	PROT	FAT	CARB
Pieces Hot Buffalo Wing	1 oz	140	2	7	17
Pretzel Sandwich Peanut Butter	1 oz	140	4	7	16
Rods	1 oz	120	3	1	24
Snaps	1 oz	120	3	1	25
Sourdough Unsalted	1 oz	100	3	0	22
Sticks 12 Multi Grain	1 oz	130	3	2	22
Superpretzel					
Mozzarella	2 (1.8 oz)	130	6	4	20
Pretzelfils Pizza	2 (1.8 oz)	130	5	2	22
Soft	1 (2.25 oz)	160	5	1	34
Soft Bites	5 (1.9 oz)	150	31	1	32
Softstix	2 (1.8 oz)	130	4	3	22
Tom Sturgis					
Little Cheesers	17 (1 oz)	120	3	2	22
Little Ones	17 (1 oz)	110	2	2	22
Utz					
Braided Twists Baked Honey Wheat	1 oz	110	3	2	23
Chocolate Covered	6 (1.1 oz)	140	2	5	22
Hard	1	90	2	0	18
Special	1 oz	110	3	1	21
Special Multigrain	1 oz	110	3	1	21
Sticks Organic Whole Grain	1 oz	120	3	2	22
PRUNE JUICE					
jarred	1 cup	182	2	tr	45
Lakewood					
Organic	8 oz	165	1	0	40
Old Orchard					
Healthy Balance	8 oz	70	0	0	12
Sunsweet					
100% Juice	8 oz	180	2	0	43
PlumSmart	8 oz	160	0	0	39
Tree Of Life					
Organic 100% Juice	8 oz	180	1	0	43
PRUNES					
cooked w/o sugar	½ cup	133	1	tr	35
dried	1	20	tr	tr	5
Earthbound Farms					
Organic Dried Plums	5	110	1	0	25

FOOD	PORTION	CALS	PROT	FAT	CARB
Love'n Bake					
Prune Lekvar	2 tbsp	90	0	0	21
Sunsweet					
Pitted	5 (1.5 oz)	100	1	0	24
PUDDING					
READY-TO-EAT					
Jell-O					
100 Calorie Pack Fat Free Chocolate Vanilla Swirl	1 pkg (4 oz)	100	2	0	23
100 Calorie Pack Fat Free Tapioca	1 pkg (4 oz)	100	1	0	23
Sugar Free Dulce De Leche	1 pkg (3.7 oz)	60	1	1	13
Vanilla	1 serv (4 oz)	110	1	2	23
Kozy Shack					
Black Forest	1 pkg (4 oz)	120	3	3	22
Lifeway					
Organic Chocolate	½ cup	170	4	4	30
Organic Rice	½ cup	140	4	4	22
Organic Vanilla	½ cup	150	3	4	24
SoYummi					
GoLite Bavarian Cream	1 pkg (3.5 oz)	86	3	3	12
Mousse All Flavors	1 pkg (4.4 oz)	137	4	4	21
Swiss Miss					
Chocolate	1 pkg	150	3	4	27
Low Fat Chocolate	1 pkg	130	3	2	26
Pie Lover's Banana Cream	1 pkg	130	2	4	23
Pie Lover's Lemon Meringue	1 pkg	140	0	3	28
Swirl Chocolate Vanilla	1 pkg	140	2	4	27
ZenSoy					
Banana	1 pkg (4 oz)	100	2	1	21
Chocolate	1 pkg (4 oz)	130	3	1	29
Vanilla	1 pkg (4 oz)	110	2	1	23
TAKE-OUT					
blancmange	1 serv (4.7 oz)	154	4	5	25
bread w/ raisins	1 cup	306	11	9	47
coconut	1 cup	291	8	9	45
corn	1 cup	328	11	13	43
indian pudding	½ cup	156	5	4	25
noodle pudding kugel	1 cup	297	9	10	44
plum pudding	1 slice (1.5 oz)	125	2	5	20

FOOD	PORTION	CALS	PROT	FAT	CARB
queen of puddings	1 serv (4.4 oz)	266	6	10	41
rice pudding	1 cup	302	8	4	60
sweet potato	½ cup	107	2	3	19
tapioca	1 cup	236	10	7	35
yorkshire	1 serv (3 oz)	177	6	8	22
PUFFERFISH					
raw	3 oz	72	17	0	0
PUMMELO					
fresh	1	228	5	tr	59
sections	1 cup	71	1	tr	18
PUMPKIN					
butter	1 tbsp	32	0	0	8
canned	½ cup	41	1	tr	10
cooked mashed	½ cup	24	1	tr	6
flowers cooked	½ cup	10	1	tr	2
flowers raw	1	0	tr	0	tr
leaves cooked	½ cup	7	1	tr	1
leaves raw	½ cup	4	1	tr	tr
raw cubed	½ cup	15	1	tr	4
Jake & Amos					
Pumpkin Butter	1 tbsp (0.5 oz)	5	0	0	1
Tree Of Life					
Organic Puree	½ cup (4.3 oz)	50	1	0	10
TAKE-OUT					
indian sago	1 serv (2.3 oz)	75	2	5	6
PUMPKIN SEEDS					
dried	1 oz	154	7	13	5
roasted	¼ cup	296	19	24	8
salted & roasted	¼ cup	296	19	24	8
whole roasted	1 oz	127	5	6	15
whole roasted	¼ cup	71	3	3	9
whole salted roasted	¼ cup	71	3	3	9
Mrs. May's					
Pumpkin Crunch	1 oz	164	9	11	8
Tree Of Life					
Seeds Roasted & Salted	¼ cup (2 oz)	300	13	24	8
PURSLANE					
cooked	1 cup	21	2	tr	4
fresh	1 cup	7	1	tr	1

FOOD	PORTION	CALS	PROT	FAT	CARB
QUAIL					
cooked bone removed	1 (2.7 oz)	177	19	11	0
QUICHE					
Mrs. Smith's					
Pour-A-Quiche Bacon & Onion	1 serv (4.3 oz)	230	14	16	6
TAKE-OUT					
cheese pie	⅛ (9 in)	566	17	44	27
lorraine pie	⅛ (9 in)	568	17	44	27
mushroom	1 slice (3 oz)	256	9	18	17
spinach pie	⅛ (9 in)	342	11	26	17
QUINCE					
fresh	1	53	tr	tr	14
QUINOA					
cooked	1 cup (6.5 oz)	222	8	4	39
quinoa not prep	¼ cup (1.5 oz)	156	6	3	27
Alti Plano Gold					
Natural	1 pkg	170	6	3	30
Ancient Harvest Quinoa					
Flakes not prep	¼ cup	159	5	2	28
Organic Inca Red not prep	¼ cup	163	6	3	29
Organic Traditional not prep	¼ cup	172	6	3	31
TruRoots					
Organic not prep	¼ cup (1.6 oz)	172	5	3	31
RABBIT					
domestic w/o bone roasted	3 oz	167	25	7	0
wild w/o bone stewed	3 oz	147	28	3	0
RACCOON					
roasted	3 oz	217	25	12	0
RADICCHIO					
raw shredded	½ cup	5	tr	tr	1
RADISHES					
chinese dried	½ cup	157	5	tr	37
chinese raw	1 (12 oz)	62	2	tr	14
chinese raw sliced	½ cup	8	tr	tr	2
chinese sliced cooked	½ cup	13	tr	tr	3
daikon dried	½ cup	157	5	tr	37
daikon raw	1 (12 oz)	62	2	tr	14

FOOD	PORTION	CALS	PROT	FAT	CARB
daikon raw sliced	½ cup	8	tr	tr	2
daikon sliced cooked	½ cup	13	tr	tr	3
red raw	10	7	tr	tr	2
red sliced	½ cup	10	tr	tr	2
white icicle raw	1 (0.5 oz)	2	tr	tr	tr
white icicle raw sliced	½ cup	7	1	tr	1
Cadis					
Fresh	6 (2.6 oz)	12	1	tr	2
TAKE-OUT					
korean kimchee	½ cup	31	2	1	6
moo namul saengche korean salad	1 serv (3.7 oz)	34	1	tr	8

RAISINS

FOOD	PORTION	CALS	PROT	FAT	CARB
cinnamon coated	¼ cup	108	1	tr	29
cooked	¼ cup	162	1	tr	42
golden seedless	¼ cup	109	1	tr	29
jumbo golden	¼ cup	130	1	0	31
milk chocolate coated	28 (1 oz)	109	1	4	19
milk chocolate coated	¼ cup	176	2	7	31
seedless	55 (1 oz)	86	1	tr	23
sultanas	1 oz	88	1	0	23
Amazin' Raisin					
All Flavors	1 pkg (1 oz)	84	1	0	22
Bob's Red Mill					
Unsulfured	⅓ cup	130	1	0	31
Earthbound Farms					
Organic Jumbo Flame Seedless	¼ cup	120	1	0	32
Emily's					
Milk Chocolate Covered	29 (1.4 oz)	180	2	8	26
Fool					
Cinnamon Raisin Spread	1 tbsp	20	0	0	5
Godiva					
Milk Chocolate Covered	1 pkg (1.2 oz)	150	2	7	21
Revolution Foods					
Organic	1 pkg (1.2 oz)	100	1	0	28
Sun-Maid					
Chocolate Covered	30 (1.4 oz)	170	2	6	26
Golden	¼ cup (1.4 oz)	130	1	0	31
Jumbo	¼ cup (1.4 oz)	130	1	0	31
Seedless	¼ cup (1.4 oz)	130	1	0	31
Snack Box	1 (1 oz)	90	1	0	22

FOOD	PORTION	CALS	PROT	FAT	CARB
RAMBUTAN					
canned in syrup	1 (0.3 oz)	7	tr	tr	2
canned in syrup	1 cup (4.3 oz)	123	1	tr	31
puerto rican fresh	5 (1.6 oz)	34	tr	tr	8
Polar					
In Syrup	½ cup	68	0	0	17
RASPBERRIES					
black fresh	1 cup	70	2	1	16
canned in heavy syrup	½ cup	116	1	tr	30
canned water pack	1 cup	43	1	1	10
fresh	1 cup	64	1	1	15
fresh	1 pt	162	4	2	37
frzn sweetened	1 cup	129	1	tr	33
frzn unsweetened	1 cup	65	2	1	15
C&W					
Ultimate Red	¾ cup	70	2	0	15
Cascadian Farm					
Organic frzn	1¼ cup	60	1	0	17
Oregon					
In Heavy Syrup	½ cup	120	tr	0	30
Stoneridge Orchards					
Dried Whole	⅓ cup (1.4 oz)	130	1	1	32
RASPBERRY JUICE					
Old Orchard					
Organic 100% Juice	8 oz	120	0	0	29
RED BEANS					
Allens					
Red Beans	½ cup	100	6	1	19
RELISH					
hamburger	1 tbsp	19	tr	tr	5
hamburger	½ cup	158	1	1	42
hot dog	½ cup	111	2	1	28
hot dog	1 tbsp	14	tr	tr	4
piccalilli	1.4 oz	13	tr	tr	2
sweet	½ cup	159	tr	1	43
sweet	1 tbsp	19	tr	tr	5
tomato	¼ cup (2.8 oz)	119	1	tr	28

FOOD	PORTION	CALS	PROT	FAT	CARB
Cascadian Farm					
Organic Sweet Relish	1 tbsp (0.5 oz)	15	1	0	4
Claussen					
Sweet Pickle	1 tbsp (0.5 oz)	15	0	0	3
Gedney					
Hot Dog	1 tbsp	18	0	0	4
Organic Sweet	1 tbsp	15	0	0	4
Patak's					
Brinjal Eggplant Sweet Spicy	1 tbsp	70	0	4	8
Garlic	1 tbsp	45	0	3	4
Lime Mild	1 tbsp	30	0	3	0
Mango Mild	1 tbsp	40	0	4	1
Peloponnese					
Sun Dried Tomato	1 tbsp	25	0	2	2
Texas Sassy					
Pickle Relish	1 tbsp (0.5 oz)	30	0	0	7
Tree Of Life					
Organic Sweet Pickle	1 tbsp (0.5)	15	0	0	4
RENNIN					
tablet	1 (0.9 g)	1	0	0	tr
RHUBARB					
fresh	½ cup	13	1	tr	3
frozen	½ cup	60	tr	tr	3
frzn as prep w/ sugar	½ cup	139	tr	tr	37
RICE (see also RICE CAKES, WILD RICE)					
arborio	½ cup	100	2	0	22
brown long grain cooked	1 cup (6.8 oz)	216	5	2	45
brown medium grain cooked	1 cup (6.8 oz)	218	5	2	46
glutinous cooked	1 cup (6.1 oz)	169	4	tr	37
starch	1 oz	98	tr	0	24
white long grain cooked	1 cup (5.5 oz)	205	4	tr	45
white long grain instant cooked	1 cup (5.8 oz)	162	3	tr	35
white medium grain cooked	1 cup (6.5 oz)	242	4	tr	53
white short grain cooked	1 cup (6.5 oz)	242	4	tr	53
Amy's					
Bowls Brown Rice Black-Eyed Peas & Veggies	1 pkg (8.9 oz)	290	11	11	38
Bowls Brown Rice & Vegetables	1 pkg (9.9 oz)	260	9	9	36

FOOD	PORTION	CALS	PROT	FAT	CARB
Arrowhead Mills					
Organic Brown Basmati not prep	¼ cup	140	3	2	31
Organic Long Grain Brown not prep	¼ cup	160	3	1	32
Betty Crocker					
Bowl Appetit! Teriyaki Rice	1 bowl (2.5 oz)	260	7	3	54
Carolina					
Saffron Yellow Mix not prep	1 serv	190	4	0	43
Country Crock					
Cheddar Broccoli Rice	1 cup (7 oz)	270	8	11	35
Green Giant					
Rice Pilaf	1 pkg (9.9 oz)	200	5	3	40
White & Wild & Green Beans	1 pkg (9.9 oz)	260	6	5	48
Knorr					
Asian Side Dish Chicken Fried Rice as prep	1 cup	240	7	1	48
Rice Sides Rice Medley as prep	1 cup	250	6	5	45
Rice Sides Sesame Chicken w/ Whole Grains as prep	⅔ cup	300	7	9	51
Lundberg					
Eco-Farmed Black Japonica not prep	¼ cup	170	5	2	38
Eco-Farmed California Brown Basmati not prep	¼ cup	160	4	2	34
Eco-Farmed White California Arborio not prep	¼ cup	160	6	0	43
Organic Brown Golden Rose not prep	¼ cup	160	3	1	34
Organic Rice Sensations Ginger Miso not prep	½ cup	116	3	1	24
Organic Risotto Porcini Mushroom not prep	½ cup	143	4	1	35
Organic White Sushi Rice not prep	¼ cup	150	4	0	36
Organic Wild Blend not prep	¼ cup	150	4	2	35
RiceXpress Chicken Herb	½ pkg (4.4 oz)	250	4	5	47
RiceXpress Santa Fe Grill	½ pkg (4.4 oz)	260	5	5	50

FOOD	PORTION	CALS	PROT	FAT	CARB
Risotto Butternut Squash not prep	½ cup	143	4	1	31
Marrakesh Express					
Pilaf Tomato & Basil as prep	1 cup	190	6	0	41
Risotto Parmesan as prep	1 cup	200	5	1	42
Minute					
Boil-In-Bag White as prep	1 cup	180	4	0	41
Brown as prep	1 cup	150	3	2	34
Ready To Serve Brown	1 pkg (4.4 oz)	170	3	5	28
Ready To Serve White	1 pkg (4.4 oz)	190	3	4	34
Ready To Serve Yellow	1 pkg (4.4 oz)	190	3	4	35
White as prep	1 cup	200	5	0	45
Near East					
Long Grain & Wild Original as prep	1 cup	220	5	4	43
Pilaf Curry as prep	1 cup	220	4	4	44
Pilaf Original as prep	1 cup	220	4	4	43
Pilaf Sesame Ginger as prep	1 cup	270	5	4	55
Pilaf Spanish Rice as prep	1 cup	310	5	7	54
Whole Grains Brown Rice as prep	1 cup	210	5	4	41
Patak's					
Basmati	1 pkg	430	9	5	87
Coconut	1 pkg	500	10	12	87
Yellow	1 pkg	440	10	5	89
Rice A Roni					
Beef as prep	1 cup	310	7	9	51
Chicken as prep	1 cup	310	7	9	51
Express Asian Fried	1 cup	280	6	6	51
Fried Rice as prep	1 cup	320	7	11	49
Garden Vegetable as prep	1 cup	270	6	10	41
Long Grain & Wild as prep	1 cup	250	5	7	43
Lower Sodium Chicken as prep	1 cup	270	7	5	51
Parmesan Chicken as prep	1 cup	370	8	15	51
Red Beans & Rice as prep	1 cup	290	8	7	51
Savory Whole Grain Blends Spanish as prep	1 cup	250	5	8	42
Spanish as prep	1 cup	260	6	7	44
Success					
Boil-In-Bag Brown as prep	1 cup	150	4	1	33

FOOD	PORTION	CALS	PROT	FAT	CARB
Boil-In-Bag Jasmine as prep	¾ cup	150	3	0	36
Boil-In-Bag White as prep	1 cup	190	4	0	43
Ready To Serve Brown	1 cup	170	3	5	28
Ready To Serve White	1 pkg	190	3	4	34
Ready To Serve Yellow Rice Mix	1 pkg	190	3	4	35
Whole Grain Herb Roasted Chicken as prep	1 cup	290	7	10	43
Whole Grain Multigrain Pilaf as prep	1 cup	230	7	3	43
Whole Grain Portobello Mushroom as prep	1 cup	220	6	2	45
TastyBite					
Pilaf Multigrain	½ pkg (5 oz)	200	9	5	33
Pilaf Tandoori	½ pkg (5 oz)	183	3	3	37
Thai Kitchen					
Jasmine not prep	2 tbsp (1.5 oz)	160	3	0	36
Uncle Ben's					
Long Grain & Wild Herb Roasted Chicken as prep	1 cup	190	5	1	39
Long Grain & Wild Sun-Dried Tomato Florentine as prep	1 cup	180	6	1	39
Zatarain's					
Black Beans & Rice as prep	1 cup	230	8	1	47
Caribbean Rice Mix as prep	1 cup	160	3	2	34
Yellow as prep	½ cup	110	3	0	23
TAKE-OUT					
coconut rice	1 serv	500	6	42	30
congee	½ cup (4.1 oz)	44	1	–	10
dirty rice w/ chicken giblets	1 cup (6.9 oz)	291	11	10	38
nasi goreng indonesian rice & vegetables	1 cup (4.9 oz)	130	4	0	28
pea palau rice & peas fried in ghee	1 serv	144	4	5	21
pilaf	½ cup	84	4	3	11
risotto	1 serv (6.6 oz)	426	6	18	65
spanish	¾ cup	363	11	27	19

RICE CAKES
Hain

FOOD	PORTION	CALS	PROT	FAT	CARB
Mini Munchies Apple Cinnamon	9 (0.5 oz)	60	1	1	14

FOOD	PORTION	CALS	PROT	FAT	CARB
Lundberg					
Eco-Farmed Apple Cinnamon	1 (0.7 oz)	80	2	1	18
Eco-Farmed Brown Rice Salt Free	1 (0.7 oz)	70	1	0	14
Eco-Farmed Toasted Sesame	1 (0.7 oz)	70	2	0	15
Organic Caramel Corn	1 (0.7 oz)	80	1	1	18
Organic Green Tea w/ Lemon	1 (0.7 oz)	80	1	0	17
Organic Mochi Sweet	1 (0.7 oz)	70	1	0	15
Quaker					
Mini Delights Chocolatey Drizzle	1 pkg (0.7 oz)	90	1	4	14
Riceworks					
Sweet Chili	10 (1 oz)	140	2	6	19
Wasabi	10 (1 oz)	140	2	6	19
ROCKFISH					
pacific cooked	1 fillet (5.2 oz)	180	36	3	0
pacific cooked	3 oz	103	20	2	0
pacific raw	3 oz	80	16	1	0
ROE (see also individual fish names)					
fresh baked	1 oz	58	8	2	1
ROLL					
FROZEN					
Joy Of Cooking					
Ciabatta Olive Oil Rosemary	1 (1.7 oz)	120	4	2	21
French Baguettes Mini	1 (1.6 oz)	100	3	0	20
Pillsbury					
Dinner Rolls Crusty French	1 (1.2 oz)	90	3	1	15
Dinner Rolls Crusty Sourdough	1 (1.2 oz)	90	4	1	17
Dinner Rolls Whole Wheat	1 (1.2 oz)	90	4	1	17
READY-TO-EAT					
bialy	1 (2.2 oz)	138	14	0	32
brioche sweet roll	1 (3.5 oz)	410	10	23	41
cheese	1 (2.3 oz)	238	5	12	29
cinnamon raisin	1 (2.1 oz)	223	4	10	31
dinner	1 (1 oz)	78	3	1	14
egg	1 (1.2 oz)	107	3	2	18
french	1 (1.3 oz)	105	3	2	19
garlic	1 (1.5 oz)	133	5	3	22
hamburger or hot dog	1 (1.5 oz)	120	4	2	21

FOOD	PORTION	CALS	PROT	FAT	CARB
hamburger or hot dog multi grain	1 (1.5 oz)	113	4	3	19
hamburger or hot dog reduced calorie	1 (1.5 oz)	84	4	1	18
hamburger or hot dog whole wheat	1 (1.5 oz)	114	4	2	22
hard	1 (2 oz)	167	6	2	30
hoagie or submarine roll whole wheat	1 (4.7 oz)	359	12	6	69
hot cross bun	1	202	5	4	38
mexican bolillo	1 (4.1 oz)	305	10	2	60
oat bran	1 (1.2 oz)	78	3	2	13
oatmeal	1 (1.3 oz)	103	3	2	17
pumpernickel	1 (1.3 oz)	100	4	1	19
rye	1 med (1.3 oz)	103	4	1	19
sourdough	1 (1.6 oz)	130	5	1	25
wheat	1 (1 oz)	76	2	2	13
whole wheat	1 med (1.3 oz)	96	3	2	18
Arnold					
Whole Grains Sandwich 100% Whole Wheat	1 (2.2 oz)	160	8	2	26
Calise					
Kaiser 100% Whole Wheat	1 (2.5 oz)	190	8	3	33
Ecce Panis					
Focaccia	1 (3.2 oz)	260	8	5	49
French Meadow Bakery					
Gluten Free Italian	1 (4.4 oz)	340	3	9	63
J.J. Cassone					
Sandwich	1 (2.5 oz)	190	7	2	38
Mrs Baird's					
Home Bake	1 (1 oz)	80	2	2	13
Natural Ovens					
Better Wheat Buns	1 (2.2 oz)	170	7	3	30
Nature's Own					
100% Whole Grain Sugar Free	1 (1.9 oz)	110	6	2	23
Butter Buns	1 (1.7 oz)	120	5	2	23
Pepperidge Farm					
Hamburger 100% Whole Wheat	1	120	6	2	18
Hoagie Soft w/ Sesame Seeds	1	210	7	6	35

FOOD	PORTION	CALS	PROT	FAT	CARB
Hot & Crusty Sourdough	1	100	4	1	21
Hot Dog	1	140	5	3	26
Hot Dog Whole Grain White	1	110	6	1	21
Parker House Dinner	1	80	3	2	14
Premium Wheat	1	220	8	5	36
Sandwich Buns Sesame Seeds	1 (1.6 oz)	130	5	3	22
Rudi's Organic Bakery					
100% Whole Wheat	1 (2.3 oz)	160	7	2	29
Hot Dog Spelt	1 (2 oz)	140	5	2	28
Hot Dog Wheat	1 (2 oz)	150	5	2	28
Hot Dog White	1 (2 oz)	150	5	2	28
S. Rosen's					
Brat & Sausage Rolls	1 (2.1 oz)	160	6	3	28
Klassic Kaiser	1 (2.6 oz)	230	6	3	46
Stroehmann					
Hot Dog Wheat	1 (1.8 oz)	140	5	3	25
Weight Watchers					
Sandwich Wheat	1 (2 oz)	140	6	2	28
REFRIGERATED					
crescent	1 (1 oz)	78	3	1	14
Pillsbury					
Crescent Big & Buttery	1 (1.7 oz)	170	3	10	20
Crescent Butter Flake	1 (1 oz)	110	2	6	11
Crescent Original	1 (1 oz)	110	2	6	11
Crescent Reduced Fat	1 (1 oz)	90	2	5	12
ROSE APPLE					
fresh	3.5 oz	32	1	tr	7
ROSE HIP					
fresh	1 oz	26	1	0	5
ROSELLE					
fresh	1 cup	28	1	tr	6
ROSEMARY					
dried	1 tsp	4	tr	tr	1
fresh	1 tbsp	1	tr	tr	tr
ROUGHY					
orange baked	3 oz	75	16	1	0

RUBS (*see* HERBS/SPICES)

FOOD	PORTION	CALS	PROT	FAT	CARB
RUTABAGA					
cooked mashed	1 cup	94	3	1	21
cubed cooked	1 cup	66	2	tr	14
Glory					
Cut Fresh	1 cup	50	2	0	11
Sunshine					
Diced	½ cup	30	tr	0	7
SABLEFISH					
baked	3 oz	213	15	17	0
fillet baked	5.3 oz	378	26	30	0
smoked	3 oz	218	15	17	0
smoked	1 oz	72	5	6	0
SAFFLOWER					
seeds dried	1 oz	147	5	11	10
SAFFRON					
dried	1 tsp	2	tr	tr	tr
SAGE					
ground	1 tsp	2	tr	tr	tr
SALAD (see also SALAD TOPPINGS)					
Dole					
Field Greens	1½ cups (3 oz)	20	1	0	4
Earthbound Farms					
Organic Baby Arugula Salad	2 cups	20	2	0	3
Organic Baby Lettuce Salad	2 cups	15	1	0	3
Organic Baby Spinach Salad	2 cups	10	2	0	7
Organic Fresh Herb Salad	2 cups	15	2	0	4
Organic Mixed Baby Greens	2 cups	15	2	0	4
Fresh Express					
50/50 Mix	3 cups	10	2	0	5
Asian Supreme w/ Dressing as prep	2½ cups	170	3	10	17
Caesar Lite w/ Dressing as prep	2½ cups	100	2	7	8
Caesar w/ Dressing as prep	2½ cups	150	2	13	8
Fancy Field Greens	3 cups	20	1	0	3
Gourmet Cafe Caribbean Chicken as prep	1 pkg (3.5 oz)	120	4	6	14
Gourmet Cafe Chicken Caesar w/ Crostini as prep	1 pkg (3.5 oz)	150	8	11	5

FOOD	PORTION	CALS	PROT	FAT	CARB
Gourmet Cafe Chopped Turkey Chef as prep	1 pkg (3.5 oz)	120	5	9	7
Gourmet Cafe Orchard Harvest as prep	1 pkg (3.5 oz)	230	5	18	13
Gourmet Cafe Tuscan Pesto Chicken as prep	1 pkg (3.5 oz)	130	7	8	6
Gourmet Cafe Waldorf Chicken as prep	1 pkg (3.5 oz)	190	7	10	19
More Carrots American	1½ cups	15	1	0	3
Organic Italian	2½ cups	15	1	0	3
Original Iceberg Garden With Zip	1½ cups	15	1	0	3
Pacifica! Veggie Supreme w/ Dressing as prep	3 cups	220	4	15	18
Spring Mix	3 cups	15	1	0	3
Sweet Baby Greens	3 cups	10	1	0	2
Veggie Lover's	2 cups	20	1	0	4
Lifestyle Foods					
Asian w/ Chicken	1 pkg (8.9 oz)	340	13	16	36
Casear	1 pkg (5 oz)	210	5	11	22
Garden	1 pkg (6.6 oz)	180	4	12	14
Greek	1 pkg (6 oz)	130	3	11	6
Mann's					
Rainbow	3 oz	25	2	0	5
TAKE-OUT					
7-layer salad	2 cups	557	11	51	15
caesar	4 cups	734	22	61	28
chef salad w/o dressing	3 cups	535	52	32	9
cobb w/ dressing	4 cups	645	32	49	23
greek w/ dressing	4 cups	424	28	29	14
mixed salad greens shredded	1 cup	9	1	tr	2
somen w/ lettuce egg fish pork	2 cups	550	40	17	57
spinach w/o dressing	4 cups	429	20	19	45
tossed w/ avocado w/o dressing	2 cups	90	2	6	9
tossed w/ chicken w/o dressing	3 cups	194	33	4	5
tossed w/ egg w/o dressing	2 cups	93	7	5	6
tossed w/ seafood w/o dressing	3 cups	120	19	1	8
tossed w/ shrimp & egg w/o dressing	3 cups	185	30	5	5

FOOD	PORTION	CALS	PROT	FAT	CARB
tossed w/o dressing	2 cups	22	1	tr	5
waldorf	1 cup	242	2	21	15
wilted lettuce w/ bacon dressing	1 cup	99	3	8	3

SALAD DRESSING (see also SALAD TOPPINGS)
MIX
Good Seasons
Italian as prep	2 tbsp	130	0	13	3
Italian not prep	⅛ pkg (3 g)	5	0	0	1

READY-TO-EAT
blue cheese	1 tbsp	77	1	8	1
french	1 tbsp	67	tr	6	3
french reduced calorie	1 tbsp	22	0	1	4
italian	1 tbsp	69	tr	7	2
italian reduced calorie	1 tbsp	16	tr	2	1
russian	1 tbsp	76	tr	8	2
russian reduced calorie	1 tbsp	23	tr	1	5
sesame seed	1 tbsp	68	1	7	1
thousand island	1 tbsp	59	tr	6	2
thousand island reduced calorie	1 tbsp	24	tr	2	3

Bernstein's
Chunky Blue Cheese	2 tbsp	120	1	13	2
Creamy Caesar	2 tbsp	120	0	13	1
Italian Restaurant Recipe	2 tbsp	120	1	12	1
Light Fantastic Roasted Garlic Balsamic	2 tbsp	45	0	4	3
Red Wine & Garlic Italian	2 tbsp	110	0	1	2

Bragg
Ginger & Sesame	2 tbsp	150	0	12	2
Organic Vinaigrette	2 tbsp	150	0	15	3

Cains
Caesar Creamy	2 tbsp	170	0	19	1
Caesar Fat Free	2 tbsp	30	0	0	6
Caesar Light	2 tbsp	70	2	6	5
Chianti Vinaigrette	2 tbsp	130	0	12	5
Creamy Dill Cucumber Fat Free	2 tbsp	35	0	0	8
French	2 tbsp	120	0	11	6
French Light	2 tbsp	80	0	5	10
Greek	2 tbsp	160	0	17	2

FOOD	PORTION	CALS	PROT	FAT	CARB
Italian Fat Free	2 tbsp	15	0	0	4
Ranch	2 tbsp	180	0	19	1
Ranch Light	2 tbsp	80	0	6	6
Follow Your Heart					
Lemon Herb	2 tbsp (1 oz)	100	0	11	1
Sesame Miso	2 tbsp (1 oz)	64	1	6	3
Thousand Island	2 tbsp (1 oz)	80	0	8	3
Gotta Luv It					
Chipotle Lime	2 tbsp	110	0	11	3
Raspberry Balsamic Vinaigrette	2 tbsp	150	0	14	6
Sweet & Tangy Italian	2 tbsp	140	0	15	2
Kraft					
Honey Dijon	2 tbsp	100	0	9	6
Italian Creamy	2 tbsp	100	0	11	2
Light Done Right Caesar	2 tbsp	60	1	5	3
Light Done Right Red Wine Vinaigrette	2 tbsp	45	0	4	3
Ranch Garlic	2 tbsp	120	0	12	3
Special Collection Classic Italian Vinaigrette	2 tbsp	60	0	4	5
Special Collection Parmesan Romano	2 tbsp	140	1	14	2
Special Collection Tangy Tomato Bacon	2 tbsp	100	0	6	10
Thousand Island w/ Bacon	2 tbsp	100	0	8	7
LiteHouse					
Bleu Cheese Bacon	2 tbsp	150	1	16	1
Organic Vinaigrette Raspberry Lime	2 tbsp	40	0	2	5
Ranch Homestyle	2 tbsp	120	0	12	2
Ranch Lite	2 tbsp	70	0	6	2
Sesame Ginger	2 tbsp	35	0	0	8
Spinach Salad	2 tbsp	50	1	0	11
Vinaigrette Huckleberry	2 tbsp	20	0	0	4
Vinaigrette Lite Honey Dijon	2 tbsp	130	0	13	3
Lucini					
Delicate Cucumber & Shallots	2 tbsp (1 oz)	120	0	12	2
Fig & Walnut Savory Balsamic	2 tbsp (1 oz)	110	0	10	4
Roasted Hazelnut & Extra Virgin Olive Oil	2 tbsp (1 oz)	120	1	11	3

FOOD	PORTION	CALS	PROT	FAT	CARB
Marie's					
Blue Cheese Lite Chunky	2 tbsp	80	1	6	7
Blue Cheese Vinaigrette	2 tbsp	120	2	11	4
Caesar	2 tbsp	170	1	19	1
Coleslaw	2 tbsp	120	0	13	8
Creamy Ranch	2 tbsp	170	1	19	1
Red Wine Vinaigrette	2 tbsp	60	0	5	6
Sesame Ginger	2 tbsp	70	0	8	7
Milo's					
Gorgonzola Pear Riesling	2 tbsp	70	0	7	2
Pomegranate Port	2 tbsp	90	0	7	6
Naturally Fresh					
Balsamic Vinaigrette	2 tbsp	10	0	0	2
Bleu Cheese	2 tbsp	170	1	18	1
Bleu Cheese Bacon	2 tbsp	170	1	18	1
Bleu Cheese Lite	2 tbsp	100	1	10	1
Buffalo Ranch	2 tbsp	110	0	10	4
Classic Oriental	2 tbsp	100	0	11	9
Ginger	2 tbsp	70	1	7	1
Greek Feta	2 tbsp	100	0	12	1
Honey French	2 tbsp	100	0	11	5
Honey Mustard	2 tbsp	140	1	13	5
Orange Miso	2 tbsp	100	0	9	4
Ranch Classic	2 tbsp	150	1	16	1
Ranch Lite	2 tbsp	80	1	8	2
Slaw	2 tbsp	90	0	10	6
Newman's Own					
Lighten Up Light Balsamic Vinaigrette	2 tbsp (1 oz)	45	0	4	2
OrganicVille					
Herbs De Provence	2 tbsp (1 oz)	100	0	11	tr
Miso Ginger	2 tbsp (1 oz)	100	0	10	1
Orange Cranberry	2 tbsp (1 oz)	100	0	10	3
Pomegranate	2 tbsp (1 oz)	100	0	10	2
Ranch Non Dairy	2 tbsp (1 oz)	90	tr	9	1
Sesame Goddess	2 tbsp (1 oz)	130	1	13	2
Petrini's					
Italian Original	2 tbsp (1 oz)	106	tr	12	tr
Italian Ranch	2 tbsp (1 oz)	140	0	14	1

FOOD	PORTION	CALS	PROT	FAT	CARB
School House Kitchen					
Balsamic Vinaigrette Basico	2 tbsp	160	0	17	3
Soy Vay					
Cha-Cha Chinese Chicken	3 tbsp	190	2	15	11
Texas Sassy					
Vinaigrette	2 tbsp (1 oz)	80	0	8	4
Three Acre Kitchen					
Balsamic Vinaigrette	2 tbsp (1.1 oz)	130	0	14	3
Vino De Milo					
Gorgonzola Pear Riesling	2 tbsp	80	0	7	2
Pomegranate Port	2 tbsp	90	0	7	5
Wild Thymes Farm					
Salad Refreshers Black Currant	1 tbsp	36	tr	3	3
Salad Refreshers Meyer Lemon	1 tbsp	35	0	3	3
Salad Refreshers Morello Cherry	1 tbsp	34	tr	3	3
Salad Refreshers Pomegranate	1 tbsp	33	0	3	3
Vinaigrette Mandarin Orange Basil	1 tbsp	43	0	4	2
Vinaigrette Raspberry Pear	1 tbsp	43	0	4	1
Vinaigrette Roasted Apple Shallot	1 tbsp	42	0	4	2
Vinaigrette Toasted Sesame Wasabi	1 tbsp	42	tr	4	1
Wishbone					
Bountifuls Berry Delight	2 tbsp	35	0	0	8
Bountifuls Tuscan Romano Basil	2 tbsp	25	0	1	4
Western	2 tbsp (1 oz)	160	0	12	11
Western Fat Free	2 tbsp (1 oz)	50	0	0	12
Western Light Just 2 Good	2 tbsp (1 oz)	70	0	2	13
TAKE-OUT					
vinegar & oil	1 tbsp	72	0	8	tr
SALAD TOPPINGS					
Fresh Gourmet					
Wonton Strips Wasabi Ranch	2 tbsp	35	1	2	4
Naturally Fresh					
Fruit & Nut Mix	½ tbsp	45	1	4	2
Glazed Almond & Pecan Pieces	½ tbsp	40	1	3	3

FOOD	PORTION	CALS	PROT	FAT	CARB
SALBA					
Salba Smart					
Ground	2 tbsp	65	3	4	5
Whole Grain	1 tbsp	65	3	4	5
SALMON					
CANNED					
w/ bone	½ cup	106	15	5	0
Polar					
Pink	¼ cup	90	12	5	0
Sockeye Red	¼ cup	110	13	7	0
FRESH					
atlantic farmed baked	4 oz	233	25	14	0
coho wild poached	4 oz	209	31	9	0
pink baked	4 oz	169	29	5	0
roe raw	1 oz	59	7	3	tr
sockeye baked	4 oz	245	31	12	0
FROZEN					
Dr. Praeger's					
Salmon Cakes	1 (2.9 oz)	190	10	10	15
Gorton's					
Fillets Classic Grilled	1 (3 oz)	100	15	3	2
SMOKED					
lox	1 oz	33	5	1	0
TAKE-OUT					
guisado salmon stew	1 serv (7.4 oz)	320	26	16	18
roulette w/ spinach stuffing	1 serv (4 oz)	160	13	6	10
salmon cake	1 (4.2 oz)	264	16	16	14
salmon loaf	1 slice (3.7 oz)	206	16	11	9
SALSA					
black bean & corn	2 tbsp	15	1	0	3
citrus	2 tbsp (1 oz)	10	0	0	2
peach	2 tbsp	15	0	0	4
tomatoless corn & chile	2 tbsp	45	1	0	10
Amy's					
Organic Black Bean & Corn	2 tbsp (1 oz)	15	1	0	3
Organic Medium	2 tbsp (1 oz)	10	0	0	2
Bone Suckin'					
Fat Free Gluten Free	2 tbsp	40	0	0	10

FOOD	PORTION	CALS	PROT	FAT	CARB
Chi-Chi's					
Fiesta Mild	2 tbsp	10	0	0	2
Chukar Cherries					
Peach Cherry	1 tbsp	13	0	0	3
Clint's					
Texas Medium	2 tbsp (1 oz)	5	0	0	1
Dave's Gourmet					
Insanity	2 tbsp (1 oz)	15	tr	0	2
Dei Fratelli					
Casera Mild	2 tbsp (1.1 oz)	5	0	0	2
DelGrosso					
Chunky Hot	2 tbsp (1.1 oz)	10	0	0	3
Chunky Mild	2 tbsp (1.1 oz)	10	0	0	3
Emerald Valley					
Organic Fiesta	1 tbsp (1 oz)	20	tr	0	4
Organic Green	2 tbsp (1 oz)	10	0	0	2
Jala-Fresca					
Green Stuff Medium	2 tbsp	10	0	0	2
Muir Glen					
Organic Medium	2 tbsp	10	0	0	3
Number 9					
Black Bean & Corn	2 tbsp (1.1 oz)	20	1	0	4
Hot	2 tbsp (1.1 oz)	15	1	0	2
Mild	2 tbsp (1.1 oz)	15	1	0	2
OrganicVille					
Mild	2 tbsp (1 oz)	15	0	0	3
Pineapple	2 tbsp (1 oz)	15	0	0	4
Pace					
Black Bean & Corn	2 tbsp	25	1	0	5
Organic Picante	2 tbsp	10	0	0	2
Thick & Chunky	2 tbsp	10	0	0	2
Robert Rothchild Farm					
Tomatillo & Pepper	2 tbsp	20	0	0	5
Salba Smart					
Organic Omega-3 Enriched	2 tbsp	12	0	0	2
Snyder's Of Hanover					
Sweet	2 tbsp	20	0	0	5
Utz					
Sweet	2 tbsp	10	0	0	2

FOOD	PORTION	CALS	PROT	FAT	CARB
Walnut Acres					
Organic Fiesta Cilantro	2 tbsp	10	0	0	2
Organic Sweet Southwestern Peach	2 tbsp	20	0	0	5
SALSIFY					
fresh sliced cooked	½ cup	46	2	tr	10
SALT SUBSTITUTES					
gomasio sesame salt	2 tsp	34	1	3	2
AlsoSalt					
Butter Flavored	¼ tsp	1	0	0	0
Garlic Flavored	¼ tsp	1	0	0	0
Original	¼ tsp	1	0	0	0
French's					
No Salt	¼ cup	0	0	0	0
Nu-Salt					
Salt Substitute	1 pkg (1 g)	0	0	0	0
SALT/SEASONED SALT					
kosher	¼ tsp	0	0	0	0
salt	1 dash (0.4 g)	0	0	0	0
salt	1 tbsp (0.6 oz)	0	0	0	0
salt	1 tsp (6 g)	0	0	0	0
sea salt coarse	1 tsp	0	0	0	0
sea salt fine	¼ tsp	0	0	0	0
BaconSalt					
Original	¼ tsp	0	0	0	0
Peppered	¼ tsp	0	0	0	0
Bob's Red Mill					
Garlic Salt Blend	¼ tsp	0	0	0	0
Sea Salt	¼ tsp	0	0	0	0
Maine Coast					
Sea Salt w/ Sea Veg	¼ tsp	0	0	0	0
Morton					
Iodized	¼ tsp	0	0	0	0
Ocean's Flavor					
Natural Sea Salt	¼ tsp	0	0	0	0
Spice Hunter					
Celery Salt	¼ tsp	0	0	0	0
Garlic Salt	¼ tsp	0	0	0	0

FOOD	PORTION	CALS	PROT	FAT	CARB
SANDWICHES					
Alexia					
Panini Tuscan Four Cheese w/ Roasted Tomato & Basil	1 pkg (6 oz)	380	18	15	42
Panini Tuscan Grilled Chicken w/ Mozzarella	1 pkg (6 oz)	400	23	18	37
Panini Tuscan Grilled Steak w/ Mushrooms & Onions	1 pkg (6 oz)	370	22	12	43
Panini Tuscan Smoked Chicken w/ Fire Roasted Vegetables & Parmesan	1 pkg (6 oz)	410	22	19	37
Amy's					
Pocket Sandwich Tofu Scramble	1 (4 oz)	180	11	6	23
Pocket Sandwich Vegetable Pie	1 (5 oz)	300	8	9	45
Wrap Indian Somosa	1 (5 oz)	250	8	9	35
Aunt Jemima					
Biscuit Sausage Egg & Cheese	1 (4 oz)	340	12	21	27
Croissant Sausage Egg & Cheese	1 (4 oz)	350	13	23	22
Griddlecake Sausage Egg & Cheese	1 (4.4 oz)	350	13	20	30
Aunt Trudy's					
Fillo Pocket Cheese & Tomato	1 (5 oz)	320	11	15	36
Fillo Pocket Classic Samosa	1 (5 oz)	280	6	10	43
Fillo Pocket Mediterranean Olive & Veggies	1 (5 oz)	270	6	10	41
Organic Fillo Pocket Roasted Sweet Potato	1 (5 oz)	310	5	12	45
Cedarlane					
Wrap Low Fat Couscous & Vegetable Veggie	1 (6 oz)	220	14	3	36
DiGiorno					
Flatbread Melts Chicken Parmesan	1 (6 oz)	380	19	14	45
Fillo Factory					
Organic Fillo Pocket Asian Vegetable	1 (5 oz)	240	5	10	34
Gardenburger					
Wrap Black Bean Chipotle	1 (4.7 oz)	240	13	8	32
Wrap Pizza 100% Meatless Margherita	1 (4.7 oz)	240	12	8	34

FOOD	PORTION	CALS	PROT	FAT	CARB
Guiltless Gourmet					
Wrap Black Bean Chipotle	1 (5.7 oz)	270	9	3	51
Wrap California Veggie	1 (5.7 oz)	300	10	5	53
Wrap Mediterranean Spinach	1 (5.7 oz)	270	10	5	45
Hot Pockets					
Bacon Egg & Cheese	1 (2.2 oz)	160	6	8	17
Barbecue Beef	1 (4.5 oz)	310	11	10	42
Biscuit Sausage Egg & Cheese	1 (4.5 oz)	270	10	11	32
Calzone Four Meat & Four Cheese	½ (4.2 oz)	300	11	13	35
Calzone Pepperoni & Three Cheese	½ (4.2 oz)	330	11	15	39
Chicken Melt	1 (4.5 oz)	300	12	11	36
Croissant Chicken Parmesan	1 (4.5 oz)	340	9	15	41
Croissant Turkey Bacon Club	1 (4.5 oz)	320	12	15	34
Ham & Cheese	1 (4.5 oz)	290	11	11	36
Meatballs & Mozzarella	1 (4.5 oz)	300	11	12	36
Philly Steak & Cheese	1 (4.5 oz)	270	12	9	34
Steak Fajita	1 (4.5 oz)	280	10	12	33
Turkey & Ham w/ Cheese	1 (4 .5 oz)	280	12	10	35
Jimmy Dean					
Bagel Sausage Egg & Cheese	1 (4.8 oz)	380	13	21	34
Biscuit Sausage Egg & Cheese	1 (4.5 oz)	440	13	31	27
Croissant Sausage Egg & Cheese	1 (4.5 oz)	430	13	29	30
D-Lights Croissants Turkey Sausage Egg White & Cheese	1 (4.8 oz)	300	17	12	31
D-Lights Honey Wheat Muffin Canadian Bacon Egg White & Cheese	1 (4.5 oz)	230	15	6	30
Muffin Sausage Egg & Cheese	1 (4.6 oz)	350	13	21	28
Lean Pockets					
Bacon Egg & Cheese	1 (2.2 oz)	150	6	5	18
Barbecue Beef	1 (4.5 oz)	290	11	7	46
Chicken Cheddar & Broccoli	1 (4.5 oz)	260	11	7	40
Chicken Fajita	1 (4.5 oz)	240	10	7	35
Chicken Parmesan	1 (4.5 oz)	290	11	7	45
Ham & Cheese	1 (4.5 oz)	270	12	7	39
Meatballs & Mozzarella	1 (4.5 oz)	260	14	7	35
Philly Steak & Cheese	1 (4.5 oz)	270	11	7	38
Sausage Egg & Cheese	1 (2.2 oz)	140	6	5	18

FOOD	PORTION	CALS	PROT	FAT	CARB
Steak Fajita	1 (4.5 oz)	250	10	7	36
Three Cheese & Chicken Quesadilla	1 (4.5 oz)	260	13	7	34
Turkey & Ham w/ Cheddar	1 (4.5 oz)	280	12	7	40
Turkey Broccoli & Cheese	1 (4.5 oz)	270	10	7	39
Lunchables					
Chicken Dunks	1 pkg	310	12	6	52
Cracker Stackers Bologna & American	1 pkg (4.1 oz)	390	14	22	34
Cracker Stackers Ham & Swiss	1 pkg (4.5 oz)	340	20	18	23
Sub Ham + American	1 pkg	350	13	11	49
Sub Turkey + Cheddar	1 pkg	360	11	8	62
Oscar Mayer					
Deli Creations Honey Ham & Swiss	1 pkg (6.8 oz)	440	28	14	51
Deli Creations Steakhouse Cheddar	1 pkg (7.1 oz)	450	29	15	50
Deli Creations Turkey & Cheddar Dijon	1 pkg (6.7 oz)	430	26	15	48
PBJammerz					
Peanut Butter & Jelly All Flavors	1 (2 oz)	220	8	13	22
Pillsbury					
Toaster Scrambles Cheese Egg & Bacon	1 (1.6 oz)	180	4	12	15
Toaster Scrambles Cheese Egg & Sausage	1 (1.6 oz)	180	4	12	15
Stouffer's					
Corner Bistro Panini Philly Style Steak & Cheese	1 pkg (6 oz)	340	20	16	33
Corner Bistro Panini Southwestern Chicken	1 pkg (6 oz)	360	20	16	31
Van's					
Breakfast In A Pocket Sandwich Ham Egg & Cheese	1 (4.5 oz)	370	11	22	30
Breakfast In A Pocket Sandwich Veggie Egg & Cheese	1 (4.5 oz)	340	10	19	31
Breakfast Panini Huevos Rancheros	1 (4.5 oz)	270	11	11	33
Breakfast Panini Sausage Egg & Cheese	1 (4.5 oz)	290	14	13	28

FOOD	PORTION	CALS	PROT	FAT	CARB
TAKE-OUT					
bacon & egg	1 (6.2 oz)	388	21	21	28
bacon lettuce & tomato w/ mayo	1 (5.8 oz)	344	12	17	35
beef barbecue w/ bun	1 (6.7 oz)	417	32	12	42
calzone beef & cheese	1 (14 oz)	1476	62	76	131
calzone cheese	1 (15 oz)	1632	80	93	117
chicken fillet	1 (6.4 oz)	515	24	29	39
chicken fillet w/ cheese	1 (8 oz)	632	29	39	42
chicken salad	1 (5 oz)	333	19	16	28
crab cake w/ bun	1	308	21	8	36
crispy chicken fillet w/ lettuce tomato & mayo	1 (7.7 oz)	537	27	26	49
croque monsieur	1 (12.4 oz)	765	41	46	43
egg salad	1 (5.6 oz)	485	14	35	28
french dip w/ roll	1 (6.8 oz)	357	26	13	34
fried egg	1 (3.4 oz)	226	10	9	26
grilled cheese	1 (2.9 oz)	290	9	16	28
gyro	1 (13.7 oz)	593	44	12	74
ham & egg	1 (4.4 oz)	272	15	11	27
ham w/ cheese lettuce & mayo	1 (5.4 oz)	369	19	18	32
hot turkey w/ gravy	1	389	40	10	32
peanut butter & banana	1	617	10	14	43
peanut butter & jelly	1 (3.3 oz)	327	10	14	42
reuben w/ sauerkraut & cheese	1 (6.4 oz)	463	21	29	30
roast beef w/ gravy	1 (7.8 oz)	386	30	16	30
sloppy joe pork on bun	1 (6.5 oz)	318	23	9	34
tuna melt	1 (5.3 oz)	350	20	16	30
tuna salad w/ lettuce	1 (5.9 oz)	289	19	7	37
turkey w/ mayo	1 (5 oz)	329	29	11	26
SAPODILLA					
fresh	1	140	1	2	34
fresh cut up	1 cup	199	1	3	48
SAPOTES					
fresh	1	301	5	1	76
SARDINES					
CANNED					
atlantic in oil w/ bone	2	50	6	3	0
atlantic in oil w/ bone	1 can (3.2 oz)	192	23	11	0

FOOD	PORTION	CALS	PROT	FAT	CARB
pacific in tomato sauce w/ bone	1 can (13 oz)	658	61	44	0
pacific in tomato sauce w/ bone	1 (1.3 oz)	68	6	5	0
King Oscar					
In Olive Oil	1 can (3.75 oz)	150	14	11	0
Skinless Boneless In Soya Oil	3 pieces (1.9 oz)	120	13	7	0
Polar					
In Mustard	1 can (4.5 oz)	170	17	7	10
In Tomato Sauce	1 can (4.5 oz)	120	17	4	5
In Water	1 can (3 oz)	100	20	3	tr
FRESH					
raw	3.5 oz	135	19	5	0

SAUCE (see also BARBECUE SAUCE, GRAVY, SPAGHETTI SAUCE)

FOOD	PORTION	CALS	PROT	FAT	CARB
adobo fresco	2 tbsp	81	1	8	7
bearnaise	1 oz	177	1	19	1
cheese mix as prep w/ milk	1 cup	307	16	17	23
curry mix as prep	1 cup	120	3	6	14
curry mix as prep w/ milk	1 cup	270	11	15	26
enchilada sauce green	¼ cup	46	1	4	3
enchilada sauce red	¼ cup	79	1	8	2
fish sauce chinese	1 tbsp	9	2	0	tr
fish sauce vietnamese nuoc mam	1 tbsp	6	1	0	1
hoisin	1 tbsp	35	1	1	7
moroccan tagine	½ cup (4 oz)	70	2	3	10
mushroom mix as prep w/ milk	1 cup	228	11	10	24
oyster	1 tbsp	8	tr	0	2
plum sauce	0.5 oz	42	0	0	10
satay peanut sauce	1 oz	77	2	6	3
sour cream mix as prep w/ milk	1 cup	509	19	30	45
stroganoff mix as prep	1 cup	271	12	11	34
sweet & sour mix as prep	1 cup	294	1	tr	73
teriyaki	1 tbsp	15	1	0	3
teriyaki mix as prep	1 cup	131	4	1	28
white sauce mix as prep w/ milk	1 cup	241	10	13	21
Ahh!Gourmet					
Perky Savory Coffee Sauce	4 tbsp	71	tr	0	17
Ritzy Kumquat Plum Sauce	4 tbsp	98	tr	0	24
Spicy Garlicky Sweet Sauce Paste	4 tbsp	101	2	4	16
Spicy Ginger Soy Sauce Paste	4 tbsp	137	2	8	15

FOOD	PORTION	CALS	PROT	FAT	CARB
Asian Creations					
Marvelous Mango	¼ cup	20	0	0	6
Pad Thai Pizzazz	2 oz	110	2	6	14
Peanut Passion	¼ cup	130	4	9	12
Bear-Man					
Sap-Happy Golden Bear	2 tbsp	60	0	0	20
Bone Suckin'					
Hiccuppin' Hot	1 tsp	10	0	0	2
Yaki Stir Fry	1 tbsp	30	0	0	7
Burbon Chicken					
Marinade Original	1 tbsp (0.6 oz)	5	0	0	1
Cains					
Tartar	2 tbsp	160	0	16	2
Chef Hymie Grande					
New Mexico Sweet Basting Sauce	2 tbsp (1.2 oz)	35	0	0	8
China Pride					
Duck Sauce Sweet & Pungent	2 tbsp	80	0	0	19
Dave's Gourmet					
Hot Sauce Roasted Garlic	1 tsp (5 g)	0	0	0	0
Insanity Sauce	1 tsp (5 g)	10	0	1	0
Jammin' Jerk	1 tsp (5 g)	5	0	0	1
Steak Sauce	1 tbsp (0.6 oz)	20	0	0	5
Dei Fratelli					
Sloppy Joe Sauce	¼ cup (2.2 oz)	35	1	0	9
DelGrosso					
Sloppy Joe Sauce	¼ cup (2.2 oz)	60	1	1	13
D'Oni					
Happy Together Orange Chili Garlic	2 tbsp	50	0	0	12
Ethnic Gourmet					
Punjab Saag Spinach	4 oz	60	2	3	6
Simmer Sauce Calcutta Masala	4 oz	90	2	5	10
Simmer Sauce Delhi Korma	4 oz	100	2	7	9
Fortun's					
Asian Style Pepper	¼ cup (2 oz)	40	1	1	5
Lemon Dill Caper w/ White Wine	¼ cup (2 oz)	20	0	1	3
Marsala & Mushroom	¼ cup (2 oz)	40	1	1	5
Spicy Mustard w/ Brandy	¼ cup (2 oz)	35	0	2	2
Stroganoff	¼ cup (2 oz)	45	1	3	3

FOOD	PORTION	CALS	PROT	FAT	CARB
Frank's					
RedHot Chile & Lime Sauce	1 tsp	0	0	0	0
RedHot Original Cayenne Pepper Sauce	1 tsp	0	0	0	0
RedHot X-tra Hot	1 tsp	0	0	0	0
French's					
Worcestershire	1 tsp	0	0	0	1
Good Clean Food					
Simmer Sauce Balsamic Mushroom	⅜ cup (3 oz)	100	2	6	9
Simmer Sauce Cacciatore	⅜ cup (3 oz)	70	2	4	7
Simmer Sauce Creole	⅜ cup (3 oz)	45	2	2	7
Simmer Sauce Dill	⅜ cup (3 oz)	60	2	4	5
Simmer Sauce French Tarragon	⅜ cup (3 oz)	90	2	6	8
Simmer Sauce Mediterranean	⅜ cup (3 oz)	50	1	3	6
House Of Tsang					
General Tsao	1 tsp	45	0	1	10
Hoisin	1 tsp	15	0	0	4
Kobe Steak Grill	1 tbsp	50	0	4	2
Korean Teriyaki Stir Fry	1 tbsp	35	0	2	5
Peanut Sauce Bangkok Padang	1 tbsp	45	1	3	4
Spicy Brown Bean	1 tbsp	15	0	0	3
Sweet & Sour	1 tbsp	35	0	0	8
Sweet Ginger Sesame	1 tbsp	40	0	1	8
Thai Peanut	1 tbsp	50	1	3	4
Knorr					
Alfredo Mix as prep	2 oz	60	2	3	5
Bearnaise Mix as prep	2 oz	35	2	1	5
Curry Indian Madras	1 oz	30	tr	2	2
Curry Thai	1 oz	35	tr	3	3
Demi-Glace Mix as prep	2 oz	30	1	1	4
Green Peppercorn Mix as prep	2 oz	35	1	1	5
Hollandaise Mix as prep	2 oz	35	2	1	5
Mango Habanero	1 oz	20	tr	0	6
Sweet Red Chili	1 oz	80	1	0	19
White Mix as prep	2 oz	20	tr	1	3
La Choy					
Sweet & Sour	2 tbsp (1.2 oz)	60	0	0	14
Teriyaki	1 tbsp (0.6 oz)	40	tr	0	10

FOOD	PORTION	CALS	PROT	FAT	CARB
Latino Chef					
Chimichurri Sun Dried Tomato	2 tbsp	120	2	10	8
Sofrito	2 tbsp	20	0	1	3
Lea & Perrins					
Worcestershire	1 tsp (0.2 oz)	5	0	0	1
Manwich					
Sloppy Joe Original	¼ cup (2.2 oz)	30	1	0	7
Milo's					
Simmer Sauce Bombay Cabernet	3 oz	35	1	0	7
Naturally Fresh					
Seafood Cocktail	2 tbsp	25	0	0	5
Tartar Sauce	2 tbsp	130	0	14	2
Old El Paso					
Enchilada Mild	¼ cup	25	0	1	4
OrganicVille					
Island Teriyaki	1 tbsp (0.5 oz)	25	tr	1	4
Pace					
Taco Sauce Green	1 tbsp	5	0	0	1
Taco Sauce Red	2 tbsp	10	0	0	2
Patak's					
Jalfrezi Sweet Peppers & Coconut	½ cup	140	2	8	15
Korma Rich Creamy Coconut	½ cup	240	2	20	13
Rogan Josh Spicy Tomato & Cardamon	½ cup	90	2	4	12
Tikka Masala Tangy Lemon & Cilantro	½ cup	120	1	8	12
Road's End Organics					
Alfredo Style Dairy Free Gluten Free	⅓ pkg	35	3	0	5
Cheddar Style Dairy Free	⅓ pkg	35	2	0	6
Robert Rothchild Farm					
Anne Mae's Smoky Sweet Chipotle	2 tbsp	35	tr	0	9
Simply Boulder					
Coconut Peanut	2 tbsp (1 oz)	90	2	7	6
Lemon Pesto	2 tbsp (1 oz)	50	0	5	3
Zesty Pineapple	2 tbsp (1 oz)	45	0	3	7

FOOD	PORTION	CALS	PROT	FAT	CARB
Soy Vay					
Hoisin Garlic Asian Glaze & Marinade	1 tbsp	40	1	1	7
Veri Veri Teriyaki	1 tbsp	35	0	1	6
Tabasco					
Pepper Sauce	1 tsp	0	0	0	0
Texas Sassy					
Marinade Salsa	1 tbsp (0.5 oz)	15	0	0	3
Pickle Sauce	1 tbsp (0.5 oz)	30	0	0	7
Thai Kitchen					
Premium Fish Sauce	1 tbsp (0.5 oz)	10	2	0	0
The Gracious Gourmet					
Pesto Lemon Artichoke	2 tbsp (1 oz)	50	1	5	2
The Wizard's					
Organic Worcestershire Vegetarian Wheat Free	1 tsp	0	0	0	1
Three Acre Kitchen					
Marinade Balsamic w/ Juniper & Rosemary	1 tbsp (0.5 oz)	50	0	5	2
Wild Thymes Farm					
Marinade Hawaiian Teryaki	1 tbsp	19	1	1	3
Marinade Korean Ginger Scallion	1 tbsp	20	tr	1	3
Marinade New Orleans Creole	1 tbsp	11	tr	0	3
WildWood					
Aioli	1 tbsp	80	0	9	0
Pesto Basil & Pine Nuts	¼ cup	230	5	23	2
Wingers					
Hotter Than Hot	1 tsp	0	0	0	0
World Harbors					
Buccaneer Blends Pirate's Original	1 tbsp (0.6 oz)	20	0	0	4
Chimichurri	2 tbsp (1.2 oz)	40	0	0	9
Fajita	2 tbsp (1.1 oz)	45	0	0	10
Jerk	2 tbsp (1 oz)	70	0	0	18
Lemon Pepper & Garlic	2 tbsp (1 oz)	35	0	0	8
Thai	2 tbsp (1 oz)	40	0	0	8
Zatarain's					
Cocktail	¼ cup	70	1	0	17
Etouffee Base as prep	½ cup	35	1	0	7

FOOD	PORTION	CALS	PROT	FAT	CARB
TAKE-OUT					
cucumber yogurt sauce	1½ tbsp	20	2	0	3
SAUERKRAUT					
canned	½ cup	22	1	tr	5
Ba-Tampte					
Kosher	2 tbsp (1 oz)	5	0	0	1
Dei Fratelli					
Sauerkraut	2 tbsp (1 oz)	5	0	0	1
Gedney					
Sauerkraut	½ cup	15	0	0	3
Tree Of Life					
Organic	½ cup (3.6 oz)	15	0	0	3
SAUSAGE					
beef & pork	1 link (2.3 oz)	196	8	17	1
beef & pork w/ cheddar cheese	1 link (2.7 oz)	228	10	20	2
bierschinken	3.5 oz	174	18	11	tr
bierwurst	3.5 oz	258	16	21	0
blutwurst uncooked	3.5 oz	424	13	39	0
bockwurst	3.5 oz	276	12	25	0
bratwurst chicken cooked	1 (3 oz)	148	16	9	0
bratwurst pork cooked	1 link (2.5 oz)	226	10	19	2
brotwurst pork & beef	1 link (2.5 oz)	226	10	19	2
chipolata	3.5 oz	342	14	32	1
chorizo	1 link (2.1 oz)	273	14	23	1
fleischwurst	3.5 oz	305	12	29	0
free range chicken breakfast	2 links (2.7 oz)	110	14	6	1
gelbwurst uncooked	3.5 oz	363	12	33	0
italian pork cooked	1 (2.4 oz)	230	13	18	3
jagdwurst	3.5 oz	211	16	16	0
knockwurst pork & beef	1 (2.5 oz)	221	8	20	2
mettwurst uncooked	3.5 oz	483	13	45	0
plockwurst uncooked	3.5 oz	312	19	45	0
polish kielbasa	2 oz	127	7	10	2
pork cooked	2 links (1.7 oz)	163	9	14	0
regensburger uncooked	3.5 oz	354	13	31	0
turkey italian smoked	1 (2 oz)	88	8	5	3
vienna canned	1 link (0.5 oz)	37	2	3	tr
vienna canned	1 can (4 oz)	260	12	22	3
weisswurst uncooked	3.5 oz	305	11	27	0
zungenwurst (tongue)	3.5 oz	285	17	24	0

FOOD	PORTION	CALS	PROT	FAT	CARB
Applegate Farms					
Organic Andouille	1 (3 oz)	120	13	6	3
Organic Spinach & Feta	1 (3 oz)	120	13	7	2
Armour					
Sizzle & Serve Turkey	3 (1.8 oz)	130	9	9	2
Banquet					
Brown'N Serve Lite Original	3 (2.1 oz)	120	9	9	2
Brown'N Serve Lite Maple	3 (2 oz)	130	9	9	4
Butterball					
Bratwurst Turkey	1 (3.2 oz)	140	17	8	1
Breakfast Turkey	3 (3 oz)	130	15	7	0
Polska Kielbasa Turkey	2 oz	100	8	6	4
Sweet Italian Turkey	1 (3.2 oz)	140	16	8	1
Healthy Ones					
Smoked	2 oz	80	7	3	6
Honeysuckle White					
Turkey Roll Mild Italian	2.5 oz	100	13	5	1
Jimmy Dean					
Fully Cooked Original Links	3 (2.4 oz)	240	9	22	1
Fully Cooked Original Patties	2 (2.4 oz)	240	9	23	1
Fully Cooked Turkey Links	3 (2.4 oz)	120	13	7	1
Fully Cooked Turkey Patties	2 (2.4 oz)	120	13	7	1
Original Links	3 (2 oz)	170	7	14	1
Original Patties cooked	2 (2.4 oz)	240	9	23	1
Pork All Natural cooked	2 oz	190	12	15	1
Pork Light cooked	2 oz	140	9	11	1
Johnsonville					
Bratwurst Original	1 (3 oz)	270	15	22	2
Breakfast Patty Original	2 (2 oz)	180	10	15	1
Grilling Chorizo	1 (3 oz)	280	16	22	3
Italian Mild	1 (3 oz)	270	15	22	3
Original Summer	1 (2 oz)	170	9	15	1
Polish	1 (2.7 oz)	240	9	21	2
Pork	2 oz	180	10	15	1
Smoked Turkey	1 (3 oz)	110	10	6	4
Jones					
All Natural Light	3 (2.1 oz)	130	9	9	3
Libby's					
Vienna Sausage BBQ	3	140	5	12	4

FOOD	PORTION	CALS	PROT	FAT	CARB
Organic Prairie					
Bratwurst Pork	1 (3 oz)	210	13	19	1
Perdue					
Turkey Breakfast	2 oz	80	9	5	0
Turkey Sweet Italian cooked	1 link (2.8 oz)	150	15	8	4
Wampler					
Bratwurst as prep	1 (2.5 oz)	230	12	20	0
Breakfast Links as prep	2 (1.2 oz)	130	7	11	0
Breakfast Patties as prep	1 (1.1 oz)	120	5	11	0
Italian as prep	1 (2.5 oz)	230	12	20	0
SAUSAGE DISHES					
TAKE-OUT					
italian sausage w/ peppers & onions	1 cup	210	17	11	14
sausage roll	1 (2.3 oz)	311	5	24	22
SAUSAGE SUBSTITUTES					
meatless	1 patty (1.3 oz)	98	7	7	4
meatless	1 link (0.9 oz)	64	5	5	2
Gardenburger					
Veggie Breakfast	1 patty (1.5 oz)	45	5	3	3
Morningstar Farms					
Breakfast Patties	1 (1.3 oz)	80	8	3	4
Worthington					
Saucettes Breakfast Links	1 (1.3 oz)	90	6	6	1
Yves					
Veggie Brats Classic	1 (3.3 oz)	160	19	5	5
SAVORY					
ground	1 tsp	4	tr	tr	1
SCALLOP					
raw	3 oz	75	14	1	2
Mrs. Paul's					
Fried	13 (3.7 oz)	260	12	11	28
TAKE-OUT					
breaded & fried	2 lg	67	6	3	3
SCONE					
TAKE-OUT					
apricot	1	232	5	7	39
blueberry	1 (3 oz)	270	7	9	41

FOOD	PORTION	CALS	PROT	FAT	CARB
cheese	1 (3.5 oz)	364	10	18	44
orange poppy	1 (3 oz)	260	6	6	47
plain	1 (3.5 oz)	362	8	14	54
raisin	1 (3 oz)	270	6	8	43

SCUP
fresh baked	3 oz	115	21	3	0

SEA BASS (see BASS)

SEA CUCUMBER
dried	1 oz	74	14	1	1
fresh	1 oz	20	5	tr	tr

SEA TROUT (see TROUT)

SEA URCHIN
canned	1 oz	39	4	1	3
fresh	1 oz	36	4	1	3
roe paste	1 tbsp	19	2	tr	3

SEAWEED
agar dried	1 oz	87	2	tr	23
agar fresh	1 oz	tr	tr	tr	2
hijiki dried	1 tbsp	9	1	0	2
irishmoss fresh	1 oz	14	tr	tr	4
kelp fresh	1 oz	12	tr	tr	3
kombu fresh	1 oz	12	tr	tr	3
laver fresh	1 oz	10	2	tr	1
nori fresh	1 oz	10	2	tr	1
nori sheet dried	1 (8 x 8 in)	5	1	0	1
seahair dried	1 tbsp	13	1	0	3
spirulina dried	1 oz	83	16	2	7
spirulina fresh	1 oz	7	2	tr	1
tangle fresh	1 oz	12	tr	tr	3
wakame fresh	1 oz	13	1	tr	3
Maine Coast					
Organic Alaria Whole Leaf	1/3 cup	18	1	tr	3
Organic Dulse Granules	1 tsp	6	0	0	2
Organic Dulse Whole Leaf	1/2 cup	19	2	tr	3
Organic Kelp Granules	1/2 tsp	5	0	0	2
Organic Kelp Whole Leaf	1/3 cup	17	1	tr	3
Organic Laver Whole Leaf	1/3 cup	22	2	tr	3

FOOD	PORTION	CALS	PROT	FAT	CARB
SEITAN (see WHEAT)					
SEMOLINA					
dry	1 cup (5.9 oz)	601	21	2	122
SESAME					
seeds	1 tsp	16	1	2	tr
sesame butter	1 tbsp	95	3	8	4
sesame crunch candy	20 pieces (1.2 oz)	181	4	12	18
sesame crunch candy	1 oz	146	3	9	14
tahini from roasted & toasted kernels	1 tbsp	89	3	8	3
tahini from stone ground kernels	1 tbsp	86	3	7	4
tahini from unroasted kernels	1 tbsp	85	3	8	3
Arrowhead Mills					
Organic Seeds	¼ cup	210	9	19	3
Organic Tahini	2 tbsp	190	8	18	3
Mrs. May's					
Black Sesame Crunch	1 oz	165	4	11	14
Peloponnese					
Tahini	1 tbsp	100	4	9	2
Tree Of Life					
Organic Sesame Tahini	2 tbsp	108	5	15	8
Seeds	¼ cup (1.3 oz)	210	6	18	8
SESBANIA					
flower	1	1	tr	0	tr
flowers	1 cup	5	tr	tr	1
flowers cooked	1 cup	23	1	tr	5
SHAD					
american baked	3 oz	214	18	15	0
cooked	1 oz	55	7	3	1
roe baked w/ butter & lemon	1 oz	36	6	1	tr
SHALLOTS (see ONION)					
SHARK					
fin dried	1 oz	32	7	tr	–
raw	3 oz	111	18	4	0

FOOD	PORTION	CALS	PROT	FAT	CARB
TAKE-OUT					
batter-dipped & fried	3 oz	194	16	12	5
SHEEPSHEAD FISH					
cooked	3 oz	107	22	1	0
cooked	1 fillet (6.5 oz)	234	48	3	0
raw	3 oz	92	17	2	0
SHELLFISH (see individual names, SHELLFISH SUBSTITUTES)					
SHELLFISH SUBSTITUTES					
crab imitation	1 cup (4.4 oz)	144	17	1	16
scallop imitation	3 oz	84	11	tr	9
shrimp imitation	3 oz	86	11	1	8
surimi	3 oz	84	13	1	6
surimi	1 oz	28	4	tr	2
TAKE-OUT					
crab salad	1 cup	395	18	26	21
SHELLIE BEANS					
canned	½ cup	37	2	tr	8
SHERBET					
orange	1 bar (2.75 fl oz)	91	1	1	20
orange	½ cup (4 fl oz)	132	1	2	29
orange	½ gal	2158	17	31	469
Ciao Bella					
Lemon	1 pkg (3.5 oz)	120	0	0	31
Mango	1 pkg (3.5 oz)	100	0	0	25
Raspberry	1 pkg (3.5 oz)	110	1	0	28
Dippin' Dots					
Lemon Lime	½ cup	97	1	1	22
Hershey's					
Lemon	½ cup (3.4 oz)	100	tr	1	23
Orange	½ cup (3.4 oz)	100	tr	1	23
Strawberry	½ cup (3.4 oz)	110	tr	1	25
Hola Fruta					
Bar Pomegranate & Blueberry	1 (2.5 oz)	100	1	1	22
Mango	½ cup	130	1	0	31
Margarita	½ cup	140	1	1	30
Peach	½ cup	130	8	1	30
Pomegranate	½ cup	140	1	1	32

FOOD	PORTION	CALS	PROT	FAT	CARB
Land O' Lakes					
Orange	½ cup (3.2 oz)	130	2	2	28
Turkey Hill					
Fruit Rainbow	½ cup	120	0	1	26
Orange Grove	½ cup	120	1	1	26
SHRIMP					
CANNED					
canned	1 can (6 oz)	136	26	2	1
chinese shrimp paste	1 tbsp	46	1	0	10
Polar					
Tiny Peeled	¼ cup (2 oz)	44	10	0	1
DRIED					
dried	10	15	3	tr	tr
FRESH					
broiled	6 med	46	7	2	tr
steamed	6 med	41	8	1	tr
FROZEN					
Blue Horizon Organic					
Garlic Shrimp	1 serv (3.5 oz)	160	15	2	21
Panko Shrimp	1 serv (3.5 oz)	160	15	2	22
Popcorn Shrimp	1 serv (3.5 oz)	160	15	2	21
Tempura Shrimp	1 serv (3.5 oz)	160	15	2	21
Contessa					
Orange Shrimp	11 to 13 (6 oz)	250	14	8	33
Ragin' Cajun	8 to 10 (4 oz)	170	11	10	9
Shrimp Scampi	8 to 10 (4 oz)	290	9	27	4
Gorton's					
Popcorn Crunchy Golden	20 (3.2 oz)	240	8	12	24
Temptations Breaded Butterfly	5 (3.5 oz)	250	11	11	27
Temptations Scampi Sauced	1 serv (4 oz)	120	10	6	8
Mrs. Paul's					
Butterfly	7 (4 oz)	250	12	11	27
Van de Kamp's					
Battered	6 (4 oz)	200	14	6	22
Breaded Popcorn	20 (4 oz)	260	11	11	30
TAKE-OUT					
breaded & fried	6 med (2.3 oz)	162	14	8	8
curried	1 cup	295	27	14	14
jambalaya	1 cup	309	27	9	28
scampi	1 cup	310	26	22	1

FOOD	PORTION	CALS	PROT	FAT	CARB
shrimp cocktail w/ sauce	4 shrimp	87	11	1	7
shrimp newburg	1 serv (6.4 oz)	456	22	37	8
shrimp salad	¾ cup	212	20	12	4
shrimp w/ crab stuffing	5	158	16	8	5

SMELT
rainbow cooked	3 oz	106	19	3	0
rainbow raw	3 oz	83	15	2	0

SMOOTHIES (see also FRUIT DRINKS, YOGURT DRINKS)
Arthur's
Carrot Energizer	1 bottle (11 oz)	200	2	1	47
Green Energy	1 bottle (11 oz)	230	2	1	53

Bolthouse Farms
Green Goodness	8 oz	140	2	0	33
Mango Lemonade	8 oz	120	tr	0	30
Passion Fruit Apple Carrot Juice	8 oz	120	2	0	29

C&W
Berry Blend	½ cup	90	2	2	15
Peach	½ cup	80	2	2	15

Horizon Organic
Tropical Punch	1 bottle (6.2 oz)	120	4	0	25

Kidz Dream
Orange Cream	1 box	120	4	2	21

Nutiva
Organic HempShake Amazon Acai not prep	4 tbsp	100	9	3	15
Organic HempShake Chocolate not prep	4 tbsp	80	7	2	19

Odwalla
Bluberry B Monster	8 oz	140	0	0	33
Citrus C Monster	8 oz	150	2	0	36
Mango Tango	8 oz	150	1	1	34

Sambazon
Acai Amazon Cherry	8 oz	156	5	0	16
Acai Mango Banana	8 oz	190	2	5	38
Acai Mango Uprising	8 oz	190	2	5	38
Acai Protein Warrior Vanilla	8 oz	215	8	6	33

FOOD	PORTION	CALS	PROT	FAT	CARB
Acai Shaman's Immunity	8 oz	90	1	0	24
Acai Soy Energy	8 oz	210	6	6	25
Acai Strawberry Sensation	8 oz	210	1	4	42
Acai Supergreens Revolution	8 oz	200	2	4	40
Organic Acai	1 bottle	155	1	3	31
Soy Fusion					
Berry	1 box (8.45 oz)	120	2	1	24
Matcha Green Tea	1 box (8.45 oz)	110	3	2	19
Tropicana					
Fruit Smoothie Mixed Berry	1 bottle (11 oz)	220	1	0	54
Fruit Smoothie Tropical Fruit	1 bottle (11 oz)	220	1	0	53
V8					
Splash Tropical Colada	8 oz	100	3	0	21
SNACKS					
cheese puffs	1 oz	122	2	3	21
oriental mix	1 oz	155	6	12	9
pork skins	1 oz	154	17	9	0
pork skins barbecue	1 oz	152	16	9	1
Barbara's Bakery					
Cheese Puffs Bakes Original	¾ cup	160	2	11	13
Cheese Puffs Original	¾ cup (1 oz)	150	2	10	16
Carole's					
Soycrunch Cinnamon & Raisins	½ cup	110	6	1	19
Soycrunch Original	½ cup	120	5	2	16
Soycrunch Toffee	½ cup	110	7	2	15
Cheetos					
Crunchy	1 pkg (1.25 oz)	200	2	13	19
Cheez It					
Right Bites Party Mix	1 pkg (0.74 oz)	100	2	4	15
Lance					
Cheese Puffs	9 (1 oz)	170	2	12	13
Gold-N-Chees	1 oz	150	2	8	17
Lifestyle Foods					
Awake	1 pkg (5 oz)	170	3	0	55

FOOD	PORTION	CALS	PROT	FAT	CARB
Essential	1 pkg (5.6 oz)	200	9	10	21
Miami	1 pkg (7.5 oz)	180	5	0	36
Power Up	1 pkg (6.7 oz)	670	18	33	77
Medora Snacks					
Corners Sea Salt	1 oz	130	2	3	22
Pucci Garlic	1 oz	120	4	4	17
Pucci Tomato Basil	1 oz	120	4	4	17
Sotos Cheese Olive Oil & Lemon	1 oz	120	2	4	19
Michael Season's					
Cheese Puffs & Curls	1½ cups	180	3	13	13
Robert's American Gourmet					
Booty Barbeque	1 oz	130	2	5	20
Booty Pirate's	1 oz	130	2	5	18
Booty Veggie	1 oz	130	1	6	17
Smart Puffs	1 oz	130	2	6	17
Tings	1 oz	160	1	8	17
Silhouette Solution					
Puffs BBQ	1 pkg (1.06 oz)	120	15	4	8
Snikiddy					
Puffs Grilled Cheese	1 pkg (0.6 oz)	80	2	3	10
Puffs Rockin' Ranch	1 pkg (0.6 oz)	83	1	0	11
Snyder's Of Hanover					
CheddAirs	1 oz	130	3	5	20
MultiGrain Cheese Puffs	1 oz	130	2	6	19
Sweet Emotions					
Chocolate Passion	1 pkg (0.5 oz)	60	1	3	10
Cinnamon Joy	1 pkg (0.5 oz)	60	1	3	10
T.G.I. Friday's					
Mozzarella Sticks	20 (1 oz)	150	2	9	14
Utz					
Cheese Balls	50 (1 oz)	150	2	9	16
Cheese Curls	18 (1 oz)	150	2	9	16
Onion Rings	41 (1 oz)	130	1	5	20
Party Mix	1 oz	150	2	7	19
Pork Cracklins	0.5 oz	90	6	7	0
Pork Rinds Original	0.5 oz	80	9	5	0
SNAIL					
cooked	3 oz	233	41	1	13
raw	3 oz	117	20	tr	7

FOOD	PORTION	CALS	PROT	FAT	CARB
TAKE-OUT					
escargot cooked	5	25	4	0	1
SNAKE					
fresh	3 oz	78	17	tr	3
SNAPPER					
cooked	3 oz	109	22	1	0
cooked	1 fillet (6 oz)	217	45	3	0
raw	3 oz	85	17	1	0
SODA					
club	12 oz	0	0	0	0
cola	12 oz	151	tr	tr	39
cream	12 oz	191	0	0	49
diet cola	12 oz	2	tr	0	tr
ginger ale	12 oz	124	tr	0	32
grape	12 oz	161	0	0	42
lemon lime	12 oz	149	0	0	38
orange	12 oz	177	0	0	46
pepper type	12 oz	151	0	tr	38
quinine	12 oz	125	0	0	32
root beer	12 oz	152	tr	0	39
shirley temple	1 serv	159	0	0	41
tonic water	12 oz	125	0	0	32
Ale 8 One					
Soft Drink	1 bottle (12 oz)	120	0	0	30
Barq's					
Diet French Vanilla Creme	8 oz	1	0	0	tr
Diet Red Creme	8 oz	4	0	0	0
Diet Root Beer	8 oz	1	0	0	tr
Floatz	8 oz	127	0	0	34
French Vanilla Creme	8 oz	112	0	0	30
Red Creme	8 oz	115	0	0	31
Root Beer	8 oz	111	0	0	30
Cape Cod Dry					
Cranberry	8 oz	120	0	0	29
Diet Cranberry	8 oz	10	0	0	2
Carver's					
Ginger Ale	8 oz	94	0	0	24

FOOD	PORTION	CALS	PROT	FAT	CARB
Coca-Cola					
C2	8 oz	45	0	0	12
Classic	8 oz	97	0	0	27
W/ Lime	8 oz	98	0	0	27
Coke					
Cherry	8 oz	104	0	0	28
Diet	8 oz	1	0	0	tr
Diet Cherry	8 oz	1	0	0	tr
Diet Plus	8 oz	0	0	0	0
Diet Vanilla	8 oz	1	0	0	tr
Diet w/ Lime	8 oz	2	0	0	tr
Vanilla	8 oz	100	0	0	28
DRY					
Juniper Berry	1 bottle (12 oz)	55	0	0	15
Vanilla Bean	1 bottle (12 oz)	60	0	0	16
Fanta					
Apple	8 oz	121	0	0	33
Citrus	8 oz	91	0	0	25
Orange	8 oz	111	0	0	35
Fresca					
Soda	8 oz	2	0	0	tr
Goya					
Ginger Beer	1 bottle (12 oz)	190	0	0	43
GuS					
Dry Cola	1 bottle (12 oz)	95	0	0	24
Dry Crimson Grape	1 bottle (12 oz)	90	0	0	22
Dry Pomegranate	1 bottle (12 oz)	98	0	0	24
Star Ruby Grapefruit	1 bottle (12 oz)	90	0	0	22
Hansen's					
Blackberry	1 bottle	150	tr	0	37
Health Cola					
Soda	1 bottle (12 oz)	140	0	0	35
HotLips					
Apple	1 bottle	136	0	0	34
Boysenberry	1 bottle	152	1	0	37
Pear	1 bottle	142	tr	1	34
Inca Kola					
Diet	8 oz	1	0	0	tr
Soda	8 oz	96	0	0	26

FOOD	PORTION	CALS	PROT	FAT	CARB
Jones Soda					
Blue Bubble Gum	1 bottle (12 oz)	190	0	0	48
Cream	1 bottle (12 oz)	190	0	0	48
Crushed Melon	1 bottle (12 oz)	190	0	0	48
FuFu Berry	1 bottle (12 oz)	190	0	0	46
Green Apple	1 bottle (12 oz)	180	0	0	46
Orange Cream	1 bottle (12 oz)	180	0	0	46
Lucozade					
Soda	7 oz	136	0	0	36
Manzana Mia					
Soda	8 oz	99	0	0	27
Mello Yellow					
Diet	8 oz	3	0	0	tr
Soda	8 oz	118	0	0	32
Mr. Pibb					
Diet	8 oz	1	0	0	tr
Northern Neck					
Diet Ginger Ale	8 oz	4	0	0	0
Ginger Ale	8 oz	94	0	0	24
Nutrisoda					
Calm Sparkling Wild Berry & Citron	1 can (8.7 oz)	0	0	0	1
Flex Sparkling Black Cherry & Apple	1 can (8.7 oz)	5	0	0	1
Immune Sparkling Tangerine & Lime	1 can (8.7 oz)	15	2	0	1
Slender Sparkling Guava & Grapefruit	1 can (8.7 oz)	10	0	0	1
Oogave Natural					
All Flavors	8 oz	68	0	0	17
Orangina					
Sparkling Citrus	8 oz	100	0	0	26
Pepsi					
Cola	8 oz	100	0	0	28

FOOD	PORTION	CALS	PROT	FAT	CARB
Diet	8 oz	0	0	0	0
Diet Vanilla	8 oz	0	0	0	0
One	8 oz	1	0	0	0
Wild Cherry	8 oz	100	0	0	28
Pibb					
Zero	8 oz	2	0	0	tr
Polar					
Birch Beer	8 oz	110	0	0	28
Bitter Lemon Mixer	8 oz	120	0	0	29
Collins Mixer	8 oz	90	0	0	22
Cream	8 oz	120	0	0	30
Diet Pomegranate Dry	8 oz	10	0	0	2
Orange	8 oz	130	0	0	32
Pomegranate Dry	8 oz	120	0	0	30
Seltzer All Flavors	8 oz	0	0	0	0
Strawberry	8 oz	120	0	0	30
Tonic Water	8 oz	90	0	0	23
Vichy Water	8 oz	0	0	0	0
Red Flash					
Soda	8 oz	105	0	0	28
Reed's					
Ginger Brew Original	1 bottle (12 oz)	145	0	0	37
Santa Cruz					
Organic Cherry	1 can (12 oz)	140	0	0	34
Organic Ginger Ale	1 can (12 oz)	150	0	0	37
Organic Root Beer	1 can (12 oz)	150	0	0	36
Organic Vanilla Creme	1 can 12 oz)	160	0	0	38
Sprite					
Diet Zero	8 oz	0	0	0	0
ReMix Aruba Jam	8 oz	97	0	0	26
Soda	8 oz	96	0	0	26
Steaz					
Organic Green Tea Soda Cola	8 oz	90	0	0	23
Organic Green Tea Soda Diet Black Cherry	8 oz	20	0	0	5
Organic Green Tea Soda Ginger Ale	8 oz	90	0	0	23
Organic Green Tea Soda Lemon	8 oz	90	0	0	23

FOOD	PORTION	CALS	PROT	FAT	CARB
Stirrings					
Ginger Ale	8 oz	120	0	0	31
Tab					
Soda	8 oz	1	0	0	tr
Tava					
Sparkling Brazilian Samba	8 oz	0	0	0	0
Sparkling Mediterranean Fiesta	8 oz	0	0	0	0
Thomas Kemper					
Black Cherry	1 bottle (12 oz)	170	0	0	40
Ginger Ale	1 bottle (12 oz)	150	0	0	36
Orange Cream	1 bottle (12 oz)	170	0	0	42
Root Beer	1 bottle (12 oz)	160	0	0	41
Root Beer Low Calorie	1 bottle (12 oz)	20	0	0	5
Vanilla Cream	1 bottle (12 oz)	150	0	0	38
Tropicana					
Twister Orange	1 can (12 oz)	180	0	0	52
Vignette					
Wine Country Soda Chardonnay	1 bottle (12 oz)	130	0	0	33
Wine Country Soda Pinot Noir	1 bottle (12 oz)	130	0	0	31
Virgil's					
Micro Brewed Root Beer	1 bottle (12 oz)	160	0	0	42
SOLE					
cooked	1 fillet (4.5 oz)	148	31	2	0
cooked	3 oz	99	21	1	0
lemon raw	3.5 oz	85	17	1	0
TAKE-OUT					
breaded & fried	3.2 oz	211	13	11	15
SORGHUM					
sorghum	1 cup (6.7 oz)	651	22	6	143

FOOD	PORTION	CALS	PROT	FAT	CARB
SOUFFLE					
Heavenly Souffle					
Chocolate	1 (2.6 oz)	262	3	16	29
TAKE-OUT					
cheese	1 cup	194	9	15	6
chicken	1 cup (5.6 oz)	278	20	18	9
corn	1 cup	257	10	11	34
lime chilled	1 cup	388	11	18	48
seafood	1 cup	245	17	15	9
spinach	1 cup	124	6	8	7
SOUP					
CANNED					
Allens					
Chicken Broth	1 cup	10	1	0	1
Amy's					
Organic Butternut Squash Light In Sodium	1 cup (8.6 oz)	100	2	3	20
Organic Chunky Tomato Bisque	1 cup (8.4 oz)	120	2	4	21
Organic Chunky Tomato Bisque Light In Sodium	1 cup (8.6 oz)	120	2	4	21
Organic Cream Of Mushroom	¾ cup (6.5 oz)	150	3	9	13
Organic Lentil Light In Sodium	1 cup (8.6 oz)	180	8	5	25
Organic No Chicken Noodle Soup	1 cup (8.6 oz)	100	5	3	13
Organic Pasta & 3 Bean	1 cup (8.6 oz)	150	5	4	22
Organic Southwestern Vegetable	1 cup (8.7 oz)	140	4	4	21
Organic Split Pea	1 cup (8.6 oz)	100	7	0	19
Split Pea Light In Sodium	1 cup (8.6 oz)	100	7	0	19
Tom Kha Phak Thai Coconut	1 cup (7 oz)	140	4	10	9
Butterball					
Chicken Broth 99% Fat Free	1 cup	10	tr	0	2
Campbell's					
25% Less Sodium Chicken Noodle as prep	1 cup	60	3	2	8
25% Less Sodium Cream Of Mushroom as prep	1 cup	110	2	8	8
98% Fat Free Cream Of Broccoli as prep	1 cup	70	2	2	10

FOOD	PORTION	CALS	PROT	FAT	CARB
98% Fat Free Cream Of Celery as prep	1 cup	60	1	3	8
98% Fat Free Cream Of Chicken as prep	1 cup	70	2	3	10
Cheddar Cheese as prep	1 cup	110	2	5	12
Chicken & Stars as prep	1 cup	70	3	2	11
Chicken Alphabet as prep	1 cup	70	3	2	12
Chicken Noodle O's as prep	1 cup	90	3	3	15
Chunky Beef and Country Vegetables	1 cup	150	10	3	21
Chunky Chicken Mushroom Chowder	1 cup	210	7	12	19
Chunky Grilled Chicken w/ Vegetables & Pasta	1 cup	100	8	2	15
Chunky Hearty Vegetable w/ Pasta	1 cup	120	4	2	23
Chunky New England Clam Chowder	1 cup	210	7	9	25
Chunky Roadhouse Beef & Bean Chili	1 cup	230	15	8	25
Chunky Sirloin Burger w/ Country Vegetables	1 cup	180	10	7	20
Curly Noodle as prep	1 cup	80	4	2	11
Double Noodle Chicken as prep	1 cup	110	3	2	20
Goldfish Pasta Meatball as prep	1 cup	90	4	3	11
Healthy Request Chicken Noodle as prep	1 cup	60	3	2	8
Healthy Request Chicken Rice as prep	1 cup	70	2	2	13
Healthy Request Cream Of Chicken as prep	1 cup	80	2	3	12
Healthy Request Italian Style Wedding	1 cup	120	7	3	15
Healthy Request Minestrone as prep	1 cup	80	3	1	15
Healthy Request Tomato as prep	1 cup	90	2	2	10
Low Sodium Chicken Broth	1 can	25	4	1	1
Mega Noodle as prep	1 cup	90	3	2	15

FOOD	PORTION	CALS	PROT	FAT	CARB
Microwavable Bowl Chicken Noodle	1 cup	70	4	2	10
Microwavable Bowl Vegetable	1 cup	110	4	1	22
Select Beef w/ Roasted Barley	1 cup	130	9	1	22
Select Harvest Caramelized French Onion	1 cup (8.4 oz)	80	3	3	12
Select Harvest Chicken Tuscany	1 cup	90	7	2	12
Select Harvest Chicken w/ Egg Noodles	1 cup	100	8	3	11
Select Harvest Chicken w/ Whole Grain Pasta	1 cup (8.4 oz)	100	7	2	14
Select Harvest Italian Style Wedding	1 cup (8.4 oz)	130	7	5	13
Select Harvest Light Minestrone w/ Whole Grain Pasta	1 cup	80	4	1	14
Select Harvest Light Savory Chicken w/ Vegetables	1 cup	80	5	1	15
Select Harvest Light Southwestern Style Vegetable	1 cup	50	2	0	13
Select Harvest Light Vegetable & Pasta	1 cup	60	3	0	13
Select Harvest Tomato w/ Basil	1 cup	80	1	0	18
Select Italian Sausage w/ Pasta & Pepperoni	1 cup	150	7	6	18
Select Mexican Chicken Tortilla	1 cup	130	8	3	19
Select Potato Broccoli Cheese	1 cup	120	3	4	18
Select Savory Chicken & Long Grain Rice	1 cup	90	7	1	15
Select Split Pea w/ Roasted Ham	1 cup	160	10	1	29
Select Vegetable Beef	1 cup	110	8	2	16
Soup At Hand 25% Less Sodium Chicken w/ Mini Noodles	1 pkg (10.75 oz)	80	4	2	11
Soup At Hand Vegetable Medley	1 pkg (10.75 oz)	100	3	2	19
Soup At Hand Velvety Potato	1 pkg (10.75 oz)	160	2	7	21
V8 Garden Broccoli	1 cup	80	3	2	15
V8 Golden Butternut Squash	1 cup	140	3	2	28
V8 Sweet Red Pepper	1 cup	120	3	2	22
V8 Tomato Herb	1 cup	90	3	0	19

FOOD	PORTION	CALS	PROT	FAT	CARB
Comfort Care					
Hearty Beef Barley	1 cup (8 oz)	190	12	7	23
Savory Chicken	1 cup (8 oz)	200	13	7	25
Tomato Cheddar Jack	1 cup (8 oz)	90	8	2	13
Dr. McDougall's					
Chunky Tomato Gluten Free Vegan	1 cup (8.6 oz)	90	2	0	20
Vegetable Gluten Free Vegan	1 cup (3.3 oz)	230	4	13	25
Go Appetit					
Carrot Bisque	8 oz	110	6	5	13
Gazpacho	8 oz	100	1	7	9
Mango Melange	8 oz	150	3	5	27
Health Valley					
Beef Broth Fat Free	1 cup	10	2	0	0
Chicken Broth Fat Free	1 cup	20	5	0	0
Chicken Broth Fat Free No Salt Added	1 cup	35	5	2	0
Chicken Broth Low Fat	1 cup	35	5	2	0
Clam Chowder Manhattan	1 cup	90	3	3	13
Clam Chowder New England	1 cup	110	5	4	15
Corn & Vegetable Fat Free	1 cup	70	5	0	17
Garden Vegetable Fat Free	1 cup	80	3	0	18
Lentil & Carrot Fat Free	1 cup	100	10	0	25
Organic Black Bean	1 cup	130	7	1	25
Organic Cream Of Mushroom	1 cup	90	1	5	11
Organic Minestrone	1 cup	100	4	2	20
Organic Minestrone No Salt Added	1 cup	70	3	0	17
Organic Mushroom Barley	1 cup	70	2	0	17
Organic Mushroom Barley No Salt Added	1 cup	70	2	0	17
Organic Split Pea No Salt Added	1 cup	110	10	0	23
Organic Tomato	1 cup	80	3	0	18
Organic Tomato No Salt Added	1 cup	80	3	0	18
Tomato Vegetable Fat Free	1 cup	80	6	0	17
Vegetable Broth Fat Free	1 cup	20	0	0	5
Healthy Choice					
Bean & Ham	1 cup	180	11	2	29
Chicken & Dumplings	1 cup	140	9	3	21
Country Vegetable	1 cup (8.6 oz)	110	5	1	19

FOOD	PORTION	CALS	PROT	FAT	CARB
Old Fashioned Chicken Noodle	1 cup	100	9	2	13
Vegetable Beef	1 cup	130	9	1	22
Zesty Gumbo	1 cup	100	6	2	16
Hormel					
Bean & Ham	1 pkg (7.5 oz)	190	9	4	29
Beef Vegetable	1 pkg (7.5 oz)	100	6	1	16
Chicken Noodle	1 pkg (7.5 oz)	100	7	3	12
Chicken w/ Rice	1 pkg (7.5 oz)	110	4	3	18
New England Clam Chowder	1 pkg (7.5 oz)	140	5	5	18
Imagine					
Lobster Bisque	1 cup	130	5	5	15
Organic Bistro Cuban Black Bean Bisque	1 cup	170	8	4	30
Organic Broth Beef	1 cup	20	2	1	1
Organic Broth Free Range Chicken	1 cup	10	1	0	1
Organic Broth Vegetable	8 oz	20	2	0	2
Organic Creamy Butternut Squash	1 cup	90	0	2	18
Organic Creamy Chicken	1 cup	70	3	2	12
Organic Creamy Sweet Corn	1 cup	120	4	3	20
Organic Sweet Potato	1 cup	110	2	2	23
Lucini					
Roman Tomato Cream	1 cup (8.6 oz)	170	4	9	18
Umbrian Lentil	1 cup (8.6 oz)	160	7	5	23
Manischewitz					
Beef Broth	1 cup (8.4 oz)	150	1	1	1
Chicken Broth	1 cup (8.4 oz)	15	1	1	1
Chicken Broth Low Sodium	1 cup (8.4 oz)	15	1	1	1
Muir Glen					
Organic Garden Vegetable	1 cup	80	3	1	16
Organic Southwest Black Bean	1 cup	140	7	1	27
Original SoupMan					
Italian Wedding	1 cup	120	4	6	18
New England Clam Chowder	1 cup	290	14	19	16
Organic Butternut Squash	1 cup	250	3	13	33
Tomato Basil	1 cup	140	4	7	18
Turkey Chili	1 cup	210	18	7	18

FOOD	PORTION	CALS	PROT	FAT	CARB
Progresso					
40% Less Sodium Italian Style Wedding	1 cup (8.7 oz)	90	5	2	11
50% Less Sodium Garden Vegetable	1 cup (8.8 oz)	100	3	0	22
50% Less Sodium Zesty Chicken Gumbo	1 cup (8.7 oz)	110	7	2	18
High Fiber Creamy Tomato Basil	1 cup (8.8 oz)	130	3	4	26
Light Beef Pot Roast	1 cup (8.4 oz)	80	6	1	12
Light Chicken Vegetable Rotini	1 cup (8.3 oz)	70	6	2	10
Light Italian Style Vegetable	1 cup (8.6 oz)	60	3	0	12
Light Savory Vegetable Barley	1 cup (8.5 oz)	60	2	0	14
Light Vegetable	1 cup (8.4 oz)	60	3	0	14
Light Vegetable & Noodle	1 cup (8.7 oz)	60	2	1	12
Reduced Sodium Chicken Broth	1 cup (8.4 oz)	20	3	0	2
Rich & Hearty Beef Pot Roast	1 cup (8.7 oz)	120	8	2	20
Rich & Hearty Chicken & Homestyle Noodles	1 cup (8.6 oz)	100	7	2	14
Rich & Hearty Chicken Pot Pie	1 cup (8.6 oz)	170	8	6	21
Rich & Hearty Savory Beef Barley Vegetable	1 cup (8.6 oz)	130	8	1	22
Rich & Hearty Sirloin Steak & Vegetables	1 cup	130	8	2	21
Rich & Hearty Slow Cooked Vegetable Beef	1 cup (8.6 oz)	120	6	1	20
Rich & Hearty Steak & Roasted Russet Potatoes	1 cup (8.6 oz)	140	8	2	23
Traditional Beef & Vegetable	1 cup (8.7 oz)	120	8	2	18
Traditional Beef Barley	1 cup (8.5 oz)	120	7	2	20
Traditional Chickarina	1 cup (8.3 oz)	120	8	5	12
Traditional Chicken & Sausage Gumbo	1 cup (8.7 oz)	130	6	4	18
Traditional Chicken & Wild Rice	1 cup (8.4 oz)	100	6	2	15
Traditional Chicken Noodle	1 cup (8.3 oz)	100	7	3	12
Traditional Homestyle Chicken	1 cup (8.4 oz)	100	6	2	14
Traditional Italian Style Wedding	1 cup (8.4 oz)	100	6	4	12
Traditional Manhattan Clam Chowder	1 cup (8.4 oz)	100	3	2	17

FOOD	PORTION	CALS	PROT	FAT	CARB
Traditional New England Clam Chowder	1 cup (8.4 oz)	110	4	2	20
Traditional Potato Broccoli & Cheese	1 cup (8.8 oz)	180	5	10	18
Traditional Split Pea w/ Ham	1 cup (8.5 oz)	140	9	1	24
Traditional Turkey Noodle	1 cup (8.4 oz)	80	5	2	12
Vegetable Classics Creamy Mushroom	1 cup (8.1 oz)	130	2	3	9
Vegetable Classics French Onion	1 cup (8 oz)	50	1	2	8
Vegetable Classics Hearty Black Bean w/ Bacon	1 cup (8.5 oz)	160	8	1	29
Vegetable Classics Hearty Tomato	1 cup (8.6 oz)	110	2	1	23
Vegetable Classics Lentil	1 cup (8.5 oz)	150	9	2	28
Vegetable Classics Vegetable	1 cup (8.4 oz)	80	3	1	16
Snow's					
Clam Chowder	1 cup (8.4 oz)	200	5	15	13
Swanson					
50% Low Sodium Beef Broth	1 cup	15	3	0	1
Beef Broth	1 cup	15	2	0	1
Beef Stock	1 cup	30	4	0	3
Chicken Broth	1 cup	10	1	0	1
Chicken Stock	1 cup	20	4	0	1
Vegetable Broth	1 cup	15	0	0	3
FROZEN					
Kettle Cuisine					
Angus Beef Steak Chili w/ Beans Gluten Free Dairy Free	1 pkg (10 oz)	250	19	12	17
Chicken w/ Rice Noodles Gluten Free	1 pkg (10 oz)	140	15	3	12
New England Clam Chowder Gluten Free	1 pkg (10 oz)	330	15	18	26
Roasted Vegetable Gluten Free Dairy Free	1 pkg (10 oz)	140	3	6	19
Tabatchnick					
Barley Mushroom	1 serv (7.5 oz)	80	3	1	17
Chicken w/ Dumplings	1 serv (7.5 oz)	150	5	6	19
Cream Of Broccoli	1 serv (7.5 oz)	130	4	5	18

FOOD	PORTION	CALS	PROT	FAT	CARB
Macaroni & Cheese	1 serv (7.5 oz)	250	9	8	34
Minestrone	1 serv (7.5 oz)	100	5	2	18
No Salt Pea	1 serv (7.5 oz)	140	13	0	34
Old Fashioned Potato	1 serv (7.5 oz)	100	3	2	21
Southwest Bean	1 serv (7.5 oz)	220	11	5	35
Split Pea	1 serv (7.5 oz)	140	13	0	34
Vegetable	1 serv (7.5 oz)	90	3	2	17
Vegetarian Chili	1 serv (7.5 oz)	180	12	4	28
Wild Rice	1 serv (7.5 oz)	80	3	1	16
MIX					
beef broth cube	1 cube	6	1	tr	1
chicken broth cube	1 cube (4.8 g)	9	1	tr	1
Edward & Sons					
Bouillon Cubes Not-Beef	½ cube	20	1	2	1
Bouillon Cubes Not-Chicken	½ cube	15	1	2	1
Veggie Low Sodium	½ cup	20	1	2	1
HamBeens					
15 Bean as prep	½ cup	120	8	1	20
15 Bean Beef as prep	½ cup	120	8	1	20
15 Bean Cajun as prep	½ cup	120	8	1	20
15 Bean Chicken as prep	½ cup	120	8	1	20
Spanish American Black Bean as prep	½ cup	120	7	1	22
Health Valley					
Chicken Noodles w/ Vegetables	1 cup	110	5	0	24
Creamy Potato w/ Broccoli Fat Free	1 cup	80	4	0	17
Leahey Gardens					
No Beef Noodle	1½ cups	89	7	1	16
No Chicken Noodle	1½ cups	94	7	1	16
Manischewitz					
Lentil as prep	1 cup	150	7	0	29
Matzo Ball Soup	1 cup	40	1	1	9
Southwestern Black Bean as prep	1 cup	90	4	1	16
Split Pea w/ Barley as prep	1 cup	110	7	0	21
Vegetable & Pasta as prep	1 cup	90	4	0	17
Miso-Cup					
Golden Vegetable as prep	1 cup	30	2	1	3

FOOD	PORTION	CALS	PROT	FAT	CARB
Japanese Restaurant Style as prep	1 cup	60	4	2	7
Organic Traditional w/ Tofu as prep	1 cup	35	2	1	4
Reduced Sodium as prep	1 cup	25	2	1	3
Savory Seaweed as prep	1 cup	30	3	1	3
Nissin					
Chicken Vegetable as prep	1 pkg	290	6	13	38
White Cheddar as prep	1 pkg	290	6	13	38
Silhouette Solution					
Mediterranean Tomato	1 pkg (1.16 oz)	110	15	3	8
Newbury Chicken Cream	1 pkg (1.3 oz)	110	15	3	8
Streit's					
Matzo Ball as prep	1 cup	50	tr	0	12
Thai Kitchen					
Rice Noodle Bowl Lemongrass & Chili as prep	½ pkg	110	2	2	23
Rice Noodle Bowl Thai Ginger as prep	½ pkg	120	2	2	23
REFRIGERATED					
Moosewood					
Organic Creamy Potato & Corn Chowder	1 cup (8.4 oz)	170	5	6	28
Organic Hungarian Vegetable Noodle	1 cup (8.4 oz)	80	2	2	13
Organic Savannah Sweet Potato Bisque	1 cup (8.4 oz)	200	6	11	20
Organic Texas Two Bean Chili	1 cup (8.4 oz)	200	9	4	34
Organic Tuscan White Bean & Vegetable	1 cup (8.4 oz)	130	6	2	24
Organic Classics					
French Onion w/ Croutons	1 cup	140	3	6	17
Seafood Chowder	1 cup	160	11	6	17
TAKE-OUT					
ban mien fish head	1 serv (10 oz)	277	20	10	27
beef stew soup	1 cup (8.8 oz)	221	23	5	20
bird's nest	1 cup (8.6 oz)	112	13	3	8
black bean turtle soup	1 cup	241	15	1	45
broccoli cheese	1 cup	165	6	9	15
brunswick stew soup	1 cup (8.5 oz)	232	27	6	17

FOOD	PORTION	CALS	PROT	FAT	CARB
caldo de res beef soup	1 cup	143	12	5	12
corn & cheese chowder	¾ cup	215	9	12	21
duck soup	1 cup (8.6 oz)	412	16	37	2
egg drop	1 cup	73	8	4	1
gazpacho	1 cup	46	1	tr	5
greek lemon	¾ cup	63	4	2	7
hot & sour	1 serv (14 oz)	173	14	9	9
matzo ball soup	1 cup	118	7	5	10
minestrone	1 cup	233	9	13	22
miso w/ tofu	1 cup	84	6	3	8
onion soup gratinee	1 serv	492	25	27	38
oxtail	1 cup	68	3	2	9
pasta e fagioli	1 cup (8.8 oz)	194	9	5	30
ratatouille	1 cup (7.5 oz)	266	2	25	12
shark fin	1 bowl (10 oz)	164	15	9	9
shrimp bisque	1 cup	263	22	14	13
sopa de albondigas	1 cup	171	10	11	9
thai lemon grass	1 bowl	100	10	4	5
vietnamese pho beef noodle	1 serv (7.8 oz)	480	15	12	78
wonton soup	1 cup	183	14	7	14
zupa koprowa polish dill soup	1 bowl	54	11	2	6
SOUR CREAM					
sour cream	1 tbsp (0.4 oz)	26	tr	3	1
sour cream	1 cup (8 oz)	493	7	48	10
Breakstone's					
Sour Cream	2 tbsp (1 oz)	60	tr	5	1
Cabot					
Light	2 tbsp	35	1	3	2
No Fat	2 tbsp	20	1	0	3
Sour Cream	2 tbsp	50	1	5	1
Friendship					
All Natural	2 tbsp (1 oz)	60	1	5	1
Light	1 tbsp (1 oz)	40	1	3	3
Nonfat	2 tbsp (1 oz)	25	2	0	4
Horizon Organic					
Lowfat	2 tbsp	35	1	2	3
Sour Cream	2 tbsp	60	1	5	1
Land O' Lakes					
Fat Free	2 tbsp (1.1 oz)	20	1	0	3
Light	2 tbsp (1.1 oz)	40	1	3	2
Sour Cream	2 tbsp (1.1 oz)	60	1	6	2

FOOD	PORTION	CALS	PROT	FAT	CARB
Nancy's					
Organic	2 tbsp	60	1	6	2
Organic Valley					
Lowfat	2 tbsp	40	1	2	1
SOUR CREAM SUBSTITUTES					
nondairy	1 oz	59	1	6	2
nondairy	1 cup	479	6	45	15
Vegan Gourmet					
Alternative Sour Cream	2 tbsp (1 oz)	50	0	5	3
SOURSOP					
fresh	1	416	6	2	105
fresh cut up	1 cup	150	2	1	38

SOY (*see also* CHEESE SUBSTITUTES, ICE CREAM AND FROZEN DESSERTS, MILK SUBSTITUTES, MISO, SMOOTHIES, SOY SAUCE, SOYBEANS, TEMPEH, TOFU, YOGURT FROZEN)

FOOD	PORTION	CALS	PROT	FAT	CARB
Bob's Red Mill					
Protein Powder	1 tbsp	20	5	0	0
I.M. Healthy					
SoyNut Butter Chocolate	2 tbsp	190	6	14	12
SoyNut Butter Honey Creamy	2 tbsp	170	7	11	10
SoyNut Butter Original Chunky	2 tbsp	170	7	11	10
SoyNut Butter Original Creamy	2 tbsp	170	7	11	10
SoyNut Butter Unsweetened Creamy	2 tbsp	190	9	15	6
Simple Food					
Soynut Butter Chocolate	2 tbsp	190	10	12	8
Soynut Butter No Sugar No Salt	2 tbsp	200	10	14	8
South Beach					
Soy Nuts Dark Chocolate	1 pkg (0.7 oz)	100	3	6	9
Soy Wonder					
Creamy Spread	2 tbsp	170	8	11	10
SoyButter					
Spread	2 tbsp	200	7	15	8

SOY DRINKS (*see* MILK SUBSTITUTES, SMOOTHIES)

SOY SAUCE

FOOD	PORTION	CALS	PROT	FAT	CARB
shoyu	1 tbsp	9	1	tr	2
soy sauce	1 tbsp	7	tr	tr	1
tamari	1 tbsp	11	2	tr	1

FOOD	PORTION	CALS	PROT	FAT	CARB
Angostura					
Lite Soy	1 tbsp (0.5 oz)	10	1	0	2
Soy Sauce	1 tbsp (0.5 oz)	10	1	0	1
Dave's Gourmet					
Soyabi Sauce	1 tbsp (0.6 oz)	30	0	2	4
House Of Tsang					
Ginger Soy Sauce	1 tbsp	20	0	0	4
Less Sodium	1 tbsp	5	0	0	0
La Choy					
Lite	1 tbsp (0.5 oz)	15	1	0	2
Mitsukan					
Ponzu Citrus Seasoned	1 tbsp (0.5 oz)	10	0	0	1
Soy Vay					
Wasabiyaki	1 tbsp	35	tr	1	6
Tree Of Life					
Organic Shoyu	1 tbsp (0.5 oz)	15	2	0	1
Organic Tamari Wheat Free	1 tbsp (0.5 oz)	15	2	0	1
SOYBEANS					
dried cooked	1 cup	298	29	15	17
dry roasted	½ cup	387	34	19	28
green cooked	½ cup	127	11	6	10
roasted	½ cup	405	30	22	29
roasted & toasted	1 cup	490	40	26	33
roasted & toasted salted	1 cup	490	40	26	33
sprouts raw	½ cup	43	5	2	3
sprouts steamed	½ cup	38	4	2	3
sprouts stir fried	1 cup	125	13	7	9
Arrowhead Mills					
Organic Dried not prep	¼ cup	160	14	8	11
C&W					
In the Pod	½ cup	110	9	4	12
KooLoos					
Soy Nuts & Flaxseed BBQ	1 pkg (1 oz)	130	7	4	16
Soy Nuts & Flaxseed Original	1 pkg (1 oz)	140	7	5	15
Seapoint Farms					
Edamame Dry Roasted Goji Blend	¼ cup	120	11	3	15
Edamame Dry Roasted Lightly Salted	¼ cup	130	14	4	10
Edamame Dry Roasted Wasabi	¼ cup	130	14	5	9

FOOD	PORTION	CALS	PROT	FAT	CARB
Edamame In Pods frzn	½ cup	100	8	3	9
Edamame In Pods Lightly Salted	½ cup	100	8	3	9
Edamame Shelled	½ cup	100	8	3	9
Organic Edamame In Pods	½ cup	100	8	3	9
Organic Edamame Shelled	½ cup	100	8	3	9

SPAGHETTI (see PASTA, PASTA DINNERS, PASTA SALAD, SPAGHETTI SAUCE)

SPAGHETTI SAUCE
JARRED

FOOD	PORTION	CALS	PROT	FAT	CARB
marinara sauce	1 cup	171	4	8	25
spaghetti sauce	1 cup	272	12	12	40
Amy's					
Organic Family Marinara	½ cup (4.4 oz)	80	1	5	10
Organic Marinara Low Sodium	½ cup (4.4 oz)	40	1	1	7
Barilla					
Arrabbiata Tomato & Spicy Pepper	½ cup	90	2	3	11
Garden Vegetable	½ cup	70	2	2	11
Green & Black Olive	½ cup	80	2	3	10
Italian Baking Sauce	¼ cup (4.4 oz)	60	2	1	12
Mushroom & Garlic	½ cup	70	3	2	12
Dave's Gourmet					
Pasta Sauce Spicy Heirloom Marinara	½ cup (4.4 oz)	45	1	2	7
Pasta Sauce Wild Mushroom	½ cup (4.4 oz)	60	2	3	7
Dei Fratelli					
Arrabbiata	½ cup (4.2 oz)	50	2	2	8
Pizza Sauce	¼ cup (2.2 oz)	30	1	2	5
DelGrosso					
Garden Style	½ cup (4.4 oz)	70	2	2	12
Mushroom	½ cup (4.4 oz)	70	3	2	11
New York Style	¼ cup (2.1 oz)	35	1	1	6
Original Meat Flavored	½ cup (4.4 oz)	80	3	2	12
Pizza Sauce Pepperoni	¼ cup (2.2 oz)	40	2	1	6
Three Cheese	½ cup (4.4 oz)	80	2	2	13
Francesco Rinaldi					
Alfredo	¼ cup (2.1 oz)	80	1	6	3
Chunky Eggplant Parmesan	½ cup (4.4 oz)	90	2	5	11
Chunky Mushroom & Pepper	½ cup (4.4 oz)	80	2	3	13

FOOD	PORTION	CALS	PROT	FAT	CARB
Hearty Mushroom Pepper & Onion	½ cup (4.4 oz)	80	2	3	12
Hearty Sweet & Tasty Tomato	½ cup (4.4 oz)	100	2	5	16
Hearty Three Cheese	½ cup (4.4 oz)	80	3	2	15
Organic Burgundy Marinara	½ cup (4.3 oz)	100	1	7	9
Premium Vodka	¼ cup (2.1 oz)	60	2	4	4
Traditional Meat Flavored	½ cup (4.4 oz)	80	2	4	12
Traditional No Salt Added	½ cup (4.4 oz)	70	2	3	12
Traditional Original	½ cup (4.4 oz)	80	2	3	12
Hunt's					
Italian Sausage	½ cup	60	3	2	10
Meat	½ cup	60	3	1	11
Traditional	½ cup	50	2	1	10
With Mushrooms	½ cup	45	2	1	10
Knorr					
W/ Meat	4 oz	110	6	5	9
Lucini					
Rustic Tomato Basil	½ cup (4.4 oz)	80	2	5	8
Spicy Tuscan	½ cup (4.4 oz)	80	2	5	8
Milo's					
Portobello Shiraz	4 oz	40	2	5	8
Muir Glen					
Organic Chunky Tomato	¼ cup	15	tr	0	4
Organic Garlic Roasted Garlic	½ cup	60	2	1	12
Organic Pizza Sauce	¼ cup	40	1	2	6
Organic Tomato Sauce No Salt Added	¼ cup	25	1	0	5
Pomi					
Marinara	½ cup	80	1	4	5
Prego					
100% Natural Roasted Garlic Parmesan	½ cup	100	3	1	20
Heart Smart Traditional Italian	½ cup	100	2	3	15
Italian	½ cup	70	2	2	13
Italian Marinara	½ cup	100	2	5	11
Italian Meat	½ cup	130	2	4	19
Italian Roasted Red Pepper & Garlic	½ cup	90	2	4	13
Italian Three Cheese	½ cup	80	3	2	14
Italian Tomato Basil & Garlic	½ cup	80	2	3	12
Organic Mushroom	½ cup	90	2	3	13

FOOD	PORTION	CALS	PROT	FAT	CARB
Progresso					
Lobster Sauce	½ cup (4.3 oz)	100	3	7	6
Red Clam w/ Tomato & Basil	½ cup (4.4 oz)	60	4	1	8
White Clam w/ Garlic & Herb	½ cup (4.4 oz)	120	4	10	4
Ragu					
Fresh Italian	4 oz	110	2	3	19
Marinara	4 oz	100	1	3	16
Old World Style Margherita	½ cup (4.4 oz)	70	2	2	10
Old World Style Sweet Tomato Basil	½ cup (4.4 oz)	60	2	2	10
Pizza Quick Fresh Italian	2 oz	35	1	1	5
Robert Rothchild Farm					
Artichoke	½ cup	80	2	5	8
S&W					
Tomato Sauce	¼ cup (2.1 oz)	20	1	0	4
Vino De Milo					
Mediterranean Pinot Grigio	½ cup	90	2	4	12
Portobello Shiraz	½ cup	40	1	1	9
Walnut Acres					
Organic Garlic Garlic	½ cup	125	2	1	10
Organic Marinara & Zinfandel	½ cup	125	2	1	9
Organic Roasted Garlic	½ cup	125	2	1	11
Organic Tomato & Basil	½ cup	125	2	1	9
TAKE-OUT					
bolognese	5 oz	195	11	15	4

SPANISH FOOD

FROZEN

FOOD	PORTION	CALS	PROT	FAT	CARB
Amy's					
Bowl Mexican Casserole	1 pkg (9.4 oz)	470	11	16	70
Burrito Black Bean	1 (6 oz)	280	9	8	44
Burrito Cheddar Cheese	1 (6 oz)	300	11	9	43
Burrito Southwestern	1 (5.5 oz)	300	12	10	43
Enchilada Black Bean Vegetable	1 (4.7 oz)	180	5	6	26
Cedarlane					
Organic Burrito Low Fat Rice & Cheese	1 (6 oz)	260	13	1	48
Organic Enchilada Low Fat Black Bean & Tofu	1 (9 oz)	220	10	3	42
Roasted Chile Relleno	1 pkg (10 oz)	400	23	20	37
Zone Burrito Beans & Cheese	1 (6 oz)	350	27	13	37

FOOD	PORTION	CALS	PROT	FAT	CARB
Contessa					
Fajitas Shrimp	2 (8 oz)	230	11	4	37
Paella w/ Chicken & Seafood	1½ cups	200	17	3	28
Seafood Veracruz not prep	1¾ cups	180	15	2	27
El Monterey					
Burrito Bean & Cheese	1 (5 oz)	280	10	8	43
Burrito Beef & Bean	1 (5 oz)	370	10	17	42
Burrito Half Pound Spicy Red Hot Beef & Bean	1 (8 oz)	600	17	29	68
Burrito Supreme Breakfast Egg Cheese & Sausage	1 (4.5 oz)	300	10	13	34
Burrito Supreme Shredded Steak & Cheese	1 (5 oz)	290	12	9	41
Burrito XX Large Bean & Cheese	1 (10 oz)	590	21	17	88
Burrito XX Large Beef & Bean	1 (10 oz)	730	22	35	83
Cruncheros Cheese & Beef	3 (4.5 oz)	330	10	16	35
Cruncheros Taco Beef & Cheese	4 (5.6 oz)	460	12	29	38
Enchiladas Cheese w/ Sauce	1 serv (8 oz)	250	11	15	22
Enchiladas Shredded Beef w/ Sauce	1 serv (4 oz)	140	6	6	15
Quesadillas Chicken & Cheese	2 (6 oz)	380	17	15	43
Quesadillas Steak & Cheese	2 (6 oz)	400	21	15	42
Tamales Chicken	1 (4.5 oz)	240	8	12	27
Tamales Shredded Beef	1 (4.5 oz)	310	9	19	27
Taquitos Corn Shredded Beef	3 (4.5 oz)	300	11	13	31
Taquitos Flour Char-Broiled Chicken Breast	3 (5 oz)	380	15	19	36
Taquitos Flour Chicken & Cheese	3 (4.5 oz)	350	10	18	36
Taquitos Southwest Chicken In A Seasoned Batter	2 (2.8 oz)	175	6	8	20
Tornados Apple Cinnamon	1 (3 oz)	180	4	5	31
Tornados Sausage Egg & Cheese	1 (3 oz)	230	6	13	23
Tornados Shredded Beef	1 (3 oz)	210	7	10	23
Tornados Steak Egg & Cheese	1 (3 oz)	170	7	6	22
Tornados XXL Southwest Chicken	1 (4.2 oz)	210	7	10	28

FOOD	PORTION	CALS	PROT	FAT	CARB
Health Is Wealth					
Vegetarian Hot Tamale Munchees	6 (3 oz)	160	6	3	26
Helen's Kitchen					
Cheese Enchiladas w/ Tofu Steaks In Spicy Red Sauce	½ pkg (5 oz)	150	5	9	20
Jose Ole					
Burrito Chicken	1 (5 oz)	270	9	7	41
Chimichanga Shredded Beef	1 (5 oz)	350	13	15	39
Patio					
Burrito Bean & Cheese	1	280	8	8	44
Burrito Beef & Bean Mild	1	300	10	10	44
Enchilada Beef	1 meal	380	11	12	55
Enchilada Cheese	1 meal	390	12	13	58
Enchilada Combo Dinner	1 meal	380	11	12	57
Enchilada & Beef Tamale	1 meal	460	13	14	69
Stouffer's					
Chicken Enchilada w/ Cheese Sauce & Rice	1 pkg (7.13 oz)	280	12	12	30
Tyson					
Meal Kit Chicken Fajita	1 (3.8 oz)	130	8	4	17
Meal Kit Quesadilla Chicken	1 (4 oz)	250	15	10	26
READY-TO-EAT					
taco shell corn	1 (6.5 inch)	98	2	5	13
taco shell flour	1 (7 inch)	173	3	9	19
TAKE-OUT					
arroz con coco	1 cup	532	7	38	46
burrito w/ beans	1 med (5 oz)	295	10	8	45
burrito w/ beans & rice	1 (3.5 oz)	221	7	5	37
burrito w/ beef	1 sm (3.4 oz)	297	18	13	25
burrito w/ beef & beans	1 med (5 oz)	331	17	13	36
burrito w/ beef beans & cheese	1 med (5 oz)	379	21	19	30
burrito w/ chicken & beans	1 med (5 oz)	295	18	9	34
burrito w/ pork & beans	1 med (5 oz)	320	18	12	35
chiles rellenos meat & cheese filled	1 (5 oz)	213	10	16	9
chimichanga w/ bean cheese lettuce & tomato	1 (4.1 oz)	271	8	18	22
chimichanga w/ beef & rice	1 (10 oz)	634	19	36	58

FOOD	PORTION	CALS	PROT	FAT	CARB
chimichanga w/ beef beans lettuce & tomato	1 (4.1 oz)	254	9	15	22
chimichanga w/ beef cheese lettuce & tomato	1 (4.1 oz)	337	13	24	19
chimichanga w/ chicken sour cream lettuce & tomato	1 (4 oz)	277	9	20	17
empanada fruit filled	1 (3.8 oz)	452	4	25	55
empanada meat & vegetable	1 (7.8 oz)	881	18	61	66
empanada sweet potato	1 (7.8 oz)	546	8	23	76
enchilada w/ beans	1 (4.1 oz)	179	6	6	27
enchilada w/ beans & cheese	1 (4.6 oz)	233	9	11	25
enchilada w/ beef	1 (4 oz)	214	11	10	21
enchilada w/ beef & beans	1 (4 oz)	195	8	8	25
frijoles	1 cup	278	18	2	49
frijoles w/ cheese	1 cup	225	11	8	29
nachos w/ beans & cheese	1 serv (9.4 oz)	616	25	33	57
nachos w/ beef beans cheese & sour cream	1 serv (19 oz)	1620	59	97	133
paella	1 serv (7 oz)	308	23	16	17
pupusa meat filled	1 (3.6 oz)	187	8	6	26
quesadilla w/ cheese	1 (5 oz)	498	20	28	40
quesadilla w/ meat & cheese	1 (6.5 oz)	605	32	35	40
taco de jueye w/ crab meat	1 (4.2 oz)	266	16	14	18
taco w/ beans lettuce tomato & salsa	1 (2.8 oz)	117	4	5	16
taco w/ chicken lettuce tomato & salsa	1 (2.5 oz)	114	8	5	10
taco w/ fish lettuce tomato & salsa	1 (2.7 oz)	101	8	4	10
tostada w/ beef lettuce tomato & salsa	1 (2.7 oz)	143	8	8	11

SPICES (see individual names, HERBS/SPICES)

SPINACH
CANNED
drained	1 cup	49	6	1	7
Freshlike					
Cut Leaf	½ cup	45	5	1	5
Popeye					
Leaf Spinach	½ cup	30	3	0	4
Leaf Spinach No Salt Added	½ cup	40	4	1	5

FOOD	PORTION	CALS	PROT	FAT	CARB
S&W					
Leaf	½ cup (4 oz)	30	2	0	4
FRESH					
baby raw	2 cups	20	1	0	5
cooked	1 cup	41	5	tr	7
malabar cooked	1 cup	10	1	tr	1
mustard cooked	1 cup	29	3	tr	5
new zealand cooked	1 cup	22	2	tr	4
raw	1 cup	7	1	tr	1
Fresh Express					
Baby Spinach	3 cups	20	2	0	3
Organic Baby Spinach	3 cups	35	2	0	9
FROZEN					
chopped cooked	1 cup	30	4	tr	5
Birds Eye					
Chopped	⅓ cup	20	2	0	2
Birds Eye					
Creamed	½ cup (4.4 oz)	90	3	4	9
C&W					
Baby Chopped	1 cup	30	2	0	3
Creamed	½ cup	100	4	7	6
Cascadian Farm					
Organic Cut	⅓ cup	25	2	0	3
Cedarlane					
Organic Spanakopita Spinach & Feta Pie	½ pkg (5 oz)	260	12	8	38
Dr. Praeger's					
Spinach Bites	2 (2 oz)	110	3	3	17
Fillo Factory					
Spanakopita Spinach & Cheese Fillo Appetizers	3 (3 oz)	190	6	9	20
Health Is Wealth					
Creamed	½ pkg (4.5 oz)	100	5	4	27
Spinach Munchees	6 (3 oz)	180	7	7	25
Stouffer's					
Creamed	½ pkg (4.5 oz)	200	5	16	8
TAKE-OUT					
indian saag	1 serv	28	2	2	2
spanakopita spinach pie	1 serv (3 oz)	148	5	11	8

FOOD	PORTION	CALS	PROT	FAT	CARB
SPINACH JUICE					
juice	7 oz	14	2	0	2
SPORTS DRINKS (see ENERGY DRINKS)					
SPOT					
baked	3 oz	134	20	5	0
SPROUTS					
kidney bean	½ cup	27	4	tr	4
lentil sprouts	½ cup	40	3	tr	8
mung bean	½ cup	16	2	tr	3
mung bean canned	½ cup	8	1	tr	1
mung bean cooked	½ cup	13	1	tr	3
pea	½ cup	77	5	tr	17
radish	½ cup	8	1	tr	1
La Choy					
Bean Sprouts	⅔ cup	15	tr	0	3
TAKE-OUT					
mung bean stir fried	½ cup	31	3	tr	7
SQUAB					
boneless baked	1 (4 oz)	242	26	14	0
SQUASH (see also SQUASH SEEDS, ZUCCHINI)					
CANNED					
crookneck sliced	½ cup	14	1	tr	3
Sunshine					
Slice Yellow	½ cup	25	0	0	5
FRESH					
acorn cooked mashed	½ cup	41	1	tr	11
acorn cubed baked	½ cup	57	1	tr	15
butternut baked	½ cup	41	1	tr	11
crookneck sliced cooked	½ cup	18	1	tr	4
hubbard baked	½ cup	51	3	tr	11
hubbard cooked mashed	½ cup	35	2	tr	8
scallop sliced cooked	½ cup	14	1	tr	3
spaghetti cooked	½ cup	23	1	tr	5
Glory					
Yellow Sliced	¾ cup	20	1	0	3
FROZEN					
butternut cooked mashed	½ cup	47	1	tr	12
crookneck sliced cooked	½ cup	24	1	tr	5

FOOD	PORTION	CALS	PROT	FAT	CARB
C&W					
Butternut	½ cup	45	1	0	10
McKenzie's					
Southland Butternut	½ cup	70	1	3	10
TAKE-OUT					
fritter	1 (0.8 oz)	81	2	5	8
squash pie	1 slice (5.4 oz)	291	6	12	40
SQUASH SEEDS					
roasted	1 oz	148	9	12	4
salted & roasted	1 oz	148	9	12	4
seeds dried	1 oz	154	7	13	5
seeds whole roasted	1 oz	127	5	6	15
SQUID					
baked	1 cup	192	26	6	5
canned in its own ink	1 can (4 oz)	122	21	2	4
dried	1 sm (1.5 oz)	147	25	2	5
pickled	1 oz	26	4	tr	1
steamed	1 cup	147	25	2	5
Contessa					
Calamari + Sauce	13 pieces + 2 tbsp sauce	160	5	6	21
Van de Kamp's					
Fried Calamari	15 pieces (4 oz)	270	10	13	26
TAKE-OUT					
arroz con calamares	1 cup	400	14	17	47
calamari breaded & fried	1 cup	296	26	12	17
SQUIRREL					
roasted	3 oz	147	26	4	0
STARFRUIT					
fresh	1	42	1	tr	10
STRAWBERRIES					
canned in heavy syrup	½ cup	117	1	tr	30
fresh halves	1 cup	49	1	tr	12
fresh whole	1 cup	46	1	tr	11
fresh whole	1 pint	114	2	1	27
frzn sweetened sliced	½ cup	122	1	tr	33
frzn sweetened whole	1 cup	199	1	tr	54

FOOD	PORTION	CALS	PROT	FAT	CARB
frzn whole unsweetened	1 cup	77	1	tr	20
organic fresh whole	8 med	45	1	0	12
C&W					
Ultimate Sliced frzn	⅔ cup	50	0	0	12
Chukar Cherries					
Dried	¼ cup	120	tr	0	29
Emily's					
Dark Chocolate Covered	6 (1.4 oz)	170	1	8	28
FruitziO					
Freeze-Dried	1 pkg (0.9 oz)	100	2	0	22
LiteHouse					
Glaze Sugar Free	3 tbsp	35	0	0	8
Marie's					
Glaze	2 tbsp	40	0	0	10
Polar					
Strawberries In Syrup	½ cup	90	1	0	21
Stoneridge Orchards					
Dried	⅓ cup (1.4 oz)	140	0	0	35

STUFFING/DRESSING

FOOD	PORTION	CALS	PROT	FAT	CARB
Fresh Gourmet					
All Natural Multi-Grain w/ Cranberries not prep	⅓ cup (1 oz)	110	3	3	19
Organic Seasoned not prep	⅓ cup (1 oz)	110	3	3	19
Pepperidge Farm					
Corn Bread	¾ cup	170	4	2	33
Cube	¾ cup	140	4	1	28
Herb Seasoned	¾ cup	170	5	2	33
One Step Turkey	½ cup	170	4	7	23
Zatarain's					
Creole Chicken as prep	½ cup	100	3	1	20
French Bread as prep	½ cup	100	3	1	20
TAKE-OUT					
bread	1 cup	352	6	17	44
cornbread	½ cup	179	3	9	22
kishke stuffed derma	1 piece (1.3 oz)	166	2	12	13
oyster	1 cup	304	7	18	29
sausage	½ cup	292	8	11	40

FOOD	PORTION	CALS	PROT	FAT	CARB
STURGEON					
broiled	3 oz	115	18	4	0
roe raw	1 oz	59	7	3	tr
smoked	1 oz	49	9	1	0
TAKE-OUT					
breaded & fried	4 oz	252	19	15	9
SUCKER					
white baked	3 oz	101	18	3	0
SUGAR (see also FRUCTOSE, SYRUP)					
brown organic	1 tsp	17	0	0	4
brown packed	1 cup (7.7 oz)	828	0	0	214
brown unpacked	1 cup (5.1 oz)	547	0	0	141
cinnamon sugar	1 tsp	16	tr	tr	4
cube	1 (2 g)	9	0	0	2
maple	1 piece (1 oz)	99	tr	tr	25
powdered	1 tbsp (0.3 oz)	31	0	0	8
powdered unsifted	1 cup (4.2 oz)	467	tr	tr	119
raw	1 pkg (5 g)	19	0	0	5
sugarcane stem	3 oz	54	1	0	14
white	1 tsp (4 g)	15	0	0	4
white	1 tbsp (0.4 oz)	49	0	0	13
white	1 cup (7 oz)	773	0	0	200
white	1 packet (3 g)	12	0	0	3
Bob's Red Mill					
Date Sugar	1 tsp	11	0	0	3
Turbinado	1 tsp	10	0	0	3
Domino					
Dark Brown	1 tsp (4 g)	15	0	0	4
Demerara Raw Cane	1 tsp	15	0	0	4
Equinox					
Organic Maple Flakes	2 tsp	15	0	0	4
Sugar In The Raw					
Turbinado Sugar	1 pkg (5 g)	20	0	0	5
Tree Of Life					
Date Sugar	1 tsp (4 g)	10	0	0	3
Organic Cane Juice Dehydrated	1 tsp (3.5 g)	15	0	0	3
Turbinado	1 tsp (4 g)	15	0	0	4

FOOD	PORTION	CALS	PROT	FAT	CARB
Wholesome Sweeteners					
Organic Fair Trade Dark Brown Sugar	1 tsp	15	0	0	4
Organic Fair Trade Powdered	¼ cup	120	0	0	30
Organic Fair Trade Sucanat	1 tsp	15	0	0	4
Organic Turbinado	1 tsp	15	0	0	4
SUGAR SUBSTITUTES					
Equal					
Packet	1 pkg	0	0	0	tr
Fructevia					
All Natural	1 tsp (4 g)	5	0	0	2
Fruit Sweetness					
Sugar Substitute	1 serv (0.9 oz)	0	0	0	0
Nature's Family					
Sun Crystals	1 pkg (4.5 g)	4	0	0	1
Nevella					
No Calorie Sweetener	1 tsp	0	0	0	tr
Neway					
Sweet Sensation	¼ tsp	0	0	0	tr
PureVia					
All Natural	1 pkg (2 g)	0	0	0	2
Splenda					
Brown Sugar Blend	½ tsp (2 g)	10	0	0	2
Cafe Sticks	1 pkg (1 g)	0	0	0	tr
Flavor Accents Sticks	1 pkg (1 g)	0	0	0	tr
Flavors For Coffee	1 pkg (1 g)	0	0	0	tr
No Calorie Granulated	1 tsp (0.5 g)	0	0	0	tr
No Calorie Sweetener w/ Fiber	1 pkg	0	0	0	2
Sugar Blends	½ tsp (2 g)	10	0	0	2
Stevia In The Raw					
100% Natural Sweetener	1 pkg (1 g)	0	0	0	0
Steviva					
Blend	1 tbsp (0.4 oz)	2	0	0	0
Sun Crystals					
Natural Sweetener	1 pkg (5 g)	4	0	0	5
Susta					
Natural Sweetener	1 pkg (2 g)	5	0	0	2
Sweet Fiber					
All Natural	1 pkg	0	0	0	tr

FOOD	PORTION	CALS	PROT	FAT	CARB
Sweete					
Sugar Free	1 pkg	0	0	0	tr
Truvia					
Calorie Free Sweetener	1 pkg (3.5 g)	0	0	0	3
Whey Low					
Gold	1 tsp	4	0	0	4
Granular	1 tsp	4	0	0	4
Maple Buzz	¼ cup	57	0	0	57
Wholesome Sweeteners					
Organic Zero	1 pkg (6 g)	0	0	0	6
ZSweet					
All Natural	1 pkg (1 g)	0	0	0	tr
SUGAR-APPLE					
fresh	1	146	3	tr	37
fresh cut up	1 cup	236	5	1	59
SUNCHOKE					
fresh raw sliced	½ cup	57	2	tr	13
SUNFISH					
pumpkinseed baked	3 oz	97	21	1	0
SUNFLOWER					
seeds dry roasted w/ salt	¼ cup	186	6	16	8
seeds dry roasted w/o salt	¼ cup	186	6	16	8
seeds w/ hulls dried	¼ cup	66	3	6	2
Arrowhead Mills					
Organic Seeds	¼ cup	170	7	15	6
Bob's Red Mill					
Seeds Roasted & Salted	3 tbsp	186	6	15	6
Dakota Gourmet					
Seeds Honey Roasted	¼ cup (1 oz)	170	5	12	8
Lance					
Shelled Seeds	1 pkg (1.8 oz)	300	6	25	14
SunButter					
Creamy	2 tbsp	200	7	16	7
Organic	2 tbsp	203	8	16	7
SunGold					
Seeds Roasted Salted	1 oz	172	7	15	4
Tree Of Life					
Seeds Kernels Raw	¼ cup (1.3 oz)	210	8	18	7

FOOD	PORTION	CALS	PROT	FAT	CARB
SUSHI					
TAKE-OUT					
cucumber roll	1 (1.1 oz)	43	1	0	9
inari	1 sm	46	1	1	9
prawn cooked	1 (1.1 oz)	36	1	0	8
roll california	1 (1.2 oz)	48	1	1	8
roll fresh salmon	4 pieces	250	11	7	37
roll preserved radish	3 (1 oz)	27	0	0	6
roll seaweed	1 (1.1 oz)	43	1	1	9
roll tuna	1 (1.1 oz)	37	3	0	6
roll vegetable	1 (1.2 oz)	27	1	1	5
roll yellowtail	1 (0.6 oz)	25	1	1	3
saba	1 (0.8 oz)	33	1	1	5
sashimi	1 serv (6 oz)	198	24	7	4
scallop cooked	1 (1 oz)	43	2	tr	8
seasoned jellyfish	1 (1.2 oz)	58	2	1	11
sweet beancurd	1 (1.2 oz)	64	2	2	10
unagi	1 (1 oz)	54	2	2	8
vinegared ginger	⅓ cup (1.6 oz)	48	1	tr	12
wasabi	2 tsp (0.3 oz)	5	tr	tr	1
SWAMP CABBAGE					
chopped cooked w/o salt	1 cup	20	2	tr	4
SWEET POTATO (*see also* YAM)					
baked w/ skin w/o salt	1 lg (6.3 oz)	162	4	tr	37
baked w/ skin w/o salt	1 med (4 oz)	103	2	tr	24
canned in syrup	½ cup	106	1	tr	25
canned mashed	½ cup	129	3	tr	30
leaves cooked w/o salt	1 cup	22	1	tr	5
paste dulce de calabaza	1 oz	82	tr	tr	21
Diner's Choice					
Mashed	⅔ cup	160	3	3	33
Dr. Praeger's					
Sweet Potato Bites	2 (2 oz)	110	3	3	20
Glory					
Casserole	½ cup	180	2	0	43
Cut Fresh	1 serv (5 oz)	140	2	0	36
Sweet Potatoes	⅔ cup	160	3	0	37
Green Giant					
Candied	¾ cup	240	2	7	41

FOOD	PORTION	CALS	PROT	FAT	CARB
Health Is Wealth					
Southern Style	½ pkg (5 oz)	190	2	5	36
Mann's					
Fresh Cubes	1 serv (3 oz)	60	1	0	15
Mrs. Paul's					
Candied	1 serv (5 oz)	300	1	1	73
Princella					
In Light Syrup	⅔ cup	160	0	0	39
Mashed	⅔ cup	120	1	0	28
Royal Prince					
Candied	½ cup	210	1	0	50
Trappey's					
Sugary Sam Cut Sweet	⅔ cup	160	0	0	39
Tree Of Life					
Organic Puree	½ cup (4.5 oz)	130	3	0	30
TAKE-OUT					
candied	1 serv (3.7 oz)	151	1	3	29
white fried batata blanca frita	1 serv (8 oz)	792	7	29	129
SWEETBREAD (PANCREAS)					
beef braised	3 oz	230	23	15	0
lamb braised	3 oz	199	19	13	0
pork braised	3 oz	186	24	9	0
veal braised	3 oz	218	25	12	0
Rumba					
Beef	4 oz	260	14	23	0
SWISS CHARD					
cooked	½ cup	18	2	tr	4
raw chopped	½ cup	3	tr	tr	1
SWORDFISH					
cooked	3 oz	132	22	4	0
raw	3 oz	103	17	3	0
SYRUP					
corn dark & light	¼ cup	240	0	tr	65
date syrup	1 tbsp	63	tr	tr	15
maple	1 cup (11.1 oz)	824	tr	1	212
maple	1 tbsp	52	0	0	13
raspberry	1 oz	76	tr	0	19
rose hip	1 oz	9	0	0	2

FOOD	PORTION	CALS	PROT	FAT	CARB
sorghum	1 cup (11.6 oz)	957	0	0	247
sorghum	1 tbsp (0.7 oz)	61	0	0	16
sugar syrup	¼ cup	76	0	0	20
Cary's					
Maple	¼ cup	210	0	0	53
Sugar Free	¼ cup	30	0	0	12
Hershey's					
Caramel	2 tbsp (1.4 oz)	110	tr	0	27
Strawberry	2 tbsp (1.4 oz)	100	0	0	26
Strawberry Sugar Free	2 tbsp (1 oz)	10	0	0	4
Lundberg					
Organic Sweet Dreams Brown Rice	2 tbsp	110	1	0	31
Navitas Naturals					
Yacon	2 tbsp	90	0	0	22
Nesquik					
Strawberry Calcium Fortified	2 tbsp (1.4 oz)	110	0	0	27
Neway					
Sweet Sensation Luo Han Guo Syrup	1 tsp	8	0	0	2
Tree Of Life					
Maple Grade A	¼ cup	200	0	0	53
Wholesome Sweeteners					
Organic Blue Agave	1 tbsp	60	0	0	16
Organic Corn Syrup	2 tbsp	120	0	0	30

TAHINI (*see* SESAME)

TAMARIND

dried sweetened pulpitas	1 piece (0.8 oz)	56	1	tr	15
dried sweetened pulpitas	½ cup	279	3	1	73
fresh	1 (2 g)	5	tr	tr	1
fresh cut up	1 cup	143	2	tr	38

TAMARIND JUICE

nectar	1 cup	143	tr	tr	37

TANGERINE
CANNED

in light syrup	1 cup	154	1	tr	41
juice pack	1 cup	92	2	tr	24

FOOD	PORTION	CALS	PROT	FAT	CARB
FRESH					
fresh	1 sm (2.7 oz)	40	1	tr	10
fresh	1 med (3.1 oz)	47	1	tr	12
fresh	1 lg (4.2 oz)	64	1	tr	16
sections	1 cup	103	2	1	26
Noble					
Florida Tangerines	1 (3.8 oz)	50	1	1	15
River Pride					
Sweet	1 (3.8 oz)	50	1	1	15
TANGERINE JUICE					
canned sweetened	1 cup	124	1	1	30
fresh	1 cup	106	1	tr	25
Natalie's Orchid Island Juice					
100% Juice	8 oz	106	1	0	25
Odwalla					
100% Juice	8 oz	110	1	0	25
Santa Cruz					
Organic Sparkling	8 oz	110	0	0	26
SSips					
Drink	1 box (7 oz)	120	0	0	31
TAPIOCA					
pearl dry	¼ cup (1.3 oz)	136	tr	tr	34
starch	1 oz	98	17	tr	24
Let's Do Organic					
Granulated	1 tbsp	35	0	0	9
Starch	1 tbsp	0	0	0	9
TARO					
chips	10 (0.8 oz)	115	1	6	16
leaves cooked	½ cup	18	2	tr	3
raw sliced	½ cup	56	1	tr	14
shoots sliced cooked	½ cup	10	1	tr	2
sliced cooked	½ cup (2.3 oz)	94	tr	tr	23
tahitian sliced cooked	½ cup	30	3	tr	5
TARPON					
fresh	3 oz	87	17	2	0
TARRAGON					
dried crumbled	1 tsp	2	tr	tr	tr
ground	1 tsp	5	tr	tr	1

FOOD	PORTION	CALS	PROT	FAT	CARB
TEA/HERBAL TEA (*see also* ICED TEA)					
HERBAL					
chamomile brewed	1 cup	2	0	tr	tr
Celestial Seasonings					
Chamomile as prep	1 cup	0	0	0	0
REGULAR					
brewed tea	1 cup (6 oz)	2	0	0	1
Daily Detox					
Original	1 tea bag	0	0	0	0
Oregon Chai					
Chai Tea Latte Original Caffeine Free Concentrate	½ cup	78	0	0	18
Chai Tea Latte Original Concentrate	½ cup	78	0	0	19
Chai Tea Latte Spiced Original Mix	1 pkg	100	2	1	20
Chai Tea Latte Vanilla Mix	1 pkg	120	2	2	25
Organic Chai Cider Concentrate	½ cup	110	0	0	26
Organic Chai Nog Concentrate	½ cup	90	0	0	15
Red Rose					
English Breakfast Tea Bag as prep	1 cup	0	0	0	0
TAKE-OUT					
chai spiced latte decaf	1 cup	130	2	3	23
TEMPEH					
tempeh	½ cup	165	16	6	14
White Wave					
Five Grain	⅓ block (2.7 oz)	160	12	6	15
WildWood					
Organic Nori Seaweed	3 oz	170	13	7	16
TESTICLES					
prairie oysters cooked	1 pair (6.8 oz)	241	44	6	0
THYME					
dried crumbled	1 tsp	3	tr	tr	1
fresh	1 tsp	1	tr	tr	tr
ground	1 tsp	4	tr	tr	1

FOOD	PORTION	CALS	PROT	FAT	CARB
TILAPIA					
Gorton's					
Fillets Crunchy Breaded frzn	1 (3 oz)	80	14	3	tr
High Liner					
Loins	1 fillet (4 oz)	110	23	2	0
Van de Kamp's					
Lightly Breaded Fillets	1 (4 oz)	240	16	11	17
TAKE-OUT					
battered & fried	1 fillet (4 oz)	206	21	9	8
breaded & fried	1 fillet (4 oz)	300	26	14	16
broiled w/o fat	1 fillet (3.5 oz)	128	26	3	0
TILEFISH					
cooked	3 oz	125	21	4	0
cooked	½ fillet (5.3 oz)	220	37	7	0
raw	3 oz	81	15	2	0
TOFU					
firm	¼ block (3 oz)	118	13	7	3
firm	½ cup	183	20	11	5
fresh fried	1 piece (0.5 oz)	35	2	3	1
fuyu salted & fermented	1 block (⅓ oz)	13	1	1	1
koyadofu dried frozen	1 piece (½ oz)	82	8	5	2
okara	½ cup	47	2	1	8
regular	¼ block (4 oz)	88	9	6	2
regular	½ cup	94	6	6	2
Amy's					
Organic Tofu Scramble w/ Hash Browns & Veggies	1 pkg (8.9 oz)	320	19	19	19
House					
Atsu-Age Cutlet	1 (2.5 oz)	100	11	5	2
Cut-Age Shredded Fried	1 serv (0.5 oz)	50	4	4	0
Ganmodoki Fritter Small	3 (1.6 oz)	120	7	9	2
Medium Firm	3 oz	60	7	3	1
Organic Extra Firm	3 oz	90	11	5	0
Organic Firm	3 oz	60	8	3	0
Soft Silken	3 oz	50	5	3	2
Steak Cajun	1 (3 oz)	40	12	1	1
Steak Grilled	1 (3 oz)	90	9	5	2
Sukui	3 oz	45	5	2	2

FOOD	PORTION	CALS	PROT	FAT	CARB
Tokusen Kinugoshi	1 piece (5 oz)	90	10	4	3
Yaki Broiled	3 oz	90	9	5	2
TofuTown					
Tofu Tenders Havana Black Bean	½ pkg (5 oz)	210	15	8	18
Tofu Tenders Mediterranean Tahini	½ pkg (5 oz)	240	15	13	16
Tofu Tenders Sesame Ginger Teriyaki	½ pkg (5 oz)	240	15	9	24
Tree Of Life					
Organic Firm	½ block (3.2 oz)	110	11	5	4
White Wave					
Baked Garlic Herb Italian	1 piece (2 oz)	90	9	5	2
Baked Sesame Peanut Thai	1 piece (2 oz)	90	9	5	2
Baked Zesty Lemon Pepper	1 piece (2 oz)	90	9	5	3
Extra Firm	⅕ block (3.2 oz)	110	11	6	3
Organic Extra Firm	⅕ block (3.2 oz)	110	11	6	3
Organic Firm	⅓ block (3.2 oz)	110	11	6	3
Organic Soft	⅕ block (3.2 oz)	110	10	6	3
Reduced Fat	⅕ block (3.2 oz)	90	10	4	4
WildWood					
Organic Baked Aloha	1 piece (3.5 oz)	180	20	5	15
Organic Calcium Rich Medium	3 oz	70	7	4	2
Organic Golden Pineapple Teriyaki	3 oz	160	13	12	5
Organic High Protein Super Firm	3 oz	100	14	4	5
Organic Smoked Mild Szechuan	3 oz	150	14	6	11
TAKE-OUT					
breaded deep fried w/ soy sauce japanese style	1 piece (0.4 oz)	15	0	1	1
soy sauce marinated & grilled	1 serv (4 oz)	181	19	11	6

FOOD	PORTION	CALS	PROT	FAT	CARB
TOMATILLO					
fresh	1 (1.2 oz)	11	tr	tr	2
fresh chopped	½ cup (2.3 oz)	21	1	1	4
TOMATO					
CANNED					
green pickled	½ cup (2.5 oz)	26	1	tr	6
green whole pickled	1 (2.6 oz)	27	1	tr	6
paste	1 can (6 oz)	139	7	1	32
paste	¼ cup (2.3 oz)	54	3	tr	12
paste no salt added	1 can (6 oz)	139	7	1	32
puree	1 can (28 oz)	312	14	2	74
puree	1 cup (8.8 oz)	95	4	1	22
puree w/o salt	1 can (28 oz)	312	14	2	74
sauce	1 cup (8.6 oz)	59	3	tr	13
sauce no salt added	1 cup (8.6 oz)	102	3	tr	21
stewed	1 cup (8.9 oz)	66	2	tr	16
Cento					
Paste	2 tbsp (1.2 oz)	30	1	0	7
Contadina					
Paste Italian Herbs	2 tbsp	35	1	1	7
Dei Fratelli					
Chopped Italian Tomatoes	½ cup (4.3 oz)	40	1	1	8
Del Monte					
Diced w/ Garlic & Onion	½ cup	40	2	1	8
Organic Tomato Paste	2 tbsp	30	2	0	6
Hunt's					
Diced w/ Basil Garlic & Oregano	½ cup	35	1	0	7
Paste No Salt Added	2 tbsp (1.2 oz)	30	1	0	6
Muir Glen					
Organic Chunky Tomato & Herb	½ cup	60	2	1	11
Organic Diced Fire Roasted	½ cup	30	1	0	6
Organic Diced w/ Basil & Garlic	½ cup	30	1	0	6
Polar					
Grape	½ cup	50	0	0	12
Pomi					
Chopped	½ cup	20	1	0	4
Progresso					
Crushed w/ Added Puree	¼ cup (2.1 oz)	20	1	0	4
Diced	½ cup (4.4 oz)	25	1	0	5
Puree	¼ cup (2.2 oz)	25	1	0	5
Whole Peeled w/ Basil	½ cup (4.2 oz)	20	1	0	4

FOOD	PORTION	CALS	PROT	FAT	CARB
Redpack					
Crushed In Puree	¼ cup	20	0	0	4
Diced In Juice	½ cup	25	1	0	5
Petite Diced Onion Celery & Green Pepper	½ cup	45	1	0	10
S&W					
Crushed	¼ cup (2.1 oz)	20	1	0	4
Paste	2 tbsp (1.2 oz)	30	2	0	6
Petite Cut	½ cup (4.4 oz)	25	1	0	6
Puree	¼ cup (2.2 oz)	30	1	0	6
Ready-Cut Italian Recipe	½ cup (4.2 oz)	25	1	0	4
Ready-Cut No Salt Added	½ cup (4.4 oz)	25	1	0	6
Stewed No Salt Added	½ cup (4.4 oz)	35	1	0	9
Stewed Original	½ cup (4.3 oz)	35	1	0	7
Whole Peeled	½ cup (4.4 oz)	25	1	0	6
DRIED					
sun dried	1 piece (2 g)	5	tr	tr	1
sun dried	¼ cup (0.5 oz)	35	2	tr	8
sun dried in oil drained	¼ cup (1 oz)	59	1	4	6
sun dried in oil drained	1 piece (3 g)	6	tr	tr	1
tomato powder	1 oz	85	4	tr	21
FRESH					
bruschetta	¼ cup	50	2	3	6
cherry	1 (0.6 oz)	3	tr	tr	1
cherry	½ cup (2.6 oz)	13	1	tr	3
grape tomatoes	20	30	1	0	6
green	1 med (4.3 oz)	28	1	tr	6
green	1 lg (6.4 oz)	42	2	tr	9
green	1 sm (3.2 oz)	21	1	tr	5
green chopped	1 cup (6.3 oz)	41	2	tr	9
orange	1 (4 oz)	18	1	tr	4
orange chopped	1 cup (5.5 oz)	25	2	tr	5
plum	1 (2.2 oz)	11	1	tr	2
red	1 lg (6.4 oz)	33	2	tr	7
red	1 med (4.3 oz)	22	1	tr	5
red	1 sm (3.2 oz)	16	1	tr	4
red chopped	½ cup (3.2 oz)	16	1	tr	4
red slice	1 lg (0.9 oz)	5	tr	tr	1
roma	1 (2.2 oz)	11	1	tr	2
yellow	1 (7.4 oz)	32	2	1	6
yellow chopped	½ cup (2.4 oz)	10	1	tr	2

FOOD	PORTION	CALS	PROT	FAT	CARB
Earthbound Farms					
Organic Roma	1 med (5.2 oz)	35	1	1	7
TAKE-OUT					
aspic	½ cup (4 oz)	32	3	tr	6
broiled slices	2 (2.9 oz)	18	1	tr	4
broiled whole	1 med (3.7 oz)	23	1	tr	5
bruschetta on toasted italian bread	1 slice	106	4	3	18
fried slices	2 (2.5 oz)	122	2	9	8
scalloped	½ cup (4 oz)	99	2	5	12
stewed	½ cup (1.8 oz)	40	1	1	7
stuffed w/ rice	1 (5.2 oz)	110	2	3	20
stuffed w/ rice & meat	1 (5.2 oz)	142	7	6	15
TOMATO JUICE					
tomato juice	1 cup (8.5 oz)	41	2	tr	10
tomato juice w/o added salt	1 cup (8.5 oz)	41	2	tr	10
Campbell's					
Healthy Request	8 oz	50	2	0	10
Low Sodium	8 oz	50	2	0	10
Organic	8 oz	50	2	0	10
Dei Fratelli					
Tomato Juice	8 oz	40	2	0	10
Lakewood					
Organic	8 oz	35	1	0	7
Tree Of Life					
Organic 100% Juice	8 oz	50	1	0	10
TONGUE					
beef simmered	3 oz	241	16	19	0
lamb braised	3 oz	234	18	17	0
pork braised	3 oz	230	20	16	0
veal braised	3 oz	172	22	9	0
Rumba					
Beef	4 oz	250	17	18	4
TORTILLA					
corn	1 (6 in diam)	56	1	1	12
corn w/o salt	1 (6 in diam)	56	1	1	12
flour w/o salt	1 (8 in diam)	114	3	3	20
French Meadow Bakery					
Fat Flush	1 (1 oz)	100	5	1	18

FOOD	PORTION	CALS	PROT	FAT	CARB
Gluten Free	1 (1.5 oz)	120	1	1	24
Hemp	1 (1.1 oz)	90	5	3	12
La Tortilla Factory					
Carb Cutting Original	1 (1.3 oz)	60	5	2	11
Organic Yellow Corn	2 (2.4 oz)	120	3	2	25
Smart & Delicious Low Fat Low Sodium	1 (2.5 oz)	150	5	2	32
Rudi's Organic Bakery					
Spelt	1 (2 oz)	140	5	3	27
Salba Smart					
Whole Wheat Omega-3 Enriched	1 (1.5 oz)	120	4	3	21
Tumaro's					
Honey Wheat	1 (8 in)	110	3	2	23
Low In Carbs Garden Vegetable	1 (8 in)	100	7	3	12
Low In Carbs Green Onion	1 (8 in)	100	7	3	13
Low In Carbs Multi Grain	1 (8 in)	100	7	3	13
Low In Carbs Salsa	1 (8 in)	100	7	3	13
Pesto & Garlic	1 (8 in)	110	3	1	23
Premium White	1 (8 in)	120	3	2	23
Soy-full Heart 8 Grain 'N Soy	1 (1.4 oz)	100	6	0	14
Soy-full Heart Apple 'N Cinnamon	1 (1.4 oz)	90	6	3	13
Soy-full Heart Wheat Soy & Flax	1 (1.4 oz)	90	6	3	13
Spinach & Vegetables	1 (8 in)	110	3	2	23

TORTILLA CHIPS (*see* CHIPS)

TRAIL MIX

FOOD	PORTION	CALS	PROT	FAT	CARB
Back To Nature					
Bar Harbor Blend	1 oz	130	2	7	17
Harvest Blend	1 oz	150	5	10	12
Nantucket Blend	1 oz	130	3	7	15
Pacific Heights Blend	1 oz	160	4	11	13
Enjoy Life					
Gluten Free Not Nuts! Beach Bash	1 oz	130	4	7	13
Gluten Free Not Nuts! Mountain Mambo	1 oz	140	5	8	12
Kopali					
Organic Mix	½ pkg (1 oz)	130	4	6	15

FOOD	PORTION	CALS	PROT	FAT	CARB
Mrs. May's					
Coconut Almond Crunch	1 oz	183	4	15	10
Navitas Naturals					
3 Berry Cacao Nibs & Cashews	1 oz	110	3	5	16
Goji Cacao Nibs & Cashews	1 oz	120	4	6	13
Goji Golden Berry & Mulberry	1 oz	90	3	0	19
Planters					
Berry Nut & Chocolate	3 tbsp (1 oz)	120	2	5	18
SunRise					
Honey Coated	3 tbsp (1 oz)	137	5	6	14
W/ Fruit	3 tbsp (1 oz)	130	4	6	16
TREE FERN					
chopped cooked	½ cup	28	tr	tr	8
TRIPE					
beef simmered	3 oz	80	10	3	2
Rumba					
Beef Tripe	4 oz	110	15	5	0
TAKE-OUT					
mondongo w/ potatoes	1 cup	300	24	11	26
TRITICALE					
dry	½ cup (3.4 oz)	323	13	2	69
TROUT					
baked	3 oz	162	23	7	0
rainbow cooked	3 oz	129	22	4	0
sea trout baked	3 oz	113	18	4	0
TRUFFLES					
fresh	0.5 oz	4	2	tr	9
Aux Delices Des Bois					
Black Truffle Butter	0.5 oz	90	0	10	0
TUNA					
CANNED					
light in oil	1 can (6 oz)	399	50	14	0
light in oil	3 oz	169	25	7	0
light in water	3 oz	99	22	1	0
light in water	1 can (5.8 oz)	192	42	1	0
white in oil	3 oz	158	23	7	0
white in oil	1 can (6.2 oz)	331	47	14	0

FOOD	PORTION	CALS	PROT	FAT	CARB
white in water	3 oz	116	23	2	0
white in water	1 can (6 oz)	234	46	4	0
Bumble Bee					
Sensations Lemon & Pepper w/ Crackers	1 pkg (3.6 oz)	200	19	8	13
Solid White Albacore In Water	¼ cup (2 oz)	60	13	1	0
Chicken Of The Sea					
Albacore Solid In Water	2 oz	70	15	1	0
Chunk White Albacore In Water	¼ cup (2 oz)	50	11	1	0
Polar					
Albacore Solid White In Water	2 oz	70	18	1	0
Chunk Light In Water	2 oz	60	13	1	0
Progresso					
Albacore Solid White Olive Oil	¼ cup (2 oz)	90	16	3	0
Solid Light Olive Oil drained	¼ cup (2 oz)	120	15	6	0
StarKist					
Chunk Light In Water	¼ cup (2 oz)	60	13	5	0
Chunk Light In Water Flavor Pouch	1 pkg (3 oz)	90	19	1	0
Low Sodium Chunk White In Water	¼ cup (2 oz)	60	15	1	0
Solid Light In Water	2 oz	60	13	1	0
Solid White Albacore In Water	2 oz	70	15	1	0
Tuna Creations Hickory Smoked Flavor Pouch	2 oz	60	13	1	0
Tree Of Life					
Wild Light Tongol Chunk In Spring Water No Salt Added	¼ cup (2.4 oz)	50	12	0	0
FRESH					
bluefin cooked	3 oz	157	25	5	0
bluefin raw	3 oz	122	20	4	0
skipjack baked	3 oz	112	24	1	0
yellowfin baked	3 oz	118	25	1	0
MIX					
StarKist					
Lunch To-Go Chunk Light	1 pkg	310	20	9	27
Tuna Helper					
Creamy Broccoli as prep	1 cup	310	6	11	39
Creamy Pasta as prep	1 cup	320	5	12	39
Tetrazzini as prep	1 cup	290	6	10	33

FOOD	PORTION	CALS	PROT	FAT	CARB
TAKE-OUT					
tuna salad	1 cup	383	33	19	19
TURBOT					
european baked	3 oz	104	17	3	0
TURKEY (see also JERKY, TURKEY DISHES, TURKEY SUBSTITUTES)					
CANNED					
w/ broth	1 cup	220	32	9	0
Hormel					
Chunk White & Dark	2 oz	70	11	3	0
Premium Chunk White	2 oz	60	11	2	0
FRESH					
breast pre-basted w/ skin roasted	3.5 oz	126	22	3	0
breast roasted w/ skin	4 oz	212	32	8	0
breast roasted w/o skin	4 oz	212	33	4	0
dark meat w/o skin roasted	3 oz	170	26	7	0
dark meat w/o skin roasted	1 cup (5 oz)	262	40	10	0
ground cooked	3 oz	193	22	11	0
leg w/ skin roasted	1 (19 oz)	1136	152	54	0
light meat w/ skin roasted half turkey	2.3 lbs	2069	87	87	0
light meat w/o skin roasted	4 oz	183	35	4	0
neck simmered	1 (5.3 oz)	274	41	11	0
skin roasted	1 oz	141	13	13	0
skin roasted from half turkey	8.7 oz	1096	49	98	0
tail cooked	1 (2 oz)	197	13	16	0
w/ skin roasted	1 serv (4.2 oz)	249	34	12	0
w/ skin roasted	½ turkey (4 lbs)	3857	522	181	0
w/o skin roasted	1 cup (5 oz)	238	41	7	0
w/o skin roasted	1 serv (3.7 oz)	177	31	5	0
wing w/ skin roasted	1 (6.5 oz)	426	51	23	0
wing w/o skin roasted	1 (5.2 oz)	237	45	5	0
Butterball					
Burger Patties	1 (4 oz)	150	22	8	0
Cutlets	4 oz	120	28	1	0
Drumstick	4 oz	170	22	8	0
Ground 7% Fat	4 oz	150	22	8	0
Ground White	4 oz	130	26	4	0

FOOD	PORTION	CALS	PROT	FAT	CARB
Strips	4 oz	120	28	1	0
Thighs	4 oz	170	22	8	0
Wings	1 (6.3 oz)	380	36	25	0
Empire					
Gound White	4 oz	160	23	8	0
Honeysuckle White					
85% Lean Ground	4 oz	240	20	17	0
93% Lean Patties	1 (4 oz)	160	22	8	0
97% Lean Ground White	4 oz	130	26	2	0
99% Fat Free Breast Cutlets	4 oz	120	28	1	0
99% Fat Free Breast Tenderloin	4 oz	120	28	1	0
Drumettes	4 oz	180	24	8	0
Marinated Strips Asian Grill	4 oz	160	17	7	8
Necks	4 oz	150	23	6	0
Tenderloins Creamy Dijon Mustard	4 oz	140	21	4	0
Tenderloins Homestyle	4 oz	130	21	4	0
Tenderloins Teriyaki	4 oz	140	21	4	5
Thighs	4 oz	190	21	11	0
Whole Honey Roasted	4 oz	180	20	9	5
Wings	4 oz	220	23	14	0
Perdue					
Breast Fillets Boneless Skinless cooked	3 oz	110	26	1	0
Drumsticks roasted	3 oz	140	21	7	0
Ground Breast cooked	3 oz	110	25	1	0
Patties cooked	1 (3 oz)	160	20	8	0
Whole Breast	3 oz	170	23	8	0
Whole Dark Meat cooked	3 oz	190	21	11	0
Whole White Meat roasted	3 oz	150	23	7	0
Shady Brook					
Tenderloin Zesty Italian Herb	4 oz	130	21	4	4
FROZEN					
roast boneless seasoned light & dark meat roasted	3.5 oz	155	21	6	3
sticks breaded fried	1 (2.2 oz)	179	9	11	11
Butterball					
Boneless Roast	4 oz	130	22	5	0
Breast Boneless Roast	4 oz	110	21	3	1
Breast Tenderloin Teriyaki	4 oz	110	21	1	4

FOOD	PORTION	CALS	PROT	FAT	CARB
Breast Whole	4 oz	110	21	3	1
Breast Whole Smoked Cooked	3 oz	120	18	5	1
Whole Turkey	1 serv (4 oz)	170	20	10	0
Whole Turkey Baked	3 oz	130	17	7	0
Honeysuckle White					
Breast Boneless Roast	4 oz	170	21	7	0
Jennie-O					
Burger	1 (4 oz)	160	19	9	0
Organic Prairie					
Whole Young	4 oz	190	23	10	0
READY-TO-EAT					
bologna	1 slice (1 oz)	59	3	4	1
breast	1 slice (0.7 oz)	22	4	tr	1
ham	1 slice (1 oz)	35	5	1	1
pastrami	2 oz	70	9	2	2
salami	1 slice (1 oz)	48	5	3	tr
Applegate Farms					
Organic Herb	2 oz	50	11	1	0
Butterball					
Breast Honey Roasted Thick Sliced	1 slice (1 oz)	35	5	1	2
Breast Oven Roasted Extra Thin Slice	7 slices (2 oz)	70	10	2	3
Breast Smoked Thin Sliced	4 slices (1.9 oz)	70	7	2	4
Breast Strips Oven Roasted	½ pkg (3 oz)	90	18	1	2
Deep Fried Original Thick Sliced	1 slice (1 oz)	30	5	1	1
Carl Buddig					
Honey Roasted Sliced	2 oz	90	9	5	2
Turkey Sliced	2 oz	90	9	5	tr
Healthy Ones					
Oven Roasted 97% Fat Free	7 slices (2 oz)	60	9	2	2
Honeysuckle White					
Simply Done Whole Breast	4 oz	160	21	7	2
Hormel					
Natural Choice Deli Turkey Honey	4 slices (2 oz)	60	10	1	3
Natural Choice Deli Turkey Oven Roasted	4 slices (2 oz)	60	10	1	3
Natural Choice Deli Turkey Smoked	4 slices (2 oz)	60	10	1	3

FOOD	PORTION	CALS	PROT	FAT	CARB
Organic Prairie					
Roasted Breast Slices	2 oz	60	14	1	0
Oscar Mayer					
Breast Smoked Shaved	2 oz	50	8	1	2
Sara Lee					
Breast Cracked Pepper	4 slices (1.8 oz)	50	9	1	1
Breast Hardwood Smoked	4 slices (1.8 oz)	50	11	1	1
Tyson					
Breast Oven Roasted	2 slices (1.6 oz)	40	8	1	1
TURKEY DISHES					
FROZEN					
gravy & turkey	1 cup (8.4 oz)	160	14	6	11
TAKE-OUT					
boneless breast w/ cranberry apple stuffing	1 serv (5 oz)	260	32	9	10
turkey a la king	1 cup (8.5 oz)	465	24	34	16
turkey creole w/o rice	1 cup	189	29	4	9
turkey croquette	1 (2 oz)	158	10	9	8
turkey divan	1 cup	321	40	14	9
turkey fricassee	1 cup	322	29	18	8
turkey meatloaf	1 lg slice (5 oz)	243	29	9	11
turkey salad	1 cup	417	29	32	3
turkey tetrazzini	1 cup	369	19	18	29
TURKEY SUBSTITUTES					
Worthington					
Turkee Slices	3 slices (3.3 oz)	180	14	12	5
Yves					
Meatless Deli Turkey Slices	4 slices	100	16	2	5
Meatless Ground Turkey	⅓ cup	60	12	1	8
TURMERIC					
ground	1 tsp	8	tr	tr	1
TURNIPS					
canned greens	½ cup	17	2	tr	3
cooked mashed	½ cup (4.2 oz)	47	2	tr	10
cubed cooked	½ cup (3 oz)	33	1	tr	7
fresh greens chopped cooked	½ cup	15	1	tr	3
frzn greens cooked	½ cup	24	3	tr	4

FOOD	PORTION	CALS	PROT	FAT	CARB
greens raw chopped	½ cup	7	tr	tr	2
raw cubed	½ cup (2.4 oz)	25	1	tr	6
Allens					
Seasoned	½ cup	35	4	1	5
Glory					
Greens Fresh	2 cups	20	1	0	5
Greens Seasoned canned	½ cup	35	1	0	4
Root Cut Fresh	½ cup	20	1	0	4
Sensibly Seasoned Greens	½ cup	20	1	0	4
TURTLE					
raw	3.5 oz	85	18	1	0
TUSK FISH					
raw	3.5 oz	79	17	tr	0
VANILLA					
vanilla extract	1 tsp (4.2 g)	12	0	0	1
vanilla extract	1 tbsp (0.5 oz)	37	tr	tr	2
vanilla extract alcohol free	1 tsp (4.2 g)	2	0	0	1
Bob's Red Mill					
Organic Extract	1 tsp	0	0	0	0
VEAL (see also VEAL DISHES)					
breast braised	3 oz	226	23	14	0
chop cooked	1 med (6.5 oz)	230	26	13	0
chop breaded fried	1 med (6.5 oz)	290	35	12	13
cubed braised	3 oz	160	30	4	0
cutlet cooked	3 oz	141	26	4	0
ground broiled	3 oz	146	21	6	0
leg roasted	3 oz	136	24	4	0
loin roasted	3 oz	184	21	10	0
patty breaded fried	1 (2.8 oz)	211	16	13	7
shank braised	3 oz	162	27	5	0
VEAL DISHES					
TAKE-OUT					
cordon bleu	1 serv (8 oz)	490	33	35	4
parmigiana	1 serv (6.4 oz)	362	27	21	15
scallopini	1 slice + sauce (3.4 oz)	238	18	17	2
stew	1 serv (8.8 oz)	192	15	6	18
veal marengo	1 serv (8.8 oz)	274	33	9	7

FOOD	PORTION	CALS	PROT	FAT	CARB
veal marsala	1 slice + sauce (3.4 oz)	268	12	19	6
veal paprikash	1 serv (8.6 oz)	280	36	12	5
veal picatta	1 piece + sauce (3.5 oz)	154	16	9	2

VEGETABLE JUICE

FOOD	PORTION	CALS	PROT	FAT	CARB
low sodium tomato & vegetable juice	1 cup (3.5 oz)	53	1	tr	11
vegetable juice cocktail	8 oz	46	2	tr	11
Bolthouse Farms					
Vedge Tomato Carrot Celery	8 oz	60	3	0	11
Dei Fratelli					
Vegetable Juice	8 oz	45	2	2	11
Green To Go					
100% Natural Organic as prep	1 pkg (0.3 oz)	32	1	tr	6
Lakewood					
Super Veggie	6 oz	40	2	0	9
Mott's					
100% Juice Veggie Blend	1 bottle (14 oz)	90	5	1	15
V8					
100% Vegetable Essential Antioxidants	8 oz	50	2	0	11
Calcium Enriched	8 oz	50	2	0	11
High Fiber	8 oz	60	2	0	13
Low Sodium	8 oz	50	2	0	10
Organic	8 oz	50	2	0	10
Vegetable Juice	8 oz	50	0	0	10
Walnut Acres					
Organic Incredible Vegetable	8 oz	50	2	0	12

VEGETABLES MIXED
CANNED

FOOD	PORTION	CALS	PROT	FAT	CARB
mixed vegetables	½ cup	39	2	tr	8
peas & carrots	½ cup	48	3	tr	11
peas & onions	½ cup	30	2	tr	5
succotash	½ cup	102	4	1	23
Del Monte					
Savory Sides Homestyle Vegetable Medley	½ cup	70	1	3	11

FOOD	PORTION	CALS	PROT	FAT	CARB
Savory Sides Rio Grande Vegetables	½ cup	70	2	0	14
McSweet					
Giardiniera	5 pieces (1 oz)	25	0	0	6
S&W					
Mixed	½ cup (4.4 oz)	45	2	0	10
Peas & Pearl Onions	½ cup (4.3 oz)	40	3	0	11
The Gracious Gourmet					
Tapenade Fennel Blood Orange	2 tbsp (1 oz)	50	0	5	3
Veg-All					
Original Mixed	½ cup	40	1	0	8
DRIED					
Fun-Yums					
Fresh Crispy Mixed Veggies	1 serv (0.9 oz)	114	1	4	18
FRESH					
Mann's					
Broccoli & Cauliflower	1 serv (3 oz)	25	2	0	4
California Stir Fry	1 serv (3 oz)	30	2	0	6
Medley	1 serv (3 oz)	25	2	0	5
Veggies On The Go w/ Dip	1 cup + 1 tbsp dip	100	1	8	7
FROZEN					
mixed vegetables cooked	½ cup	54	3	tr	12
peas & carrots cooked	½ cup	38	3	tr	8
peas & onions cooked	½ cup	40	2	tr	8
succotash cooked	½ cup	79	4	1	17
Birds Eye					
Asparagus Gold & White Corn & Baby Carrots	⅔ cup	70	2	1	13
Italian Herb Harvest Vegetables	1¼ cups	90	2	6	6
Spring Vegetables In Citrus Sauce	1¼ cups	70	2	4	8
Steamfresh Asian Medley	1 cup (3.3 oz)	50	2	2	6
Steamfresh Broccoli Cauliflower & Carrots	¾ cup	30	1	0	5
Steamfresh Broccoli & Cauliflower	1 cup	30	1	0	4
Steamfresh Broccoli Carrots Sugar Snap Peas & Water Chestnuts	¾ cup (2.9 oz)	35	1	0	6
Steamfresh Mixed Vegetables	⅔ cup (3.2 oz)	40	2	0	12

FOOD	PORTION	CALS	PROT	FAT	CARB
C&W					
Early Harvest Peas & Baby Carrots	⅔ cup	60	3	0	10
Petite Peas & Pearl Onions	⅔ cup	60	4	0	11
Cascadian Farm					
Organic Mixed Vegetables	⅔ cup	60	2	0	12
Organic Peas & Carrots	⅔ cup	50	2	0	10
French Meadow Bakery					
Vegetarian Sweet N' Spicy Cuban Style Veggies	1 pkg (12 oz)	250	6	9	39
Green Giant					
Broccoli & Carrots w/ Garlic & Herbs as prep	½ cup	40	2	1	7
Garden Vegetable Medley as prep	½ cup	70	2	1	14
Mixed Vegetables as prep	½ cup	50	2	0	11
Southwestern Style as prep	½ cup	90	4	1	18
Szechuan Vegetables as prep	½ cup	50	2	1	9
Health Is Wealth					
Veggie Munchees Vegan	6 (3 oz)	150	4	4	26
La Choy					
Chop Suey Vegetables	½ cup (2.2 oz)	15	tr	0	3
Fancy Chinese Mixed Vegetables	½ cup (2.9 oz)	15	1	2	3
Stir Fry Vegetables	½ cup	15	tr	0	3
Melrose Made Gourmet					
Vegetable Souffle Fat Free	1 serv (4 oz)	70	12	0	5
Seapoint Farms					
Organic Veggie Blends w/ Edamame Eat Your Greens	¾ cup	60	5	2	7
Veggie Blends w/ Edamame Garden	¾ cup	60	4	2	7
Veggie Blends w/ Edamame Oriental	¾ cup	60	4	1	8
TAKE-OUT					
buddha's delight	1 serv (16 oz)	174	17	5	17
pakoras	4 (1.7 oz)	57	2	2	7
ratatouille	1 serv (3.5 oz)	96	2	7	7
samosa	1 (2.4 oz)	206	4	11	22
stir fry mixed vegetables	1 serv (4 oz)	66	3	5	3

FOOD	PORTION	CALS	PROT	FAT	CARB
succotash	½ cup	111	5	1	23
tapenade grilled vegetables	¼ cup	40	0	3	4

VENISON (see also JERKY)

FOOD	PORTION	CALS	PROT	FAT	CARB
roasted	4 oz	215	41	4	0

VINEGAR

FOOD	PORTION	CALS	PROT	FAT	CARB
balsamic	1 tbsp	14	tr	0	3
cider	1 tbsp	3	0	0	tr
red wine	1 tbsp	3	tr	0	tr
white	1 tbsp	3	0	0	tr
Barengo					
Balsamic	1 tbsp (0.5 oz)	15	0	0	4
Red Wine	1 tbsp (0.5 oz)	0	0	0	0
Carapelli					
Balsamic	1 tbsp	15	0	0	4
Red Wine	1 tbsp	5	0	0	0
White Wine	1 tbsp	5	0	0	0
Gedney					
Apple Cider	1 tbsp	3	0	0	0
Distilled White	1 tbsp	3	0	0	0
Gourme Mist					
Balsamic Of Modena	1 sec spray	1	0	0	0
Balsamic Vinegar + Raspberry	1 sec spray	1	0	0	0
Holland House					
Malt	1 tbsp (0.5 oz)	0	0	0	0
Red Wine	1 tbsp (0.5 oz)	0	0	0	0
Latino Chef					
Lulo	1 tbsp	35	1	3	1
Passion Fruit	1 tbsp	40	0	3	2
Lucini					
Balsamic 10 Year Gran Reserve	1 tbsp (0.5 oz)	20	0	0	4
Balsamic Dark Cherry Infused	1 tbsp	30	0	0	7
Italian Wine Pinot Noir	1 tbsp (0.5 oz)	tr	0	0	0
Mitsukan					
Rice	1 tbsp (0.5 oz)	0	0	0	0
Rice Seasoned	1 tbsp (0.5 oz)	25	0	0	5
Nakano					
Natural Rice	1 tbsp (0.5 oz)	0	0	0	0
Red Wine Italian Herb Seasoned	1 tbsp (0.5 oz)	20	0	0	5

FOOD	PORTION	CALS	PROT	FAT	CARB
Rice Pesto Seasoned	1 tbsp (0.5 oz)	20	0	0	5
Rice Red Pepper Seasoned	1 tbsp (0.5 oz)	20	0	0	5
Progresso					
Balsamic	2 tbsp (0.5 oz)	10	0	0	2
Tree Of Life					
Organic Apple Cider Raw Unfiltered	1 tbsp	0	0	0	tr
WAFFLES					
FROZEN					
Aunt Jemima					
Blueberry	2 (2.5 oz)	190	4	5	32
Low Fat	2 (2.5 oz)	160	4	3	30
Kashi					
Heart To Heart Honey Oat	2 (3 oz)	160	6	3	31
Lifestream					
Organic Fig + Flax	2 (2.8 oz)	210	5	0	29
Organic Pomegran Plus	2 (2.8 oz)	190	5	5	31
Van's					
Belgian Multigrain	2 (2.7 oz)	190	4	8	25
Mini Homestyle	4 (2.8 oz)	210	4	8	32
Organic Flax	2 (2.7 oz)	190	4	9	24
Organic Homestyle	2 (2.7 oz)	200	4	9	25
Original 97% Fat Free	2 (2.7 oz)	140	4	2	26
Original Buttermilk	2 (2.7 oz)	220	4	9	31
Wheat Free Buckwheat	2 (3 oz)	230	2	9	36
Wheat Free Flax	2 (3 oz)	210	3	8	33
MIX					
plain as prep 7 in diam	1 (2.6 oz)	218	6	11	25
READY-TO-EAT					
Kashi					
GoLean Blueberry	2 (3 oz)	170	8	3	33
GoLean Original	2 (3 oz)	170	8	3	33
TAKE-OUT					
belgian	1 (4.7 oz)	412	10	13	65
blueberry 9 in sq	1 (7 oz)	556	13	16	90
round 10 in diam	1 (6.8 oz)	598	14	18	94
square 9 in	1 (7 oz)	620	15	19	98
whole wheat 9 in sq	1 (7 oz)	534	18	22	67

FOOD	PORTION	CALS	PROT	FAT	CARB
WALNUTS					
black chopped	¼ cup	193	8	18	3
english chopped	¼ cup	191	4	19	4
english ground	¼ cup	131	3	13	3
english halves	14 (1 oz)	185	4	18	4
english in shell	7 (1 oz)	183	4	18	4
honey roasted	¼ cup	172	4	16	7
Back To Nature					
Unroasted Unsalted	1 oz	190	4	18	4
Diamond					
Chopped	¼ cup	200	5	20	4
WASABI (see HORSERADISH)					
WATER					
ice cubes	3	0	0	0	0
tap water	8 oz	0	0	0	0
Acquafibre					
Fiber Enhanced All Flavors	1 bottle (11.15 oz)	5	0	0	0
Adirondack					
Sparkling All Flavors	8 oz	0	0	0	0
Aloe Breeze					
Organic All Flavors	8 oz	0	0	0	0
Apple & Eve					
Water Fruits All Flavors	1 bottle (10 oz)	90	0	0	21
Aqua Pacific					
Water	1 liter	0	0	0	0
Aquafina					
Alive Wellness Berry Pomegranate	8 oz	10	0	0	2
Ayala's					
Herbal All Flavors	1 bottle	0	0	0	0
Bot					
Fortified All Flavors	1 bottle (12 oz)	40	0	0	10
Dasani					
Purified Water	8 oz	0	0	0	0
Dox					
Cardio Water	1 bottle (12 oz)	20	0	0	5
Evian					
Spring Water	1 liter	0	0	0	0

FOOD	PORTION	CALS	PROT	FAT	CARB
Fiji					
Natural Artesian	1 liter	0	0	0	0
Gerolsteiner					
Sparkling Mineral	8 oz	0	0	0	0
H 10 O					
Citrus Sport For Men	1 bottle (15.9 oz)	0	0	0	0
Peach Mango Tea For Women	1 bottle (15.9 oz)	0	0	0	0
H2Odwalla					
Enhanced Tropical Orange	1 bottle (20 oz)	120	0	0	33
Organic Enhanced Blueberry Tea	1 bottle (20 oz)	120	0	0	29
Organic Enhanced Jasmine Lime	1 bottle (20 oz)	120	0	0	30
Hawaiian Springs					
Naturally Pure	1 liter	0	0	0	0
Highland Spring					
Spring Water	1 liter	0	0	0	0
IQ					
H2O Orange Mango	8 oz	40	0	0	10
Island Chill					
Artesian Water	1 liter	0	0	0	0
Jana					
Natural European Artesian	1 liter	0	0	0	0
Joint Juice					
Fitness Water All Flavors	1 bottle (18 oz)	10	0	0	1
Jones Soda					
24C Multi Vitamin Enhanced All Flavors	1 bottle	100	0	0	24
Klear Splash					
Mini Sip	1 pkg (4 oz)	0	0	0	0
Life Water					
B-Strong	1 bottle (20 oz)	100	0	0	42
Enlighten	1 bottle (20 oz)	100	0	0	41
Zingseng	1 bottle (20 oz)	100	0	0	41
Liquid Salvation					
Ultra Hydrating	1 bottle	0	0	0	0

FOOD	PORTION	CALS	PROT	FAT	CARB
Nui					
All Natural Kid Water	10 oz	90	0	0	21
O Water					
Hydrate Black Raspberry	8 oz	25	0	0	7
Replenish Lemon Lime	8 oz	25	0	0	7
Vitalize Peach Mango	8 oz	25	0	0	7
San Benedetto					
Sparkling Mineral Water	1 liter	0	0	0	0
Skinny Water					
Hi-Energy Acai Grape Blueberry	8 oz	0	0	0	0
Total-V Passionfruit Lemonade	8 oz	0	0	0	0
Snapple					
Antioxidant Water Awaken Dragonfruit	8 oz	50	0	0	12
Antioxidant Water Restore Agave Melon	8 oz	60	0	0	13
Lyte Water	8 oz	0	0	0	0
SoNu					
Water All Flavors	8 oz	45	0	0	13
Special K2O					
Protein Water All Flavors	1 bottle (16.6 oz)	50	5	0	8
Trim Water					
Purified	1 bottle (20 oz)	10	0	0	3
Twist					
Organics All Flavors	8 oz	10	0	0	2
Vitamin + Fiber Water					
All Fruit Flavors	8 oz	50	0	0	13
VitaminWater					
XXX Acai Blueberry Pomegranate	8 oz	50	0	0	13
WaterPlus					
Antioxidants Acai Berry	8 oz	50	0	0	13
Electrolytes Fruit Punch	8 oz	50	0	0	13
Extra-C Orange Tangerine	8 oz	50	0	0	13
Vitamins Dragonfruit Kiwi	8 oz	50	0	0	13
WATER CHESTNUTS					
chinese sliced canned	½ cup	35	1	tr	9
fresh sliced	½ cup	66	1	tr	15

FOOD	PORTION	CALS	PROT	FAT	CARB
La Choy					
Sliced	½ cup	25	1	0	5
Polar					
Sliced	2 tbsp	10	1	0	3
WATERCRESS					
cooked w/o fat	1 cup	15	3	tr	2
raw chopped	1 cup	4	1	tr	tr
WATERMELON					
cut up	1 cup	46	1	tr	12
seeds dried	¼ cup	150	8	13	4
wedge	1 sm (2.5 oz)	21	tr	tr	5
wedge	1 med (10 oz)	86	2	tr	22
wedge	1 lg (20 oz)	172	3	1	43
whole melon	1 (9 lb)	1227	25	6	309
WATERMELON JUICE					
juice	8 oz	71	1	tr	18
WHALE					
beluga dried	1 oz	93	20	2	0
beluga raw	3.5 oz	111	27	1	0
WHEAT					
sprouted	1 cup (3.8 oz)	214	8	1	46
starch	3.5 oz	348	tr	tr	86
Amazing Grass					
Organic Wheat Grass	1 tbsp (0.3 oz)	35	2	0	4
Arrowhead Mills					
Whole Grain Wheat	¼ cup (1.6 oz)	150	7	1	31
Bob's Red Mill					
Vital Wheat Gluten	¼ cup	120	23	1	6
Near East					
Taboule Wheat Salad as prep	⅔ cup (3.5 oz)	120	3	3	24
White Wave					
Seitan Chicken Meat Of Wheat	3 oz	130	24	0	9
Seitan Traditional	3 oz	90	18	1	3
Seitan Vegetarian Stir Fry Strips	3 oz	110	22	2	2
WHEAT GERM					
plain	¼ cup	108	8	3	14

FOOD	PORTION	CALS	PROT	FAT	CARB
Bob's Red Mill					
Wheat Germ	2 tbsp	59	4	2	7
Kretschmer					
Original Toasted	¼ cup (0.6 oz)	35	3	1	10
Tree Of Life					
Toasted	3 tbsp (0.8 oz)	100	9	3	12
WHEY					
acid dry	1 tbsp	10	tr	tr	2
sweet dry	1 tbsp	26	1	tr	6
sweet fluid	½ cup	33	1	tr	6
whey cheese	1 oz	126	4	8	9
Action Whey					
Dream Shake All Flavors	1 scoop (0.8 oz)	90	15	3	3
Bob's Red Mill					
Protein Concentrate	¼ cup	80	16	1	1
Sweet Dairy	1 tbsp	30	1	0	6
Wellements					
Whey Protein Chocolate	1 scoop (1 oz)	120	22	2	4
Whey Protein Vanilla	1 scoop (1 oz)	120	22	2	4
WHIPPED TOPPINGS					
cream pressurized	1 tbsp (3 g)	8	tr	tr	tr
cream pressurized	1 cup (2.1 oz)	154	2	13	7
nondairy frzn	1 tbsp	13	tr	1	1
nondairy powdered as prep w/ whole milk	1 cup	151	3	10	13
nondairy pressurized	1 tbsp (4 g)	11	tr	1	1
nondairy pressurized	1 cup	184	1	16	11
Cool Whip					
Chocolate	2 tbsp	25	0	2	2
Free	2 tbsp	15	0	0	3
Regular	2 tbsp	25	0	2	2
Strawberry	2 tbsp	25	0	2	2
TruWhip					
Whipped Topping	2 tbsp (0.4 oz)	130	0	2	3
WHITE BEANS					
canned	1 cup	306	19	1	58
dried regular cooked	1 cup	249	17	1	45
dried small cooked	1 cup	253	16	1	46

FOOD	PORTION	CALS	PROT	FAT	CARB
WHITEFISH					
baked	3 oz	146	21	6	0
smoked	3 oz	92	20	1	0
smoked	1 oz	39	7	tr	0
WHITING					
broiled w/o fat	3 oz	99	20	1	0
fillet broiled w/o fat	1 (2.5 oz)	84	17	1	0
fillet steamed w/o fat	1 (2.6 oz)	84	17	1	0
hake raw	3.5 oz	84	17	1	0
TAKE-OUT					
fillet battered & fried	1 (3.1 oz)	157	15	7	6
fillet breaded & fried	1 (3.1 oz)	191	17	10	7
WILD RICE					
cooked	1 cup (5.8 oz)	166	7	1	35
Lundberg					
Organic Quick not prep	¼ cup	150	6	1	33
WINE					
chianti	1 serv (5 oz)	125	tr	0	4
chinese cooking	1 bottle (15 oz)	559	0	0	3
cooking	¼ cup (2 oz)	29	tr	0	4
haiku	1 serv	93	tr	0	3
japanese plum	3 oz	139	tr	tr	16
japanese sake	2 oz	78	tr	0	3
kir	1 serv	78	tr	0	3
madeira	3.5 oz	169	0	0	10
muscat	1 serv (5 oz)	123	tr	0	8
nonalcoholic	1 serv (5 oz)	9	1	0	2
port	1 serv (3.5 oz)	165	tr	0	14
red barbera	1 serv (5 oz)	125	tr	0	4
red burgundy	1 serv (5 oz)	127	tr	0	5
red cabernet franc	1 serv (5 oz)	122	tr	0	4
red claret	1 serv (5 oz)	122	tr	0	4
red gamay	1 serv (5 oz)	115	tr	0	4
red mouvedre	1 serv (5 oz)	129	tr	0	4
red pinot noir	1 serv (5 oz)	121	tr	0	3
red syrah	1 serv (5 oz)	122	tr	0	4
red zinfandel	1 serv (5 oz)	129	tr	0	4
sake screwdriver	1 serv	175	2	tr	23

FOOD	PORTION	CALS	PROT	FAT	CARB
sangria	1 serv	88	tr	tr	6
sangria blanco	1 serv	155	1	tr	24
sherry	2 oz	84	tr	0	5
wassail wine	1 serv	142	1	tr	22
white	1 serv (5 oz)	121	tr	0	4
white fume blanc	1 serv (5 oz)	121	tr	0	3
white pinot blanc	1 serv (5 oz)	119	tr	0	3
white pinot grigio	1 serv (5 oz)	122	tr	0	3
white riesling	1 serv (5 oz)	118	tr	0	6
white sauvignon blanc	1 serv (5 oz)	119	tr	0	3
wine cooler	1 (7 oz)	116	tr	tr	14
wine spritzer	1 serv (7 oz)	73	tr	0	2
Holland House					
Cooking Wine Marsala	2 tbsp (1 oz)	45	0	0	4
Cooking Wine Red	2 tbsp (1 oz)	20	0	0	1
Cooking Wine Sherry	2 tbsp (1 oz)	45	0	0	2
Cooking Wine Vermouth	2 tbsp (1 oz)	35	0	0	2
Cooking Wine White	2 tbsp (1 oz)	20	0	0	0

WINGED BEANS

FOOD	PORTION	CALS	PROT	FAT	CARB
dried cooked w/o salt	1 cup	253	18	10	26

WRAPS (see BREAD, SANDWICHES)

YACON
Navitas Naturals

FOOD	PORTION	CALS	PROT	FAT	CARB
Slices Dried	1 oz	90	1	0	22

YAM (see also SWEET POTATO)
CANNED
Glory

FOOD	PORTION	CALS	PROT	FAT	CARB
Candied	½ cup	210	1	0	52
S&W					
Candied	½ cup (4.9 oz)	170	2	0	46
FRESH					
mountain yam hawaii cooked w/o salt	1 cup	119	3	tr	29
yam cooked w/o salt	1 cup	158	2	tr	38
Earthbound Farms					
Organic	1 med (4.6 oz)	130	2	0	33
House					
Black Ita Konnyaku Yam Cake	1 serv (2 oz)	5	0	0	1

FOOD	PORTION	CALS	PROT	FAT	CARB
YARDLONG BEANS					
sliced cooked w/o salt	1 cup	49	3	tr	10
YAUTIA (see MALANGA)					
YEAST					
baker's compressed	1 cake (0.6 oz)	18	1	tr	3
baker's dry	1 tbsp	35	5	1	5
baker's dry	1 pkg (7 g)	21	3	tr	3
brewer's dry	1 tbsp	35	5	1	5
Bob's Red Mill					
Active Dry	1 tbsp	25	0	1	5
YELLOW BEANS					
fresh cooked w/o salt	1 cup	44	2	tr	10
fresh raw	1 cup	34	2	tr	8
YELLOWTAIL					
baked	4 oz	199	32	7	0
YOGURT (see also YOGURT DRINKS, YOGURT FROZEN)					
plain lowfat	8 oz	143	12	4	16
plain nonfat	8 oz	127	13	tr	17
plain whole milk	8 oz	138	8	7	11
tofu yogurt	1 cup	246	9	5	42
Better Whey					
All Fruit Flavors	1 pkg (6 oz)	145	15	1	23
Plain	1 pkg (6 oz)	130	17	1	17
Breyers					
Creme Savers Orange & Creme	1 pkg (8 oz)	240	7	4	45
Creme Savers Raspberries & Creme	1 pkg (8 oz)	240	7	4	45
Light! Probiotic Plus Apple Cinnamon	1 pkg (8 oz)	100	8	2	15
Light! Probiotic Plus Blueberries 'N Cream	1 pkg (8 oz)	110	8	2	15
Light! Probiotic Plus Lemon Chiffon	1 pkg (8 oz)	100	8	2	14
Light! Probiotic Plus Peaches 'N Cream	1 pkg (8 oz)	100	8	2	15
Light! Probiotic Plus Strawberry Banana	1 pkg (8 oz)	110	8	2	16

FOOD	PORTION	CALS	PROT	FAT	CARB
Light! Probiotic Plus Strawberry Cheesecake	1 pkg (8 oz)	110	8	2	16
Smart! w/ DHA Black Cherry	1 pkg (6 oz)	170	6	2	35
Smart! w/ DHA Mixed Berry	1 pkg (6 oz)	170	6	2	34
Smart! w/ DHA Peach	6 oz	170	6	2	34
Smart! w/ DHA Pineapple	1 pkg (6 oz)	170	6	2	34
Smart! w/ DHA Strawberry	1 pkg (6 oz)	170	6	2	34
Smart! w/ DHA Strawberry Banana	1 pkg (6 oz)	170	6	2	34
Smooth & Creamy Peaches 'N Cream	1 pkg (8 oz)	240	7	2	48
Smooth & Creamy Strawberry	1 pkg (8 oz)	230	7	2	46
Smooth & Creamy Vanilla Cream	1 pkg (8 oz)	240	7	2	47
YoCrunch Blueberry w/ Granola	1 pkg	240	7	3	49
YoCrunch Cookie N' Cream w/ Oreo	1 pkg	240	5	6	41
YoCrunch Naturals Strawberry Banana w/ Granola	1 pkg	245	10	3	50
YoCrunch Naturals Strawberry w/ Dark Chocolate Chips	1 pkg	280	8	9	46
YoCrunch Raspberry w/ Granola	1 pkg	240	7	3	49
YoCrunch Strawberry w/ Granola	1 pkg	240	7	3	49
YoCrunch Vanilla Nestle	1 pkg	260	7	7	44
YoCrunch Vanilla w/ Butterfinger	1 pkg	260	7	7	45
YoCrunch Light Cookies N' Cream w/ Oreo	1 pkg	170	6	5	24
YoCrunch Light Strawberry w/ Granola	1 pkg	170	6	2	33
Cabot					
Greek	1 pkg (6 oz)	210	7	17	9
Greek 2%	1 pkg (6 oz)	160	13	3	25
Non Fat Berry Banana	1 cup	130	8	0	24
Non Fat Black Cherry	1 cup	130	8	0	24
Non Fat French Vanilla	1 cup	130	8	0	24
Non Fat Plain	1 cup	100	10	0	19
Non Fat Raspberry	1 cup	130	8	0	24

FOOD	PORTION	CALS	PROT	FAT	CARB
Chobani					
Greek Yogurt Blueberry Nonfat	1 pkg (6 oz)	140	14	0	20
Greek Yogurt Honey Nonfat	1 pkg (6 oz)	150	16	0	20
Greek Yogurt Peach Nonfat	1 pkg (6 oz)	140	14	0	20
Greek Yogurt Pineapple	1 pkg (6 oz)	160	13	3	21
Greek Yogurt Plain Lowfat	1 pkg (6 oz)	130	17	4	7
Greek Yogurt Plain Nonfat	1 pkg (6 oz)	100	18	0	7
Greek Yogurt Pomegranate Nonfat	1 pkg (6 oz)	140	14	0	21
Greek Yogurt Raspberry Nonfat	1 pkg (6 oz)	120	14	0	22
Greek Yogurt Strawberry Banana	1 pkg (6 oz)	160	14	3	19
Greek Yogurt Strawberry Nonfat	1 pkg (6 oz)	140	14	0	20
Greek Yogurt Vanilla Nonfat	1 pkg (6 oz)	120	16	0	13
Dannon					
Activia Vanilla Light Fat Free	4 oz	70	5	0	13
All Natural Blended Mini Blueberry	1 (3.3 oz)	110	5	1	20
All Natural Blended Mini Strawberry	1 (3.3 oz)	110	5	1	20
Creamy Fruit Blends Raspberry	6 oz	170	7	2	32
Fruit On The Bottom Apple Cinnamon	6 oz	150	6	2	28
Fruit On The Bottom Peach	6 oz	150	6	2	28
Fruit On The Bottom Pineapple	6 oz	150	6	2	28
Fruit On The Bottom Raspberry	6 oz	150	6	2	28
La Creme Vanilla	4 oz	140	5	5	19
La Creme Mousse French Vanilla	1 (2.6 oz)	110	3	5	14
Light & Fit 0% Fat Plus Vanilla	4 oz	50	3	0	10
Light & Fit Carb & Sugar Control Blueberries 'N Cream	4 oz	60	5	3	3
Light & Fit Nonfat Cherry Vanilla	6 oz	60	5	0	11
Light & Fit Nonfat Lemon Chiffon	6 oz	60	5	0	10
Light & Fit Nonfat Raspberry	6 oz	60	5	0	11
Light & Fit Nonfat White Chocolate Raspberry	6 oz	90	5	0	10

FOOD	PORTION	CALS	PROT	FAT	CARB
Fiber One					
Creamy Nonfat Vanilla	1 pkg (4 oz)	80	4	0	19
Friendship					
Plain	1 cup	150	12	3	18
Horizon Organic					
Fat Free Peach	1 pkg (6 oz)	140	7	0	27
Fat Free Vanilla	1 cup	180	9	0	33
Kids Strawberry	1 pkg (4 oz)	110	4	1	20
Lowfat Blended Blueberry	1 pkg (6 oz)	160	7	2	30
Tube Lowfat Blueberry	1 (2 oz)	70	2	1	12
Whole Milk Plain	1 cup	160	10	7	14
La Yogurt					
Lowfat Blueberries 'N' Cream	1 pkg (6 oz)	200	7	2	39
Lowfat Fruit On The Bottom Cherry	1 pkg (8 oz)	230	6	3	47
Lowfat Fruit On The Bottom Probiotic Peach	1 pkg (6 oz)	160	6	2	31
Lowfat Fruit On The Bottom Strawberry	1 pkg (8 oz)	220	9	2	43
Lowfat Peaches 'N' Cream	1 pkg (6 oz)	200	7	2	39
Lowfat Pina Colada	1 pkg (6 oz)	160	5	2	30
Lowfat Probiotic Pina Colada	1 pkg (6 oz)	160	5	2	30
Lowfat Probiotic Plain	1 pkg (6 oz)	100	9	2	12
Lowfat Probiotic Vanilla	1 pkg (6 oz)	150	8	2	26
Lowfat Vanilla 'N' Cream	1 pkg (6 oz)	200	7	2	39
Nonfat Banana Cream	1 pkg (6 oz)	100	6	0	18
Nonfat Probiotic Cherry	1 pkg (6 oz)	100	6	0	17
Nonfat Probiotic Peach	1 pkg (6 oz)	90	6	0	16
Nonfat Probiotic Raspberry	1 pkg (6 oz)	90	6	0	15
Nonfat Probiotic Vanilla	1 pkg (6 oz)	90	6	0	15
Sabor Latino Lowfat Dulce De Leche	1 pkg (6 oz)	190	7	2	36
Sabor Latino Lowfat Guava	1 pkg (6 oz)	190	7	2	37
Sabor Latino Lowfat Horchata	1 pkg (6 oz)	210	7	2	41
Sabor Latino Lowfat Papaya	1 pkg (6 oz)	190	7	2	37
Land O' Lakes					
Strawberry Light	1 pkg (8 oz)	80	8	0	38
Strawberry Lowfat	1 pkg (8 oz)	190	8	2	36
Nancy's					
Lowfat Maple	1 pkg (8 oz)	180	10	3	26

FOOD	PORTION	CALS	PROT	FAT	CARB
Lowfat Plain	1 pkg (8 oz)	150	11	3	16
Lowfat Vanilla	1 pkg (8 oz)	140	10	3	15
Nonfat Fruit On The Top Cherry	1 pkg (8 oz)	140	10	1	25
Nonfat Plain	1 pkg (8 oz)	120	12	0	17
Nonfat Vanilla	1 pkg (8 oz)	220	12	0	40
Organic Soy Kiwi Lime	1 pkg (8 oz)	160	5	3	31
Organic Soy Plain	1 pkg (8 oz)	150	5	3	25
Organic Soy Vanilla	1 pkg (8 oz)	120	4	3	19
Whole Milk Fruit On The Top Peach	1 pkg (8 oz)	220	8	5	38
Whole Milk Honey	1 pkg (8 oz)	170	10	8	17
Oikos					
Organic Vanilla	1 pkg (5.3 oz)	110	15	0	12
Organic Honey	1 pkg (5.3 oz)	120	13	0	18
Organic Plain	1 pkg (5.3 oz)	90	15	0	6
Rachel's					
Essence Berry Jasmine w/ Zinc	1 pkg (6 oz)	160	8	3	28
Essence Plum Honey Lavender	1 pkg (6 oz)	160	8	3	28
Essence Pomegranate Acai	1 pkg (6 oz)	170	8	3	29
Exotic Kiwi Passion Fruit Lime	1 pkg (6 oz)	160	8	3	28
Exotic Orange Strawberry Mango	1 pkg (6 oz)	160	8	3	28
Exotic Pomegranate Blueberry	1 pkg (6 oz)	170	8	3	29
Siggi's					
Icelandic Skyr Vanilla 0% Milkfat	1 pkg (6 oz)	120	16	0	12
Silk					
Soy Blueberry	1 pkg (6 oz)	150	4	2	29
Soy Key Lime	1 pkg (6 oz)	150	4	2	30
Soy Plain	1 cup (8 oz)	150	6	4	22
Soy Vanilla	1 pkg (6 oz)	150	5	3	25
Strawberry	1 pkg (6 oz)	160	4	2	31
SoDelicious					
Coconut Milk Plain	1 pkg (6 oz)	130	1	7	16
Coconut Milk Vanilla	1 pkg (6 oz)	150	1	6	22
Dairy Free Cinnamon Bun	1 pkg (6 oz)	160	6	3	29
Dairy Free Raspberry	1 pkg (6 oz)	150	6	3	29
Straus					
Organic Maple Nonfat	1 pkg (8 oz)	170	12	0	30
Organic Maple Whole Milk	1 pkg (8 oz)	210	10	6	28

FOOD	PORTION	CALS	PROT	FAT	CARB
Organic Plain Lowfat	1 pkg (8 oz)	150	14	2	21
Organic Plain Nonfat	1 pkg (8 oz)	110	12	0	16
Organic Plain Whole Milk	1 pkg (8 oz)	160	10	7	13
The Greek Gods					
Honey	1 pkg (6 oz)	250	6	14	23
Plain Nonfat	1 pkg (6 oz)	60	6	0	10
Plain Traditional	1 pkg (4 oz)	130	4	11	5
Pomegranate	1 pkg (6 oz)	230	6	17	14
Vanilla Cinnamon Orange Reduced Fat	1 pkg (6 oz)	170	7	6	24
Wallaby					
Organic Banana Vanilla	1 pkg (6 oz)	150	6	3	25
Organic Lemon	1 pkg (6 oz)	150	6	3	25
Organic Maple	1 pkg (6 oz)	150	6	3	26
Organic Plain	1 cup	150	11	5	18
Organic Raspberry	1 pkg (6 oz)	150	7	3	25
Organic Vanilla	1 pkg (6 oz)	150	6	3	25
Organic Nonfat Mango Lime	1 pkg (6 oz)	140	7	0	28
Organic Nonfat Plain	1 cup	130	12	0	19
Organic Nonfat Vanilla Bean	1 pkg (6 oz)	140	7	0	28
WildWood					
Organic Soyogurt Low Fat Peach	1 pkg (6 oz)	160	5	3	29
Organic Soyogurt Low Fat Vanilla	1 pkg (6 oz)	160	5	3	30
Organic Soyogurt Plain Unsweetened	1 pkg (6 oz)	110	6	4	14
Yofarm					
YoSmooth Apricot	1 pkg	220	6	6	36
YoSmooth Peach	1 pkg	220	6	6	35
YoSmooth Raspberry	1 pkg	230	6	6	36
Yoplait					
Yo Plus All Flavors	1 pkg (4 oz)	110	4	2	21
YOGURT DRINKS (see also SMOOTHIES)					
lassi	7 oz	78	0	5	8
Dahlicious					
Lassi Green Tea	1 bottle	110	7	0	21
Lassi Mango	1 bottle	130	8	0	27
Lassi Plain	1 bottle	110	7	0	21

FOOD	PORTION	CALS	PROT	FAT	CARB
Dannon					
DanActive Plain	1 bottle (3.3 oz)	90	3	2	15
DanActive Vanilla	1 bottle (3.3 oz)	90	3	2	17
Danimals Rockin' Raspberry	1 bottle (3.1 oz)	70	2	1	15
Danimals Strawberry Explosion	1 bottle (3.1 oz)	70	2	1	15
Danimals Strikin' Strawberry Kiwi	1 bottle (3.1 oz)	70	2	1	15
Frusion Cherry Berry Blend	1 bottle (10 oz)	260	8	4	50
Frusion Pina Colada	1 bottle (10 oz)	260	8	4	50
Frusion Strawberry Blend	1 bottle (10 oz)	260	7	4	50
Light & Fit Carb & Sugar Control Berries 'N Cream	1 bottle (7 oz)	60	6	3	4
Light & Fit Smoothie Peach Passion	1 bottle (7 oz)	70	5	0	13
Light & Fit Smoothie Strawberry Banana	1 bottle (7 oz)	70	5	0	13
Lifeway					
Lassi Lowfat All Flavors	8 oz	174	14	2	25
Promise					
Activ All Flavors	1 bottle (3.5 oz)	70	1	4	9
Yo On The Go					
All Flavors	1 box (8 oz)	180	6	3	31
YOGURT FROZEN					
chocolate soft serve	1 cup	230	6	9	36
vanilla soft serve	1 cup	236	6	8	35
Dippin' Dots					
Strawberry Cheesecake	½ cup	100	4	0	21
Haagen-Dazs					
Lowfat Coffee	½ cup (3.7 oz)	200	8	5	31
Lowfat Tart Natural	½ cup (3.6 oz)	180	9	3	30
Lowfat Vanilla	½ cup (3.7 oz)	200	9	5	31
Lowfat Wildberry	½ cup (3.7 oz)	180	7	2	34
Turkey Hill					
Fudge Ripple	½ cup	100	3	0	21
Neapolitan	½ cup	90	3	0	19

FOOD	PORTION	CALS	PROT	FAT	CARB
Smoothie Orange Cream Swirl	½ cup	100	2	0	22
Smoothie Peach Mango	½ cup	90	2	0	21
Vanilla Bean	½ cup	100	3	0	19
ZUCCHINI					
baby raw	1 (0.5 oz)	3	tr	tr	1
canned italian style	1 cup	66	2	tr	16
fresh	1 sm (4.1 oz)	19	1	tr	4
pickled	¼ cup	16	tr	tr	4
raw sliced	1 cup	19	1	tr	4
sliced cooked w/o salt	1 cup	29	1	tr	7
C&W					
Yellow & Green	⅔ cup	20	1	0	3
TAKE-OUT					
breaded & fried	6 slices (3 oz)	141	2	11	10
indian pakora	1 serv	46	2	2	7
sticks breaded & fried	6 (2 oz)	90	1	7	6

PART TWO

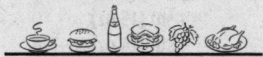

Restaurant Chains

PROTEIN POINT

**When Eating Out, Make
Smart Protein Choices**

Choose lean cuts of meat.

Choose baked or broiled chicken.

Don't order breaded fish.

*Order tofu, veggie burgers, or other meat
substitutes.*

Try an egg white omelet.

*Go easy on sauces and toppings; they contain
little protein but add on a lot of calories.*

FOOD	PORTION	CALS	PROT	FAT	CARB
A&W					
BEVERAGES					
Coke	1 sm (11 oz)	145	0	0	37
Diet Coke	1 sm (11 oz)	0	0	0	0
Diet Root Beer	1 sm (15 oz)	0	0	0	0
Float Diet Root Beer	1 sm (14 oz)	170	2	5	30
Float Root Beer	1 sm (14 oz)	330	2	5	70
Milkshake Chocolate	1 med	700	11	29	100
Milkshake Strawberry	1 med	670	11	29	90
Milkshake Vanilla	1 med	720	12	31	97
Root Beer	1 sm (15 oz)	220	0	0	57
DESSERTS					
Cone Vanilla	1 med	260	1	7	41
Freeze A&W Root Beer	1 med	480	25	10	89
Polar Swirl M&M	1 med	710	15	25	107
Polar Swirl Oreo	1 med	690	14	24	107
Polar Swirl Reese's	1 med	740	18	31	97
Sundae Caramel	1 med	340	8	9	57
Sundae Chocolate	1 med	320	8	8	53
Sundae Hot Fudge	1 med	350	8	11	54
Sundae Strawberry	1 med	300	7	8	47
Sundae Vanilla	1 med	310	7	8	52
MAIN MENU SELECTIONS					
Cheese Curds	1 serv	570	27	40	27
Cheese Dog	1	320	11	20	25
Cheeseburger Original Bacon	1	570	27	33	41
Cheeseburger Original Bacon Double	1	800	45	48	47
Cheeseburger Original Double	1	720	41	42	46
Chicken Strips	3	500	28	29	32
Chili Bowl	1 serv	190	12	6	22
Coney Chili Dog	1	310	13	18	24
Coney Chili Dog Cheese	1	350	13	21	27
Fries	1 lg	430	5	18	61
Fries Cheese	1 serv	380	4	19	50
Fries Chili	1 serv	370	8	16	49
Fries Chili & Cheese	1 serv	400	8	19	51
Hot Dog Plain	1	280	11	17	22
Onion Rings	1 serv	350	5	18	45
Papa Burger	1	720	41	42	46

FOOD	PORTION	CALS	PROT	FAT	CARB
Sandwich Crispy Chicken	1	590	31	29	54
Sandwich Grilled Chicken	1	440	31	19	54
SAUCES					
Dipping Sauce BBQ	1 serv (1 oz)	40	0	0	10
Dipping Sauce Honey Mustard	1 serv (1 oz)	100	0	6	12
Dipping Sauce Ranch	1 serv (1 oz)	160	0	17	2
Dipping Sauce Sweet & Sour	1 serv (1 oz)	45	0	0	12
ARBY'S					
BEVERAGES					
Dr. Pepper	1 (16 oz)	180	0	0	52
Jamocha Shake	1 reg	498	13	13	81
Pepsi	1 (16 oz)	130	0	0	34
Shake Chocolate	1 reg	507	13	13	83
Shake Orange Cream	1 (17 oz)	637	15	17	105
Shake Strawberry	1 reg	498	13	13	81
Shake Strawberry Banana Swirl	1 (17 oz)	567	15	16	87
Shake Vanilla	1 reg	437	13	13	66
Sierra Mist	1 (16 oz)	100	0	0	27
BREAKFAST SELECTIONS					
Biscuit	1	273	5	15	28
Biscuit Bacon	1	340	9	21	29
Biscuit Bacon Egg & Cheese	1	461	17	28	30
Biscuit Chicken	1	417	15	23	39
Biscuit Ham	1	316	13	17	29
Biscuit Ham Egg & Cheese	1	437	20	23	31
Biscuit Sausage	1	436	10	31	26
Biscuit Sausage Egg & Cheese	1	557	18	38	30
Biscuit Sausage Gravy	1	961	7	68	107
Breakfast Syrup	1 serv (1 oz)	78	0	0	20
Cinnamon Roll Original Gourmet	1	507	10	10	73
Croissant	1	190	3	10	21
Croissant Bacon & Egg	1	337	11	22	23
Croissant Bacon Egg & Cheese	1	378	14	22	23
Croissant Ham & Cheese	1	274	13	12	22
Croissant Ham Egg & Cheese	1	434	22	24	26
Croissant Sausage & Egg	1	433	12	32	23
Croissant Sausage Egg & Cheese	1	475	15	32	23
French Toastix	1 serv	312	6	13	44

FOOD	PORTION	CALS	PROT	FAT	CARB
Muffin Blueberry	1	320	4	12	49
Pecan Sticky Bun	1	688	12	22	91
Sourdough Bacon Egg & Cheese	1	437	20	16	40
Sourdough Egg & Cheese	1	392	17	12	40
Sourdough Ham Egg & Cheese	1	679	34	35	42
Sourdough Sausage Egg & Cheese	1	514	19	27	40
Twist Chocolate	1	250	4	12	34
Twist Cinnamon	1	260	3	14	33
Wrap Bacon Egg & Cheese	1	515	16	29	50
Wrap Ham Egg & Cheese	1	568	24	31	51
Wrap Sausage Egg & Cheese	1	689	21	45	50
CHILDREN'S MENU SELECTIONS					
Kids Meal Chicken Tenders	1 serv	289	19	14	21
Kids Meal Junior Roast Beef Sandwich	1	272	16	10	34
Market Fresh Mini Ham & Cheese Sandwich	1	228	14	5	28
Market Fresh Mini Turkey & Cheese Sandwich	1	235	17	4	28
DESSERTS					
Cookie Chocolate Chip	1 (1.6 oz)	202	2	10	26
Turnover Apple	1	377	4	16	65
Turnover Cherry	1	377	4	15	65
SALAD DRESSINGS AND SAUCES					
Arby's Sauce	1 serv (0.5 oz)	15	0	0	4
Dipping Sauce BBQ	1 pkg (1 oz)	40	0	0	11
Dipping Sauce Bronco Berry	1 serv (2 oz)	122	0	0	30
Dipping Sauce Buffalo	1 serv (1 oz)	10	0	1	2
Dipping Sauce Cool Ranch Sour Cream	1 serv (1.5 oz)	158	1	16	2
Dipping Sauce Honey Mustard	1 serv (1 oz)	129	0	12	6
Dressing Buttermilk Ranch	1 serv (2.2 oz)	325	1	34	4
Dressing Buttermilk Ranch Light	1 serv (2 oz)	112	1	6	13
Dressing Sante Fe Ranch	1 pkg (2.2 oz)	296	1	31	4
Horsey Sauce	1 pkg (0.5 oz)	62	0	5	3
Ketchup	1 pkg	13	0	0	3
Sauce Cheddar Cheese	1 serv (0.7 oz)	30	0	2	2
Sauce Spicy Three Pepper	1 serv (0.5 oz)	22	0	1	3
Sauce Tangy Southwest	1 serv (2 oz)	333	1	35	5

FOOD	PORTION	CALS	PROT	FAT	CARB
SALADS					
Chicken Club	1 serv	487	32	25	31
Martha's Vineyard	1 serv	277	26	8	24
Santa Fe	1 serv	477	29	21	42
SANDWICHES					
Arby's Melt	1	302	16	12	36
Beef'N Cheddar	1	445	22	21	44
Chicken Bacon & Swiss Crispy	1	624	36	29	52
Chicken Bacon & Swiss Grilled	1	462	38	17	38
Chicken Cordon Bleu Crispy	1	650	40	31	49
Chicken Cordon Bleu Grilled	1	488	42	19	35
Chicken Fillet Crispy	1	576	30	30	50
Chicken Fillet Grilled	1	414	32	17	36
Chicken Salad w/ Pecans	1	769	30	39	79
Corned Beef Reuben	1	606	34	33	55
Fish	1	543	21	25	61
French Dip	1	391	26	16	37
French Dip & Swiss	1	473	32	18	28
Ham & Swiss Melt	1	275	18	6	35
Roast Beef Cheddar	1	521	27	27	45
Roast Beef Regular	1	320	21	14	34
Roast Beef Super	1	398	21	19	40
Roast Beef Swiss	1	777	37	41	73
Roast Ham Swiss	1	705	36	31	75
Roast Turkey & Swiss	1	725	45	30	75
Roast Turkey Ranch & Bacon	1	834	49	38	75
Roast Turkey Reuben	1	611	44	30	56
Sourdough Melt Beef	1	355	18	14	40
Sourdough Melt Ham	1	380	19	13	39
Spicy Cajun Fish	1	603	21	32	61
Sub Toasted Classic Italian	1	828	37	46	69
Sub Toasted French Dip & Swiss	1	622	37	20	68
Sub Toasted Philly Beef	1	739	32	37	64
Sub Toasted Turkey Bacon Club	1	619	42	18	65
Swiss Melt	1	303	16	12	37
Ultimate BLT	1	779	23	45	75
Wrap Chicken Salad w/ Pecans	1	638	30	38	48
Wrap Corned Beef Reuben	1	577	38	29	42
Wrap Roast Turkey Ranch & Bacon	1	700	49	37	44

FOOD	PORTION	CALS	PROT	FAT	CARB
Wrap Roast Turkey Reuben	1	581	48	27	43
Wrap Southwest Chicken	1	567	36	29	42
Wrap Ultimate BLT	1	648	23	44	45
SIDES					
Bites Jalapeno	5	305	5	21	29
Bites Loaded Potato	5	353	11	22	27
Cheddar Fries	1 med	465	6	28	51
Chicken Tenders	3 pieces	379	25	18	28
Croutons Cheese & Garlic	1 pkg	77	2	5	7
Curly Fries	1 sm	338	4	20	39
Curly Fries	1 lg	631	8	37	73
Fruit Cup	1 serv	35	0	0	9
Homestyle Fries	1 sm	302	3	20	44
Homestyle Fries	1 lg	566	6	37	82
Mozzarella Sticks	8 pieces	849	36	56	75
Onion Petals	1 reg	331	4	23	35
Popcorn Chicken	1 reg	365	24	18	27
Potato Cakes	2	246	2	18	26
Seasoned Tortilla Strips	1 serv	71	1	3	9

AU BON PAIN
BAKED SELECTIONS

FOOD	PORTION	CALS	PROT	FAT	CARB
Bagel Asiago Cheese	1	360	15	4	64
Bagel Cinnamon Raisin	1	320	11	1	67
Bagel Everything	1	350	13	5	64
Bagel Honey 9 Grain	1	330	13	2	68
Bagel Jalapeno Double Cheddar	1	350	17	10	55
Bagel Onion Dill	1	350	13	1	72
Bagel Plain	1	290	11	1	59
Bagel Poppy Seed	1	290	11	1	59
Bagel Sesame Seed	1	330	12	5	61
Baguette Artisan Honey Multigrain Salad Size	1 (3.5 oz)	240	8	3	47
Baguette Artisan Honey Multigrain Sandwich Size	1 (4.7 oz)	310	10	3	62
Baguette Artisan Salad Size	1 (3.5 oz)	210	7	1	44
Baguette Artisan Sandwich Size	1 (4.7 oz)	290	10	1	59
Blondie	1	330	7	19	61
Bread Artisan Multigrain	1 serv (4 oz)	260	9	3	51
Bread Artisan Sundried Tomato	1 serv (4 oz)	240	8	1	49
Bread Cheese	1 serv (4.8 oz)	290	14	8	55

FOOD	PORTION	CALS	PROT	FAT	CARB
Bread Country White	1 serv (4 oz)	240	6	1	50
Bread Bowl	1 (9.24 oz)	640	28	3	127
Bread Stick Rosemary Garlic	1 (2.3 oz)	200	6	5	33
Brownie Chocolate Chip	1	380	5	17	62
Brownie Hazelnut Mocha	1	430	6	21	58
Brownie Rocky Road	1	410	6	17	62
Ciabatta	1 sm	180	7	1	37
Cinnamon Roll	1	350	7	12	53
Cookie Chocolate Chip	1 (2 oz)	260	2	12	37
Cookie Confetti	1 (2.4 oz)	310	3	14	42
Cookie English Toffee	1 (2 oz)	210	2	11	26
Cookie Gingerbread	1 (2.7 oz)	300	4	9	50
Cookie Hazelnut Fudge	1 (2.25 oz)	290	4	16	34
Cookie Oatmeal Raisin	1 (2 oz)	230	3	8	36
Cookie Shortbread	1 (2.3 oz)	310	3	9	34
Creme De Fleur	1 serv	550	12	26	71
Croissant Almond	1	560	12	36	52
Croissant Apple	1	230	4	10	31
Croissant Chocolate	1	330	6	17	42
Croissant Plain	1 (2.8 oz)	260	5	15	28
Croissant Raspberry Cheese	1	330	7	16	41
Croissant Sweet Cheese	1	320	4	16	39
Danish Cherry	1	370	7	19	44
Danish Sweet Cheese	1	380	7	20	44
Focaccia	1 piece (4.4 oz)	310	11	4	57
Lahvash	1 (4 oz)	320	15	1	62
Macaroon Chocolate Dipped Cranberry Almond	1	320	4	16	42
Mini Loaf Bacon & Cheese	1 (4.8 oz)	540	13	31	50
Muffin Blueberry	1	510	9	19	76
Muffin Carrot Walnut	1	520	8	25	66
Muffin Corn	1	460	9	16	69
Muffin Cranberry Walnut	1	500	10	24	61
Muffin Double Chocolate Chunk	1	590	10	20	83
Muffin Pumpkin	1	490	9	17	75
Muffin Raisin Bran	1	410	10	9	74
Muffin Low Fat Triple Berry	1	290	5	2	61
Pastry Hazelnut Creme	1	540	10	34	50

FOOD	PORTION	CALS	PROT	FAT	CARB
Poundcake Cappuccino	1 slice (5.2 oz)	530	3	26	68
Poundcake Chocolate	1 slice (4.7 oz)	500	7	29	58
Poundcake Lemon	1 slice (4.9 oz)	520	5	27	64
Poundcake Marble	1 slice (4.7 oz)	490	6	27	59
Roll Pecan	1	630	10	32	80
Roll Soft	1 (4.7 oz)	410	11	11	65
Scone Cinnamon	1	430	9	24	48
Scone Orange	1	410	9	20	51
Shortbread Chocolate Dipped	1	350	3	20	38
Toasts Basil Pesto Cheese	3 pieces (2 oz)	140	5	2	26
Tulip Blueberry	1	370	4	20	44
Tulip Chocolate Raspberry	1	430	5	21	55
Tulip Key Lime	1	440	5	22	55
BEVERAGES					
Blast Caramel	1 med (16 oz)	540	6	17	104
Blast Coffee	1 med (16 oz)	440	8	21	71
Blast Mocha	1 med (16 oz)	440	7	17	80
Blast Vanilla	1 med (12 oz)	540	6	17	104
Caffe Americano	1 sm (12 oz)	5	0	0	1
Caffe Latte	1 sm (12 oz)	200	11	11	17
Cappuccino	1 sm (12 oz)	120	6	7	10
Caramel Macchiato	1 sm (12 oz)	350	10	10	53
Chai Latte	1 sm (12 oz)	290	11	11	38
Chocolate Milk	1 (12 oz)	320	10	9	54
Hot Chocolate	1 sm (12 oz)	350	12	11	58
Iced Caffe Latte	1 sm (12 oz)	110	6	6	19
Iced Caramel Macchiato	1 sm (12 oz)	290	7	7	49
Iced Chai Latte	1 sm (12 oz)	190	5	5	31
Iced Mocha Latte	1 sm (12 oz)	210	6	11	27
Iced Tea Peach	1 med (22 oz)	120	0	0	30
Iced Vanilla Latte	1 sm (12 oz)	240	5	5	44
Iced White Chocolate Latte	1 sm (12 oz)	250	5	11	35
Lemonade	1 med (22 oz)	300	0	0	72
Mocha Latte	1 sm (12 oz)	300	11	16	35
Orange Juice	1 (8 oz)	110	2	0	26
Smoothie Peach	1 med (16 oz)	310	4	1	69
Smoothie Strawberry	1 med (16 oz)	310	4	1	66
Vanilla Latte	1 sm (12 oz)	320	9	9	50
White Chocolate Latte	1 sm (12 oz)	310	9	14	41

FOOD	PORTION	CALS	PROT	FAT	CARB
MAIN MENU SELECTIONS					
Fruit Cup	1 sm (6 oz)	70	1	0	16
Harvest Rice Bowl Cajun Shrimp	1 (20 oz)	520	16	17	69
Harvest Rice Bowl Cajun Shrimp w/ Brown Rice	1 (20 oz)	560	14	20	73
Harvest Rice Bowl Mayan Chicken	1 (19.25 oz)	490	25	14	67
Harvest Rice Bowl Mayan Chicken w/ Brown Rice	1 (19.25 oz)	540	23	16	71
Harvest Rice Bowl Steak Teriyaki	1 (19.25 oz)	530	30	15	72
Harvest Rice Bowl Steak Teriyaki w/ Brown Rice	1 (19.25 oz)	570	28	18	76
Macaroni & Cheese	1 med (12 oz)	440	19	26	31
Stew Beef	1 med (12 oz)	300	18	16	25
Stew Chicken Vegetable	1 med (12 oz)	290	11	17	26
SALAD DRESSINGS AND SPREADS					
Artichoke Aioli	1 serv (1 oz)	130	1	14	1
Basil Pesto	1 serv (1 oz)	140	2	15	1
Chili Dijon	1 serv (1 oz)	120	1	12	3
Cream Cheese Honey Pecan	1 serv (2 oz)	120	4	10	5
Cream Cheese Honey Walnut	1 serv (2 oz)	140	3	9	12
Cream Cheese Lite	1 serv (2 oz)	120	4	9	5
Cream Cheese Plain	1 serv (2 oz)	170	3	16	4
Cream Cheese Strawberry	1 serv (2 oz)	180	3	15	9
Cream Cheese Sundried Tomato	1 serv (2 oz)	120	4	10	5
Cream Cheese Vegetable	1 serv (2 oz)	170	3	16	3
Dressing Balsamic Vinaigrette	1 serv (2.25 oz)	190	9	16	11
Dressing Blue Cheese	1 serv (1.75 oz)	230	2	24	2
Dressing Caesar	1 serv (2 oz)	280	2	28	4
Dressing Fat Free Raspberry Vinaigrette	1 serv (2.25 oz)	70	0	0	17
Dressing Light Honey Mustard	1 serv (2.25 oz)	180	1	11	21
Dressing Light Olive Oil Vinaigrette	1 serv (2.25 oz)	130	0	10	9

FOOD	PORTION	CALS	PROT	FAT	CARB
Dressing Light Ranch	1 serv (2.25 oz)	150	2	15	3
Dressing Thai Peanut	1 serv (2.25 oz)	230	5	13	24
Guacamole	1 serv (1 oz)	60	1	6	2
Honey Mustard	1 serv (2.5 oz)	210	1	13	23
Hummus Roasted Red Pepper	1 serv (2 oz)	80	2	5	6
Mayonnaise	1 serv (1 oz)	200	0	22	0
Mayonnaise Herb	1 serv (1 oz)	210	0	23	1
Mayonnaise Jalapeno	1 serv (1 oz)	140	2	15	0
Mayonnaise Tarragon Sauce	1 serv (2 oz)	420	0	45	2
Mustard	1 tsp	0	0	0	0
Spread Herb Bagel	1 serv (2 oz)	130	4	11	5
Spread Sundried Tomato	1 serv (0.53 oz)	70	1	6	4
SALADS					
Caesar Asiago	1 serv	210	11	12	18
Caesar Asiago Grilled Chicken	1 (8.5 oz)	340	29	13	19
Caesar Asiago Side	1 (3.2 oz)	120	6	6	12
Chef's	1 serv	230	22	14	7
Garden	1 (7 oz)	80	4	2	14
Garden Side	1 (3.6 oz)	50	2	1	10
Mediterranean Chicken	1 (9.75 oz)	330	24	16	12
Riviera	1 (9.5 oz)	260	7	7	46
Thai Peanut Chicken	1 (11 oz)	250	22	8	22
Tuna Garden	1 (10.5 oz)	350	21	25	14
Turkey Medallion Cobb	1 (11 oz)	340	27	19	15
Turkey Spinach Sonoma	1 (12.3 oz)	310	29	13	22
SANDWICHES					
Arizona Chicken	1 (12 oz)	750	49	29	61
Baguette Turkey & Swiss	1 (12.3 oz)	770	41	38	65
Baja Turkey	1 (13 oz)	700	41	32	61
Breakfast Asiago Bagel Prosciutto & Egg	1 (9.6 oz)	660	40	25	67
Breakfast Asiago Bagel Sausage Egg & Cheddar	1 (10.2 oz)	770	36	45	55
Breakfast Bagel & Bacon	1 (4.2 oz)	340	15	6	56
Breakfast Egg On A Bagel	1 (6.8 oz)	370	21	4	62
Breakfast Egg On A Bagel w/ Bacon	1 (7.2 oz)	410	25	8	58

FOOD	PORTION	CALS	PROT	FAT	CARB
Breakfast Egg On A Bagel w/ Bacon Cheese	1 (7.9 oz)	500	30	15	59
Breakfast Egg On A Bagel w/ Cheese	1 (7.6 oz)	450	26	10	62
Breakfast Onion Dill Bagel Smoked Salmon & Wasabi	1 (7.1 oz)	490	18	11	77
Caprese	1 (11.8 oz)	700	28	35	65
Chicken Mozzarella	1 (14.5 oz)	800	50	27	71
Chicken Pesto	1 (12.5 oz)	700	44	23	62
Chicken Tarragon	1 (11 oz)	720	40	29	61
Ciabatta Bacon & Egg Melt	1 (7 oz)	400	26	15	40
Ciabatta Ham & Cheddar	1 (12 oz)	650	40	20	80
Club Smoked Turkey	1 (11.6 oz)	780	43	43	56
Croissant Ham & Cheese	1 (4.2 oz)	350	14	18	34
Croissant Spinach & Cheese	1	250	8	14	25
Hot BBQ Chicken On Farmhouse Roll	1 (14.3 oz)	970	50	44	78
Hot Eggplant & Mozzarella	1 (12.4 oz)	710	26	37	68
Hot Steakhouse On Ciabatta	1 (13 oz)	800	43	41	70
Melt Tuna	1 (12.5 oz)	760	40	41	60
Melt Turkey	1 (12.2 oz)	890	45	47	70
Portobello & Goat Cheese	1 (10 oz)	610	18	33	61
Portobello Egg & Cheddar	1 (8.5 oz)	590	22	37	42
Prosciutto Mozzarella	1 (12.7 oz)	880	40	49	71
Spicy Tuna	1 (10.3 oz)	640	28	34	57
The Montana	1 (12.5 oz)	560	40	23	62
Turkey & Cranberry Chutney	1 (10.9 oz)	680	30	24	63
Wrap Chicken Caesar Asiago	1	700	42	25	69
Wrap Chopped Turkey Club	1 (12 oz)	660	35	27	70
Wrap Mediterranean	1 (12.8 oz)	670	24	28	80
Wrap Southwest Tuna	1 (14 oz)	900	46	51	72
Wrap Thai Peanut Chicken	1 (14.5 oz)	660	38	19	84
Wrap Turkey Spinach Sonoma	1 (12 oz)	630	35	19	80
Wrap Hot Cajun Shrimp	1 (14.9 oz)	700	20	24	95
Wrap Hot Mayan Chicken	1 (13.5 oz)	630	24	19	92
Wrap Hot Steak Teriyaki	1 (13.5 oz)	660	28	19	93
SOUPS					
Baked Stuffed Potato	1 med (12 oz)	350	9	21	30
Broccoli Cheddar	1 med (12 oz)	310	11	21	20
Carrot Ginger	1 med (12 oz)	130	7	5	21

FOOD	PORTION	CALS	PROT	FAT	CARB
Chicken Florentine	1 med (12 oz)	240	8	13	25
Chicken & Dumplings	1 med (12 oz)	210	11	7	28
Chicken Noodle	1 med (12 oz)	130	9	3	20
Clam Chowder	1 med (12 oz)	320	9	18	27
Corn & Green Chili Bisque	1 med (12 oz)	250	5	14	29
Corn Chowder	1 med (12 oz)	350	9	18	40
Curried Rice & Lentil	1 med (12 oz)	150	9	2	30
French Moroccan Tomato Lentil	1 med (12 oz)	180	10	2	32
French Onion	1 med (12 oz)	130	4	5	19
Garden Vegetable	1 med (12 oz)	80	3	2	14
Harvest Pumpkin	1 med (12 oz)	190	8	10	26
Hearty Cabbage	1 med (12 oz)	110	4	5	14
Italian Wedding	1 med (12 oz)	170	8	7	10
Jamaican Black Bean	1 med (12 oz)	180	16	1	45
Mediterranean Pepper	1 med (12 oz)	100	5	3	18
Old Fashioned Tomato Rice	1 med (12 oz)	120	4	1	24
Pasta E Fagioli	1 med (12 oz)	240	11	8	36
Portuguese Kale	1 med (12 oz)	120	5	5	15
Potato Cheese	1 med (12 oz)	250	7	14	25
Potato Leek	1 med (12 oz)	300	5	20	28
Red Beans Italian Sausage & Rice	1 med (12 oz)	200	15	5	28
Southern Black Eyed Pea	1 med (12 oz)	180	12	2	31
Southwest Tortilla	1 med (12 oz)	200	4	11	24
Southwest Vegetable	1 med (12 oz)	160	4	3	17
Split Pea	1 med (12 oz)	210	18	2	42
Thai Coconut Curry	1 med (12 oz)	150	3	7	20
Tomato Basil Bisque	1 med (12 oz)	210	6	8	29
Tomato Cheddar	1 med (12 oz)	240	12	15	17
Tomato Florentine	1 med (12 oz)	120	5	3	19
Tuscan Vegetable	1 med (12 oz)	170	7	5	24
Vegetable Beef Barley	1 med (12 oz)	140	9	3	21
Vegetarian Chili	1 med (12 oz)	230	12	3	40
Vegetarian Lentil	1 med (12 oz)	140	10	2	32
Vegetarian Minestrone	1 med (12 oz)	120	5	2	21
Wild Mushroom Bisque	1 med (12 oz)	190	5	9	23
YOGURT					
Blueberry w/ Fruit	1 sm (7.5 oz)	220	6	2	44
Blueberry w/ Granola & Fruit	1 sm (8.5 oz)	310	10	6	56
Strawberry w/ Blueberries	1 sm (7.5 oz)	220	6	2	44

FOOD	PORTION	CALS	PROT	FAT	CARB
Strawberry w/ Granola & Blueberries	1 sm (8.5 oz)	310	10	6	56
Vanilla w/ Blueberries	1 sm (7.5 oz)	190	10	2	32
Vanilla w/ Granola & Blueberries	1 sm (8.5 oz)	310	10	6	56

AUNTIE ANNE'S
BEVERAGES

FOOD	PORTION	CALS	PROT	FAT	CARB
Dutch Ice Blue Raspberry	1 (14 oz)	165	0	0	38
Dutch Ice Grape	1 (14 oz)	180	0	0	43
Dutch Ice Kiwi Banana	1 (14 oz)	190	0	0	44
Dutch Ice Lemonade	1 (14 oz)	315	0	0	77
Dutch Ice Lemonade Strawberry	1 (14 oz)	330	0	0	81
Dutch Ice Mocha	1 (14 oz)	400	0	10	74
Dutch Ice Orange Creme	1 (14 oz)	280	0	0	64
Dutch Ice Pina Colada	1 (14 oz)	220	0	0	53
Dutch Ice Strawberry	1 (14 oz)	220	0	0	50
Dutch Ice Watermelon	1 (14 oz)	200	0	0	50
Dutch Ice Wild Cherry	1 (14 oz)	210	0	0	48
Dutch Latte Caramel	1 (14 oz)	350	4	15	49
Dutch Latte Coffee	1 (14 oz)	290	4	14	38
Dutch Latte Mocha	1 (14 oz)	160	5	17	47
Dutch Shake Chocolate	1 (14 oz)	580	10	27	75
Dutch Shake Coffee	1 (14 oz)	590	10	27	77
Dutch Shake Strawberry	1 (14 oz)	610	10	27	78
Dutch Shake Vanilla	1 (14 oz)	510	10	27	58
Dutch Smoothie Blue Raspberry	1 (14 oz)	230	3	8	34
Dutch Smoothie Grape	1 (14 oz)	230	3	8	36
Dutch Smoothie Kiwi Banana	1 (14 oz)	240	3	8	38
Dutch Smoothie Lemonade	1 (14 oz)	300	3	8	53
Dutch Smoothie Mocha	1 (14 oz)	330	3	13	50
Dutch Smoothie Orange Creme	1 (14 oz)	280	3	8	46
Dutch Smoothie Pina Colada	1 (14 oz)	260	3	8	44
Dutch Smoothie Strawberry	1 (14 oz)	250	3	8	40
Dutch Smoothie Wild Cherry	1 (14 oz)	250	3	8	41
Lemonade	1 (22 oz)	180	0	0	43
Lemonade Strawberry	1 (22 oz)	190	0	0	48

DIPPING SAUCES

FOOD	PORTION	CALS	PROT	FAT	CARB
Caramel Dip	1 serv (1.5 oz)	135	1	3	27

FOOD	PORTION	CALS	PROT	FAT	CARB
Cheese Sauce	1 serv (1.25 oz)	100	3	8	4
Cream Cheese Light	1 serv (1.25 oz)	70	3	6	1
Hot Salsa Cheese	1 serv (1.25 oz)	100	2	8	4
Marinara Sauce	1 serv (1.25 oz)	10	0	0	4
Sweet	1 serv (1.4 oz)	40	0	0	10
Sweet Mustard	1 serv (1.25 oz)	60	tr	2	8
PRETZELS					
Almond	1	400	9	8	72
Almond w/o Butter	1	350	9	2	72
Cinnamon Raisin w/o Butter	1	350	9	2	74
Cinnamon Sugar	1	450	8	9	83
Garlic	1	350	9	5	68
Garlic w/o Butter	1	320	9	1	66
Glazin' Raisin	1	510	11	4	107
Glazin' Raisin w/o Butter	1	470	11	1	104
Jalapeno	1	310	8	5	59
Jalapeno w/o Butter	1	270	8	1	58
Original	1	370	10	4	72
Original w/o Butter	1	340	10	1	72
Pretzel Dog	1	290	10	16	25
Sesame	1	410	12	12	64
Sesame w/o Butter	1	350	11	6	63
Sour Cream & Onion	1	340	9	5	66
Sour Cream & Onion w/o Butter	1	310	9	1	66
Stix	6	370	10	4	72
Stix w/o Butter	6	340	10	1	72
Whole Wheat	1	370	11	5	72
Whole Wheat w/o Butter	1	350	11	2	72

BABS DELI
BAGELS

FOOD	PORTION	CALS	PROT	FAT	CARB
Apple Cinnamon	1	332	12	2	70
Banana Nut	1	340	12	2	68
Blueberry	1	330	12	2	68
Blueberry Cobbler	1	392	10	8	70
Cheddar Herb	1	352	14	6	60
Cheddar Nacho	1	352	14	6	60
Chocolate Chip	1	348	12	2	68
Cinnamon Apple Pie	1	386	10	8	68

FOOD	PORTION	CALS	PROT	FAT	CARB
Cinnamon Bun	1	400	10	8	70
Cinnamon Danish	1	396	10	8	72
Cinnamon Raisin	1	336	12	2	70
Cinnamon Sugar	1	350	12	2	74
Cranberry Walnut	1	352	12	2	72
Egg	1	328	12	2	66
Everything	1	336	12	2	68
French Toast	1	372	12	4	74
Garlic	1	330	12	2	68
Honey Oat	1	320	12	2	68
Jalapeno	1	350	14	6	30
Onion	1	336	12	2	70
Plain	1	334	12	2	68
Poppy	1	344	12	2	68
Pumpernickel	1	332	12	2	68
Quiche Lorraine	1	354	16	8	54
Salt	1	324	12	2	66
Sesame	1	358	14	4	66
Spinach	1	356	14	2	72
Strawberry	1	342	12	2	72
Strawberry White Chocolate	1	364	12	4	72
Swiss Melt	1	368	18	8	58
Tomato Basil	1	322	12	2	66
Vegetable	1	318	12	2	66
Wheat	1	330	12	2	78
White Chocolate Swirl	1	396	10	8	70
BEVERAGES					
Americano	1 (16 oz)	12	0	0	2
Cafe Caramello	1 (16 oz)	212	2	8	31
Cappuccino 2% Milk	1 (16 oz)	195	13	7	20
Cappuccino Fat Free Milk	1 (16 oz)	133	12	1	18
Coffee Black Forest	1 (16 oz)	198	1	5	37
Icepresso Caramel Decadence	1 (16 oz)	300	6	12	42
Icepresso Classic	1 (16 oz)	300	8	5	52
Icepresso Java Chip	1 (16 oz)	360	6	18	48
Icepresso Latte	1 (16 oz)	300	6	12	42
Icepresso Mocha	1 (16 oz)	300	6	12	42
Icepresso Strawberry	1 (16 oz)	340	2	12	56
Italiano 2% Milk	1 (16 oz)	131	9	5	13
Italiano Fat Free Milk	1 (16 oz)	89	8	1	12

FOOD	PORTION	CALS	PROT	FAT	CARB
Jittery Monkey 2% Milk	1 (16 oz)	482	13	11	82
Jittery Monkey Fat Free Milk	1 (16 oz)	429	12	6	80
Latte 2% Milk	1 (16 oz)	212	14	7	22
Latte Cinnamon Toast 2% Milk	1 (16 oz)	299	13	7	45
Latte Cinnamon Toast Fat Free Milk	1 (16 oz)	240	11	1	44
Latte Creme Caramel 2% Milk	1 (16 oz)	303	13	7	47
Latte Creme Caramel Fat Free Milk	1 (16 oz)	244	11	1	45
Latte Fat Free Milk	1 (16 oz)	145	13	1	20
Latte Oregon Chai Tea 2% Milk	1 (16 oz)	274	9	5	48
Latte Oregon Chai Tea Fat Free Milk	1 (16 oz)	231	8	1	47
Latte Raspberry Cheesecake 2% Milk	1 (16 oz)	319	13	7	51
Latte Raspberry Cheesecake Fat Free Milk	1 (16 oz)	259	11	1	50
Latte Vanilla Creme 2% Milk	1 (16 oz)	275	13	7	39
Mocha Whipped Cream 2% Milk	1 (16 oz)	454	15	12	71
Mocha Whipped Cream Fat Free Milk	1 (16 oz)	392	14	6	70
Turtle Mocha Fat Free Milk	1 (16 oz)	522	12	12	90
MUFFINS					
My Favorite Banana Nut	2 mini	195	4	11	21
My Favorite Blueberry	2 mini	168	2	8	22
My Favorite Blueberry Cheesecake	2 mini	199	3	12	20
My Favorite Boston Cream Pie	2 mini	176	2	7	26
My Favorite Cherry Cheesecake	2 mini	170	2	10	19
My Favorite Chocolate Cheesecake	2 mini	202	2	12	22
My Favorite Chocolate Chip	2 mini	211	3	11	27
My Favorite Cinnamon Crumb Cake	2 mini	212	3	13	21
My Favorite Cinnamon Swirl Cheesecake	2 mini	214	2	11	28
My Favorite Deep Dish Apple	2 mini	177	2	8	25
My Favorite Double Chocolate	2 mini	210	2	9	28
My Favorite Fat Free Blueberry	2 mini	108	2	0	26

FOOD	PORTION	CALS	PROT	FAT	CARB
My Favorite Fat Free Cherry Pie	2 mini	109	2	0	26
My Favorite Fat Free Chocolate Marble	2 mini	125	2	0	29
My Favorite Fat Free Cinnamon Bun	2 mini	168	1	0	42
My Favorite Fat Free Raspberry Amaretto	2 mini	127	2	0	31
My Favorite Golden Corn Bread	2 mini	197	3	9	26
My Favorite Lemon Poppyseed	2 mini	201	3	10	25
My Favorite Pumpkin Spice	2 mini	181	2	8	26
SALADS					
Calypso Chicken	1 (13.6 oz)	637	20	49	34
Calypso Chicken w/ Lite Italian	1 (13.6 oz)	317	20	17	22
Chicken Caesar	1 (11.5 oz)	524	23	41	15
Chicken Caesar w/ Lite Italian	1 (11.5 oz)	268	20	12	17
Classic Caesar	1 (8.4 oz)	414	9	36	12
Classic Caesar Cafe	1 (4.3 oz)	225	5	19	9
Classic Ceasar w/ Lite Italian	1 (8.4 oz)	158	6	8	14
Garden Mix	1 (12.4 oz)	197	9	9	18
Garden Mix Cafe	1 (6.5 oz)	100	5	5	9
Grilled Chicken Club	1 (17.9 oz)	820	35	69	16
Grilled Chicken Club w/ Lite Italian	1 (17.9 oz)	500	35	31	18
Low Carb Tuna Salad Plate	1 serv (8.9 oz)	356	28	25	3
Mediterranean Bread	1 (18.8 oz)	973	30	73	52
Mediterranean Bread w/ Lite Italian	1 (18.8 oz)	626	30	32	55
SANDWICHES					
Breakfast BLT	1	704	22	31	83
Breakfast Lox & Cream Cheese	1	602	29	21	78
Breakfast Morning Classic	1	486	23	11	73
Breakfast Northern Omelette	1	699	31	31	73
Breakfast So Tradition w/ Bacon	1	566	27	18	73
Breakfast So Tradition w/ Ham	1	547	29	15	73
Breakfast So Tradition w/ Sausage	1	696	31	31	73
Build Your Own Ham	1	495	27	9	77
Build Your Own Roast Beef	1	480	29	6	77
Build Your Own Tuna	1	547	27	14	77
Build Your Own Turkey	1	465	32	3	77

FOOD	PORTION	CALS	PROT	FAT	CARB
Enchilada Bagellata	1	522	22	11	84
Gourmet Classic Turkey	1	552	32	14	74
Gourmet Holey Guacamole	1	476	33	5	76
Gourmet Kick-N Roast Beef	1	579	29	15	79
Gourmet Mediterranean Veg-Out	1	506	20	9	90
Overstuffed Classic Reuben	1	962	60	43	57
Overstuffed Corned Beef	1	661	43	19	77
Overstuffed Ham & Cheese	1	889	60	36	79
Overstuffed Manhattan Club	1	1122	69	40	120
Overstuffed Pastrami	1	661	43	19	77
Overstuffed TD Classic California	1	759	49	12	113
Overstuffed TD Classic Club	1	1110	61	43	122
Overstuffed TD Clubhouse	1	1079	69	37	117
Pizzaah Bruschetta	1 piece	162	7	12	7
Pizzaah Cheese	1 piece	189	10	7	23
Pizzaah Grilled Chicken Bruschetta	1 piece	343	17	21	24
Pizzaah Sausage	1 piece	211	11	17	6
Pizzaah Veggie	1 piece	238	12	10	32
Specialty All American Duo	1	752	46	28	78
Specialty Big Apple Club	1	797	41	37	75
Specialty Chicken Caesar	1	611	31	19	78
Specialty Roma Italian	1	764	40	34	76
Specialty Turkey Club	1	782	43	34	75
Toasted Cafe Chicken Melt	1	815	51	32	80
Toasted Deli Style Turkey	1	732	48	25	76
Toasted Roast Beef Parmesan Grinder	1	583	36	15	76
Toasted Spicy Italian Sub	1	770	40	34	77
Toasted Tuna Melt	1	641	32	23	75
SOUPS					
Beef Barley Mushroom	1 serv (8 oz)	100	6	3	12
Boston Clam Chowder	1 serv (8 oz)	210	2	13	20
Chicken & Wild Rice	1 serv (8 oz)	190	5	9	22
Chicken Gumbo	1 serv (8 oz)	130	8	3	19
Cream Of Potato	1 serv (8 oz)	240	4	14	24
Hearty Vegetable Beef	1 serv (8 oz)	100	5	1	16
New England Clam Chowder	1 serv (8 oz)	220	6	13	21

FOOD	PORTION	CALS	PROT	FAT	CARB
Split Pea w/ Ham	1 serv (8 oz)	90	5	2	15
Wisconsin Cheese	1 serv (8 oz)	210	8	11	20
SPREADS					
Cream Cheese	2 tbsp	90	1	9	2
Cream Cheese Cheddar Jalapeno	2 tbsp	90	1	8	2
Cream Cheese Garden Vegetable	2 tbsp	90	1	9	2
Cream Cheese Lite	2 tbsp	60	2	5	3
Cream Cheese Onion Chive	2 tbsp	80	1	8	2
Cream Cheese Strawberry	2 tbsp	90	1	5	5
Cream Cheese Whipped	2 tbsp	70	1	7	1
Cream Cheese Whipped Brown Sugar Cinnamon	2 tbsp	70	tr	5	5
Cream Cheese Whipped Reduced Fat Spring Veggie	2 tbsp	60	1	5	2
BAJA FRESH					
CHILDREN'S MENU SELECTIONS					
Kid's Mini Burrito Bean & Cheese	1 serv	540	18	14	84
Kid's Mini Burrito Bean & Cheese w/ Chicken	1 serv	590	28	15	84
Kid's Mini Quesadilla Cheese	1 serv	610	19	26	72
Kid's Mini Quesadilla Cheese w/ Chicken	1 serv	650	28	27	72
Kid's Taquitos Chicken	1 serv	630	18	33	60
MAIN MENU SELECTIONS					
Black Beans	1 serv	360	23	3	61
Burrito Baja Breaded Fish	1 serv	850	40	44	78
Burrito Baja Carnitas	1 serv	830	45	45	67
Burrito Baja Chicken	1 serv	790	52	38	65
Burrito Baja Mahi Mahi	1 serv	780	51	38	66
Burrito Baja Shrimp	1 serv	760	47	37	66
Burrito Baja Steak	1 serv	850	49	46	67
Burrito Bare Carnitas	1 serv	600	37	14	99
Burrito Bare Chicken	1 serv	640	45	7	97
Burrito Bare Steak	1 serv	700	41	15	99
Burrito Bare Veggie & Cheese	1 serv	580	19	10	101
Burrito Bean & Cheese Breaded Fish	1 serv	1030	54	41	108

FOOD	PORTION	CALS	PROT	FAT	CARB
Burrito Bean & Cheese Carnitas	1 serv	1010	59	42	98
Burrito Bean & Cheese Chicken	1 serv	970	67	35	96
Burrito Bean & Cheese Mahi Mahi	1 serv	960	65	35	96
Burrito Bean & Cheese No Meat	1 serv	840	39	33	96
Burrito Bean & Cheese Shrimp	1 serv	950	61	34	96
Burrito Bean & Cheese Steak	1 serv	1030	64	43	97
Burrito Dos Manos Breaded Fish	1 serv	890	39	33	107
Burrito Dos Manos Carnitas	1 serv	780	34	30	95
Burrito Dos Manos Chicken	1 serv	760	38	26	94
Burrito Dos Manos Mahi Mahi	1 serv	780	42	26	95
Burrito Dos Manos Shrimp	1 serv	780	41	26	95
Burrito Dos Manos Steak	1 serv	795	36	30	95
Burrito Grilled Veggie	1 serv	506	32	33	94
Burrito Mexicano Breaded Fish	1 serv	850	37	19	129
Burrito Mexicano Carnitas	1 serv	830	42	20	119
Burrito Mexicano Chicken	1 serv	790	50	13	117
Burrito Mexicano Mahi Mahi	1 serv	790	49	13	117
Burrito Mexicano Shrimp	1 serv	770	44	13	117
Burrito Mexicano Steak	1 serv	860	47	21	118
Burrito Ultimo Breaded Fish	1 serv	940	41	42	96
Burrito Ultimo Carnitas	1 serv	920	46	44	86
Burrito Ultimo Chicken	1 serv	880	54	36	84
Burrito Ultimo Mahi Mahi	1 serv	880	52	36	84
Burrito Ultimo Shrimp	1 serv	860	48	36	85
Burrito Ultimo Steak	1 serv	950	50	44	85
Chips & Guacamole	1 serv	1340	21	83	141
Chips & Salsa Baja	1 serv	810	13	37	98
Fajitas Corn Tortillas Breaded Fish	1 serv	1060	51	37	130
Fajitas Corn Tortillas Carnitas	1 serv	920	50	34	108
Fajitas Corn Tortillas Chicken	1 serv	860	61	24	105
Fajitas Corn Tortillas Mahi Mahi	1 serv	840	57	23	105
Fajitas Corn Tortillas Shrimp	1 serv	840	55	23	106
Fajitas Corn Tortillas Steak	1 serv	960	58	36	107
Fajitas Flour Tortillas Breaded Fish	1 serv	1340	59	46	172
Fajitas Flour Tortillas Carnitas	1 serv	1190	58	43	150
Fajitas Flour Tortillas Chicken	1 serv	1140	69	33	147

FOOD	PORTION	CALS	PROT	FAT	CARB
Fajitas Flour Tortillas Mahi Mahi	1 serv	1120	64	32	147
Fajitas Flour Tortillas Shrimp	1 serv	1120	62	32	148
Fajitas Flour Tortillas Steak	1 serv	960	58	36	170
Guacamole Side	1 (3 oz)	110	2	13	5
Nachos Breaded Fish	1 serv	2090	78	116	176
Nachos Carnitas	1 serv	2060	83	117	166
Nachos Cheese	1 serv	1890	63	108	163
Nachos Chicken	1 serv	2020	91	110	164
Nachos Mahi Mahi	1 serv	2020	90	110	164
Nachos Shrimp	1 serv	2000	85	110	164
Nachos Steak	1 serv	2120	96	118	163
Pico De Gallo Side	1 serv (8 oz)	50	2	1	12
Pinto Beans	1 serv	320	19	1	56
Pronto Guacamole Side	1 serv (6 oz)	560	9	34	60
Quesadilla Breaded Fish	1 serv	1400	62	86	96
Quesadilla Carnitas	1 serv	1370	67	87	86
Quesadilla Cheese	1 serv	1200	47	78	84
Quesadilla Chicken	1 serv	1330	75	80	84
Quesadilla Mahi Mahi	1 serv	1330	73	79	84
Quesadilla Shrimp	1 serv	1310	69	79	84
Quesadilla Steak	1 serv	1430	80	87	84
Quesadilla Veggie	1 serv	1260	48	78	96
Rice	1 serv	280	5	4	55
Rice & Beans Plate	1 serv	420	18	5	72
Salsa Baja Side	1 serv (8 oz)	70	2	3	7
Salsa Roja Side	1 serv (8 oz)	70	3	1	13
Salsa Verde Side	1 serv (8 oz)	50	2	0	11
Soup Tortilla w/ Chicken	1 serv (13.6 oz)	320	17	14	29
Soup Tortilla w/o Chicken	1 serv (12.4 oz)	270	8	14	29
Taco Grilled Mahi Mahi	1 serv	230	12	9	26
Taco Baja Breaded Fish	1 serv	250	8	13	27
Taco Baja Chicken	1 serv	210	12	5	28
Taco Baja Shrimp	1 serv	200	11	5	28
Taco Baja Steak	1 serv	230	11	8	28
Taco Soft Breaded Fish	1 serv	240	10	11	23
Taco Soft Carnitas	1 serv	250	13	12	21
Taco Soft Chicken	1 serv	230	16	10	20
Taco Soft Mahi Mahi	1 serv	240	17	10	20

FOOD	PORTION	CALS	PROT	FAT	CARB
Taco Soft Shrimp	1 serv	230	15	10	21
Taco Soft Steak	1 serv	260	15	13	21
Taquitos Chicken w/ Beans	3	780	39	40	68
Taquitos Chicken w/ Rice	3	740	30	40	66
Veggie Mix	1 serv	110	3	0	24
SALAD DRESSINGS					
Chipotle Vinaigrette	1 serv (2.5 oz)	110	0	9	0
Fat Free Salsa Verde	1 serv (2.5 oz)	15	0	0	3
Olive Oil Vinaigrette	1 serv (2.5 oz)	290	0	31	2
Ranch	1 serv (2.5 oz)	260	2	26	4
SALADS					
Baja Ensalada Chicken	1 serv	310	46	7	18
Baja Ensalada Shrimp	1 serv	230	28	6	18
Baja Ensalada Steak	1 serv	450	54	18	18
Chipotle w/ Carnitas	1 serv	640	38	30	56
Chipotle w/ Chicken	1 serv	590	47	22	54
Chipotle w/ Steak	1 serv	700	54	31	54
Side By Side Carnitas	1 serv	570	46	40	16
Side By Side Chicken	1 serv	500	60	27	12
Side By Side Steak	1 serv	620	55	42	14
Side Salad	1 (6.5 oz)	130	5	6	16
Tostada Breaded Fish	1 serv	1200	47	61	111
Tostada Carnitas	1 serv	1180	52	62	100
Tostada Chicken	1 serv	1140	60	55	98
Tostada Mahi Mahi	1 serv	1130	59	55	99
Tostada No Meat	1 serv	1010	32	53	98
Tostada Shrimp	1 serv	1120	55	55	99
Tostada Steak	1 serv	1230	65	63	98

BASKIN-ROBBINS

BEVERAGES

FOOD	PORTION	CALS	PROT	FAT	CARB
Cappuccino Blast w/ Whipped Cream	1 sm (16 oz)	330	6	14	48
Shake Chocolate Chip	1 sm (16 oz)	660	14	32	78
Shake Chocolate Chip Cookie Dough	1 sm (16 oz)	750	14	31	99
Shake Mint Chocolate Chip	1 sm (16 oz)	680	14	33	83
Shake Vanilla	1 sm (16 oz)	670	13	33	80
FROZEN YOGURT					
Cherries Jubilee	1 scoop (4 oz)	240	4	12	30
Vanilla Fat Free	1 scoop (4 oz)	150	6	0	32

FOOD	PORTION	CALS	PROT	FAT	CARB
ICE CREAM					
Butter Almond Crunch Reduced Fat No Sugar Added	1 scoop (4 oz)	220	7	11	31
Butter Pecan	1 scoop (4 oz)	280	5	18	24
Cabana Berry Banana Reduced Fat No Sugar Added	1 scoop (4 oz)	150	4	6	27
Chocolate	1 scoop (4 oz)	260	5	14	33
Chocolate Chip	1 scoop (4 oz)	270	5	16	28
Chocolate Chip Cookie Dough	1 scoop (4 oz)	310	5	15	36
Chocolate Overload Reduced Fat No Sugar Added	1 scoop (4 oz)	190	6	8	37
Gold Medal Ribbon	1 scoop (4 oz)	260	5	13	34
Mint Chocolate Chip	1 scoop (4 oz)	270	5	16	28
Nutty Coconut	1 scoop (4 oz)	300	6	20	28
Oreo Cookies 'N Cream	1 scoop (4 oz)	280	5	15	32
Peanut Butter 'N Chocolate	1 scoop (4 oz)	320	7	20	31
Pistachio Almond	1 scoop (4 oz)	290	7	19	25
Pralines 'N Cream	1 scoop (4 oz)	280	5	14	35
Reese's Peanut Butter Cup	1 scoop (4 oz)	300	6	18	31
Rocky Road	1 scoop (4 oz)	290	5	15	36
Sundae Caramel Soft Serve	1 (10 oz)	580	13	21	89
Sundae Hot Fudge Soft Serve	1 (10 oz)	610	14	25	86
Sundae Strawberry Soft Serve	1 (10 oz)	450	12	18	59
Tax Crunch	1 scoop (4 oz)	330	5	20	32
Vanilla	1 scoop (4 oz)	260	4	16	26
Vanilla Soft Serve	1 serv (6 oz)	280	8	11	37
Very Berry Strawberry	1 scoop (4 oz)	320	4	11	28
ICES					
Sherbet Rainbow	1 scoop (4 oz)	160	1	2	34
Sorbet Lemon	1 scoop (4 oz)	130	0	0	33
Sorbet Mango	1 scoop (4 oz)	120	0	0	32
Sorbet Strawberry	1 scoop (4 oz)	130	0	0	34
BEAR ROCK CAFE					
SANDWICHES					
Colorado Turkey Club	1	855	38	37	95
Coop's Chicken Salad Croissant	1	439	24	31	46
Garden Grill Ciabatta	1	406	12	25	55
Giant Panda Wrap	1	556	31	23	68
Hoot Owl	1	641	34	42	32
Rising Sunflower	1	596	35	35	35

FOOD	PORTION	CALS	PROT	FAT	CARB
Roast Turkey & Bacon	1	522	32	30	31
Rockslide Focaccia	1	958	43	62	57
The Moose	1	976	54	54	64

BEN & JERRY'S
FROZEN YOGURT

Low Fat Cherry Garcia	½ cup	170	4	3	32
Low Fat Chocolate Fudge Brownie	½ cup	190	5	3	35
Low Fat Half Baked	½ cup	190	5	3	35
Phish Food	½ cup	220	4	5	41

ICE CREAM

Bar Cherry Garcia	1	270	4	19	29
Bar Half Baked	1	340	5	16	46
Bar Vanilla	1	300	4	20	26
Bar Vanilla Almond	1	340	5	23	30
Black & Tan	½ cup	230	4	13	24
Brownie Batter	½ cup	310	5	18	32
Butter Pecan	½ cup	280	4	21	20
Cherry Garcia	½ cup	250	4	14	26
Chocolate	½ cup	260	4	16	25
Chocolate Chip Cookie Dough	½ cup	270	4	15	32
Chocolate Fudge Brownie	½ cup	260	5	13	32
Chubby Hubby	½ cup	330	7	20	31
Chunky Monkey	½ cup	300	5	18	30
Coffee	½ cup	240	4	15	21
Coffee Heath Bar Crunch	½ cup	290	4	18	29
Dave Matthews Band Magic Brownies	½ cup	250	4	13	29
Dublin Mudslide	½ cup	270	4	16	28
Everything But The	½ cup	310	5	19	30
Fossil Fuel	½ cup	280	4	17	30
Fudge Central	½ cup	300	4	18	31
Half Baked	½ cup	280	5	14	34
In A Crunch	½ cup	350	6	23	30
Karamel Sutra	½ cup	280	4	15	32
Marsha Marsha Marshmallow	½ cup	300	4	17	33
Mint Chocolate Cookie	½ cup	260	4	16	26
Neapolitan Dynamite	½ cup	250	4	13	29
New York Super Fudge Chunk	½ cup	310	5	20	29
Oatmeal Cookie Chunk	½ cup	270	4	15	31

FOOD	PORTION	CALS	PROT	FAT	CARB
Organic Chocolate Fudge Brownie	½ cup	270	4	13	30
Organic Strawberry	½ cup	210	3	12	21
Organic Sweet Cream & Cookies	½ cup	250	4	15	24
Organic Vanilla	½ cup	220	3	14	18
Peanut Butter Cup	½ cup	360	7	26	27
Phish Food	½ cup	280	4	13	37
Pistachio Pistachio	½ cup	260	5	17	21
Sandwich Wich Ice Cream Cookie	1	350	4	18	45
Strawberry	½ cup	230	4	13	26
The Godfather	½ cup	270	4	14	32
Turtle Soup	½ cup	280	4	15	30
Uncanny Cashew	½ cup	290	4	19	27
Vanilla Caramel Fudge	½ cup	280	4	15	31
Vanilla Heath Bar Crunch	½ cup	290	4	18	29
Vermonty Python	½ cup	310	4	19	30
SORBETS					
Berried Treasure	½ cup	110	0	0	29
Jamaican Me Crazy	½ cup	130	0	0	33
Strawberry Kiwi Swirl	½ cup	110	0	0	28

BILLY'S BURGER HUT

FOOD	PORTION	CALS	PROT	FAT	CARB
BEVERAGES					
Shake Chocolate	1 (20 oz)	420	9	10	63
Shake Vanilla	1 (20 oz)	320	8	10	49
MAIN MENU SELECTIONS					
Big Billy's Roast Beef Sub	1	843	51	54	62
Billyburger	1	426	20	22	35
Billyburger w/ Cheese	1	498	23	35	35
Billy's Best Red Potato Salad	1 serv	190	2	9	12
Billy's Biggest Burger ½ Pounder w/ Everything	1	852	70	58	61
Billy's Famous 7 Layer Salad	1 serv	558	10	49	18
Billy's Seafood Sandwich	1	399	21	18	43
Caesar Side Salad	1 serv	360	11	28	12
Chili w/ Cheese & Onion	1 serv	380	33	12	35
Cowboy Cobb Salad	1 serv	735	29	45	25
Cowboy Coleslaw	1 serv	180	1	9	11
French Fries	1 reg	230	5	12	25

FOOD	PORTION	CALS	PROT	FAT	CARB
Onion Rings	1 serv	250	2	10	37
Super Billy Burger w/ Bacon	1	663	35	41	39

BLIMPIE
DESSERTS

FOOD	PORTION	CALS	PROT	FAT	CARB
Cookie Chocolate Chunk	1 (1.5 oz)	200	2	10	25
Cookie Oatmeal Raisin	1 (1.5 oz)	180	2	7	27
Cookie Peanut Butter	1 (1.5 oz)	210	3	13	21
Cookie Sugar	1 (2.5 oz)	320	3	16	42
Cookie White Chocolate Macadamia Nut	1 (1.5 oz)	200	2	11	25

SALAD DRESSINGS AND SAUCES

FOOD	PORTION	CALS	PROT	FAT	CARB
Dressing Blue Cheese	1 serv (1.5 oz)	230	2	24	2
Dressing Buttermilk Ranch	1 serv (1.5 oz)	230	1	24	2
Dressing Buttermilk Ranch Light	1 serv (1.5 oz)	70	1	4	8
Dressing Creamy Caesar	1 serv (1.5 oz)	210	1	21	2
Dressing Creamy Italian	1 serv (1.5 oz)	180	0	18	4
Dressing Dijon Honey Mustard	1 serv (1.5 oz)	180	1	17	8
Dressing Italian Light	1 serv (1.5 oz)	20	0	1	2
Dressing Peppercorn	1 serv (1.5 oz)	240	1	26	1
Dressing Thousand Island	1 serv (1.5 oz)	210	0	20	6
Guacamole	1 serv (1 oz)	45	0	4	2
Italian Fat Free	1 serv (1.5 oz)	25	0	0	5
Mayonnaise	1 serv (1 oz)	200	0	22	0
Mustard Yellow Deli	1 serv (0.5 oz)	15	0	0	0
Oil Blend	1 serv (0.5 oz)	130	0	14	0
Sauce Blimpie Special	1 serv (0.5 oz)	40	0	5	0
Sauce Red Hot Original	1 serv (1 oz)	10	0	0	2

SALADS

FOOD	PORTION	CALS	PROT	FAT	CARB
Antipasto	1 serv (11.6 oz)	254	20	14	12
Buffalo Chicken	1 serv (7.7 oz)	220	25	9	10
Chicken Caesar	1 serv (9.4 oz)	190	25	8	6
Cole Slaw	1 side (4 oz)	160	1	9	20
Garden	1 serv (6.5 oz)	30	2	0	6
Macaroni	1 side (5 oz)	330	5	22	28
Northwest Potato	1 side (5 oz)	260	3	17	22
Potato	1 side (4.7 oz)	230	3	12	28
Tuna	1 serv (9.4 oz)	270	18	19	6
Ultimate Club	1 serv (10.1 oz)	280	23	14	10

FOOD	PORTION	CALS	PROT	FAT	CARB
SANDWICHES					
6 Inch Sub Blimpie Best	1 (10.4 oz)	450	24	17	49
6 Inch Sub Blimpie Best Super Stacked	1 (12.8 oz)	550	36	22	52
6 Inch Sub Blimpie Trio Super Stacked	1 (13.5 oz)	510	40	15	51
6 Inch Sub BLT	1 (7.2 oz)	430	15	22	43
6 Inch Sub BLT Super Stacked	1 (8.4 oz)	640	22	41	43
6 Inch Sub Chicken Cheddar Bacon Ranch	1 (12.1 oz)	600	36	29	48
6 Inch Sub Chicken Teriyaki	1 (8.7 oz)	450	33	12	52
6 Inch Sub Club	1 (10.2 oz)	410	23	13	49
6 Inch Sub Cuban	1 (8.2 oz)	410	29	11	43
6 Inch Sub French Dip	1 (13.4 oz)	410	30	11	46
6 Inch Sub Ham & Swiss	1 (10 oz)	420	23	14	49
6 Inch Sub Hot Pastrami	1 (7.2 oz)	430	30	16	42
6 Inch Sub Meatball	1 (10 oz)	580	27	31	50
6 Inch Sub Reuben	1 (9.2 oz)	530	34	20	52
6 Inch Sub Roast Beef & Provolone	1 (10.8 oz)	430	28	14	46
6 Inch Sub Roast Beef & Provolone On Wheat	1 (11.3 oz)	430	32	16	44
6 Inch Sub Super Stacked Hot Pastrami	1 (10.1 oz)	570	46	23	43
6 Inch Sub Tuna	1 (8.9 oz)	470	24	21	43
6 Inch Sub Turkey & Provolone	1 (10.8 oz)	410	24	13	49
6 Inch Sub Turkey & Provolone On Wheat	1 (11.3 oz)	420	27	14	47
6 Inch Sub VegiMax	1 (10.2 oz)	520	28	20	56
Blimpie Burger	1 (6 oz)	460	21	24	42
Blimpie Dog	1 (6.3 oz)	510	17	29	45
Ciabatta Buffalo Chicken	1 (11.3 oz)	540	31	23	49
Ciabatta French Dip	1 (13.8 oz)	430	31	11	49
Ciabatta Grilled Chicken Caesar	1 (10.1 oz)	580	34	20	62
Ciabatta Mediterranean	1 (10.1 oz)	450	26	8	65
Ciabatta Roast Beef Turkey & Cheddar	1 (10 oz)	520	25	24	51
Ciabatta Sicilian	1 (10 oz)	590	29	22	66
Ciabatta Spicy Chicken & Pepperoni	1 (10.1 oz)	710	33	34	65

FOOD	PORTION	CALS	PROT	FAT	CARB
Ciabatta Tuscan	1 (9.9 oz)	570	28	20	65
Ciabatta Ultimate Club	1 (7.4 oz)	520	27	24	47
Wrap Chicken Caesar	1 (9.7 oz)	220	30	8	56
Wrap Southwestern	1 (10 oz)	530	23	22	61
SOUPS					
Bean w/ Ham	1 serv (8.6 oz)	140	8	1	23
Chicken Noodle	1 serv (8.6 oz)	130	7	4	18
Chicken w/ White & Wild Rice	1 serv (8.6 oz)	250	14	10	15
Cream Of Broccoli w/ Cheese	1 serv (8.6 oz)	250	7	19	13
Cream Of Potato	1 serv (8.6 oz)	190	5	9	24
Garden Vegetable	1 serv (8.6 oz)	80	5	1	14
Grande Chili w/ Bean & Beef	1 serv (8.6 oz)	310	20	9	31
Tomato Basil w/ Raviolini	1 serv (8.6 oz)	110	4	1	22
Vegetable Beef	1 serv (8.6 oz)	80	4	2	13

BOB EVANS
BREAKFAST SELECTIONS

FOOD	PORTION	CALS	PROT	FAT	CARB
Bacon	1 piece	36	1	4	0
Benedict Ham & Cheese	1 serv	826	44	52	44
Country Benedict Sausage	1 serv	936	44	66	40
Country Benedict Spinach Bacon & Tomato	1 serv	729	30	48	42
Country Biscuit Breakfast	1 serv	659	24	45	40
Egg Hardcooked	1	60	6	4	1
Egg Over Easy	1	101	7	8	1
Egg Scrambled	1 serv	255	20	17	2
Egg Beaters	1 serv	173	28	12	3
French Toast	1 slice	131	3	2	13
French Toast Stuffed Plain	1 serv	599	11	20	53
Fruit & Yogurt Plate	1 serv	403	9	2	93
Grits	1 serv	178	3	7	28
Ham Smoked	1 slice	87	14	2	2
Hotcake Blueberry	1	328	6	9	55
Hotcake Buttermilk	1	318	6	9	53
Hotcake Cinnamon	1	417	6	15	66
Hotcake Multigrain	1	322	7	10	52
Mush	1 serv	79	1	3	11
Oatmeal	1 serv	172	6	3	32
Omelette Bacon & Cheese	1 serv	825	40	66	6
Omelette Border Scramble	1	756	42	58	15

FOOD	PORTION	CALS	PROT	FAT	CARB
Omelette Egg Beaters Bacon & Cheese	1 serv	615	57	47	7
Omelette Egg Beaters Border Scramble	1 serv	517	48	37	16
Omelette Egg Beaters Farmer's Market	1 serv	569	49	41	14
Omelette Egg Beaters Garden Harvest	1 serv	444	40	31	14
Omelette Egg Beaters Ham & Cheddar	1 serv	426	51	29	5
Omelette Egg Beaters Sausage & Cheddar	1 serv	502	49	40	4
Omelette Egg Beaters Three Cheese	1 serv	435	43	34	5
Omelette Farmer's Market	1	778	42	60	13
Omelette Garden Harvest	1 serv	654	33	50	13
Omelette Ham & Cheddar	1 serv	634	44	48	3
Omelette Sausage & Cheddar	1 serv	741	42	61	3
Omelette Three Cheese	1 serv	645	35	52	4
Omelette Western	1 serv	654	44	48	8
Pot Roast Hash	1 serv	652	38	39	34
Sausage Gravy Bowl	1 serv	268	7	17	21
Sausage Link	1	125	5	11	0
Skillet Sunshine	1 serv	842	37	60	36
Waffles Sweet Cream	1 serv	598	15	12	100
CHILDREN'S MENU SELECTIONS					
Fruit & Yogurt Dippers	1 serv	275	7	2	61
Hotcakes	1 serv	501	9	17	79
Kid's Macaroni & Cheese	1 serv	320	11	11	45
Kid's Pasta	1 serv	113	3	5	15
Mini Cheeseburgers	1 serv	306	12	19	21
Smiley Face Potatoes	1 serv	524	5	31	57
Sundae Fudge Blast	1 serv	244	3	11	33
Sundae Reese's I'm Smiling	1 serv	330	5	17	41
MAIN MENU SELECTIONS					
Seniors Chicken Parmesan	1 serv	522	38	26	33
Seniors Garden Vegetable Alfredo	1 serv	363	11	23	29
Seniors Garden Vegetable Alfredo Chicken	1 serv	452	26	26	29

FOOD	PORTION	CALS	PROT	FAT	CARB
Seniors Steak Tips & Noodles	1 serv	422	33	22	23
Seniors Stir-Fry Chicken	1 serv	368	21	13	44
SOUPS					
Bean	1 cup	144	10	3	19
Cheddar Baked Potato	1 cup	294	10	20	19
Sausage Chili	1 cup	268	16	17	18
Vegetable Beef	1 cup	135	6	5	17
BOJANGLES					
Biscuit	1	243	4	12	29
Biscuit Sandwich Bacon	1	290	8	17	26
Biscuit Sandwich Bacon Egg Cheese	1	550	17	42	27
Biscuit Sandwich Cajun Filet	1	454	20	21	46
Biscuit Sandwich Country Ham	1	270	9	15	26
Biscuit Sandwich Egg	1	400	8	30	26
Biscuit Sandwich Sausage	1	350	9	23	26
Biscuit Sandwich Smoked Sausage	1	380	10	26	27
Biscuit Sandwich Steak	1	649	14	49	37
Botato Rounds	1 serv	235	3	11	31
Buffalo Bites	1 serv	180	27	5	5
Cajun Pintos	1 serv	110	6	0	18
Cajun Spiced Breast	1 serv	278	18	17	12
Cajun Spiced Leg	1 serv	264	19	16	11
Cajun Spiced Thigh	1 serv	310	15	23	11
Cajun Spiced Wing	1 serv	355	21	25	11
Chicken Supremes	1 serv	337	21	16	26
Corn On The Cob	1 serv	140	5	2	34
Dirty Rice	1 serv	166	5	6	24
Green Beans	1 serv	25	0	0	5
Macaroni & Cheese	1 serv	198	7	14	12
Marinated Cole Slaw	1 serv	136	1	3	26
Potatoes w/o Gravy	1 serv	80	2	1	16
Sandwich Cajun Filet w/ Mayo	1	437	22	22	41
Sandwich Cajun Filet w/o Mayo	1	337	22	11	41
Sandwich Grilled Filet w/ Mayo	1	335	23	16	25
Sandwich Grilled Filet w/o Mayo	1	235	23	5	25
Seasoned Fries	1 serv	344	5	19	39
Southern Style Breast	1 serv	261	16	16	12

FOOD	PORTION	CALS	PROT	FAT	CARB
Southern Style Leg	1 serv	254	19	15	11
Southern Style Thigh	1 serv	308	16	21	14
Southern Style Wing	1 serv	337	17	21	19
Sweet Biscuit Bo Berry	1	320	4	18	37
Sweet Biscuit Cinnamon	1	320	4	18	37

BOSTON MARKET
DESSERTS

FOOD	PORTION	CALS	PROT	FAT	CARB
Apple Pie	1 slice	420	3	20	56
Brownie Chocolate Chip Fudge	1	580	9	23	81
Chocolate Cake	1 serv	600	5	32	75
Cookie Chocolate Chip	1	370	4	19	49
Cornbread	1 piece	180	2	5	31

MAIN MENU SELECTIONS

FOOD	PORTION	CALS	PROT	FAT	CARB
Broccoli w/ Garlic Butter	1 serv	80	3	6	6
Butternut Squash	1 serv	140	2	5	25
Carver Boston Chicken	1	700	44	29	68
Carver Boston Meatloaf	1	940	49	45	96
Carver Boston Sirloin Dip	1	1000	67	51	70
Carver Boston Turkey	1	770	66	27	68
Carver Boston Turkey Dip	1	770	66	27	67
Cinnamon Apples	1 serv	210	0	3	47
Cranberry Walnut Relish	1 serv	140	1	2	30
Creamed Spinach	1 serv	280	9	23	12
Dip Spinach Artichoke	1 serv	100	3	8	3
Family Meals Boneless Turkey Breast	1 serv (5 oz)	180	38	3	0
Family Meals Roasted Turkey	1 serv (5 oz)	180	38	3	0
Family Meals Rotisserie Chicken	1 serv (6 oz)	290	39	14	4
Family Meals Spiral Sliced Ham	1 serv (8 oz)	450	40	26	13
Family Meals Whole Turkey	1 serv (6.7 oz)	310	40	18	0
Fresh Vegetable Stuffing	1 serv	190	3	8	25
Garden Fresh Coleslaw	1 serv	170	2	9	21
Garlic Dill New Potatoes	1 serv	140	3	3	24
Green Bean Casserole	1 serv	60	2	2	9
Green Beans	1 serv	60	2	4	7
Individual Meal ¼ White Rotisserie Chicken	1 serv	290	45	11	4
Individual Meals 1 Thigh & 1 Drumstick	1 serv	300	32	17	6

FOOD	PORTION	CALS	PROT	FAT	CARB
Individual Meals ¼ White Rotisserie Chicken No Skin	1 serv	210	42	2	6
Individual Meals 3 Piece Dark	1 serv	380	45	19	7
Individual Meals 3 Piece Dark Skinless	1 serv	240	37	8	7
Individual Meals Award Winning Roasted Sirloin	1 serv	290	39	15	0
Individual Meals Meatloaf	1	480	29	33	23
Individual Meals Roasted Turkey	1 serv	180	38	3	0
Macaroni & Cheese	1 serv	330	14	12	39
Mashed Potatoes	1 serv	210	4	9	29
Pot Pie Pastry Topped Chicken	1	780	29	47	60
Poultry Gravy	1 serv (4 oz)	15	1	1	4
Seasonal Fresh Fruit Salad	1 serv	60	1	0	15
Spinach w/ Garlic Butter Sauce	1 serv	130	5	9	9
Squash Casserole	1 serv	320	9	24	21
Steamed Fresh Vegetables	1 serv	60	2	2	8
Sweet Corn	1 serv	170	6	4	37
Sweet Potato Casserole	1 serv	460	4	17	77
SALADS					
Entree Caesar	1	500	13	45	12
Entree Caesar w/o Dressing	1	140	11	8	8
Entree Market Chopped	1	580	10	48	30
Entree Market Chopped w/o Dressing	1	210	10	9	28
Side Caesar	1	400	5	40	7
Side Caesar w/o Dressing	1 serv	40	3	2	3
Side Market Chopped	1	440	4	43	12
Side Market Chopped w/o Dressing	1	80	3	4	10
SOUPS					
Chicken Noodle	1 serv	170	13	5	17
Chicken Tortilla w/ Toppings	1 serv	340	12	22	24
Tortilla Soup w/o Toppings	1 serv	80	5	5	7

BOSTON PIZZA
CHILDREN'S MENU SELECTIONS

Baked Salmon w/ Caesar Salad	1 serv	330	23	14	13
Bug N' Cheese	1 serv	500	21	13	73

FOOD	PORTION	CALS	PROT	FAT	CARB
Chicken Fingers w/ Fries	1 serv	390	26	19	28
Pizza Pint Size	1	390	19	7	64
Quesadilla Bacon Double Cheeseburger w/ Caesar Salad	1 serv	540	26	27	49
Reduced Size Fruit Cup	1 serv	80	0	0	18
Sandwich Grilled Chicken w/ Garden Greens	1 serv	600	10	38	45
Super Spaghetti	1 serv	440	12	13	68
Wrap Ham & Cheese w/ Fries	1 serv	550	16	28	60
DESSERTS					
Blondie Maple	1	850	7	43	111
Blondie Maple Bite Size	1	430	4	21	58
Brownie Chocolate Addiction	1	490	5	13	92
Brownie Chocolate Addiction Bite Size	1	200	2	7	35
Cheesecake New York	1 slice	620	11	33	80
Cheesecake Vanilla Bean	1 slice	770	9	52	70
Chocolate Explosion	1 serv	890	11	50	103
Tarte Au Sucre	1 serv	310	4	21	71
MAIN MENU SELECTIONS					
Angus Beef Sirloin Steak w/ Spaghetti	1 serv	1260	72	70	83
Baked 3 Cheese Penne	1 half order	460	21	14	62
Baked Seven Cheese Ravioli	1 half order	310	17	14	28
Baked Shrimp & Feta Penne	1 half order	480	28	19	54
Boston's Lasagne	1 half order	340	18	10	45
Boston's Smokey Mountain Spaghetti	1 order	1290	59	47	161
Chicken & Mushroom Fettuccini	1 half order	710	23	38	72
Chicken Parmesan w/ Seasonal Vegetables	1 serv	1060	47	74	55
Fries	1 serv	430	7	25	45
Garlic Mashed Potatoes	1 serv	730	6	60	42
Garlic Toast	1 slice	150	3	6	20
Homestyle Lasagna	1 order	590	39	33	37
Jambalaya Fettuccini	1 half order	860	33	51	71
Lemon Baked Salmon w/ Fries	1 serv	1150	50	74	61
Mama Meata Penne	1 half order	940	35	62	66

FOOD	PORTION	CALS	PROT	FAT	CARB
Mushroom Chicken w/ Garlic Mashed Potatoes	1 serv	1030	68	62	53
Pad Thai w/ Chicken	1 serv	2110	77	47	356
Pad Thai w/ Shrimp	1 serv	2090	77	45	358
Pollo Pomodoro Spaghetti	1 serv	520	26	14	73
Salmon Filet Lemon Baked	1 serv	430	51	13	33
Scallop & Prawn Fettuccini	1 half order	710	21	41	67
Seasoned Vegetables	1 serv	70	0	0	10
Shrimp Skewers Lime & Parmesan	1 serv	190	15	7	20
Sicilian Penne	1 half order	720	20	48	55
Sirloin Steak w/ Prawns & Fries	1 serv	1480	78	104	58
Slow Roasted Pork Back Ribs w/ Fries	1 serv	1680	68	123	78
Spaghetti w/ Alfredo Sauce	1 half order	440	15	11	70
Spaghetti w/ Bolognese	1 half order	400	15	5	73
Spaghetti w/ Creamy Tomato Sauce	1 half order	410	14	11	66
Spaghetti w/ Pomodoro Sauce	1 half order	450	13	14	68
Spicy Italian Penne	1 half order	980	30	61	81
Starter Baked Raviolo Bites	1 serv	450	20	22	45
Starter Basket Garlic Twist	1 serv	1140	32	39	165
Starter Basket Three Cheese Toast	1 serv	730	33	34	72
Starter Boston's Poutine	1 serv	740	23	45	53
Starter Bruschetta Sun Dried Tomato	1 serv	470	10	21	59
Starter Cactus Cuts Potatoes & Dip	1 serv	1150	15	89	72
Starter Chicken Fingers	1 serv	360	46	14	12
Starter Chicken Fingers Buffalo Style	1 serv	370	46	14	14
Starter Cracked Pepper Dry Ribs	1 serv	380	69	41	3
Starter Nachos Cactus w/ Cactus Dip	1 serv	1830	59	128	111
Starter Nachos Spicy Chicken w/ Sour Cream & Salsa	1 serv	1430	73	72	126
Starter Nachos Taco Beef w/ Sour Cream & Salsa	1 serv	1560	73	86	129

FOOD	PORTION	CALS	PROT	FAT	CARB
Starter Nachos w/ Sour Cream & Salsa	1 serv	1320	53	71	126
Starter Panzerotti Roll	1	820	41	32	94
Starter Pizza Bread Bandera w/ Santa Fe Ranch Dip	1 serv	960	32	54	89
Starter Pizza Bread w/o Sauce	1 serv	500	15	12	84
Starter Potato Skins	1 serv	650	22	46	39
Starter Quesadilla Oven Roasted Chicken	1 serv	900	43	39	96
Starter Quesadilla Southwest w/ Sour Cream & Salsa	1 serv	770	55	27	77
Starter Shrimp Stuffed Mushroom Caps	1 serv	490	23	41	12
Starter Team Platter w/ Dips & Sauces	1 serv	3030	153	205	144
Starter Thai Chicken Bites	1 serv	540	46	15	55
Starter Wings Breaded BBQ	1 serv	930	72	52	28
Starter Wings Breaded Honey Garlic	1 serv	940	72	52	31
Starter Wings Breaded Mild	1 serv	880	72	52	17
Starter Wings Breaded Teriyaki	1 serv	940	73	52	30
Starter Wings Breaded Thai	1 serv	1110	73	52	73
Starter Wings Oven Roasted BBQ	1 serv	670	54	42	19
Starter Wings Oven Roasted Honey Garlic	1 serv	700	54	42	26
Starter Wings Oven Roasted Hot	1 serv	620	53	42	9
Starter Wings Oven Roasted Teriyaki	1 serv	670	54	42	20
Starter Wings Oven Roasted Thai Chili	1 serv	770	52	40	50
The Ribber w/ Spaghetti	1 serv	970	49	43	96
Tortellini w/ Alfredo Sauce	1 half order	340	12	15	37
Tortellini w/ Bolognese	1 half order	300	13	9	40
Tortellini w/ Creamy Tomato Sauce	1 half order	310	11	14	33
Tortellini w/ Pomodoro Sauce	1 half order	340	10	18	35
Veal Parmesan w/ Spaghetti	1 serv	1020	44	72	106

FOOD	PORTION	CALS	PROT	FAT	CARB
PIZZA					
Bacon Double Cheeseburger Individual	1 pie	1140	73	54	94
Bacon Double Cheeseburger Slice	1 med	280	18	12	25
BBQ Chicken Individual	1 pie	730	37	24	93
BBQ Chicken Slice	1 med	190	10	6	25
Boston Royal Individual	1 pie	840	53	27	98
Boston Royal Slice	1 med	210	13	6	26
Californian Slice	1 med	280	11	15	24
Clubhouse Individual	1 pie	1040	44	56	94
Deluxe Individual	1 pie	850	55	29	94
Deluxe Slice	1 med	220	14	7	25
Great White North Slice	1 med	240	16	9	24
Hawaiian Individual	1 pie	780	49	20	101
Hawaiian Slice	1 med	210	13	5	27
Indy California	1 (11.3 oz)	440	16	12	69
La Quebecoise Individual	1 pie	770	42	27	93
La Quebecoise Slice	1 med	200	11	7	25
Meateor Individual	1 pie	950	63	37	91
Meateor Slice	1 med	260	17	10	25
Pepperoni Individual	1 pie	750	40	27	89
Pepperoni Slice	1 med	200	10	7	24
Pepperoni & Mushroom Individual	1 pie	750	41	27	90
Pepperoni & Mushroom Slice	1 med	200	10	7	24
Popeye Individual	1 pie	720	41	22	93
Popeye Slice	1 med	200	11	7	25
Rustic Italian Individual	1 pie	950	49	39	102
Rustic Italian Slice	1 med	260	13	10	28
Spicy Perogy Individual	1 pie	980	46	45	99
Spicy Perogy Slice	1 med	280	13	13	28
Szechuan Individual	1 pie	750	39	17	99
Szechuan Slice	1 med	200	10	4	27
Tandoori Individual	1 med	730	40	24	90
Tandoori Slice	1 med	200	11	6	25
Thai Chicken Individual	1 pie	840	45	28	108
Thai Chicken Slice	1 med	240	12	8	30
The Basic Individual	1 pie	620	34	16	88
The Basic Slice	1 med	160	9	4	24

FOOD	PORTION	CALS	PROT	FAT	CARB
Tropical Chicken Individual	1 pie	970	59	39	97
Tropical Chicken Slice	1 med	260	15	10	26
Tuscan Individual	1 pie	940	50	37	106
Tuscan Slice	1 med	250	13	10	29
Ultimate Pepperoni Individual	1 pie	870	46	37	89
Ultimate Pepperoni Slice	1 med	230	12	9	24
Vegetarian Individual	1 pie	680	37	16	101
Vegetarian Slice	1 med	180	9	4	26
Zorba The Greek Individual	1 pie	800	43	29	97
Zorba The Greek Slice	1 med	210	11	8	26
SALAD DRESSINGS AND TOPPINGS					
House Dressing	1 serv (2 oz)	270	1	28	4
Ketchup	1 serv (2 oz)	60	1	1	15
Salsa	1 serv (2 oz)	20	1	1	3
Sour Cream	1 serv (2 oz)	100	2	9	3
SALADS					
Chipotle Chicken & Bacon	1 serv	630	28	41	40
Crispy Chicken Pecan	1 serv	1100	62	86	25
Entree Caesar	1 serv	500	13	38	29
Entree Spinach	1 serv	450	13	41	9
Garden Greens w/ House Dressing	1 serv	310	3	29	13
Garden Greens w/ Low Fat Raspberry Vinagrette	1 serv	130	2	6	19
Side Caesar	1 serv	170	5	11	13
Starter Spinach	1 serv	250	9	22	6
Taco Salad Beef w/o Sour Cream & Salsa	1 serv	610	31	33	50
Taco Salad Chicken w/o Sour Cream & Salsa	1 serv	480	31	19	48
Thai Chicken Salad	1 serv	1060	61	40	117
SANDWICHES					
Beef Dip w/ Fries & Au Jus	1 serv	1340	77	62	118
Boston Cheesesteak w/ Caesar Salad & Au Jus	1 serv	1300	86	66	90
Boston Brute w/ Caesar Salad & Au Jus	1 serv	820	40	30	99
Buffalo Chicken w/ Fries	1 serv	1220	55	53	130
Chicken Parmesan w/ Fries	1 serv	1370	53	81	107

FOOD	PORTION	CALS	PROT	FAT	CARB
Ciabatta Chicken w/ Caesar Salad	1 serv	920	40	53	73
New York Steak w/ Garden Greens & Au Jus	1 serv	660	43	39	32
Stromboli Bacon Double Cheeseburger w/ Caesar Salad	1 serv	910	34	38	111
Stromboli Chicken Santa Fe w/ Caesar Salad	1 serv	750	33	22	106
Stromboli Smoked Ham & Chicken w/ Caesar Salad	1 serv	880	52	31	99
Wrap Thai Chicken	1	570	26	9	98
SOUPS					
Baked French Onion	1 serv	330	17	14	40
Clam Chowder	1 serv	260	9	14	18

BRUEGGER'S BAGELS
BAGELS

FOOD	PORTION	CALS	PROT	FAT	CARB
Asiago Parmesan	1	330	14	4	62
Baked Apple	1	370	12	3	77
Blueberry	1	330	11	2	67
Chocolate Chip	1	350	12	5	64
Cinnamon Sugar	1	330	11	2	69
Cranberry Orange	1	330	11	2	68
Everything	1	320	12	2	64
Garlic	1	320	12	2	65
Honey Grain	1	330	13	3	65
Jalapeno Bagel	1	320	12	2	64
Multi-Grain	1	350	12	4	68
Onion	1	320	12	2	64
Plain	1	320	12	2	64
Poppy	1	320	12	3	64
Pumpernickel	1	330	12	3	67
Pumpkin	1	330	11	2	68
Rosemary Olive Oil	1	350	12	7	64
Salt	1	320	12	2	64
Sesame	1	360	13	3	68
Sourdough	1	340	13	2	68
Square Asiago Parmesan	1	360	15	5	66
Square Everything	1	320	12	2	64
Square Plain	1	350	13	3	70
Square Sesame	1	360	13	3	68

FOOD	PORTION	CALS	PROT	FAT	CARB
Sun Dried Tomato	1	320	12	2	64
Whole Wheat	1	390	16	6	73
DESSERTS					
Brownie Chocolate Chunk	1	330	4	18	40
Cake Lemon Pound	1 slice	320	5	13	48
Cookie Chocolate Chip	1	500	5	22	71
Cookie Oatmeal Raisin	1	460	5	19	71
Cookie Peanut Butter	1	480	8	23	63
Cookie Triple Chocolate Chunk	1	560	6	28	71
Cookie White Chocolate Macadamia	1	580	6	31	70
Luscious Lemon Bar	1	300	3	16	36
Marshmallow Chew	1	280	2	6	55
Muffin Blueberry	1	450	8	19	64
Muffin Chocolate	1	460	6	24	57
Oreo Dream Bar	1	470	5	28	49
Pecan Chocolate Chunk	1 slice	310	3	19	32
Raspberry Sammies	1 slice	340	3	16	44
Seven Layer Bar	1	650	10	43	58
Toffee Almond Bar	1	400	4	19	53
SALADS					
Caesar w/ Dressing	1 serv	270	9	17	22
Tossed Chicken Caesar w/ Dressing	1 serv	370	27	20	23
Tossed Mandarin Medley	1 serv	340	8	17	36
Tossed Sesame Chicken	1 serv	480	22	28	30
SANDWICHES					
BLT w/ Mayo	1	570	20	23	72
Chicken Breast	1	660	47	11	87
Chicken Fajita	1	530	30	11	81
Chicken Salad w/ Mayo	1	630	28	26	73
Cranberry Gobbler	1	620	32	21	78
Cuban Chicken	1	680	44	25	74
Denver Egg	1	460	30	18	74
Egg Cheese	1	420	23	18	71
Egg Cheese Bacon	1	460	28	23	65
Egg Cheese Ham	1	460	31	18	73
Egg Cheese Sausage	1	640	32	38	72
Ham	1	460	27	7	76
Herby Turkey	1	560	30	14	78

FOOD	PORTION	CALS	PROT	FAT	CARB
Leonardo Da Veggie	1	480	21	12	74
Radishy Roast Beef	1	560	35	18	73
Roadhouse Chicken	1	710	50	19	84
Roast Beef	1	730	30	36	71
Santa Fe Turkey	1	490	30	9	75
Smoked Salmon	1	490	28	10	74
Softwich BLT w/ Mayo	1	600	22	25	73
Softwich Chicken Breast	1	630	47	11	81
Softwich Chicken Fajita	1	570	39	10	81
Softwich Chicken Salad	1	670	32	27	76
Softwich Cranberry Gobbler	1	730	40	28	80
Softwich Cuban Chicken	1	810	56	32	77
Softwich Garden Veggie	1	380	15	3	76
Softwich Ham	1	510	29	6	85
Softwich Herby Turkey	1	580	33	14	80
Softwich Hummus	1	540	20	13	85
Softwich Leonardo De Veggie	1	550	25	15	79
Softwich Mediterranean	1	790	30	33	90
Softwich Peanut Chicken	1	590	36	12	82
Softwich Radishy Roast Beef	1	670	43	26	75
Softwich Roadhouse Chicken	1	670	50	19	74
Softwich Roast Beef	1	750	33	40	72
Softwich Roasted Turkey	1	550	32	15	74
Softwich Smoked Salmon	1	520	30	11	76
Softwich Supreme Club w/o Mayo	1	880	55	39	79
Softwich Tuna Salad	1	720	26	34	76
Softwich Western Wheat	1	820	30	58	76
Supreme Club w/o Mayo	1	470	28	9	72
Tuna Salad	1	620	23	27	73
Turkey	1	510	26	14	70
Wrap Classic w/ Bacon	1	520	36	45	52
Wrap Classic w/ Ham	1	510	40	41	54
Wrap Classic w/ Sausage	1	660	38	60	52
Wrap Rio Grande Bacon	1	560	34	49	55
Wrap Rio Grande Ham	1	630	31	34	55
Wrap Rio Grande Sausage	1	510	27	47	53
Wrap Sesame Chicken Salad	1	770	31	36	80
Wrap Tossed Chicken Caesar	1	660	36	28	73

FOOD	PORTION	CALS	PROT	FAT	CARB
Wrap Tossed Mandarin Medley Salad	1	630	17	25	87
SOUPS					
Chicken Pot Pie	1 cup	250	10	19	12
Chicken Spaetzle	1 cup	120	9	5	12
Chicken Wild Rice	1 cup	260	2	19	16
Creamy Tomato	1 cup	150	5	9	16
Hearty Mushroom Barley	1 cup	110	5	2	18
Italian Wedding	1 cup	160	8	8	15
Minestrone	1 cup	120	7	2	21
Moroccan Stew	1 cup	140	4	3	26
New England Clam	1 cup	300	10	18	23
Sweet Potato Cheddar	1 cup	200	6	11	20
SPREADS					
Cream Cheese Bacon Scallion	1 scoop (1.5 oz)	140	3	12	5
Cream Cheese Cucumber Dill	1 scoop (1.5 oz)	140	3	13	3
Cream Cheese Garden Veggie	1 scoop (1.5 oz)	130	3	11	5
Cream Cheese Honey Walnut	1 scoop (1.5 oz)	150	3	12	8
Cream Cheese Jalapeno	1 scoop (1.5 oz)	140	3	13	4
Cream Cheese Light Garden Veggie	1 scoop (1.5 oz)	90	6	6	3
Cream Cheese Light Herb Garlic	1 scoop (1.5 oz)	100	6	6	4
Cream Cheese Light Plain	1 scoop (1.5 oz)	100	3	6	4
Cream Cheese Olive Pimento	1 scoop (1.5 oz)	140	3	13	3
Cream Cheese Onion & Chive	1 scoop (1.5 oz)	140	3	13	3
Cream Cheese Plain	1 scoop (1.5 oz)	130	3	11	6
Cream Cheese Pumpkin	1 scoop (1.5 oz)	120	3	11	4
Cream Cheese Strawberry	1 scoop (1.5 oz)	140	3	13	4

FOOD	PORTION	CALS	PROT	FAT	CARB
Cream Cheese Wildberry	1 scoop (1.5 oz)	140	3	12	5
Hummus	1 scoop (2 oz)	110	5	6	10

BURGER KING
BEVERAGES

FOOD	PORTION	CALS	PROT	FAT	CARB
Apple Juice	1 (6.67 oz)	90	0	0	23
BK Joe Regular	1 sm	5	1	0	1
BK Joe Turbo	1 sm (12 oz)	10	1	0	1
Chocolate Milk 1% Low Fat	1 (9 oz)	180	9	3	31
Coke Classic	1 sm (16 oz)	140	0	0	39
Diet Coke	1 sm (16 oz)	0	0	0	0
Dr Pepper	1 sm (16 oz)	140	0	0	39
Frozen Coke	1 sm (16 oz)	110	0	0	31
Iced Coffee Mocha BK Joe	1 (16 oz)	380	6	10	66
Iced Minute Maid Cherry	1 sm (16 oz)	110	0	0	31
Milk 1% Low Fat	1	110	8	3	13
Minute Maid Orange Juice	8 oz	140	2	0	33
Shake Chocolate	1 sm (16 oz)	470	8	14	75
Shake Oreo Sundae Chocolate	1 sm (16 oz)	680	9	24	105
Shake Oreo Sundae Strawberry	1 sm (16 oz)	660	9	23	103
Shake Oreo Sundae Vanilla	1 sm (16 oz)	610	9	24	87
Shake Strawberry	1 sm (16 oz)	460	7	14	73
Shake Vanilla	1 sm (16 oz)	400	8	15	57
Sprite	1 sm (16 oz)	140	0	0	39
Water Nestle Pure Life	1 bottle (16 oz)	0	0	0	0

BREAKFAST SELECTIONS

FOOD	PORTION	CALS	PROT	FAT	CARB
Biscuit Bacon Egg & Cheese	1	410	16	25	31
Biscuit Ham Egg & Cheese	1	390	16	22	31
Biscuit Sausage	1	390	12	26	28
Biscuit Sausage Egg & Cheese	1	530	20	37	31
Croissan'wich Bacon Egg & Cheese	1	340	15	20	26
Croissan'wich Double w/ Bacon Egg & Cheese	1	430	21	27	27
Croissan'wich Double w/ Ham Bacon Egg & Cheese	1	420	24	24	27
Croissan'wich Double w/ Ham Egg & Cheese	1	420	27	23	27
Croissan'wich Double w/ Ham Sausage Egg & Cheese	1	550	28	37	27

FOOD	PORTION	CALS	PROT	FAT	CARB
Croissan'wich Double w/ Sausage Bacon Egg & Cheese	1	550	25	39	27
Croissan'wich Double w/ Sausage Egg & Cheese	1	680	29	51	26
Croissan'wich Egg & Cheese	1	300	12	17	26
Croissan'wich Ham Egg & Cheese	1	340	18	18	26
Croissan'wich Sausage & Cheese	1	370	14	25	23
Croissan'wich Sausage Egg & Cheese	1	470	19	32	26
French Toast Sticks	3 pieces	240	4	13	26
Hash Browns	1 sm	260	2	17	25
Hash Browns	1 lg	620	5	40	60
Omelet Sandwich Enormous	1	730	37	45	44
Omelet Sandwich Ham	1	290	13	13	33
DESSERTS					
Cini-minis	1 serv	390	7	18	51
Dutch Apple Pie	1 serv	300	2	13	45
Hershey Sundae Pie	1	310	3	19	32
MAIN MENU SELECTIONS					
BK Chicken Fries	6 pieces	260	12	15	18
BK Stacker Double	1	610	34	39	32
BK Stacker Quad	1	1000	62	68	34
BK Stacker Triple	1	800	48	54	33
BK Veggie Burger	1	420	23	16	46
Cheeseburger	1	330	17	16	31
Cheeseburger Double	1	500	30	29	31
Chicken Sandwich Original	1	660	24	40	52
Chicken Sandwich Tendercrisp	1	790	33	44	68
Chicken Sandwich Tendergrill	1	510	37	19	49
Chicken Tenders	5 pieces	210	12	12	13
Chick'n Crisp Spicy Sandwich	1	480	15	31	36
Double Cheeseburger	1	410	25	21	30
French Fries No Salt Added	1 sm	230	2	13	26
French Fries Salted	1 sm	230	2	13	26
French Fries Salted	1 lg	500	5	28	57
Hamburger	1	290	15	12	30
Onion Rings	1 sm	140	2	7	18

FOOD	PORTION	CALS	PROT	FAT	CARB
Onion Rings	1 lg	440	6	22	53
Sandwich BK Big Fish	1	640	24	32	67
The Angus Steak Burger	1	640	33	33	55
Whopper	1	670	28	39	51
Whopper w/ Cheese	1	760	33	47	52
Whopper Double	1	900	47	57	51
Whopper Double w/ Cheese	1	990	52	64	52
Whopper Jr.	1	370	15	21	31
Whopper Jr. w/ Cheese	1	410	18	24	32
Whopper Triple	1	1130	67	74	51
Whopper Triple w/ Cheese	1	1230	71	82	52
SALAD DRESSINGS AND TOPPINGS					
Breakfast Syrup	1 serv (1 oz)	80	0	0	21
Croutons Garlic Parmesan	1 serv	60	1	2	9
Dipping Sauce Barbecue	1 serv (1 oz)	40	0	0	11
Dipping Sauce Honey Mustard	1 serv (1 oz)	90	0	6	8
Dipping Sauce Ranch	1 serv (1 oz)	140	1	15	1
Dipping Sauce Sweet And Sour	1 serv (1 oz)	40	0	0	11
Dressing Ken's Creamy Caesar	1 serv (2 oz)	210	3	21	4
Dressing Ken's Fat Free Ranch	1 serv (2 oz)	60	0	0	15
Dressing Ken's Honey Mustard	1 serv (2 oz)	270	1	23	15
Dressing Ken's Ranch	1 serv (2 oz)	190	1	20	2
Jam Grape	1 serv	30	0	0	7
Jam Strawberry	1 serv	30	0	0	7
Ketchup	1 pkg	10	0	0	3
Mayonnaise	1 pkg	80	0	9	1
SALADS					
Chicken Garden Tendercrisp	1	410	29	22	26
Chicken Garden Tendergrill w/o Dressing or Croutons	1	240	33	9	8
Side Garden w/o Dressing	1	15	1	0	3
BURGERVILLE					
BEVERAGES					
Barq's Root Beer	1 (20 oz)	180	0	0	49
Coca Cola	1 (20 oz)	161	0	0	44
Diet Coke	1 (20 oz)	0	0	0	0
Hot Chocolate Ghirardelli	1 (12 oz)	230	4	0	38
House Coffee	1 (10 oz)	5	0	0	1
Iced Tea	1 (20 oz)	0	0	0	0
Iced Tea Nestea Raspberry	1 (20 oz)	127	0	0	34

FOOD	PORTION	CALS	PROT	FAT	CARB
Lemonade Odwalla	1 (20 oz)	240	0	0	65
Milk 2%	1 (8 oz)	121	8	5	12
Orange Juice Odwalla	1 (10 oz)	138	3	0	31
Pibb Xtra	1 (20 oz)	163	0	0	42
Sprite	1 (20 oz)	158	0	0	42
BREAKFAST SELECTIONS					
Bagel	1	310	12	1	63
Bagel Bacon And Egg	1	490	23	16	64
Bagel Ham And Egg	1	490	28	13	65
Bagel Sausage And Egg	1	640	27	31	64
Breakfast Platter w/ Bacon	1 serv	730	25	49	55
Breakfast Platter w/ Ham	1 serv	725	30	46	56
Breakfast Platter w/ Sausage	1 serv	880	29	64	56
Hash Browns	1 serv	230	2	15	22
Toaster Biscuit	1	320	5	9	31
Toaster Biscuit Bacon And Egg	1	450	16	29	32
Toaster Biscuit Ham And Egg	1	440	21	26	33
Toaster Biscuit Sausage And Egg	1	600	20	44	32
DESSERTS					
Cone Vanilla	1	250	5	11	32
Cone YoCream Frozen Yogurt	1	190	4	0	39
Cookie Chocolate Chunk	1	320	4	14	48
Cookie Oatmeal Raisin	1	290	4	8	50
Cookie Sugar	1	305	3	15	39
Cookie White Chocolate Macadamia	1	340	4	16	46
Strawberry Shortcake	1 serv	440	6	15	72
Sundae Caramel	1	380	6	15	56
Sundae Fresh Strawberry	1	340	6	14	48
Sundae Hot Fudge	1	380	7	18	51
Sundae Triple Berry	1	340	6	14	46
Sundae YoCream Caramel	1	260	4	1	56
Sundae YoCream Hot Fudge	1	260	5	4	51
Sundae YoCream Strawberry	1	220	4	0	48
Sundae YoCream Triple Berry	1	200	4	0	43
MAIN MENU SELECTIONS					
Apple Slices	1 serv	29	0	0	9
Cheeseburger	1	350	14	19	29
Cheeseburger Colossal	1	520	30	30	31
Cheeseburger Double Beef	1	430	22	25	29

FOOD	PORTION	CALS	PROT	FAT	CARB
Cheeseburger Tillamook	1	630	34	40	31
Cheeseburger Tillamook Pepper Bacon	1	690	39	46	28
Chicken Strips	5	320	23	14	26
French Fries	1 serv	410	6	18	57
Gardenburger Spicy Black Bean	1	550	24	32	45
Gardenburger The Original	1	450	18	19	52
Halibut	3 pieces	320	21	16	24
Hamburger	1	300	12	15	29
Hamburger Burgerville Classic	1	510	27	30	30
Onion Rings Walla Walla	1 serv	810	12	48	83
Sandwich Crispy Chicken	1	490	21	19	59
Sandwich Deluxe Crispy Chicken	1	590	27	30	56
Sandwich Halibut	1	480	18	27	41
Sandwich Low Fat Grilled Chicken	1	320	24	5	44
Sandwich Nine Grain Turkey Club	1	550	27	32	38
Sweet Potato Fries	1 serv	530	4	29	60
Turkey Burger Seasoned	1	540	36	29	33
Yukon Golds	1 serv	450	5	21	59
SALAD DRESSINGS AND TOPPINGS					
Burgerville Spread Cups	1	280	0	30	4
Cream Cheese	1 serv	100	2	10	1
Cream Cheese Light	1 serv	70	3	5	2
Dip BBQ Sauce	1 serv	60	1	1	13
Dressing Blue Cheese	1 serv	240	1	24	3
Dressing Caesar	1 serv	220	1	22	2
Dressing Honey Mustard	1 serv	210	0	20	6
Dressing Ranch	1 serv	195	0	21	2
Sauce Sweet And Sour	1 serv	90	0	4	12
Tartar Cups	1	260	0	28	2
Vinaigrette Honey Lime	1 serv	250	0	23	10
Vinaigrette Raspberry	1 serv	45	0	2	6
SALADS					
Grilled Chicken	1	430	32	27	16
Rogue River Smokey Blue	1	290	9	11	38
Side Salad	1	50	3	3	4

FOOD	PORTION	CALS	PROT	FAT	CARB
Wild Smoked Salmon & Hazelnuts	1	440	30	28	19

CARL'S JR.
BEVERAGES

FOOD	PORTION	CALS	PROT	FAT	CARB
Malt Chocolate	1 (15 oz)	780	17	35	98
Malt Oreo Cookie	1 (15 oz)	790	18	39	91
Malt Strawberry	1 (15 oz)	770	17	35	97
Malt Vanilla	1 (15 oz)	760	17	35	99
Shake Chocolate	1 (14 oz)	710	14	33	85
Shake Oreo Cookie	1 (14 oz)	720	16	37	79
Shake Strawberry	1 (14 oz)	700	14	33	84
Shake Vanilla	1 (14 oz)	710	14	33	86

BREAKFAST SELECTIONS

FOOD	PORTION	CALS	PROT	FAT	CARB
Breakfast Burger	1	830	37	47	65
Burrito Bacon & Egg	1	570	30	33	37
Burrito Loaded Breakfast	1	820	38	51	52
Burrito Steak & Egg	1	660	40	36	44
French Toast Dips w/o Syrup	5	430	9	18	58
Hash Brown Nuggets	1 serv	330	3	21	32
Sandwich Sourdough Breakfast	1 serv	460	28	21	39
Sunrise Croissant Sandwich	1	560	20	41	27

DESSERTS

FOOD	PORTION	CALS	PROT	FAT	CARB
Cheesecake Strawberry Swirl	1 serv	290	6	17	30
Chocolate Cake	1 serv	300	3	12	48
Cookie Chocolate Chip	1	350	3	18	46

MAIN MENU SELECTIONS

FOOD	PORTION	CALS	PROT	FAT	CARB
Burger Jalapeno	1	720	27	45	50
Burger Teriyaki	1	660	28	34	61
Cheeseburger Double Western Bacon	1	970	62	52	71
Cheeseburger Western Bacon	1	710	32	33	70
Chicken Breast Strips	3	420	23	25	28
Chicken Stars	4	170	9	11	10
CrissCut Fries	1 serv	410	5	24	43
Famous Star w/ Cheese	1	660	27	39	53
Fish & Chips	1 serv	630	26	28	68
French Fries	1 sm	290	5	14	37
Fried Zucchini	1 serv	320	6	19	31
Hamburger Big	1	470	24	17	54
Hamburger Kid's	1	460	24	17	53

FOOD	PORTION	CALS	PROT	FAT	CARB
Onion Rings	1 serv	430	6	21	53
Sandwich Bacon Swiss Crispy Chicken	1	720	35	35	64
Sandwich Carl's Catch Fish	1	660	22	31	75
Sandwich Charbroiled BBQ Chicken	1	360	34	5	48
Sandwich Charbroiled Chicken Club	1	550	40	25	43
Sandwich Charbroiled Santa Fe Chicken	1	610	37	32	43
Sandwich Spicy Chicken	1	560	15	30	59
Six Dollar Burger The Bacon Cheese	1	1070	46	76	50
Six Dollar Burger The Guacamole Bacon	1	1140	43	86	54
Six Dollar Burger The Jalapeno	1	1030	39	74	52
Six Dollar Burger The Low Carb	1	490	33	37	6
Six Dollar Burger The Original	1	1010	40	68	60
Six Dollar Burger The Western Bacon	1	1130	47	66	83
Super Star w/ Cheese	1	930	47	59	54
SALAD DRESSINGS					
Blue Cheese	1 serv (2 oz)	320	2	34	1
House	1 serv (2 oz)	220	1	22	2
Italian Fat Free	1 serv (2 oz)	15	0	0	4
Low Fat Balsamic	1 serv (2 oz)	35	0	15	5
Thousand Island	1 serv (2 oz)	240	0	23	7
SALADS					
Charbroiled Chicken	1	260	34	7	16
Side	1	50	3	3	5
CARVEL					
Brown Bonnet	1	370	3	21	40
Cake Ice Cream	1 slice	270	4	14	33
Carvelanche Cake Mix	1 reg (16 oz)	720	13	27	106
Carvelanche Cookies & Cream	1 reg (16 oz)	550	7	30	64
Carvelanche Triple Fudge Cake Mix	1 reg (16 oz)	900	16	41	134
Chipsters	1	330	4	16	44
Cone Cake Chocolate	1 sm	260	6	13	32
Cone Cake Chocolate	1 lg	600	13	30	71

FOOD	PORTION	CALS	PROT	FAT	CARB
Cone Cake Vanilla	1 sm	280	4	16	31
Cone Cake Vanilla	1 lg	650	9	36	68
Cone Sugar Chocolate	1 sm	300	7	13	40
Cone Sugar Vanilla	1 sm	320	5	15	39
Cone Waffle Chocolate	1 sm	330	7	13	47
Cone Waffle Chocolate	1 lg	660	15	30	86
Cone Waffle Vanilla	1 sm	350	5	16	46
Cone Waffle Vanilla	1 lg	710	10	36	83
Dashers Banana Barge	1	940	17	46	121
Dashers Bananas Foster	1	600	6	24	90
Dashers Fudge Brownie	1	810	9	42	98
Dashers Mint Chocolate Chip	1	720	8	39	85
Dashers Peanut Butter Cup	1	1090	20	63	97
Dashers Strawberry Shortcake	1	590	8	29	78
Flying Saucer 98% Fat Free Chocolate	1	180	5	3	34
Flying Saucer 98% Fat Free Vanilla	1	180	5	3	35
Flying Saucer Chocolate	1	230	4	10	33
Flying Saucer Deluxe Sprinkles	1	330	4	15	47
Flying Saucer Vanilla	1	240	4	11	33
Ice Cream Chocolate	1 sm (4 oz)	250	6	13	29
Ice Cream Vanilla	1 sm (4 oz)	240	3	14	25
Ice Cream No Fat Chocolate	1 sm (4 oz)	160	3	0	37
Ice Cream No Fat Vanilla	1 sm (4 oz)	160	5	0	33
Sherbet All Flavors	1 sm (4 oz)	180	1	2	39
Sinful Love Bar	1	460	4	29	47
Sprinkle Cup	1	230	2	15	28
Sundae Bittersweet Fudge	1 reg	690	8	38	77
Sundae Caramel	1 reg	670	8	34	81
Sundae Hot Fudge	1 reg	670	8	38	73
Sundae Strawberry	1 reg	580	7	33	63
Sundae Mini Chocolate Syrup	1	200	2	9	27
Thick Shake Chocolate	1 reg (16 oz)	650	14	27	93
Thick Shake Vanilla	1 reg (16 oz)	610	10	28	81
Thinny Thin Classic Sundae No Fat Fudge	1 reg	380	8	2	81
Thinny Thin Classic Sundae No Fat Strawberry	1 reg	320	8	0	69

FOOD	PORTION	CALS	PROT	FAT	CARB
Thinny Thin Miniature Sundae No Fat	1	190	4	0	45
Thinny Thin Miniature Sundae No Sugar Added	1	200	5	3	42
Thinny Thin No Fat Carvelanche Strawberry	1 (16 oz)	430	12	0	91
Thinny Thin No Fat Chocolate	1 sm	160	3	0	37
Thinny Thin No Fat Vanilla	1 sm	160	5	0	33
Thinny Thin No Sugar Added Vanilla	1 sm	180	7	3	34
Thinny Thin Parfait No Fat	1	190	4	0	42
Thinny Thin Shake No Fat Chocolate	1 (16 oz)	440	5	0	104
Thinny Thin Shake No Fat Mocha	1 (16 oz)	440	10	0	97
Thinny Thin Shake No Fat Vanilla	1 (16 oz)	300	9	0	62
CHIPOTLE					
Barbacoa	1 serv (4 oz)	228	27	13	1
Black Beans	1 serv (4 oz)	130	9	1	22
Carnitas	1 serv (4 oz)	227	29	12	0
Cheese	1 serv (1 oz)	110	7	9	tr
Chicken	1 serv (4 oz)	219	29	11	0
Chips	1 serv (4 oz)	490	7	19	71
Crispy Taco Shells	3	180	3	7	26
Fajita Vegetables	1 serv (3 oz)	100	1	8	6
Flour Tortilla	1 (6 inch)	300	9	8	48
Flour Tortilla	1 (13 inch)	330	9	8	55
Guacamole	1 serv (4 oz)	170	2	15	8
Lettuce	1 serv (1 oz)	5	tr	0	tr
Pinto Beans	1 serv (4 oz)	138	9	1	23
Rice	1 serv (3.5 oz)	168	3	5	28
Salsa Corn	1 serv (4 oz)	100	3	1	22
Salsa Tomato	1 serv (4 oz)	25	1	0	6
Sour Cream	1 serv (2 oz)	120	2	10	2
Steak	1 serv (4 oz)	230	29	12	2
Tomatillo Green	1 serv (2 oz)	15	1	tr	3
Tomatillo Red	1 serv (2 oz)	28	1	1	4
Vinaigrette	1 serv (2 oz)	282	0	26	11

FOOD	PORTION	CALS	PROT	FAT	CARB
CHURCH'S CHICKEN					
DESSERTS					
Pie Apple	1 pie (3 oz)	280	2	11	39
Pie Edward's Double Lemon	1 pie (3 oz)	300	5	14	39
Pie Edward's Strawberry Cream Cheese	1 pie (2.8 oz)	280	4	15	32
MAIN MENU SELECTIONS					
Biscuit Honey Butter	1	240	3	12	28
Cajun Rice	1 reg	130	1	7	16
Chicken Fried Steak w/ White Gravy	1 serv (7.5 oz)	610	24	43	31
Cole Slaw	1 reg	150	1	10	15
Corn On The Cob	1 ear	140	4	3	24
Country Fried Steak w/ White Gravy	1 serv (5.8 oz)	470	21	28	36
Crunchy Tenders	1 (2 oz)	120	12	6	6
French Fries	1 reg	290	3	14	38
Jalapeno Cheese Bombers	4 (4 oz)	240	8	10	29
Macaroni & Cheese	1 reg	210	8	11	23
Mashed Potatoes & Gravy	1 reg	70	2	2	12
Okra	1 reg	350	3	22	36
Original Breast	1	200	22	11	3
Original Leg	1	110	10	6	3
Original Thigh	1	330	21	23	8
Original Wing	1	300	27	19	7
Sandwich Bigger Better Chicken w/ Cheese	1	510	20	27	46
Sandwich Country Fried Steak	1	490	13	32	38
Sandwich Spicy Fish	1	320	10	20	25
Spicy Breast	1	320	21	20	12
Spicy Crunchy Tenders	1 (2 oz)	135	11	7	7
Spicy Fish Fillet	1 piece (2.3 oz)	160	7	9	13
Spicy Leg	1	180	12	11	8
Spicy Thigh	1	480	22	35	20
Spicy Wing	1	430	29	27	17
Sweet Corn Nuggets	1 reg	600	7	29	72
Whole Jalapeno Peppers	2	10	0	0	2
SAUCES					
BBQ	1 pkg	30	0	0	7

FOOD	PORTION	CALS	PROT	FAT	CARB
Creamy Jalapeno	1 pkg	100	0	11	1
Honey	1 pkg	27	0	0	7
Honey Mustard	1 pkg	110	0	11	4
Hot Sauce	1 pkg	0	0	0	0
Ketchup	1 pkg	18	0	0	5
Purple Pepper	1 pkg	45	0	0	12
Ranch	1 pkg	130	0	13	1
Sweet & Sour	1 pkg	30	0	0	8
CICI'S					
EXTRAS					
Apple Pizza	1 slice	149	3	4	26
Brownie	1	143	1	6	22
Cinnamon Roll	1	139	2	6	20
Garlic Bread	1 slice	99	4	5	10
PIZZA					
Buffet 12 Inch Alfredo	1 slice	139	8	5	18
Buffet 12 Inch Bacon Cheddar	1 slice	145	6	5	18
Buffet 12 Inch Bar-B-Que	1 slice	172	8	6	21
Buffet 12 Inch Beef	1 slice	170	9	7	18
Buffet 12 Inch Cheese	1 slice	152	7	5	20
Buffet 12 Inch Ham & Pineapple	1 slice	141	7	4	19
Buffet 12 Inch Ole	1 slice	108	5	4	13
Buffet 12 Inch Pepperoni	1 slice	175	8	7	21
Buffet 12 Inch Pepperoni & Jalapeno	1 slice	163	8	6	20
Buffet 12 Inch Sausage	1 slice	197	8	7	19
Buffet 12 Inch Spinach Alfredo	1 slice	151	7	5	20
Buffet 12 Inch Zesty Ham & Cheese	1 slice	153	6	6	18
Buffet 12 Inch Zesty Pepperoni	1 slice	157	6	7	18
Buffet 12 Inch Zesty Tomato Alfredo	1 slice	136	6	5	18
Buffet 12 Inch Zesty Veggie	1 slice	124	5	4	17
To-Go 15 Inch Bar-B-Que	1 slice	289	13	10	36
To-Go 15 Inch Cheese	1 slice	223	11	8	28
To-Go 15 Inch Ham & Pineapple	1 slice	225	11	8	27
To-Go 15 Inch Ole	1 slice	169	7	4	26
To-Go 15 Inch Pepperoni	1 slice	240	11	10	27
To-Go 15 Inch Spinach Alfredo	1 slice	243	11	8	32
To-Go 15 Inch Zesty Pepperoni	1 slice	246	10	12	26
To-Go 15 Inch Zesty Veggie	1 slice	213	9	9	25

FOOD	PORTION	CALS	PROT	FAT	CARB
CINNABON					
BAKED SELECTIONS					
Caramel Pecanbon	1	1100	16	56	141
Cinnabon Bites	6	520	8	16	78
Cinnabon Classic	1	813	15	32	117
Cinnabon Stix	1	379	6	21	41
Cinnamon Filled Churro	1	281	5	11	39
Minibon	1	339	6	13	49
BEVERAGES					
Caramelatta Chill	1 (16 oz)	520	12	19	76
Chillatta Cappuccino	1 (16 oz)	330	5	11	56
Chillatta Caramel	1 (16 oz)	480	8	18	72
Chillatta Chocolate Mocha	1 (16 oz)	460	8	14	72
Chillatta Mango	1 (16 oz)	340	6	11	57
Chillatta Strawberry	1 (16 oz)	330	5	11	54
Chillatta Strawberry Banana	1 (16 oz)	350	5	11	58
Chillatta Tropical Blast	1 (16 oz)	330	2	7	69
Mochalatta Chill	1 (16 oz)	450	11	18	66
CORNER BAKERY					
BREAKFAST SELECTIONS					
Baked French Toast	1 serv	570	13	15	86
Buckhead Cheese Grits	1 serv	350	11	22	19
Oatmeal	1 serv	280	12	7	41
Oatmeal Crunchy Honey Banana	1 serv	380	12	3	78
Oatmeal Swiss	1 serv	330	4	1	79
Panini Ham & Cheddar	1	720	42	34	57
Panini Smoked Bacon & Cheddar	1	680	33	34	56
Scrambler All American w/o Potatoes & Bread	1 serv	310	23	22	3
Scrambler Anaheim w/o Potatoes & Bread	1 serv	490	30	36	10
Scrambler Farmer's w/o Potatoes & Bread	1 serv	430	31	31	6
The Commuter Croissant	1	720	29	46	44
PASTA					
Chicken Carbonara	1 serv	740	51	28	70
Half Moon Cheese Ravioli	1 serv	550	28	21	63
Penne w/ Marinara	1 serv	550	20	11	92
Pesto Cavatappi	1 serv	930	52	40	93

FOOD	PORTION	CALS	PROT	FAT	CARB
SALAD DRESSINGS					
Caesar	1 serv	310	1	32	2
House	1 serv	280	0	27	8
Ranch	1 serv	160	2	16	2
Vinaigrette Balsamic	1 serv	300	0	31	4
SALADS					
Caesar	1 serv	520	11	44	19
Caesar w/ Roasted Chicken & Croutons	1 serv	640	27	49	8
Chopped w/o Bread	1 serv	810	40	61	27
Harvest	1 serv	860	19	68	53
Harvest w/ Roasted Chicken	1 serv	980	37	72	53
Santa Fe Ranch	1 serv	680	19	44	56
Santa Fe Ranch w/ Roasted Chicken	1 serv	800	37	49	56
Side Cucumber Tomato	1 (6 oz)	120	1	9	9
Side Egg	1 (6 oz)	570	16	53	2
Side Roasted Potato Bacon	1 (6 oz)	370	8	23	29
Side Seasonal Fruit Medley	1 (6 oz)	90	1	0	22
Side Tomato Mozzarella Pasta	1 (6 oz)	205	7	8	24
Side Tuna	1 (6 oz)	310	34	16	3
SANDWICHES					
Bavarian w/ Ham	1	720	40	25	78
Bavarian w/ Turkey	1	690	39	22	78
Chicken Pesto	1	840	41	41	75
Panini California Grille	1	700	29	41	59
Panini Chicken Pomodori	1	890	47	45	74
Panini Club	1	900	50	48	72
Panini Corned Beef Reuben	1	930	44	48	76
Panini Grilled Ham & Swiss	1	880	45	44	75
Southwest Roast Beef	1	840	44	37	78
Tomato Mozzarella	1	670	28	26	73
Tuna Salad On Olive Bread	1	450	29	16	42
Turkey Derby	1	650	39	29	60
Turkey Frisco	1	850	44	38	79
Uptown Turkey	1	660	39	29	61
SOUPS					
Big Al's Chili w/ Cheddar Cheese	1 (10 oz)	380	23	17	29
Bread Bowl	1	420	12	30	21

FOOD	PORTION	CALS	PROT	FAT	CARB
Cheddar	1 (10 oz)	310	9	23	16
Chicken Wild Mushroom Brie Stew	1 (10 oz)	260	11	14	20
Loaded Baked Potato w/ Garnish	1 (10 oz)	420	13	29	29
Mom's Chicken Noodle	1 (10 oz)	170	8	4	23
Old Fashioned Beef Stew	1 (10 oz)	260	7	13	20
Roasted Poblano Corn Chowder	1 (10 oz)	330	4	21	34
Roasted Tomato Basil w/o Garnish	1 (10 oz)	170	3	5	27
Zesty Chicken Tortilla w/ Tortilla Strips	1 (10 oz)	230	8	11	26

D'ANGELO
CHILDREN'S MENU SELECTIONS

FOOD	PORTION	CALS	PROT	FAT	CARB
D'Lite Turkey	1	217	19	3	30
Sub Cheeseburger	1	294	15	13	28
Sub Ham & Cheese	1	227	14	5	32
Sub Kidz Tuna	1	438	15	29	30
Sub Meatball	1	330	15	15	37

SALAD DRESSINGS

FOOD	PORTION	CALS	PROT	FAT	CARB
Bleu Cheese	1 serv	152	1	15	3
Caesar	1 serv	397	6	43	6
Caesar Fat Free	1 serv	57	0	0	9
Creamy Italian	1 serv	340	0	37	9
Greek w/ Feta Cheese	1 serv	227	0	26	6
Honey Mustard	1 serv	150	0	142	7
Olive Oil Vinaigrette	1 serv	170	0	17	9
Ranch Lite	1 serv	240	2	19	6

SALADS

FOOD	PORTION	CALS	PROT	FAT	CARB
Antipasto	1 serv	284	16	18	17
Caesar w/ Dressing	1 serv	474	15	39	25
Chicken Caesar w/ Dressing	1 serv	533	35	38	19
Chicken Stir Fry w/o Dressing	1 serv	168	25	3	11
Cobb w/o Dressing	1 serv	292	27	17	11
Greek	1 serv	290	11	23	17
Lobster w/o Dressing	1 serv	376	26	26	12
Roast Beef w/o Dressing	1 serv	131	19	3	10
Steak Tip Caesar	1 serv	661	32	50	21
Tossed Garden w/o Dressing	1 serv	49	3	1	11
Turkey w/o Dressing	1 serv	157	26	2	10

FOOD	PORTION	CALS	PROT	FAT	CARB
SANDWICHES					
D'Lite Chicken Caesar Salad	1	374	34	7	43
D'Lite Chicken Stir Fry	1	426	37	6	57
D'Lite Classic Veggie	1	362	15	7	63
D'Lite Fresh Veggie	1	348	13	7	62
D'Lite Grilled Chicken Breast	1	388	31	7	52
D'Lite Roast Beef	1	338	25	5	51
D'Lite Turkey	1	347	28	4	51
D'Lite Turkey Cranberry	1	444	28	4	75
Pokket Big Papi	1	469	39	11	53
Pokket BLT & Cheese	1	397	22	17	38
Pokket Caesar Salad	1	616	20	39	54
Pokket Capicola & Cheese	1	362	26	13	35
Pokket Cheese	1	519	29	27	41
Pokket Cheeseburger	1	459	27	25	31
Pokket Chicken Caesar Salad	1	674	40	39	47
Pokket Chicken Club	1	526	34	28	36
Pokket Chicken Honey Dijon	1	508	41	20	40
Pokket Chicken Salad	1	623	27	42	34
Pokket Chicken Stir Fry	1	380	35	9	39
Pokket Classic Vegetable	1	368	19	13	46
Pokket Classic Veggie No Cheese	1	212	9	1	44
Pokket Greek	1	790	16	61	49
Pokket Grilled Chicken	1	303	29	5	35
Pokket Ham	1	229	17	3	35
Pokket Ham & Cheese	1	326	22	10	38
Pokket Ham & Salami	1	386	23	17	34
Pokket Hamburger	1	399	24	20	29
Pokket Italian	1	525	28	30	36
Pokket Lobster	1	530	29	31	34
Pokket Meatball	1	574	26	31	52
Pokket Mortadella & Cheese	1	410	21	21	35
Pokket Number 9	1	407	31	18	31
Pokket Pastrami	1	438	24	25	33
Pokket Pepperoni	1	407	21	20	35
Pokket Roast Beef	1	247	23	3	33
Pokket Salad	1	196	8	1	40
Pokket Salami & Cheese	1	509	25	30	33
Pokket Seafood Salad	1	449	14	22	50

FOOD	PORTION	CALS	PROT	FAT	CARB
Pokket Steak	1	305	25	12	24
Pokket Steak & Cheese	1	377	29	17	26
Pokket Steak Bomb	1	631	43	32	44
Pokket Steak Tip	1	452	27	16	45
Pokket Tuna	1	664	24	49	33
Pokket Turkey	1	256	26	2	33
Pokket Turkey Club	1	332	34	7	32
Sub Big Papi	1 sm	525	40	15	60
Sub BLT & Cheese	1 sm	463	23	19	51
Sub Capicola & Cheese	1 sm	408	25	13	48
Sub Cheese	1 sm	589	30	28	55
Sub Cheeseburger	1 sm	526	29	26	44
Sub Chicken Club	1	593	35	29	49
Sub Chicken Honey Dijon	1	575	42	22	53
Sub Chicken Salad	1 sm	692	29	44	48
Sub Chicken Stir Fry	1 sm	449	37	11	53
Sub Classic Veggie	1 sm	462	21	15	64
Sub Grilled Chicken	1 sm	369	30	7	48
Sub Ham	1 sm	302	18	5	49
Sub Ham & Cheese	1 sm	395	24	11	52
Sub Ham & Salami	1 sm	456	25	19	48
Sub Hamburger	1 sm	466	25	22	42
Sub Italian	1 sm	614	30	31	54
Sub Lobster	1 sm	598	30	33	48
Sub Meatball	1 sm	644	28	33	66
Sub Meatballs & Cheese	1 sm	750	36	41	67
Sub Mortadella & Cheese	1 sm	479	23	23	49
Sub Number 9	1 sm	450	31	19	41
Sub Pastrami	1 sm	613	34	34	47
Sub Pepperoni	1 sm	603	28	33	49
Sub Roast Beef	1 sm	320	25	5	48
Sub Salad	1 sm	281	10	3	57
Sub Salami & Cheese	1 sm	579	27	32	47
Sub Seafood Salad	1 sm	498	14	23	61
Sub Steak	1 sm	373	27	14	37
Sub Steak & Cheese	1 sm	446	31	19	40
Sub Steak Bomb	1 sm	670	43	33	52
Sub Steak Tip	1 sm	545	29	18	63
Sub Tuna	1	685	24	46	47
Sub Turkey Club	1 sm	401	33	9	49

FOOD	PORTION	CALS	PROT	FAT	CARB
Sub Toasted Italian Bistro	1 sm	585	29	31	49
Sub Toasted Pastrami Reuben	1 sm	750	30	47	55
Sub Toasted Roast Beef & Cheddar	1 sm	564	35	26	51
Sub Toasted Spicy Meatball	1 sm	933	61	57	71
Sub Toasted Tuna & Swiss	1 sm	796	32	54	49
Sub Toasted Turkey Thanksgiving	1 sm	705	32	20	80
Sub Toasted Turkey & Ham	1 sm	532	33	24	49
Wrap Big Papi	1	593	41	23	56
Wrap BLT & Cheese	1	544	24	26	54
Wrap Buffalo Chicken Salad	1	823	40	44	67
Wrap Caesar Salad	1	711	20	44	65
Wrap Capicola & Cheese	1	494	25	20	53
Wrap Cheese	1	675	30	35	59
Wrap Cheeseburger	1	609	30	33	48
Wrap Chicken Caesar Salad	1	830	42	47	65
Wrap Chicken Cobb	1	931	36	55	71
Wrap Chicken Filet & Bacon	1	639	38	28	58
Wrap Chicken Honey Dijon	1	672	60	29	43
Wrap Chicken Salad	1	782	29	51	53
Wrap Chicken Stir Fry	1	535	37	17	57
Wrap Classic Veggie	1	486	24	13	68
Wrap Greek	1	765	15	61	44
Wrap Grilled Chicken	1	422	34	6	59
Wrap Ham & Cheese	1	435	26	10	60
Wrap Ham & Salami	1	513	30	18	57
Wrap Hamburger	1	509	28	21	50
Wrap Italian	1	631	32	29	59
Wrap Lobster	1	749	33	43	57
Wrap Meatball	1	687	31	31	75
Wrap Mortadella & Cheese	1	522	25	21	58
Wrap Number 9	1	517	32	24	44
Wrap Pastrami	1	550	28	25	55
Wrap Peppercorn Steak	1	702	41	40	45
Wrap Pepperoni	1	519	25	21	57
Wrap Roast Beef	1	448	26	13	58
Wrap Salad	1	324	13	2	66
Wrap Salami & Cheese	1	605	29	29	56
Wrap Seafood Salad	1	541	17	22	69

FOOD	PORTION	CALS	PROT	FAT	CARB
Wrap Steak	1	392	28	13	41
Wrap Steak & Cheese	1	464	33	18	43
Wrap Steak Bomb	1	670	43	33	52
Wrap Steak Tip	1	432	26	16	41
Wrap Tuna	1	731	27	44	56
Wrap Turkey	1	369	30	3	55
Wrap Turkey Club	1	415	34	8	52
SOUPS					
Beef Stew	1 sm	220	12	8	23
Broccoli & Cheddar Cheese	1 sm	270	9	21	11
Chicken Noodle	1 sm	110	6	3	14
Hearty Vegetable	1 sm	40	2	0	7
Italian Wedding	1 sm	120	6	6	11
Lobster Bisque	1 sm	360	8	29	16
New England Clam Chowder	1 sm	320	9	18	31
Portuguese Kale	1 sm	130	8	4	16
EL POLLO LOCO					
DESSERTS					
Caramel Flan	1 serv (5.5 oz)	290	5	12	41
Churros	2	300	3	18	32
Cone Vanilla	1	330	8	8	55
Soft Serve Vanilla	1 cup (5 oz)	300	8	8	48
MAIN MENU SELECTIONS					
BBQ Black Beans	1 serv (6 oz)	200	7	3	38
Bowl The Original Pollo	1 serv	540	37	4	85
Burrito BRC	1 (7.5 oz)	390	14	10	61
Burrito Classic Chicken	1 (10.3 oz)	500	30	14	63
Burrito Twice Grilled	1 (15 oz)	830	66	37	58
Burrito Ultimate Grilled	1 (13.6 oz)	650	38	20	80
Chicken Breast	1 (4.3 oz)	220	36	9	0
Chicken Breast Skinless	1 (4 oz)	180	35	4	0
Chicken Leg	1 (1.8 oz)	90	12	4	0
Chicken Thigh	1 (3.1 oz)	220	21	15	0
Chicken Wing	1 (1.3 oz)	90	11	5	0
Cole Slaw	1 serv (6 oz)	120	1	9	8
Corn Cobbette	1 (5 oz)	90	2	1	19
French Fries	1 serv (5.5 oz)	440	6	21	57
Fresh Vegetables w/ Margarine	1 serv (4.1 oz)	60	2	3	8
Fresh Vegetables w/o Margarine	1 serv (4 oz)	35	2	0	8

FOOD	PORTION	CALS	PROT	FAT	CARB
Gravy	1 serv (1 oz)	10	0	0	2
Loco Nachos	1 serv	170	3	14	7
Macaroni & Cheese	1 serv (5.5 oz)	280	11	17	28
Mashed Potatoes	1 serv (5 oz)	100	2	1	20
Pinto Beans	1 serv (6 oz)	140	9	0	25
Quesadilla Cheese	1 (4.5 oz)	420	19	23	35
Refried Beans w/ Cheese	1 serv (6.3 oz)	270	14	7	36
Skinless Breast Meal	1 serv	310	35	12	17
Soup Chicken Tortilla w/o Tortilla Strips	1 serv (10 oz)	140	15	6	8
Spanish Rice	1 serv (4.5 oz)	160	3	1	34
Taco Al Carbon	1 (3.1 oz)	150	11	5	17
Taco Soft Chicken	1 (4.5 oz)	270	17	13	19
Taquito Chicken	1	190	10	9	18
Tortilla Chips	1 serv (1.5 oz)	210	3	10	28
Tortilla Corn 6 Inches	2	120	2	2	24
Tortilla Flour 6.5 Inches	2	210	5	7	30
SALAD DRESSINGS AND TOPPINGS					
Creamy Cilantro	1 serv (1.5 oz)	220	1	23	1
Creamy Cilantro Light	1 pkg	70	1	5	6
Guacamole	1 serv (1 oz)	45	tr	4	4
Hot Sauce Jalapeno	1 pkg	5	0	0	1
Jack & Poblano Queso	1 serv (1.8 oz)	100	3	8	4
Ketchup	1 pkg	10	0	0	2
Light Italian	1 pkg	20	0	1	2
Pico De Gallo Medium	1 serv (1 oz)	10	0	1	1
Ranch	1 pkg	230	1	24	2
Salsa Avocado Hot	1 serv (1 oz)	30	0	3	1
Salsa Chipotle Hot	1 serv (1 oz)	5	0	0	1
Salsa House Mild	1 serv (1 oz)	5	0	0	1
Sour Cream	1 serv (1 oz)	60	1	5	1
Thousand Island	1 pkg	220	0	21	6
SALADS					
Caesar Pollo	1 (11.4 oz)	520	27	38	17
Ceasar Pollo w/o Dressing	1 (9.4 oz)	220	25	7	15
Garden	1 (4.8 oz)	120	5	4	9
Tostada Chicken	1 (17.3 oz)	840	40	40	76
Tostada Chicken w/o Shell	1 (14.7 oz)	410	33	11	42

EMERALD CITY SMOOTHIE

FOOD	PORTION	CALS	PROT	FAT	CARB
Apple Andie	1 (11 oz)	230	11	1	46

FOOD	PORTION	CALS	PROT	FAT	CARB
Berry Berry	1 (13 oz)	350	8	0	77
Blueberry Blast	1 (13 oz)	380	13	0	78
Coconut Passion	1 (11 oz)	600	24	23	80
Cranberry Delight	1 (10 oz)	550	11	1	127
Energizer	1 (10 oz)	350	18	1	62
Fruity Supreme	1 (9 oz)	280	12	1	59
Grape Escape	1 (10 oz)	480	11	1	109
Guava Sunrise	1 (13 oz)	366	12	1	80
Kiwi Kic	1 (11 oz)	400	13	1	88
Lean Body	1 (11 oz)	330	40	8	24
Lean Out	1 (11 oz)	600	56	26	35
Low Carb	1 (10 oz)	350	54	2	27
Mango Mania	1 (8 oz)	370	11	0	82
Marionberry Fuel	1 (13 oz)	380	14	0	81
Mega Mass	1 (14 oz)	610	29	10	103
Mini Mass	1 (13 oz)	520	27	11	79
Mocha Bliss	1 (10 oz)	550	34	8	63
Nutty Banana	1 (11 oz)	720	27	25	97
Orange Twister	1 (10 oz)	140	3	0	31
Pacific Splash	1 (12 oz)	240	2	0	58
PB&J	1 (14 oz)	630	22	25	77
Peach Pleasure	1 (12 oz)	270	12	0	54
Peanut Passion	1 (11 oz)	580	22	25	61
Pineapple Bliss	1 (12 oz)	210	6	1	45
Power Fuel	1 (11 oz)	450	39	3	66
Quick Start	1 (10 oz)	280	17	0	46
Raspberry Dream	1 (13 oz)	410	18	1	80
Rejuvenator	1 (10 oz)	340	17	1	62
Sambazon	1 (15 oz)	410	14	6	92
Slim N Fit	1 (10 oz)	350	25	1	60
The Builder	1 (18 oz)	1270	67	46	144
Zesty Lemon	1 (14 oz)	430	19	9	67
Zip Zip	1 (10 oz)	240	18	3	35
Zone Zinger	1 (14 oz)	430	25	3	76

EVOS
BEVERAGES

FOOD	PORTION	CALS	PROT	FAT	CARB
Shake Mango Guava	1 reg (16 oz)	180	0	0	48
Shake Multi-Berry	1 reg (20 oz)	200	1	1	52
Shake Strawberry Banana	1 reg (16 oz)	190	1	1	47
Shake Organic Cappuccino	1 reg (16 oz)	230	5	3	47
Shake Organic Vanilla	1 reg (16 oz)	180	6	3	30

FOOD	PORTION	CALS	PROT	FAT	CARB
CHILDREN'S MENU SELECTIONS					
Kids Champion Burger	1	400	29	12	48
Kids Chicken Strips	1 serv	130	14	3	13
Kids Freerange Steakburger	1	390	27	15	39
Kids Good Corn Dog	1	150	7	4	27
MAIN MENU SELECTIONS					
Airbaked Chicken Strips	1 serv	260	28	6	26
Airfries	1 reg	230	4	8	35
American Champion	1	420	30	12	53
American DeLite	1	330	22	6	53
Burger Bun	1	190	7	2	39
Cheddar Cheese Slice	1	80	5	7	0
Crispy Mesquite Chicken	1 serv	330	21	5	53
Freerange Steakburger	1	400	27	15	42
Fresh Fruit Bowl	1 serv	200	2	1	52
Good Corn Dog	1	150	7	4	22
Herb Crusted Trout	1 serv	440	21	25	62
Honey Mesquite Chicken	1 serv	290	26	3	41
Spicy Chipotle Turkey	1 serv	370	31	9	42
Veggie Chili	1 reg	110	7	2	20
Veggie Garden Grill Italian	1	350	24	5	54
Wraps Avocado Turkey	1	480	32	15	51
Wraps Crispy Buffalo Chicken	1	440	23	11	64
Wraps Crispy Thai Trout	1	660	25	20	96
Wraps Freerange Beef Taco	1	600	34	28	53
Wraps Honey Wheat	1	300	8	8	49
Wraps Southwest Soy Taco	1	500	35	25	58
Wraps Spicy Thai Chicken	1	510	30	10	76
Wraps Spinach Herb	1	310	9	8	52
Wraps Tomato Basil Chicken	1	520	25	11	82
SALAD DRESSINGS AND TOPPINGS					
Balsamic Vinegar	1 serv (0.5 oz)	5	0	0	2
Crispy Noodles	1 serv (7 g)	35	1	1	5
Croutons Multi-Grain	1 serv (7 g)	30	1	2	4
Dressing Avocado	1 serv (3 oz)	190	3	21	5
Dressing Caesar	1 serv (1.7 oz)	300	2	32	2
Dressing Fat Free Vinaigrette	1 serv (1 oz)	5	0	0	2
Dressing Raspberry	1 serv (2 oz)	50	0	0	14
Dressing Spicy Thai	1 serv (1.4 oz)	150	0	9	15
Extra Virgin Olive Oil	1 serv (1 oz)	250	0	28	0

FOOD	PORTION	CALS	PROT	FAT	CARB
Herb Spread	1 serv (0.7 oz)	30	0	3	2
Ketchup Cayenne Firewalker	1 serv (1.2 oz)	35	1	0	9
Ketchup Garlic Gravity	1 serv (1.2 oz)	35	1	0	9
Ketchup Mesquite Magic	1 serv (1.2 oz)	35	1	0	9
Mustard Mesquite Honey	1 serv (0.7 oz)	80	0	8	3
Mustard	1 serv (0.5 oz)	10	1	0	1
Southwest Sour Cream	1 serv (1.4 oz)	60	2	35	4
Spicy Chipotle Mayo	1 serv (0.7 oz)	30	0	2	2
Tomato Basil Sauce	1 serv (1.4 oz)	150	2	15	5
SALADS					
Bordeaux Bistro w/o Dressing	1	260	13	22	7
For Salads Chicken Strips	1 serv (3 oz)	130	14	3	13
For Salads Grilled Chicken	1 serv (3 oz)	90	19	1	1
Mediterranean Summer w/o Dressing	1	200	13	8	22
Santa Ana Caesar w/o Dressing	1	20	2	0	4
Side Salad w/o Dressing	1	35	2	0	8
Spicy Thai w/o Dressing	1	35	2	0	7
SUPPLEMENTS					
Fat Burner	1 serv (5 g)	16	0	0	4
Go Energy	1 serv (5 g)	15	0	0	4
Mega Protein	1 serv (0.5 oz)	45	12	0	0
Multi-Vitamin	1 serv (5 g)	10	0	0	3

FAZOLI'S
BEVERAGES

FOOD	PORTION	CALS	PROT	FAT	CARB
Lemon Ice All Flavors	1	360	0	0	90
Lemon Ice Original	1 reg	180	0	0	45
Lemon Ice Strawberry	1	320	0	0	81
CHILDREN'S MENU SELECTIONS					
Fettuccine Alfredo	1 serv	290	9	5	50
Meat Lasagna	1 serv	260	14	13	21
Ravioli w/ Marinara	1 serv	290	13	7	43
Spaghetti w/ Meatballs	1 serv	350	14	7	55
Ziti w/ Meat Sauce	1 serv	190	9	6	25
DESSERTS					
Cheesecake Original	1 slice	290	6	22	17
Cheesecake Turtle	1 slice	450	6	28	43
Cookie Chocolate Chunk	1	510	5	26	68
MAIN MENU SELECTIONS					
Breadstick	1	100	3	2	20

FOOD	PORTION	CALS	PROT	FAT	CARB
Breadstick Garlic	1	150	3	7	20
Fettuccine Alfredo	1 sm	520	16	12	83
Fettuccine w/ Marinara	1 serv	450	15	3	88
Fettuccine w/ Meat Sauce	1 serv	500	20	7	87
Oven Baked Chicken Parmesan	1 serv	960	56	33	117
Oven Baked Meat Lasagna	1 serv	510	27	25	43
Oven Baked Rigatoni Romano	1 serv	1090	11	54	101
Oven Baked Spaghetti	1 serv	680	32	22	90
Oven Baked Spaghetti w/ Meatballs	1 serv	940	46	40	100
Panini Four Cheese & Tomato	1	510	28	22	53
Panini Grilled Chicken	1	540	35	18	56
Panini Smoked Turkey	1	620	35	29	54
Penne w/ Alfredo	1 serv	520	16	12	83
Penne w/ Marinara	1 serv	450	15	3	88
Penne w/ Meat Sauce	1 serv	500	20	7	87
Pizza Slice Cheese	1	270	13	11	31
Pizza Slice Pepperoni	1	310	14	14	31
Platter Classic Sampler	1	810	34	25	110
Platter Ultimate Sampler	1	980	43	29	134
Ravioli w/ Marinara	1 serv	500	22	15	71
Ravioli w/ Meat Sauce	1 serv	550	26	20	71
Spaghetti w/ Alfredo	1 serv	520	16	12	83
Spaghetti w/ Marinara	1 sm	450	15	3	88
Spaghetti w/ Meat Sauce	1 sm	500	20	7	87
Submarinos Club	half	973	37	34	65
Submarinos Ham n'Swiss	1	680	34	30	65
Submarinos Italian Beef	half	660	46	24	68
Submarinos Original	half	940	35	58	68
Topping Broccoli	1 serv	25	3	0	5
Topping Broccoli & Tomatoes	1 serv	30	3	0	6
Topping Garlic Shrimp	1 serv	160	10	12	3
Topping Italian Sausage	1 serv	240	10	21	3
Topping Meatballs	1 serv	160	13	18	6
Topping Peppery Chicken	1 serv	70	14	1	1
Ziti w/ Meat Sauce	1 serv	480	23	15	65
SALAD DRESSINGS					
Caesar	1 serv	220	1	25	1
Fat Free Honey Mustard	1 serv	60	0	0	15
Fat Free Italian	1 serv	25	0	0	6

FOOD	PORTION	CALS	PROT	FAT	CARB
Honey French	1 serv	220	0	18	14
Italian	1 serv	160	0	14	7
Ranch	1 serv	220	1	24	2
Ranch Lite	1 serv	120	1	12	2
SALADS					
Chicken & Fruit	1	220	23	2	28
Chicken & Pasta Caesar	1	440	35	15	41
Chicken BLT Ranch	1	270	31	10	13
Parmesan Chicken	1	360	31	15	31
Side Caesar	1	40	4	2	4
Side Garden	1	25	2	0	4
Side Pasta	1	320	11	12	41

FIVE GUYS BURGERS AND FRIES
MAIN MENU SELECTIONS

FOOD	PORTION	CALS	PROT	FAT	CARB
Bacon Burger	1 (9.8 oz)	780	43	50	39
Bacon Cheese Dog	1 (7 oz)	695	26	48	41
Bacon Dog	1 (6.4 oz)	625	22	42	40
Cheese Dog	1 (6.5 oz)	615	22	41	41
Cheeseburger	1 (10.6 oz)	840	47	55	40
Cheeseburger Bacon	1 (11 oz)	920	51	62	40
Fries	1 lg (16 oz)	1464	24	71	184
Fries	1 reg (8.6 oz)	620	10	30	78
Grilled Cheese	1 (4 oz)	430	11	26	41
Hamburger	1 (9.3 oz)	700	39	43	39
Hot Dog	1 (5.9 oz)	545	18	35	40
Little Burgers Bacon Burger	1 (6.5 oz)	560	27	33	39
Little Burgers Cheeseburger	1 (6.7 oz)	550	27	32	40
Little Burgers Cheeseburger Bacon	1 (7.2 oz)	630	31	39	40
Little Burgers Hamburger	1 (6 oz)	480	23	26	39
Veggie Sandwich	1 (7.3 oz)	440	16	15	60
TOPPINGS					
A1 Steak Sauce	1 tbsp (0.6 oz)	15	0	0	3
Bacon	2 slices (0.5 oz)	80	4	7	0
BBQ Sauce	1 tbsp (0.6 oz)	60	0	8	16
Cheese	1 slice (0.7 oz)	70	4	6	tr
Green Peppers	1 serv (0.8 oz)	5	0	0	2
Hot Sauce	1 tsp (5 g)	0	0	0	0
Jalapenos	1 serv (0.4 oz)	3	0	0	tr
Ketchup	1 tbsp (0.6 oz)	15	0	0	4

FOOD	PORTION	CALS	PROT	FAT	CARB
Lettuce	1 serv (1 oz)	4	0	0	1
Mayonnaise	1 serv (0.5 oz)	100	0	11	0
Mushrooms	1 serv (0.9 oz)	10	1	0	1
Mustard	1 tbsp (0.6 oz)	0	0	0	0
Onions	1 serv (0.9 oz)	10	0	0	3
Pickle Chips	6 (1 oz)	5	0	0	1
Relish	1 serv (0.5 oz)	15	0	0	4
Tomatoes	1 serv (1.8 oz)	9	tr	0	2

GREAT STEAK & POTATO
BEVERAGES

Great Steak Lemonade	1 sm (12 oz)	180	03	0	48
Orange Juice	1 (12 oz)	118	0	0	30

BREAKFAST SELECTIONS

Potatoes Deluxe Home	1 serv (12 oz)	390	4	23	44
Potatoes Fresh Cut Home	1 serv (10.6 oz)	380	3	23	42
Sandwich Bacon Egg Cheese	1 (7.6 oz)	600	29	36	39
Sandwich Egg Cheese	1 (7 oz)	500	23	29	39
Sandwich Ham Cheese	1 (5.5 oz)	430	18	22	41
Sandwich Ham Egg Cheese	1 (9 oz)	570	31	32	42
Sandwich Sausage Egg Cheese	1 (9 oz)	700	30	47	39
Sandwich Steak Egg Cheese	1 (10 oz)	600	34	34	40

CHILDREN'S MENU SELECTIONS

Grilled Cheese w/ Fry	1 serv (8.8 oz)	530	15	28	57
Kid's Great Fry	1 (6.1 oz)	270	4	13	36
Kids Nuggets	1 serv (2.7 oz)	165	11	9	10
Slider Chicken w/ Fry	1 serv (11.5 oz)	570	23	25	60
Slider Steak w/ Fry	1 serv (11.8 oz)	580	24	28	60

MAIN MENU SELECTIONS

Baked Potato Broccoli & Cheese	1 (8.9 oz)	400	13	24	35
Baked Potato Cheese & Bacon	1 (7.8 oz)	530	25	35	29
Baked Potato Plain	1 (6 oz)	160	4	0	36
Baked Potato Sour Cream & Chive	1 (7.3 oz)	350	5	23	32
Baked Potato The King	1 (8.8 oz)	590	26	41	31
Cheeseburger	1 (10.2 oz)	640	40	35	41
Chicagoland Cheesesteak 7 Inch	1 (13.3 oz)	680	43	29	63
Coney Island Fry	1 reg (12.7 oz)	570	18	30	61

FOOD	PORTION	CALS	PROT	FAT	CARB
Great Fry	1 reg (10.2 oz)	440	7	20	60
Great Steak Cheesesteak 7 Inch	1 (13.6 oz)	740	41	37	62
Great Steak Cheesesteak Wrap	1 (13.7 oz)	820	40	43	67
Gyro	1 (12 oz)	580	29	30	52
Ham Delight 7 Inch	1 (13.1 oz)	710	36	33	71
Ham Explosion 7 Inch	1 (14 oz)	710	37	34	70
Hamburger	1 (9.7 oz)	590	37	30	40
Kansas City BBQ Cheesesteak 7 Inch	1 (12 oz)	680	40	26	71
King Fry	1 reg (11.4 oz)	630	20	39	52
Nacho Fry	1 reg (11.8 oz)	510	12	27	53
Pastrami 7 Inch	1 (13.3 oz)	790	43	41	65
Philly Buffalo Chicken 7 Inch	1 (13.8 oz)	660	37	24	65
Philly Burger	1 (14.2 oz)	820	46	50	47
Philly Original Cheesesteak 7 Inch	1 (11.8 oz)	650	40	26	62
Philly Original Chicken 7 Inch	1 (11 oz)	620	37	22	62
Philly Teriyaki Chicken	1 (14 oz)	290	40	32	65
Philly Turkey 7 Inch	1 (13 oz)	670	38	30	64
Philly Ultimate Chicken	1 (14.6 oz)	730	38	33	64
Philly Slider Chicken	1 (5.4 oz)	300	19	13	24
Philly Slider Steak	1 (5.6 oz)	310	20	15	24
Philly Wrap Original Chicken	1 (11.3 oz)	700	36	28	67
Philly Wrap Ultimate Chicken	1 (14.7 oz)	810	36	39	69
Potato Skins	1 serv (6.4 oz)	390	17	26	24
Reuben 7 Inch	1 (12 oz)	690	37	33	61
Super Steak Wrap Cheesesteak	1 (15.7 oz)	930	41	54	69
The Great Potato Chicken	1 (13 oz)	600	32	33	37
The Great Potato Ham	1 (12.8 oz)	520	29	28	43
The Great Potato Steak	1 (13.5 oz)	620	35	38	37
The Great Potato Turkey	1 (12.8 oz)	490	31	25	39
Veggi Delight 7 Inch	1 (12.2 oz)	610	20	31	66
Wacker Fry	1 reg (9.8 oz)	490	12	27	51
Wisconsin Inside-Out 7 Inch	1 (6.2 oz)	560	24	27	57
SALAD DRESSINGS AND SAUCES					
Dressing Ranch	1 oz	170	1	18	1
Dressing Thousand Island	1 oz	130	0	12	4
Mayonnaise	1 oz	200	0	22	0
Mayonnaise Dijon	1 oz	110	0	11	3
Oil	1 serv (0.3 oz)	60	0	7	0

FOOD	PORTION	CALS	PROT	FAT	CARB
Sauce Buffalo	1 oz	10	0	0	2
Sauce Marinara Dipping	2 oz	15	1	0	3
Sauce Teriyaki	1 oz	25	2	0	3
Sauce Tzatziki	1 oz	50	0	4	2
SALADS					
Chef w/o Dressing	1 (16.1 oz)	260	28	11	15
Garden w/o Dressing	1 (12 oz)	60	3	1	13
Great Salad Grilled Chicken	1 (18.8 oz)	380	31	18	18
Great Salad Grilled Ham	1 (18.8 oz)	360	24	20	28
Great Salad Grilled Steak	1 (19.3 oz)	400	33	23	18
Great Salad Grilled Turkey	1 (18.8 oz)	330	30	17	20
Side w/o Dressing	1 (6 oz)	30	2	0	6
Wedge Grilled Chicken	1 (14.8 oz)	270	24	12	11
Wedge Grilled Steak	1 (15.3 oz)	290	28	16	11
HUNGRY HOWIE'S PIZZA					
OTHER MENU SELECTIONS					
Cajun Bread	¼ bread	300	9	9	46
Chicken Tenders	2	140	13	5	11
Cinnamon Bread	¼ bread	313	9	9	59
Howie Bread	¼ bread	300	9	9	46
Howie Wings	5	180	14	13	0
Sub Deluxe Italian	½ sub	506	24	18	61
Sub Ham & Cheese	½ sub	475	26	15	61
Sub Pizza	½ sub	689	30	34	67
Sub Pizza Special	½ sub	606	29	24	68
Sub Steak & Cheese	½ sub	491	27	15	64
Sub Turkey	½ sub	466	25	13	63
Sub Turkey Club	½ sub	556	42	15	63
Sub Vegetarian	½ sub	530	22	21	64
Three Cheeser Bread	¼ bread	370	15	14	47
PIZZA					
Cheese Slice	1 sm	161	10	4	20
Cheese Slice	1 med	191	11	6	23
Cheese Slice	1 lg	208	12	5	25
Cheese Slice	1 extra lg	395	23	9	42
Cheese Slice Thin	1 med	111	7	5	10
Cheese Slice Thin	1 lg	124	8	6	11
Medium Topping Anchovies	1 serv	44	7	3	0
Medium Topping Bacon	1 serv	32	6	1	tr

FOOD	PORTION	CALS	PROT	FAT	CARB
Medium Topping Banana Peppers	1 serv	6	tr	0	1
Medium Topping Beef	1 serv	30	2	2	tr
Medium Topping Black Olives	1 serv	7	0	tr	tr
Medium Topping Ham	1 serv	7	1	tr	0
Medium Topping Mushrooms	1 serv	2	tr	0	tr
Medium Topping Pepperoni	1 serv	22	1	2	0
Medium Topping Pineapple	1 serv	5	1	0	2
Medium Topping Sausage	1 serv	27	2	2	tr
SALAD DRESSINGS AND SAUCES					
Dressing Blue Cheese	1 serv (1 oz)	150	1	16	1
Dressing Creamy Italian	1 serv (1 oz)	120	0	12	2
Dressing Fat Free Italian	1 serv (1.5 oz)	25	0	0	5
Dressing Fat Free Ranch	1 serv (1.5 oz)	45	0	0	10
Dressing French Style	1 serv (1 oz)	30	0	0	7
Dressing Greek	1 serv (1 oz)	110	0	11	2
Dressing Italian	1 serv (1 oz)	80	0	8	2
Dressing Ranch	1 serv (1 oz)	180	0	19	1
Dressing Thousand Island	1 serv (1 oz)	140	0	14	4
Sauce Dipping	1 serv (3 oz)	45	3	1	9
SALADS					
Antipasto	1 sm	115	9	7	3
Chef	1 sm	114	9	7	4
Garden	1 sm	20	1	tr	3
Greek	1 sm	126	7	7	8

IVAR'S SEAFOOD BARS

FOOD	PORTION	CALS	PROT	FAT	CARB
Chicken	3 pieces (4.5 oz)	250	22	11	14
Chowder Salmon	1 cup	220	4	13	22
Chowder White	1 cup	330	17	19	24
Clams	1 serv (5 oz)	400	17	21	33
Cocktail Sauce	¼ cup	50	1	0	12
Fish	3 pieces	220	22	9	12
French Fries	1 serv (3.5 oz)	300	4	16	34
Oysters	5	290	17	14	22
Prawns	1 serv (5 oz)	290	20	15	18
Salmon Fried	3 pieces (4.5 oz)	210	24	9	9
Scallops	1 serv (5 oz)	240	22	9	14
Tartar Sauce	2 tbsp	140	0	15	1

FOOD	PORTION	CALS	PROT	FAT	CARB
JACK IN THE BOX					
BEVERAGES					
Barq's Root Beer	1 (20 oz)	180	0	0	50
Chocolate Milk Low Fat Chug	1 (3.5 oz)	200	11	3	34
Coca Cola Classic	1 (20 oz)	170	0	0	46
Coffee Regular & Decaf	1 (11 oz)	5	0	0	1
Diet Coke	1 (20 oz)	0	0	0	0
Dr Pepper	1 (20 oz)	150	0	0	42
Fanta Orange	1 (20 oz)	150	0	0	41
Fanta Strawberry	1 (20 oz)	150	0	0	41
Iced Tea	1 (20 oz)	5	0	0	2
Lemonade	1 (20 oz)	160	0	0	42
Orange Juice	1 (10 oz)	140	2	0	32
Reduced Fat Milk Chug	1 (3.5 oz)	130	10	5	13
Shake Chocolate	1 (16 oz)	880	14	45	107
Shake Oreo	1 (16 oz)	910	14	49	102
Shake Strawberry	1 (16 oz)	880	13	44	105
Shake Vanilla	1 (16 oz)	790	13	44	83
Sprite	1 (20 oz)	160	0	0	42
BREAKFAST SELECTIONS					
Biscuit Bacon Egg Cheese	1	430	17	25	34
Biscuit Chicken	1	450	15	24	42
Biscuit Sausage	1	440	12	29	32
Biscuit Sausage Egg Cheese	1	740	27	55	35
Biscuit Spicy Chicken	1	460	21	22	44
Breakfast Jack	1	290	17	12	39
Breakfast Jack Bacon	1	300	16	14	29
Breakfast Jack Sausage	1	450	20	28	29
Breakfast Sandwich Ciabatta	1	710	36	30	63
Breakfast Sandwich Ultimate	1	570	34	27	49
Burrito Hearty Breakfast	1	480	25	29	29
Burrito Sirloin Steak & Egg w/o Salsa	1	790	37	48	52
Croissant Sausage	1	580	21	39	37
Croissant Supreme	1	450	20	25	36
French Toast Sticks	4 (4.2 oz)	470	7	23	58
French Toast Sticks Blueberry	4	450	8	20	59
Hash Browns	1 serv	150	1	10	13
Sandwich Extreme Sausage	1	670	29	48	31

FOOD	PORTION	CALS	PROT	FAT	CARB
DESSERTS					
Cake Chocolate Overload	1 serv (3.2 oz)	300	4	7	57
Cheesecake	1 serv (3.6 oz)	310	7	16	34
MAIN MENU SELECTIONS					
Bacon Cheddar Potato Wedges	1 serv (9 oz)	720	21	48	52
Cheeseburger Bacon Ultimate	1	1090	46	77	53
Cheeseburger Junior Bacon	1	430	20	25	30
Cheeseburger Sourdough Ultimate	1	950	38	73	36
Cheeseburger Ultimate	1	1010	40	71	53
Chicken Fajita Pita	1	280	21	9	30
Chicken Sandwich	1	400	15	21	38
Chicken Strips Crispy	4	500	35	25	36
Chicken Strips Grilled	4 (5 oz)	180	37	2	3
Ciabatta Chipotle w/ Grilled Chicken	1	690	44	28	65
Ciabatta Chipotle w/ Spicy Crispy Chicken	1	750	37	34	75
Ciabatta Burger Bacon 'N' Cheese	1	1120	45	76	66
Ciabatta Burger Single Bacon 'N' Cheese	1	870	31	54	66
Ciabatta Sirloin Steak 'N' Cheddar	1	770	43	38	65
Club Sourdough Grilled Chicken	1	530	36	28	34
Curly Fries Seasoned	1 sm (3 oz)	270	4	15	30
Egg Rolls	1	130	5	6	15
Fish & Chips	1 serv (7.6 oz)	570	17	30	58
Fries Natural Cut	1 sm	340	5	17	41
Fruit Cup	1 serv	90	1	0	22
Hamburger	1	310	16	14	30
Hamburger Deluxe	1	370	17	21	31
Hamburger Deluxe w/ Cheese	1	460	21	28	33
Hamburger w/ Cheese	1	350	18	17	31
Jack's Spicy Chicken	1 serv	620	25	31	61
Jack's Spicy Chicken w/ Cheese	1	700	29	37	62
Jumbo Jack	1	600	21	35	51
Jumbo Jack w/ Cheese	1	690	25	42	54
Mozzarella Cheese Sticks	3	240	11	12	21
Onion Rings	8 (4.2 oz)	500	6	30	51

FOOD	PORTION	CALS	PROT	FAT	CARB
Sampler Trio	1 serv	750	35	39	65
Sandwich Bacon Chicken	1	440	19	24	39
Sirloin Burger w/ American Cheese & Red Onion	1	1120	54	73	63
Sirloin Burger w/ Swiss & Grilled Onions	1	1070	53	71	61
Sirloin Steak Melt	1	640	36	40	34
Sourdough Jack	1	710	27	51	36
Spicy Chicken Bites	1 serv	290	18	14	21
Stuffed Jalapeno	3 (2.5 oz)	230	7	13	22
Taco Monster Beef	1	240	8	14	20
Taco Regular Beef	1	160	5	8	15
SALAD DRESSINGS AND TOPPINGS					
Asian Sesame	1 serv (2.5 oz)	230	1	17	20
Bacon Ranch	1 serv (2.5 oz)	320	2	33	4
Creamy Southwest	1 serv (2.5 oz)	270	1	27	4
Dipping Sauce Barbeque	1 serv (1 oz)	45	0	0	11
Dipping Sauce Buttermilk House	1 serv (0.9 oz)	130	0	13	3
Dipping Sauce Frank's Red Hot Buffalo	1 serv (1 oz)	10	0	0	2
Dipping Sauce Sweet & Sour	1 serv (1 oz)	45	0	0	11
Dipping Sauce Teriyaki	1 serv (1 oz)	60	1	0	13
Dipping Sauce Zesty Marinara	1 serv (0.8 oz)	15	0	0	4
Low Fat Balsamic	1 serv (2.5 oz)	40	0	2	6
Mayo Onion Sauce	1 serv (0.5 oz)	90	1	10	4
Ranch	1 serv (2.5 oz)	390	1	41	4
Ranch Lite	1 serv (2.5 oz)	190	1	18	3
Soy Sauce	1 serv (0.3 oz)	5	1	0	1
Syrup Log Cabin	1 serv (2 oz)	190	0	0	49
Taco Sauce	1 serv (0.3 oz)	0	0	0	0
Tartar Sauce	1 serv (1.5 oz)	210	0	22	2
SALADS					
Asian w/ Crispy Chicken w/o Dressing	1 (13.8 oz)	330	21	13	34
Asian w/ Grilled Chicken w/o Dressing	1 (12.8 oz)	160	22	2	18
Chicken Club w/ Crispy Chicken w/o Dressing	1 (14 oz)	480	33	27	26

FOOD	PORTION	CALS	PROT	FAT	CARB
Chicken Club w/ Grilled Chicken w/o Dressing	1 (13 oz)	320	34	16	11
Side w/o Dressing	1 (4.3 oz)	50	3	3	5
Southwest w/ Crispy Chicken w/o Dressing	1 (16 oz)	480	30	23	44
Southwest w/ Grilled Chicken w/o Dressing	1 (15 oz)	320	31	12	27

JAMBA JUICE
BEVERAGES

FOOD	PORTION	CALS	PROT	FAT	CARB
Acai Super Antioxidant	1 (16 oz)	290	4	5	59
Acai Topper	1 (12 oz)	440	8	9	86
Aloha Pineapple	1 (16 oz)	300	5	1	70
Banana Berry	1 (16 oz)	300	3	1	72
Berry Fulfilling	1 (16 oz)	160	7	1	34
Berry Topper	1 (12 oz)	420	11	9	80
Blackberry Bliss	1 (16 oz)	260	1	1	61
Boost 3G Charger Super	1 (3 g)	5	0	0	2
Boost Flax & Fiber	1 (0.4 oz)	30	1	2	7
Boost Soy Protein	1 (8.9 g)	30	8	0	0
Boost Weight Burner Super	1 (3.5 g)	30	0	3	0
Boost Whey Protein Super	1 (12 g)	45	10	0	1
Caribbean Passion	1 (16 oz)	270	2	1	63
Carrot Juice	1 (16 oz)	100	3	1	22
Chocolate Moo'd	1 (16 oz)	460	12	6	93
Chunky Strawberry Topper	1 (12 oz)	480	13	15	74
Coldbuster	1 (16 oz)	270	3	2	63
Mango Mantra	1 (16 oz)	170	7	1	36
Mango Metabolizer	1 (16 oz)	290	2	4	63
Mango Peach Topper	1 (12 oz)	450	11	9	86
Mango-A-Go-Go	1 (16 oz)	310	2	1	72
Matcha Green Tea Blast	1 (16 oz)	290	8	0	62
Mega Mango	1 (16 oz)	250	3	1	62
Orange Dream Machine	1 (16 oz)	350	8	2	75
Orange Juice	1 (16 oz)	220	3	1	52
Peach Perfection	1 (16 oz)	230	2	0	57
Peach Pleasure	1 (16 oz)	290	2	1	68
Peanut Butter Moo'd	1 (16 oz)	490	13	11	85
Pomegranate Heart Happy	1 (16 oz)	300	4	1	72
Pomegranate Paradise	1 (16 oz)	260	2	1	64
Pomegranate Pick-Me-up	1 (16 oz)	280	2	2	67

FOOD	PORTION	CALS	PROT	FAT	CARB
Protein Berry Workout w/ Soy Protein	1 (16 oz)	290	15	1	55
Protein Berry Workout w/ Whey	1 (16 oz)	300	17	0	56
Razzmatazz	1 (16 oz)	300	2	1	70
Shot Matcha Energy Orange Juice	1 (4 oz)	60	1	0	13
Shot Matcha Energy Soymilk	1 (4 oz)	70	3	0	14
Shot Wheatgrass Detox	1 oz	5	tr	0	tr
Strawberries Wild	1 (16 oz)	280	3	0	66
Strawberry Energizer	1 (16 oz)	300	2	1	71
Strawberry Nirvana	1 (16 oz)	170	7	0	36
Strawberry Surf Rider	1 (16 oz)	330	2	1	80
Strawberry Whirl	1 (16 oz)	240	1	1	59
FOOD					
Cheddar Tomato Twist	1 (3.2 oz)	240	8	5	41
Cookie Omega-3 Chocolate Brownie	1 (1.5 oz)	150	3	4	30
Cookie Omega-3 Oatmeal	1 (1.5 oz)	150	2	6	26
Loaf Reduced Fat Blueberry Lemon	1 (3 oz)	290	2	8	53
Loaf Reduced Fat Cranberry Orange	1 (3 oz)	310	6	9	52
Loaf Zucchini Walnut	1 (3 oz)	270	5	9	43
Oatcake Blueberry	1 (3.25 oz)	280	6	9	46
Oatmeal Apple Cinnamon	1 serv (9.1 oz)	290	8	4	60
Oatmeal Blueberry & Blackberry	1 serv (8.9 oz)	290	8	4	59
Oatmeal Fresh Banana	1 serv (9.6 oz)	280	9	4	57
Oatmeal w/ Brown Sugar	1 serv (7.6 oz)	220	8	4	44
Pretzel Apple Cinnamon	1 (5.2 oz)	380	11	4	76
Pretzel Sourdough Parmesan	1 (5 oz)	410	14	10	67
JIMMY JOHN'S					
BEVERAGES					
Coke	1 sm	248	0	0	68
Diet Coke	1 sm	0	0	0	0
Iced Tea	1 sm	3	0	0	1
Iced Tea Raspberry	1 sm	195	0	0	53
Lemonade	1 sm	243	0	0	65
Lemonade Light	1 sm	13	0	0	3
Sprite	1 sm	243	0	0	65

FOOD	PORTION	CALS	PROT	FAT	CARB
SANDWICHES					
Giant Club Beach	1	798	37	37	78
Giant Club Billy	1	867	48	40	77
Giant Club Bootlegger	1	720	40	28	74
Giant Club Country	1	840	47	38	75
Giant Club Gourmet Smoked Ham	1	851	45	40	76
Giant Club Gourmet Veggie	1	856	33	46	77
Giant Club Hunter's	1	854	49	38	76
Giant Club Italian Night	1	975	47	52	77
Giant Club Lulu	1	790	42	34	74
Giant Club Tuna	1	719	34	29	77
Giant Club Ultimate Porker	1	843	40	41	73
Slim Double Provolone	1	588	32	19	71
Slim Ham & Cheese	1	534	34	12	72
Slim Salami Capicola Cheese	1	624	35	21	72
Slim Tuna Salad	1	577	24	19	72
Slim Turkey Breast	1	407	27	1	70
Sub Big John	1	564	24	27	54
Sub J.J.B.L.T.	1	662	29	35	54
Sub Pepe	1	684	30	37	55
Sub Totally Tuna	1	502	21	20	57
Sub Turkey Tom	1	555	24	26	54
Sub Vegetarian	1	640	21	36	57
Sub Vito	1	579	32	25	56
The J.J. Gargantuan	1	1008	69	55	60
Unwich Hunter's Club	1	520	35	38	8
Unwich The J.J. Gargantuan	1	769	57	55	11
SIDES					
Cookie Chocolate Chunk	1	421	5	18	62
Cookie Raisin Oatmeal	1	421	7	16	65
Jimmy Chips	1 pkg	160	2	8	18
Jimmy Chips BBQ	1 pkg	160	2	9	17
Jimmy Chips Jalapeno	1 pkg	150	2	7	18
Jimmy Chips Sea Salt & Vinegar	1 pkg	140	2	8	16
Pickle Spear	1	4	0	0	1
Pickle Whole	1	15	0	0	3

KENTUCKY FRIED CHICKEN
BEVERAGES

Diet Pepsi	1 med (14 oz)	0	0	0	0

FOOD	PORTION	CALS	PROT	FAT	CARB
Mountain Dew	1 med (14 oz)	190	0	0	54
Pepsi	1 med (14 oz)	180	0	0	47
DESSERTS					
Cake Double Chocolate Chip	1 slice	330	4	16	41
Cookie Sweet Life Chocolate Chip	1 (1.2 oz)	160	2	7	23
Cookie Sweet Life Oatmeal Raisin	1 (1.2 oz)	150	2	5	24
Cookie Sweet Life Sugar	1 (1.2 oz)	160	2	6	23
Lil' Bucket Chocolate Cream	1	280	3	13	38
Lil' Bucket Lemon Creme	1 serv	410	7	15	61
Lil' Bucket Strawberry Short Cake	1 serv	210	2	7	33
Pie Mini's Apple	3 (4 oz)	370	2	20	44
Teddy Graham Cinnamon Snacks	1 serv	90	1	3	15
MAIN MENU SELECTIONS					
Baked Beans	1 serv	220	8	1	45
Biscuit	1 (2 oz)	220	4	11	24
Bowl Chicken & Biscuit	1	870	29	44	88
Bowl Mashed Potato w/ Gravy	1	740	27	36	80
Bowl Rice w/ Gravy	1	620	26	28	67
Chicken Pot Pie	1 (15 oz)	770	33	40	70
Cole Slaw	1 serv	180	1	10	22
Corn On The Cob	1 ear (3 inch)	70	2	2	13
Crispy Strips	2 (3.5 oz)	240	20	13	11
Extra Crispy Breast	1 (5.7 oz)	440	34	27	15
Extra Crispy Drumstick	1 (2 oz)	160	12	10	6
Extra Crispy Thigh	1 (4 oz)	370	18	28	12
Extra Crispy Whole Wing	1 (1.8 oz)	170	13	11	6
Green Beans	1 serv	50	2	2	7
KFC Snacker	1	290	15	13	29
KFC Snacker Buffalo	1	260	15	8	31
KFC Snacker Fish	1	330	17	15	31
KFC Snacker Fish w/o Sauce	1	290	17	12	29
KFC Snacker Honey BBQ	1	210	14	3	32
KFC Snacker Ultimate Cheese	1	280	15	11	30
Macaroni & Cheese	1 serv	180	8	8	18
Mashed Potatoes w/ Gravy	1 serv	140	2	5	20
Mashed Potatoes w/o Gravy	1 serv	110	2	4	17

FOOD	PORTION	CALS	PROT	FAT	CARB
Original Recipe Breast	1 (5.6 oz)	360	37	21	7
Original Recipe Breast w/o Skin Or Breading	1 (3.8 oz)	140	29	2	1
Original Recipe Drumstick	1 (2 oz)	130	12	8	2
Original Recipe Thigh	1 (4.4 oz)	330	20	24	8
Original Recipe Whole Wing	1 (1.6 oz)	130	11	8	4
Popcorn Chicken	1 reg (4 oz)	400	21	26	22
Potato Salad	1 serv	180	2	9	22
Potato Wedges	1 serv	260	4	13	33
Sandwich Crispy Twister	1	550	26	28	49
Sandwich Double Crunch	1	470	27	23	38
Sandwich Honey BBQ	1	280	22	4	40
Sandwich Tender Roast	1	380	37	13	29
Sandwich Tender Roast w/o Sauce	1	300	37	5	28
Seasoned Rice	1 serv	180	4	1	32
Twister Oven Roasted	1	420	28	17	40
Twister Oven Roasted w/o Sauce	1	330	28	7	39
Wings Boneless Fiery Buffalo	5	420	28	20	33
Wings Boneless Honey BBQ	5	450	28	20	41
Wings Boneless Sweet & Spicy	5	440	27	19	38
Wings Boneless Teriyaki	5	500	28	21	50
Wings Fiery Buffalo	5	380	21	24	19
Wings Honey BBQ	5	390	21	24	23
Wings Hot	5	350	20	24	14
Wings Hot & Spicy	5	400	21	24	24
Wings Teriyaki	5	480	22	25	40
SALAD DRESSINGS					
Creamy Parmesan Caesar	1 serv (2 oz)	260	2	26	4
Golden Italian Light	1 serv (1.5 oz)	45	0	3	6
Ranch	1 serv (2 oz)	200	1	20	3
Ranch Fat Free	1 serv (1.5 oz)	35	1	0	8
SALADS					
Crispy BLT w/o Dressing	1 (12 oz)	330	28	17	18
Crispy Caesar w/o Dressing & Croutons	1 (11 oz)	350	29	19	16
Croutons Parmesan Garlic	1 pkg	60	2	3	8
Roasted BLT w/o Dressing	1 (12 oz)	200	29	6	8

FOOD	PORTION	CALS	PROT	FAT	CARB
Roasted Caesar w/o Dressing & Croutons	1 (11 oz)	220	30	8	6
Side Caesar w/o Dressing & Croutons	1 (3 oz)	50	4	3	2
Side House w/o Dressing	1 (3 oz)	15	1	0	2

KOO-KOO-ROO
MAIN MENU SELECTIONS

FOOD	PORTION	CALS	PROT	FAT	CARB
Baked Yam	1 serv (6 oz)	197	3	tr	47
Black Beans	1 serv (6 oz)	125	8	3	23
Buffalo Wings	6	606	44	28	42
Burrito California Chicken	1	810	46	41	60
Burrito Fajita Chicken	1	750	40	33	70
Burrito Original Chicken	1	709	41	28	71
Butternut Squash	1 serv (6 oz)	66	2	tr	17
Chicken Bowl Chargrilled w/o Sauce	1	569	41	19	57
Chicken Bowl Spicy Garlic Ginger w/o Sauce	1	485	42	6	63
Creamed Spinach	1 serv (8 oz)	100	4	6	10
Italian Vegetable	1 serv (5.5 oz)	47	1	2	9
Kernel Corn	1 serv (4.5 oz)	105	4	1	26
Mashed Potatoes	1 serv (6.5 oz)	188	4	5	32
Original Breast	1 (4.1 oz)	187	34	6	tr
Original Chicken Dark	3 pieces (5 oz)	320	39	16	5
Roasted Garlic Potatoes	1 serv (5 oz)	133	2	5	21
Rotisserie Chicken Breast & Wing	1 serv (6.5 oz)	355	49	16	1
Rotisserie Chicken Leg & Thigh	1 serv (4.8 oz)	300	31	18	1
Rotisserie Half Chicken	1 serv (11.3 oz)	655	80	34	2
Sandwich BBQ Chicken	1	562	45	12	71
Sandwich Chicken Caesar	1	781	56	36	63
Sandwich Original Chicken	1	661	41	29	63
Sandwich Turkey Hand Carved	1	599	46	32	31
Southwestern Bowl w/o Sauce	1	570	37	19	67
Tostada Bowl w/o Sauce w/o Shell	1	528	40	22	45
Traditional Turkey Dinner	1 serv	692	42	29	67
Turkey Breast Sliced	1 serv	182	25	8	0
Turkey Pot Pie	1	883	37	44	83

FOOD	PORTION	CALS	PROT	FAT	CARB
Wrap Caesar Chicken	1	757	42	39	59
Wrap Chipotle Chicken	1	924	42	43	89
SALADS					
BBQ Chicken w/o Dressing	1	365	38	14	22
Cantaloupe & Honeydew	1 serv (5 oz)	50	1	tr	12
Chicken Caesar w/o Dressing	1	286	34	11	13
Chinese Chicken w/o Dressing	1	550	40	29	39
Creamy Coleslaw	1 serv (5 oz)	238	1	20	14
Cucumber	1 serv (4.5 oz)	41	1	tr	9
House	1	113	6	4	16
Tangy Tomato	1 serv (4.5 oz)	60	1	4	6
Tossed w/ Dressing	1 serv (3 oz)	16	1	tr	3
SOUPS					
Chicken Noodle	1 serv (5 oz)	71	6	3	4
Chicken Tortilla	1 serv (5 oz)	112	8	6	7
Ten Vegetable	1 serv (5 oz)	94	3	2	16

KRISPY KREME

BEVERAGES

FOOD	PORTION	CALS	PROT	FAT	CARB
Chillers Fruity Orange You Glad	1 (12 oz)	180	0	0	43
Chillers Fruity Very Berry	1 (12 oz)	170	0	0	43
Chillers Kremey Berries & Kreme	1 (12 oz)	620	3	28	92
Chillers Kremey Chocolate Chocolate	1 (12 oz)	970	4	29	104
Chillers Kremey Lemon Sherbert	1 (12 oz)	630	3	28	95
Chillers Kremey Lotta Latte	1 (12 oz)	670	4	28	49
Chillers Kremey Mocha Dream	1 (12 oz)	670	3	28	105
Chillers Kremey Oranges & Kreme	1 (12 oz)	630	3	28	92
DOUGHNUTS					
Apple Fritter	1	380	4	20	47
Caramel Kreme Crunch	1	380	4	19	40
Chocolate Iced Cake	1	280	3	14	36
Chocolate Iced Custard Filled	1	300	3	17	36
Chocolate Iced Glazed	1	250	3	12	33
Chocolate Iced Kreme Filled	1	350	3	20	39
Chocolate Iced w/ Sprinkles	1	270	3	12	38
Cinnamon Apple Filled	1	290	3	16	32
Cinnamon Bun	1	260	3	16	28

FOOD	PORTION	CALS	PROT	FAT	CARB
Cinnamon Twist	1	240	3	15	23
Dulce De Leche	1	300	3	18	31
Glazed Chocolate Cake	1	300	3	15	42
Glazed Cinnamon	1	210	2	12	24
Glazed Creme Filled	1	340	3	20	39
Glazed Cruller	1	240	2	14	26
Glazed Cruller Chocolate	1	290	2	15	37
Glazed Lemon Filled	1	290	3	16	36
Glazed Original	1	200	2	12	22
Glazed Pumpkin Spice	1	300	2	14	42
Glazed Raspberry Filled	1	300	3	16	36
Glazed Sour Cream	1	300	2	13	43
Holes Glazed Blueberry	4	220	3	12	27
Holes Glazed Cake	4	210	2	10	29
Holes Glazed Chocolate Cake	4	210	2	10	29
Holes Glazed Original	4	200	2	11	25
Holes Glazed Pumpkin Spice	4	210	2	10	29
Maple Iced Glazed	1	240	2	12	32
New York Cheesecake	1	340	4	20	34
Powdered Cake	1	290	3	14	37
Powdered Strawberry Filled	1	290	3	16	33
Sugar	1	200	2	12	21
Traditional Cake	1	230	3	13	25

KRYSTAL
BEVERAGES
Coca Cola Classic	1 sm (16 oz)	129	0	0	40
Coca Cola Classic frzn	1 (16 oz)	130	0	0	36
Diet Coke	1 sm (16 oz)	tr	0	0	tr
Sprite	1 sm (16 oz)	126	0	0	39

BREAKFAST SELECTIONS
4 Carb Scrambler Bacon	1 serv	370	24	29	4
4 Carb Scrambler Sausage	1 serv	600	32	51	3
Biscuit & Gravy	1	280	5	14	34
Biscuit Bacon Egg Cheese	1	390	11	23	33
Biscuit Chik	1	360	13	15	40
Biscuit Plain	1	270	5	13	33
Biscuit Sausage	1	480	12	33	33
Country Breakfast	1 serv	660	24	42	46
Kryspers	1 serv	190	1	13	17
Krystal Sunriser	1	240	12	14	14
Scrambler	1 serv	440	20	26	33

FOOD	PORTION	CALS	PROT	FAT	CARB
DESSERTS					
Fried Apple Turnover	1	220	3	10	31
Lemon Icebox Pie	1 serv	260	5	9	41
MAIN MENU SELECTIONS					
BA Burger	1	470	22	27	39
BA Burger Cheese	1	530	25	32	40
BA Burger Double Bacon Cheese	1	800	44	53	41
Chik'n Bites	1 sm	310	17	19	16
Chik'n Bites Salad	1 serv	290	20	20	12
Fries	1 reg	470	4	20	53
Fries Chili Cheese	1 serv	540	13	28	59
Krystal	1	160	7	7	17
Krystal Bacon Cheese	1	190	10	10	16
Krystal Cheese	1	180	9	9	17
Krystal Chik	1	240	11	11	24
Krystal Chili	1 serv	200	13	7	22
Krystal Double	1	260	13	13	24
Krystal Double Cheese	1	310	16	16	26
Pup Chili Cheese	1	210	9	12	17
Pup Corn	1	260	5	19	19
Pup Plain	1	170	6	9	15
MARBLE SLAB CREAMERY					
Cone Honey Wheat	1	130	3	3	24
Cone Sugar	1	130	2	3	23
Cone Vanilla Cinnamon	1	130	2	3	24
Frozen Yogurt Nonfat	½ cup	100	3	tr	22
Frozen Yogurt Nonfat No Sugar Added	½ cup	90	4	tr	17
Ice Cream Reduced Fat	1 serv (6.75 oz)	390	6	20	47
Ice Cream Superpremium	1 serv (6.75 oz)	450	8	28	44
Sorbet	½ cup	90	0	0	22
MARCO'S PIZZA					
OTHER MENU SELECTIONS					
Cheezybread Bran	1 piece	80	3	2	11
Chicken Tumblers BBQ	1	67	4	2	7
Chicken Tumblers Hot & Spicy	1	57	4	2	5

FOOD	PORTION	CALS	PROT	FAT	CARB
Chicken Tumblers Naked	1	57	4	2	5
Chicken Wings BBQ	1	71	5	4	3
Chicken Wings Hot & Spicy	1	60	5	4	0
Chicken Wings Naked	1	60	5	4	0
Cinnasquares	1 piece	60	1	2	9
Salad Chicken Ranch	1 serv	240	22	13	10
Salad Italian	1 serv	230	12	17	11
Sub Chicken Club	½	385	28	16	34
Sub Ham & Cheese	½	400	21	21	33
Sub Italian	½	430	24	23	35
Sub Steak & Cheese	½	380	29	15	33
Sub Veggie	½	355	16	16	39
PIZZA					
Cheese Large	1 slice	280	14	8	33
Cheese Medium	1 slice	210	11	6	24
Cheese Small	1 slice	200	11	6	23
Chicken Fresco Large	1 slice	350	20	13	35
Chicken Fresco Medium	1 slice	260	15	10	26
Chicken Fresco Small	1 slice	180	11	7	19
Deep Pan Cheese	1 slice	290	15	8	36
Deep Pan Pepperoni	1 slice	330	16	12	36
Deluxe Uno Large	1 slice	380	20	16	35
Deluxe Uno Medium	1 slice	280	15	12	26
Deluxe Uno Small	1 slice	200	10	9	18
Garden Large	1 slice	310	16	10	36
Garden Medium	1 slice	230	12	8	26
Garden Small	1 slice	160	8	5	19
Hawaiian Chicken Large	1 slice	380	22	15	35
Hawaiian Chicken Medium	1 slice	260	15	10	26
Hawaiian Chicken Small	1 slice	180	10	6	18
Meat Supremo Large	1 slice	430	23	21	34
Meat Supremo Medium	1 slice	300	15	15	25
Meat Supremo Small	1 slice	210	11	10	18
Pepperoni Large	1 slice	310	15	11	33
Pepperoni Medium	1 slice	230	11	9	24
Pepperoni Small	1 slice	210	10	8	23
White Cheezy Medium	1 slice	260	13	11	24
White Cheezy Small	1 slice	170	9	7	17
White Cheezy Large	1 slice	340	17	15	33

FOOD	PORTION	CALS	PROT	FAT	CARB
MAUI WOWI					
SMOOTHIES					
Fresh Fruit Banana Banana	1 (12 oz)	210	2	1	50
Fresh Fruit Black Raspberry	1 (12 oz)	240	2	0	59
Fresh Fruit Kiwi Lemon Lime	1 (12 oz)	180	3	0	42
Fresh Fruit Lemon Wave	1 (12 oz)	415	tr	tr	108
Fresh Fruit Mango Orange Banana	1 (12 oz)	240	3	1	57
Fresh Fruit Passion Papaya	1 (12 oz)	220	2	1	54
Fresh Fruit Pina Colada	1 (12 oz)	240	3	3	57
MAX & ERMA'S					
Black Bean Roll Up	1 serv	577	29	10	95
Caribbean Chicken Lunch Portion	1 serv	536	28	20	59
Fruit Smoothie	1	124	1	tr	29
Garlic Breadstick	1	156	4	6	21
Hula Bowl w/ Fat Free Honey Mustard Dressing w/o Breadsticks	1 serv	823	46	7	79
Salad Baby Greens w/o Breadsticks	1 serv	119	1	11	6
Salad Shrimp Stack	1 serv	322	20	12	116
Salad Dressing Bleu Cheese	2 tbsp	201	1	21	tr
Salad Dressing French Fat Free	2 tbsp	126	tr	tr	31
Salad Dressing Honey Mustard Fat Free	2 tbsp	60	0	0	14
Salad Dressing Italian	2 tbsp	110	0	12	1
Salad Dressing Ranch	2 tbsp	120	1	13	1
Salad Dressing Tex Mex Low Fat	2 tbsp	23	3	tr	2
MCALISTER'S DELI					
CHILDREN'S MENU SELECTIONS					
Kid's Nacho	1 serv	734	12	43	74
Mac's Dog	1	307	10	19	24
Pita Pizza	1	503	24	21	54
Sandwich Ham & Cheese	1	455	26	22	39
Sandwich PB&J	1	714	23	32	86
Sandwich Toasted Cheese	1	620	30	38	40
Sandwich Turkey & Cheese	1	451	26	21	39

FOOD	PORTION	CALS	PROT	FAT	CARB
DESSERTS					
Brownie Chocolate	1 (3.5 oz)	424	6	18	59
Brownie Delight	1 (11 oz)	917	13	48	111
Chocolate Loving Spoon Cake	1 (4 oz)	538	6	35	54
Ice Cream Vanilla Bean	1 scoop (5 oz)	160	3	10	19
Kentucky Pie	1 slice (12 oz)	807	14	64	110
New York Cheesecake	1 slice (5 oz)	505	7	35	37
Sundae Topping Caramel	2 tbsp	100	1	0	20
Sundae Topping Chocolate	1 tbsp	110	1	0	21
MAIN MENU SELECTIONS					
Appetizers Chips & Salsa	1 serv (5 oz)	87	3	5	9
Appetizers Dip Cheese & Chili	1 serv (5 oz)	572	10	35	54
Appetizers Dip Cheese & Veggie Chili	1 serv (5 oz)	552	9	31	58
Appetizers Nacho Basket	1 serv (6 oz)	579	10	33	61
Appetizers Nacho Chili	1 serv (6 oz)	564	12	37	46
Appetizers Nacho Veggie Chili	1 serv (6 oz)	537	11	31	52
Chicken Cordon Bleu	1 serv	810	59	39	53
Chili Vegetarian	1 serv (8 oz)	133	8	1	28
Cole Slaw	1 serv (4 oz)	190	1	15	14
Fruit Cup	1 serv (4 oz)	98	1	0	12
Giant Spud Cheese	1 (27 oz)	930	55	48	139
Giant Spud Grilled Chicken	1 (27 oz)	839	52	25	99
Giant Spud Just A Spud	1 (26 oz)	604	20	4	123
Giant Spud Ole	1 (30 oz)	1252	68	60	110
Giant Spud Ole w/ Chili	1 (33 oz)	1512	69	78	134
Giant Spud Ole w/ Veggie Chili	1 (33 oz)	1457	67	67	146
Giant Spud Veggie	1 (28 oz)	668	29	18	99
Macaroni & Cheese	1 serv (4 oz)	200	8	7	17
Mashed Potatoes	1 serv (4 oz)	136	2	8	19
Meatloaf w/ Gravy	1 serv	340	40	37	21
Open-Faced Roast Beef	1 serv	751	55	21	88
Pot Roast Spud	1 serv	906	38	30	121
Potato Salad	1 serv (4 oz)	200	3	11	22
Salmon Filet	1 serv	235	46	4	3
Steamed Vegetables	1 serv (4 oz)	43	1	0	7
SALAD DRESSINGS AND SAUCES					
Au Jus	1 serv (4 oz)	10	0	0	2
Comeback Gravy	1 serv (4 oz)	37	1	2	6
Dressing Blue Cheese	2 tbsp	140	0	15	1

FOOD	PORTION	CALS	PROT	FAT	CARB
Dressing Greek	2 tbsp	90	0	9	2
Dressing Parmesan Peppercorn	2 tbsp	150	0	16	2
Dressing Ranch	2 tbsp	100	0	11	1
Dressing Tomato Basil	2 tbsp	30	0	0	6
Dressing Lite Olive Oil Vinaigrette	2 tbsp	60	0	6	3
Dressing Lite Ranch	2 tbsp	100	0	10	1
Dressing Low Calorie Italian	2 tbsp	25	0	2	2
SALADS					
Caesar w/ Salmon	1 (17 oz)	800	34	53	42
Chicken Fiesta	1 (20 oz)	493	38	22	34
Chicken Grill	1 (21 oz)	840	57	15	47
Garden	1 (15 oz)	264	17	17	21
Garden w/ Chicken Salad	1 (18 oz)	537	30	45	14
Garden w/ Salmon	1 (17 oz)	315	28	10	28
Garden w/ Tuna Salad	1 (18 oz)	373	31	18	21
Greek Chicken	1 (19 oz)	584	38	32	32
Side Caesar	1 (6 oz)	328	5	24	19
Side Garden	1 (8 oz)	138	8	9	11
Taco	1 (26 oz)	641	38	40	33
Taco w/ Veggie Chili	1 (26 oz)	641	38	40	33
SANDWICHES					
BLT	1	654	28	38	50
Chicken Salad	1	677	15	43	58
Deli Corned Beef On Wheat	1	369	34	9	39
Deli Ham On Wheat	1	350	24	9	43
Deli Pastrami On Wheat	1	371	33	10	36
Deli Roast Beef On Wheat	1	398	27	12	49
Deli Salami On Wheat	1	565	27	32	43
Deli Turkey On Wheat	1	342	24	9	43
French Dip	1	676	44	34	50
Grilled Chicken Breast	1	751	50	36	56
Grilled Chicken Club	1	1234	76	64	87
Ham Melt	1	700	49	34	52
McAlister's Club	1	1225	66	69	86
Meatloaf Parmesan	1	708	47	36	49
Memphian	1	585	41	26	48
Muffuletta	¼ (8 oz)	615	36	35	40
New Yorker	1	628	50	25	50
Orange Cranberry Club	1	954	63	52	62

FOOD	PORTION	CALS	PROT	FAT	CARB
Reuben On Rye	1	492	25	30	35
Roast Beef Melt	1	635	40	32	48
Salmon	1	608	37	21	66
Submarine	1	833	50	48	53
Sweetberry Chicken On Wheatberry	1	701	53	24	67
Tuna Salad On Wheat	1	452	25	19	47
Turkey Melt	1	700	45	35	52
Veggie On Pita	1	522	15	36	33
Wrap Greek Chicken	1	630	48	25	57
Wrap Grilled Chicken Caesar	1	533	42	25	46
SOUPS					
Asiago Cheese Bisque	1 (8 oz)	240	5	17	17
Broccoli Cheddar	1 (8 oz)	213	8	15	13
Cheddar Potato	1 (8 oz)	213	5	13	19
Cheesy Chicken Tortilla	1 (8 oz)	150	10	6	13
Chicken & Sausage Gumbo	1 (8 oz)	150	8	5	17
Clam Chowder	1 (8 oz)	200	8	11	09
Country Potato	1 (8 oz)	173	4	8	23
Country Vegetable	1 (8 oz)	93	3	1	17
French Onion	1 (8 oz)	80	1	1	11
Red Beans & Rice	1 (8 oz)	107	9	3	25
Southwest Roasted Corn	1 (8 oz)	90	4	4	20

MCDONALD'S
BEVERAGES

FOOD	PORTION	CALS	PROT	FAT	CARB
Apple Juice	1 box (6.8 oz)	90	0	0	23
Chocolate Milk 1% Low Fat	8 oz	170	9	3	26
Coca Cola Classic	1 sm (16 oz)	150	0	0	40
Coffee	1 sm (12 oz)	0	0	0	0
Diet Coke	1 sm (16 oz)	0	0	0	0
Half & Half Creamer	1 pkg	20	0	2	0
Hi-C Orange Lavaburst	1 sm (16 oz)	160	0	0	44
Iced Coffee Caramel	1 sm (16 oz)	130	1	5	21
Iced Coffee Hazelnut	1 sm (16 oz)	130	1	5	21
Iced Coffee Regular	1 sm (16 oz)	140	1	5	22
Iced Coffee Vanilla	1 sm (16 oz)	130	1	5	21
Iced Tea	1 sm (16 oz)	0	0	0	0
Milk Lowfat 1%	1 pkg	100	8	3	12
Orange Juice	1 sm (12 oz)	140	2	0	33

FOOD	PORTION	CALS	PROT	FAT	CARB
Powerade Mountain Blast	1 sm (16 oz)	100	0	0	27
Shake Triple Thick Chocolate	1 sm (12 oz)	440	10	10	76
Shake Triple Thick Strawberry	1 sm (12 oz)	420	10	10	73
Shake Triple Thick Vanilla	1 sm (16 oz)	420	9	10	72
Sprite	1 sm (16 oz)	150	0	0	39
BREAKFAST SELECTIONS					
Big Breakfast Regular Biscuit	1 serv	720	27	46	49
Biscuit	1 reg	250	4	11	32
Biscuit Regular Bacon Egg Cheese	1	450	18	25	36
Biscuit Regular Sausage	1	410	11	27	33
Biscuit Regular Sausage w/ Egg	1	500	17	32	35
Burrito Sausage	1	300	12	16	26
Deluxe Breakfast Regular Biscuit w/o Syrup & Margarine	1 serv	1070	36	55	109
English Muffin	1	160	5	3	27
Hash Browns	1 serv	140	1	8	15
Hotcake Syrup	1 pkg (2 oz)	180	0	0	45
Hotcakes & Sausage w/o Syrup & Margarine	1 serv	520	15	24	61
Hotcakes w/o Syrup & Margarine	1 serv	350	8	9	60
McGriddles Bacon Egg Cheese	1	460	19	21	48
McGriddles Sausage	1	420	11	22	44
McGriddles Sausage Egg & Cheese	1	560	20	32	48
McMuffin Sausage	1	370	14	22	29
McMuffin Sausage w/ Egg	1	250	21	27	30
McSkillet Burrito w/ Sausage	1	610	27	36	44
McSkillet Burrito w/ Steak	1	570	32	30	44
Sausage Patty	1	170	7	15	1
Scrambled Eggs	2	170	15	11	1
DESSERTS					
Apple Dippers	1 pkg	35	0	0	8
Apple Pie Baked	1	270	3	12	36
Caramel Dip Low Fat	1 pkg	70	0	1	15
Cinnamon Melts	1 serv	460	6	19	66
Cookie Chocolate Chip	1	180	2	7	22
Cookie Oatmeal	1 (1.1 oz)	150	2	6	22
Cookie Sugar	1 (1.1 oz)	150	2	6	21

FOOD	PORTION	CALS	PROT	FAT	CARB
Cookies McDonaldland	1 pkg (2 oz)	250	4	8	42
Cookies McDonaldland Chocolate Chip	1 pkg	270	3	11	39
Fruit 'n Yogurt Parfait	1 serv	160	4	2	31
Ice Cream Cone Reduced Fat Vanilla	1	150	4	4	24
Kiddie Cone	1	45	1	1	8
McFlurry Oreo	1 (12 oz)	560	14	16	88
McFlurry w/ M&M's	1 (12 oz)	620	14	20	96
Peanuts For Sundae	1 serv	45	2	4	2
Sundae Hot Caramel	1	340	7	7	60
Sundae Hot Fudge	1	330	8	10	54
Sundae Strawberry	1	280	6	6	49
MAIN MENU SELECTIONS					
Apple Sauce Strawberry	1 serv	90	0	0	23
Big Mac	1	540	25	29	45
Big N' Tasty	1	460	24	24	37
Big N' Tasty w/ Cheese	1	510	27	28	38
Cheeseburger	1	300	15	12	33
Cheeseburger Double	1	440	25	23	34
Cheesy Tots	6 pieces	210	7	12	20
Chicken McNuggets	4 pieces	170	10	10	10
Chicken Selects	3 pieces	380	23	20	28
Filet-O-Fish	1	380	15	18	38
French Fries	1 lg	570	6	30	70
French Fries	1 sm	250	2	13	30
Hamburger	1	250	12	9	31
McChicken	1	360	14	16	40
McRib	1	500	22	26	44
Onion Rings	1 sm	140	2	7	18
Quarter Pounder	1	410	24	19	37
Quarter Pounder Double w/ Cheese	1	740	48	42	40
Quarter Pounder w/ Cheese	1	510	29	26	40
Sandwich Chicken Classic Crispy	1	500	27	17	61
Sandwich Chicken Classic Grilled	1	420	32	10	51
Sandwich Club Chicken Crispy	1	660	39	28	63
Sandwich Club Chicken Grilled	1	570	44	21	52

FOOD	PORTION	CALS	PROT	FAT	CARB
Sandwich Ranch BLT Chicken Crispy	1	600	35	23	64
Sandwich Ranch BLT Chicken Grilled	1	520	40	16	53
Snack Wrap Grilled w/ Chipotle BBQ	1	260	18	8	28
Snack Wrap Grilled w/ Honey Mustard	1	260	18	9	27
Snack Wrap Grilled w/ Ranch	1	270	18	10	26
Snack Wrap w/ Chipotle BBQ	1	320	14	14	35
Snack Wrap w/ Honey Mustard	1	320	14	15	34
Snack Wrap w/ Ranch	1	140	14	16	32
SALAD DRESSINGS AND SAUCES					
Dipping Sauce Buffalo	1 serv (1 oz)	80	0	8	2
Dipping Sauce Zesty Onion Ring	1 serv (1 oz)	150	0	15	3
Dressing Ken's Light Italian	1 pkg (2 oz)	120	0	11	5
Dressing Newman's Own Creamy Caesar	1 pkg (2 oz)	170	2	18	4
Dressing Newman's Own Creamy Southwest	1 pkg (1.5 oz)	100	1	6	11
Dressing Newman's Own Low Fat Balsamic Vinaigrette	1 pkg (1.5 oz)	40	0	3	4
Dressing Newman's Own Low Fat Family Recipe Italian	1 pkg (1.5 oz)	60	1	3	8
Dressing Newman's Own Low Fat Sesame Ginger	1 pkg (1.5 oz)	90	1	3	15
Dressing Newman's Own Ranch	1 pkg (2 oz)	170	1	15	9
Honey	1 pkg (0.5 oz)	50	0	0	12
Ketchup	1 pkg	15	0	0	3
Sauce Barbecue	1 pkg (1 oz)	50	0	0	12
Sauce Creamy Ranch	1 pkg (1.5 oz)	200	0	22	2
Sauce Hot Mustard	1 pkg (1 oz)	60	1	3	9
Sauce Southwestern Chipotle Barbeque	1 pkg (1.5 oz)	70	0	0	18
Sauce Spicy Buffalo	1 pkg (1.5 oz)	60	0	7	1
Sauce Sweet'N Sour	1 pkg (1 oz)	50	0	0	12
Sauce Tangy Honey Mustard	1 pkg (1.5 oz)	70	1	3	13
SALADS					
Asian w/ Crispy Chicken w/o Dressing	1 serv	380	27	17	33

FOOD	PORTION	CALS	PROT	FAT	CARB
Asian w/ Grilled Chicken w/o Dressing	1 serv	300	32	10	23
Asian w/o Chicken & Dressing	1 serv	150	8	7	15
Bacon Ranch w/ Crispy Chicken	1 serv	350	28	16	23
Bacon Ranch w/ Grilled Chicken w/o Dressing	1 serv	260	33	9	12
Bacon Ranch w/o Chicken	1 serv	140	9	7	10
Caesar w/ Crispy Chicken	1 serv	300	25	13	22
Caesar w/ Grilled Chicken	1 serv	220	30	6	12
Caesar w/o Chicken	1 serv	90	7	4	9
Croutons Butter Garlic	1 pkg	60	2	2	10
Fruit & Walnut Snack Size	1 serv	210	4	8	31
Side Salad	1 serv	20	1	0	4
Southwest w/ Crispy Chicken w/o Dressing	1 serv	400	25	16	41
Southwest w/ Grilled Chicken	1 serv	320	30	9	30
Southwest w/o Chicken & Dressing	1 serv	140	6	5	20

MIMI'S CAFE
BEVERAGES

FOOD	PORTION	CALS	PROT	FAT	CARB
Cappuccino	1 serv	86	4	5	7
Cappuccino Iced	1 serv	86	4	5	7
Espresso	1 serv	8	0	0	1
Hot Chocolate w/ Whipped Cream	1 serv	986	8	17	193
Mocha Iced	1 serv	376	6	11	70
Mocha Latte	1 serv	376	6	11	70

CHILDREN'S MENU SELECTIONS

FOOD	PORTION	CALS	PROT	FAT	CARB
Chicken Fingers	1 serv	408	30	21	21
Grilled Cheese	1 serv	273	13	19	14
Macaroni & Cheese	1 serv	353	12	13	48
Mini Burger	1 serv	554	25	28	48
Mini Corn Dogs	1 serv	460	7	32	35
Pancakes Chocolate Chip	1 serv	563	11	29	71
Pancakes Mimi Mouse	1 serv	477	11	18	69
PB&J Soldiers	1 serv	730	18	40	78
Pepperoni Pizzadillas	1 serv	617	31	38	39
Scrambled Eggs & Bacon	1 serv	216	18	16	1
Spaghetti	1 serv	343	13	5	62
Turkey Dinner	1 serv	337	11	16	25

FOOD	PORTION	CALS	PROT	FAT	CARB
DESSERTS					
Apple Crisp Cinnamon	1 serv	898	7	37	141
Bread Pudding	1 serv	819	18	55	69
Brownie Triple Chocolate	1 serv	1950	25	87	280
Cheesecake New York Style	1 serv	1075	19	42	85
Pie Banana Foster Mud	1 serv	1245	14	73	138
Pie Pecan Chocolate Chip	1 serv	1879	21	111	220
MAIN MENU SELECTIONS					
Appetizer Dip Spinach & Artichoke	1 serv	2459	90	138	191
Appetizer Fried Chicken Tenders	1 serv	800	60	33	60
Appetizer Fried Dill Pickles	1 serv	972	16	42	132
Appetizer Jazz Fest	1 serv	1252	43	72	108
Appetizer Zucchini Parmesan	1 serv	626	22	28	73
Blackened Soul w/ Shrimp Creole	1 serv	852	78	34	59
Broiled Flat Iron Steak	1 serv	1026	68	58	58
Burger Half Pound	1	684	42	34	48
Cafe Fish & Chips	1 serv	1290	69	57	119
Cajun Blackened Salmon	1 serv	919	57	55	55
Cheeseburger BBQ Ranch	1	999	58	57	62
Cheeseburger Half Pound	1	855	53	48	49
Chicken Cordon Bleu	1 serv	1360	100	81	51
Chicken Feta Penne	1 serv	1879	57	99	158
Ciabatta Chicken	1	1251	70	72	81
Ciabatta Meatloaf	1	1036	41	61	83
Ciabatta Turkey Pesto	1	1248	45	73	83
Club Cafe	1	1132	42	63	73
Country Fried Steak	1 serv	1061	42	56	107
Crab Cake Dinner	1 serv	1662	59	100	129
Diablo Center Cut Pork Chops	1 serv	1094	54	73	55
Dip Classic Beef	1	521	49	15	43
Fillet Of Soul	1 serv	636	45	26	56
French Quarter	1	1480	66	105	68
Garlic Shrimp Spaghettini	1 serv	860	37	20	109
Grilled Beef Liver	1 serv	1003	75	45	75
Grilled Chicken Tuscan Style	1 serv	880	58	36	80
Hibachi Salmon	1 serv	846	49	40	75
Mimi's Meatloaf	1 serv	910	43	53	68

FOOD	PORTION	CALS	PROT	FAT	CARB
Mimi's Pot Roast	1 serv	1291	88	78	57
Original Patty Melt	1	976	56	56	62
Parmesan Crusted Chicken Breast	1 serv	1820	91	54	211
Pasta Jambalaya	1 serv	1223	74	44	113
Pot Pie Chicken	1 serv	1403	70	87	86
Reuben West Coast	1	2015	62	138	120
Sandwich 5 Way Grilled Cheese	1	703	39	39	49
Sandwich Albacore & Avocado	1	993	33	71	58
Sandwich Bacon Lettuce & Tomato	1	586	24	34	48
Sandwich Fresh Roasted Turkey Breast	1	532	20	27	28
Sandwich Turkey Walnut Salad On Raisin Bread	1	549	7	42	36
Sandwich Veggie Stack	1	836	27	43	93
Slow Roasted Turkey Breast	1 serv	851	25	41	72
Small Bites Black & Blue Quesadilla	1 serv	1241	73	80	60
Small Bites Chicken & Fruit	1 serv	460	73	9	21
Small Bites Citrus Salmon	1 serv	699	44	43	37
Small Bites Crab Cakes	1 serv	412	18	25	27
Small Bites Smokey Chicken Enchiladas	1 serv	1154	61	72	68
Small Bites Sweet & Sour Coconut Shrimp	1 serv	608	22	50	79
Small Bites Thai Chicken Wrap	1 serv	1004	51	41	106
Top Sirloin 12 oz	1 serv	947	79	48	49
SALAD DRESSINGS					
Balsamic Vinaigrette	1 serv	316	0	32	8
Blue Cheese	1 serv	298	2	31	1
Caesar	1 serv	273	1	29	2
Chinese Sesame	1 serv	263	0	25	11
Dijon Vinaigrette	1 serv	296	0	32	3
Honey Mustard	1 serv	243	1	22	11
Non Fat French	1 serv	65	1	0	16
Ranch	1 serv	194	1	20	2
Thousand Island	1 serv	232	0	23	6
SALADS					
Asian Chopped	1 serv	751	81	22	55

FOOD	PORTION	CALS	PROT	FAT	CARB
Blue Cheese & Walnut	1 serv	728	26	53	45
Caesar Blackened Chicken	1 serv	570	59	17	41
Chopped Cobb	1 serv	524	35	32	18
Fried Chicken	1 serv	764	23	67	16
Zesty Chicken Tostada	1 serv	1046	47	57	89
SOUPS					
Broccoli Cheddar	1 serv	270	12	10	18
Chicken Gumbo	1 serv	235	7	12	25
Clam Chowder	1 serv	240	10	14	21
Corn Chowder	1 serv	196	3	9	28
Cream Of Chicken	1 serv	337	0	29	19
French Market Onion	1 serv	207	10	12	16
Red Bean & Andouille Sausage	1 serv	256	13	10	30
Split Pea	1 serv	194	14	3	29
Vegetarian Vegetable	1 serv	60	2	0	12

MR. HERO
DESSERTS

FOOD	PORTION	CALS	PROT	FAT	CARB
Eli's Cheesecake Oreo Cookie	1 slice (2.5 oz)	260	4	17	24
Eli's Cheesecake Original Plain	1 slice (2.6 oz)	280	4	19	22
Eli's Cheesecake Snickers	1 slice (2.3 oz)	270	4	18	23
Eli's Cheesecake Strawberry Swirl	1 slice (2.6 oz)	280	4	19	22
SALADS					
Garden Side	1 serv (7.3 oz)	32	1	0	7
Grilled Chicken	1 serv (13.4 oz)	166	23	3	13
Tuna Delight	1 serv (14.4 oz)	403	13	48	10
SANDWICHES					
Cheeseburger	1 (10.4 oz)	776	26	55	47
Cheesesteak Hot Buttered	1 (9.4 oz)	669	28	42	45
Chicken Grilled Philly	1 (9.1 oz)	421	34	10	48
Deli Subs Original Italian	1 (9.5 oz)	641	22	39	47
Deli Subs Tuna 'N Cheese	1 (9.7 oz)	724	21	54	44
Deli Subs Turkey	1 (9.8 oz)	468	30	20	46
Deli Subs Ultimate Italian	1 (10.3 oz)	675	27	40	46
Romanburger	1 (11.3 oz)	861	30	62	48
Steak Tuscan	1 (10.6 oz)	625	40	31	42
Steak Zesty Bacon & Swiss	1 (9.8 oz)	616	38	32	42
Subs Meatball	1 (9.3 oz)	724	30	47	47

FOOD	PORTION	CALS	PROT	FAT	CARB
Taste Buddies Cheeseburger Bacon	1 (5.9 oz)	264	15	30	33
Taste Buddies Grilled Italiano	1 (5.3 oz)	440	00	32	32
Taste Buddies Italian Sausage	1 (5.4 oz)	368	19	22	34
Taste Buddies Tuna 'N Cheese	1 (6 oz)	483	12	38	31
SIDES					
Breadsticks	2 (6 oz)	446	10	17	64
Jalapeno Poppers	1 serv (4.5 oz)	432	9	28	37
Mozzarella Sticks	1 serv (8.7 oz)	565	31	43	12
Onion Petals	1 serv (5.7 oz)	597	6	37	56
Potato Babycakes	1 serv (5.9 oz)	477	2	37	34
Potato Waffer Fries w/ Cheese Sauce	1 serv (7.2 oz)	482	4	34	42

NOAH'S BAGELS
BAGELS AND BREADS

FOOD	PORTION	CALS	PROT	FAT	CARB
Bagel Asiago Cheese Topped	1 (4.2 oz)	330	16	6	57
Bagel Blueberry	1 (3.7 oz)	270	10	1	59
Bagel Candy Cane	1 (3.7 oz)	270	9	3	54
Bagel Cheddar Stick	1 (4.2 oz)	330	14	6	57
Bagel Chocolate Chip	1 (3.7 oz)	290	9	4	60
Bagel Chopped Garlic	1 (3.9 oz)	290	11	3	58
Bagel Cinnamon Raisin	1 (3.7 oz)	270	9	1	58
Bagel Cinnamon Sugar	1 (4.1 oz)	310	10	3	64
Bagel Cracked Pepper	1 (3.7 oz)	280	9	4	55
Bagel Cranberry Orange	1 (3.5 oz)	250	9	1	54
Bagel Dutch Apple	1 (5 oz)	340	10	3	72
Bagel Egg	1 (3.7 oz)	290	12	3	57
Bagel Everything	1 (3.9 oz)	280	10	2	57
Bagel Good Grains	1 (3.9 oz)	280	12	2	58
Bagel Jalapeno Cheddar	1 (4.9 oz)	350	15	7	58
Bagel Onion	1 (3.7 oz)	270	10	2	57
Bagel Plain	1 (3.7 oz)	270	10	1	57
Bagel Poppyseed	1 (3.9 oz)	290	11	3	57
Bagel Power	1 (4 oz)	310	11	5	61
Bagel Pumpernickel	1 (3.7 oz)	260	10	2	57
Bagel Sesame Seed	1 (3.9 oz)	290	11	3	57
Bagel Six Cheese	1 (4.5 oz)	340	16	6	57
Bagel Spinach Florentine	1 (4.9 oz)	350	16	8	58
Bagel Sun Dried Tomato	1 (3.7 oz)	270	10	2	57
Bagel Whole Wheat	1 (3.7 oz)	260	11	1	57

FOOD	PORTION	CALS	PROT	FAT	CARB
Bagel Whole Wheat Sesame & Sunflower Seeds	1 (4.4 oz)	370	15	11	61
Bialy	1 (5.3 oz)	380	11	4	77
Bread Ciabatta	1 serv (4.25 oz)	290	10	3	60
Bread Corn Meal Rye	1 slice (2 oz)	150	6	2	31
Bread Harvest Grain	1 slice (2.3 oz)	180	7	2	36
Bread Marble Rye	1 slice (1.7 oz)	160	5	1	30
Bread Potato	1 slice (1.7 oz)	140	4	2	28
Challah Braided	1 serv (2 oz)	160	6	3	29
Challah Roll	1 (3 oz)	230	8	4	44
Pizza Bagel Artichoke Tomato & Red Onion	1 (11.1 oz)	550	31	20	67
Pizza Bagel Artichoke & Spinach	1 (12 oz)	670	31	32	70
Pizza Bagel Cheese	1 (6.2 oz)	420	23	11	60
Pizza Bagel Cheesy Garlic & Herb	1 (6.2 oz)	500	24	19	62
Pizza Bagel Pepperoni	1 (6.8 oz)	500	26	19	60
Pizza Bagel Spinach & Mushroom	1 (9.5 oz)	580	27	25	68
Pizza Bagel Tomato & Rosemary	1 (8.7 oz)	540	30	20	63
BEVERAGES AND EXTRAS					
Cafe Latte Low Fat	1 reg (12 oz)	160	10	7	17
Cafe Latte Nonfat	1 reg (12 oz)	110	11	0	17
Cafe Latte Whole	1 reg (12 oz)	200	10	10	16
Cappuccino Low Fat	1 reg (12 oz)	120	7	5	13
Cappuccino Nonfat	1 reg (12 oz)	90	8	0	13
Cappuccino Whole	1 reg (12 oz)	150	7	8	13
Chai Tea Low Fat Milk	1 reg (12 oz)	220	3	2	47
Chai Tea Non Fat Milk	1 reg (12 oz)	210	3	0	47
Chai Tea Whole Milk	1 reg (12 oz)	230	3	3	47
Coca Cola	8 oz	99	0	0	27
Coca Cola Cherry	8 oz	104	0	0	28
Coffee Iced Americano	8 oz	0	0	0	0
Coffee Regular & Decaf	1 (12 oz)	0	0	0	0
Diet Coke	8 oz	1	0	0	0
Espresso	1 reg (2 oz)	0	0	0	0
Fanta Orange	8 oz	106	0	0	29
Frozen Drinks Cafe Caramel	1 (18 oz)	620	8	9	100
Frozen Drinks Cafe Mocha	1 (18 oz)	510	7	8	102

FOOD	PORTION	CALS	PROT	FAT	CARB
Frozen Drinks Strawberry Cream	1 (18 oz)	450	6	19	75
Frozen Drinks Wild Berry Fat Free	1 (18 oz)	270	4	0	62
Half & Half Creamer	1 oz	40	1	3	1
Hi-C Fruit Punch	8 oz	104	0	0	28
Hot Chocolate Nonfat	1 reg (12 oz)	220	12	2	37
Hot Chocolate Whole	1 reg (12 oz)	290	10	11	35
Iced Cappuccino Nonfat	1 reg (12 oz)	90	8	0	13
Iced Mocha Low Fat	1 reg (12 oz)	230	8	5	39
Iced Tea Raspberry	8 oz	78	0	0	21
Iced Tea Unsweetened	8 oz	1	0	0	0
Lemonade	1 (16 oz)	200	1	0	24
Lemonade Blackberry	1 (16 oz)	310	2	0	74
Macchiato Nonfat	1 reg (12 oz)	230	10	0	49
Macchiato Whole	1 reg (12 oz)	290	8	8	47
Milk Low Fat	8 oz	120	8	5	12
Milk Skim	8 oz	80	7	0	15
Milk Whole	8 oz	150	8	8	11
Mocha Low Fat	1 reg (12 oz)	230	8	5	39
Mocha Nonfat	1 reg (12 oz)	190	9	0	39
Mocha Whole	1 reg (12 oz)	270	8	9	38
Mr. Pibb	8 oz	97	0	0	26
On Top Reduced Fat Topping	2 tbsp (0.3 oz)	20	0	2	2
Orange Juice	1 (10 oz)	143	1	0	34
Sprite	8 oz	97	0	0	26
Syrup Blackberry	2 tbsp (1 oz)	100	0	0	25
Syrup Caramel	2 tbsp (1 oz)	70	0	0	18
Syrup Hazelnut	2 tbsp (1 oz)	100	0	0	25
Syrup Vanilla	2 tbsp (1 oz)	100	0	0	25
Syrup Vanilla Sugar Free	2 tbsp (1 oz)	116	0	0	0
Tea Hamey & Sons All Flavors	8 oz	0	0	0	0
Whipped Cream Light	2 tbsp (1 oz)	36	0	3	2
CREAM CHEESE AND SPREADS					
Butter	1 tbsp (0.5 oz)	110	0	11	0
Cream Cheese Whipped Onion & Chive	2 tbsp (0.7 oz)	70	1	6	3
Cream Cheese Whipped Plain	2 tbsp (0.7 oz)	70	1	7	1
Cream Cheese Whipped Reduced Fat Blueberry	2 tbsp (0.7 oz)	70	1	5	6

FOOD	PORTION	CALS	PROT	FAT	CARB
Cream Cheese Whipped Reduced Fat Garden Vegetable	2 tbsp (0.7 oz)	60	1	5	3
Cream Cheese Whipped Reduced Fat Garlic Herb	2 tbsp (0.7 oz)	60	1	5	3
Cream Cheese Whipped Reduced Fat Honey Almond	2 tbsp (0.7 oz)	70	1	5	6
Cream Cheese Whipped Reduced Fat Jalapeno Salsa	2 tbsp (0.7 oz)	60	1	5	3
Cream Cheese Whipped Reduced Fat Plain	2 tbsp (0.7 oz)	60	1	5	2
Cream Cheese Whipped Reduced Fat Strawberry	2 tbsp (0.7 oz)	60	1	5	2
Cream Cheese Whipped Reduced Fat Sun Dried Tomato & Basil	2 tbsp (0.7 oz)	60	1	5	2
Cream Cheese Whipped Smoked Salmon	2 tbsp (0.7 oz)	60	1	6	2
Deli Mustard	1 tsp (5 g)	0	0	0	0
Garlic Mayo	1 serv (1.5 oz)	270	0	27	8
Grape Jam	1 serv (1 oz)	110	0	0	28
Honey	1 serv (1 oz)	90	0	0	23
Hummus	1 serv (2 oz)	90	3	4	11
Mayo	1 tbsp (0.5 oz)	110	0	12	0
DESSERTS					
Cinnamon Twists	1 serv (3.8 oz)	370	5	21	41
Coffee Cake Apple Cinnamon	1 serv (6.6 oz)	700	5	28	108
Coffee Cake Chocolate Chip	1 serv (6.1 oz)	760	6	34	110
Coffee Cake Mixed Berry	1 serv (6.9 oz)	710	5	29	110
Cookie Chocolate Mudslide	1 (2.75 oz)	320	4	17	46
Cookie Chocolate Chip	1 (2.8 oz)	360	4	18	48
Cookie Iced Sugar	1 (3.7 oz)	480	4	15	76
Cookie Oatmeal Raisin	1 (2.8 oz)	320	5	11	54
Cookie Snickerdoodle	1 (2.8 oz)	400	3	18	56
Cookie Mini Chocolate Mudslide	1 (1.38 oz)	160	2	8	23
Cookie Mini Chocolate Chip	1 (1.38 oz)	180	2	9	24
Cookie Mini Iced Sugar	1 (1.87 oz)	230	2	7	39
Cookie Mini Oatmeal Raisin	1 (1.38 oz)	160	2	5	27
Marshmallow Crispy Treat	1 (3.9 oz)	410	5	7	86
Muffin Blueberry	1 (5 oz)	480	6	22	65
Muffin Cranberry Orange	1 (4.6 oz)	460	9	22	63

FOOD	PORTION	CALS	PROT	FAT	CARB
Muffin Strawberry White Chocolate	1 (5.5 oz)	550	7	25	78
Strudel Cinnamon Walnut	1 serv (5.4 oz)	630	9	42	56
SALAD DRESSINGS					
Caesar	2 tbsp (1 oz)	150	1	16	1
Harvest Chicken Salad	2 tbsp (1 oz)	90	0	8	3
Raspberry Vinaigrette	2 tbsp	160	0	14	8
SALADS					
Caesar	1 (10.5 oz)	600	13	53	23
Caesar Side	1 (4.5 oz)	280	6	27	7
Ceasar Chicken	1 (14 oz)	720	34	54	23
City	1 (11.5 oz)	830	14	68	39
City w/ Chicken	1 (15 oz)	950	36	71	40
Southwestern Chicken	1 (15.2 oz)	710	35	41	54
SANDWICHES					
Bagel & Lox	1 (11.2 oz)	520	25	21	65
Bagel Dog Asiago	1 (7.1 oz)	510	23	21	59
Bagel Dog Everything	1 (7.1 oz)	510	22	20	59
Bagel Dog Original	1 (6.9 oz)	490	22	20	59
Bagel Plain w/ Peanut Butter & Jelly	1 (6.2 oz)	550	17	15	90
Breakfast Wrap Santa Fe	1 (14.5 oz)	750	34	34	77
Breakfast Wrap Veggie	1 (15.6 oz)	810	35	41	77
California Chicken	1 (9.9 oz)	360	31	7	49
Club Blackened Chicken	1 (10.4 oz)	630	30	33	53
Club Deli Pesto Turkey	1 (10.9 oz)	670	27	39	47
Deli Chicken Salad	1 (11 oz)	1150	17	95	61
Deli Cornbeef	1 (14 oz)	740	44	34	61
Deli Egg Salad Kosher	1 (11.5 oz)	650	26	6	68
Deli Pastrami	1 (14 oz)	750	44	34	62
Deli Roast Beef	1 (14 oz)	730	43	34	60
Deli Tuna Salad	1 (13 oz)	740	28	45	53
Deli Turkey	1 (14.5 oz)	720	29	29	67
Deli Whitefish	1 (12.2 oz)	850	25	55	68
Deli Melts Hummus	1 (10.2 oz)	570	28	19	76
Deli Melts Pastrami	1 (9.6 oz)	530	38	17	61
Deli Melts Roast Beef	1 (9.6 oz)	530	36	17	60
Deli Melts Tuna	1 (11.6 oz)	700	42	33	82
Deli Melts Turkey	1 (9.6 oz)	500	29	14	60
Deli Melts Veggie	1 (12.3 oz)	590	25	25	70

FOOD	PORTION	CALS	PROT	FAT	CARB
Egg Mit Artichoke & Tomato	1 (12 oz)	620	28	28	67
Egg Mit Bacon & Cheddar	1 (9.2 oz)	620	33	28	61
Egg Mit Cheese & Tomato	1 (10 oz)	530	27	21	61
Egg Mit Lox & Chives	1 (8.8 oz)	490	28	17	59
Egg Mit Plain	1 (7.9 oz)	450	22	14	59
Egg Mit Spinach Mushroom & Swiss	1 (9.8 oz)	530	28	20	61
Egg Mit Turkey Sausage	1 (9.9 oz)	590	34	24	61
Egg Mit Cheese	1 (8.5 oz)	520	28	20	60
Kosher Vegetarian On Plain Bagel	1 (13.9 oz)	860	49	41	79
Panini Albacore Tuna	1 (13.6 oz)	750	32	38	62
Panini Egg Spinach Bacon	1 (11.8 oz)	790	27	43	65
Panini Egg Vegetarian Omelet	1 (13.8 oz)	670	23	31	66
Panini Italian Chicken	1 (12.5 oz)	810	47	40	67
Panini Mediterranean	1 (10.6 oz)	550	11	18	77
Panini Tomato Mozzarella	1 (7.9 oz)	440	7	16	59
Panini Turkey Club	1 (12.3 oz)	610	23	21	64
Sandwich Rachel	1 (13.9 oz)	1030	51	68	53
Sandwich Reuben	1 (13.9 oz)	770	51	41	47
Sandwich Veg Out	1 (10.1 oz)	490	19	14	75
Wrap Albacore Tuna	1 (12.3 oz)	600	29	28	57
Wrap Chicken Caesar	1 (12.6 oz)	790	37	46	62
Wrap Southwestern Turkey	1 (13.5 oz)	750	25	37	74
Wrap Veggie	1 (9.8 oz)	460	12	17	64
SIDES					
Cole Slaw	1 serv (3 oz)	120	1	6	15
Egg Salad	1 serv (5 oz)	330	13	29	3
Fresh Fruit Cup	1 (11 oz)	140	2	0	36
Fruit & Yogurt Parfait	1 (12 oz)	220	13	1	43
Kosher Pickle	1	5	0	0	1
Macaroni & Cheese	1 serv (6 oz)	340	15	17	32
Redskin Potato Salad	1 serv (3 oz)	160	1	12	13
Tuna Salad	1 serv (5 oz)	280	20	20	3
SOUPS					
Broccoli Cheese	1 cup (8.7 oz)	290	14	20	16
Chicken Noodle	1 cup (8.7 oz)	110	5	4	13
Italian Wedding	1 cup (8.7 oz)	160	11	6	15
Tortilla	1 cup (8.7 oz)	300	13	19	19
Turkey Chili	1 cup (8.7 oz)	220	20	7	24

FOOD	PORTION	CALS	PROT	FAT	CARB
NOODLES & COMPANY					
MAIN MENU SELECTIONS					
Bangkok Curry	1 sm	250	5	6	42
Bangkok Curry	1 reg	490	9	13	85
Beef Braised	1 serv	190	28	10	0
Beef Sauteed	1 serv	210	25	12	0
Buttered Noodles	1 sm	310	17	8	42
Buttered Noodles	1 reg	620	33	16	84
Chicken Breast Seasoned	1 serv	130	22	3	0
Chicken Parmesan Crusted	1 serv	190	17	8	17
Ciabatta Roll	1	160	6	2	31
Flatbread	1 serv	210	7	4	37
House Marinara	1 sm	330	13	6	53
House Marinara	1 reg	650	27	12	107
Mushroom Stroganoff	1 sm	390	14	15	50
Mushroom Stroganoff	1 reg	780	28	31	100
Organic Tofu	1 serv	180	16	11	4
Pad Thai	1 sm	350	6	10	59
Pad Thai	1 reg	700	11	20	117
Pasta Fresca	1 sm	420	15	12	56
Pasta Fresca	1 reg	780	27	22	111
Penne Rosa	1 sm	420	12	13	60
Penne Rosa	1 reg	810	24	26	119
Pesto Cavatappi	1 sm	510	18	21	62
Pesto Cavatappi	1 reg	910	36	30	124
Potstickers	3	200	5	5	31
Shrimp Sauteed	1 serv	35	8	0	0
Whole Grain Tuscan Linguine	1 sm	450	15	20	54
Whole Grain Tuscan Linguine	1 reg	770	26	26	108
Wisconsin Mac & Cheese	1 sm	450	18	16	60
Wisconsin Mac & Cheese	1 reg	900	36	31	119
SALADS					
Caesar	1 sm	160	5	14	5
Caesar	1 reg	320	11	28	11
Chinese Chopped	1 sm	150	3	7	11
Chinese Chopped	1 reg	310	6	15	23
Cucumber Tomato Side Salad	1	80	2	0	18
The Med	1 sm	150	5	6	19
The Med	1 reg	310	10	13	39
Tossed Green	1	60	1	6	3

FOOD	PORTION	CALS	PROT	FAT	CARB
SOUPS					
Chicken Noodle	1 sm	150	10	2	22
Chicken Noodle	1 reg	300	20	4	44
Thai Curry	1 sm	240	0	10	35
Thai Curry	1 reg	480	0	19	70
Tomato Basil	1 sm	210	0	12	23
Tomato Basil	1 reg	420	0	23	45
PACIUGO GELATO					
Milk Base Amarena Black Cherry Swirl	1 scoop (3.5 oz)	160	4	4	30
Milk Base Banana Creme Pie	1 scoop (3.5 oz)	80	2	2	14
Milk Base Cheesecake	1 scoop (3.5 oz)	90	3	4	12
Milk Base Chocolate	1 scoop (3.5 oz)	80	3	3	14
Milk Base Chocolate Cookies'N Milk	1 scoop (3.5 oz)	90	3	3	16
Milk Base Coconut	1 scoop (3.5 oz)	80	2	3	13
Milk Base Coffee	1 scoop (3.5 oz)	75	2	3	12
Milk Base Fiordilatte	1 scoop (3.5 oz)	75	2	2	13
Milk Base French Vanilla Bean	1 scoop (3.5 oz)	80	2	3	13
Milk Base Green Tea	1 scoop (3.5 oz)	70	2	2	12
Milk Base Hazelnut	1 scoop (3.5 oz)	85	3	4	11
Milk Base Lemon Custard	1 scoop (3.5 oz)	75	3	3	12
Milk Base Mascarpone Chocolate Rum	1 scoop (3.5 oz)	95	3	5	11
Milk Base Pannacotta Wedding Cake	1 scoop (3.5 oz)	75	2	2	13
Milk Base Peppermint	1 scoop (3.5 oz)	75	2	2	14
Milk Base Rose	1 scoop (3.5 oz)	70	8	2	12

FOOD	PORTION	CALS	PROT	FAT	CARB
Milk Base Tiramisu	1 scoop (3.5 oz)	80	2	3	12
Milk Base Zabajone	1 scoop (3.5 oz)	80	3	3	12
No Sugar Added Chocolate	1 scoop (3.5 oz)	28	2	1	9
No Sugar Added Mint	1 scoop (3.5 oz)	25	1	1	9
No Sugar Added Mocha	1 scoop (3.5 oz)	28	2	1	9
No Sugar Added Strawberry Milk	1 scoop (3.5 oz)	23	1	1	8
Soy Banana	1 scoop (3.5 oz)	40	tr	2	6
Soy Blueberry	1 scoop (3.5 oz)	40	tr	2	6
Soy Chocolate	1 scoop (3.5 oz)	38	tr	2	5
Soy Coffee	1 scoop (3.5 oz)	35	tr	2	5
Soy Hazelnut	1 scoop (3.5 oz)	35	tr	2	5
Soy Strawberry	1 scoop (3.5 oz)	38	tr	2	6
Soy Wild Berries	1 scoop (3.5 oz)	40	tr	2	6
Water Base Blackberry	1 scoop (3.5 oz)	28	0	0	7
Water Base Ginger Lemon	1 scoop (3.5 oz)	25	0	0	7
Water Base Green Apple	1 scoop (3.5 oz)	28	0	0	7
Water Base Lemon Sage	1 scoop (3.5 oz)	25	0	0	7
Water Base Lychee	1 scoop (3.5 oz)	25	0	0	6
Water Base Orange Vidalia	1 scoop (3.5 oz)	25	0	0	7
Water Base Passion Fruit	1 scoop (3.5 oz)	23	0	0	6

FOOD	PORTION	CALS	PROT	FAT	CARB
Water Base Pineapple	1 scoop (3.5 oz)	28	0	0	7
Water Base Strawberry Port	1 scoop (3.5 oz)	25	0	0	6
Water Base Watermelon	1 scoop (3.5 oz)	25	0	0	7

PEI WEI ASIAN DINER
CHILDREN'S MENU SELECTIONS

FOOD	PORTION	CALS	PROT	FAT	CARB
Kid's Wei Honey Seared Chicken w/o Noodles Or Rice	1 serv	290	16	17	19
Kid's Wei Lo Mein Chicken w/o Noodles Or Rice	1 serv	180	20	7	7
Kid's Wei Teriyaki Chicken w/o Noodles Or Rice	1 serv	240	23	5	20

DESSERTS

FOOD	PORTION	CALS	PROT	FAT	CARB
Cookie Chocolate Chip	1	342	5	14	53
Cookie Fortune	1	30	0	0	7

MAIN MENU SELECTIONS

FOOD	PORTION	CALS	PROT	FAT	CARB
Bowl w/ Brown Rice Japanese Teriyaki Beef	1 serv	580	33	17	66
Bowl w/ Brown Rice Japanese Teriyaki Chicken	1 serv	460	28	7	64
Bowl w/ Brown Rice Japanese Teriyaki Shrimp	1 serv	410	20	5	64
Bowl w/ Brown Rice Japanese Teriyaki Vegetables & Tofu	1 serv	410	13	6	71
Bowl w/ White Rice Japanese Teriyaki	1 serv	560	32	16	62
Bowl w/ White Rice Japanese Teriyaki Chicken	1 serv	440	28	6	60
Bowl w/ White Rice Japanese Teriyaki Shrimp	1 serv	390	20	5	61
Bowl w/ White Rice Japanese Teriyaki Vegetables & Tofu	1 serv	390	13	5	68
Crispy Potstickers	4	130	6	7	10
Edamame	1 serv	156	14	8	12
Fried Rice Beef	1 serv	630	37	21	68
Fried Rice Chicken	1 serv	525	32	11	68
Fried Rice Shrimp	1 serv	475	24	10	67
Fried Rice Vegetable & Tofu	1 serv	440	17	7	73

FOOD	PORTION	CALS	PROT	FAT	CARB
Ginger Broccoli Beef	1 serv	450	37	22	19
Ginger Broccoli Chicken	1 serv	300	31	9	19
Ginger Broccoli Shrimp	1 serv	230	22	7	18
Ginger Broccoli Vegetables & Tofu	1 serv	170	10	4	23
Honey Seared Chicken	1 serv	420	21	15	45
Honey Seared Shrimp	1 serv	370	14	14	43
Hot & Sour Soup	1 cup	150	7	9	11
Lemon Pepper Beef	1 serv	550	38	31	32
Lemon Pepper Chicken	1 serv	440	31	20	34
Lemon Pepper Shrimp	1 serv	380	22	18	34
Lemon Pepper Vegetables & Tofu	1 serv	230	10	10	29
Mandarin Kung Pao Beef	1 serv	610	40	34	31
Mandarin Kung Pao Chicken	1 serv	450	34	21	28
Mandarin Kung Pao Shrimp	1 serv	400	25	19	28
Mandarin Kung Pao Vegetables & Tofu	1 serv	290	13	15	23
Minced Chicken w/ Cool Lettuce Wraps w/o Rice Sticks	1 serv	250	22	4	31
Mongolian Beef	1 serv	420	36	22	14
Mongolian Chicken	1 serv	280	10	9	14
Mongolian Shrimp	2 serv	210	21	6	12
Mongolian Vegetables & Tofu	2 serv	180	10	6	19
Noodles Dan Dan Chicken	1 serv	390	26	7	54
Noodles Lo Mein Beef	1 serv	570	36	21	61
Noodles Lo Mein Chicken	1 serv	460	31	11	61
Noodles Lo Mein Shrimp	1 serv	400	23	8	60
Noodles Lo Mein Vegetables & Tofu	1 serv	400	16	8	66
Noodles Thai Blazing Beef	1 serv	630	28	32	55
Noodles Thai Blazing Chicken	1 serv	520	24	22	55
Noodles Thai Blazing Shrimp	1 serv	482	16	22	55
Noodles Thai Blazing Vegetables & Tofu	1 serv	430	10	18	59
Noodles Egg	1 serv	210	7	3	39
Noodles Rice	1 serv	130	0	0	32
Orange Peel Beef	1 serv	660	42	31	52
Orange Peel Chicken	1 serv	520	6	18	52
Orange Peel Shrimp	1 serv	460	27	16	51

FOOD	PORTION	CALS	PROT	FAT	CARB
Orange Peel Vegetables & Tofu	1 serv	330	14	10	46
Pad Thai Beef	1 serv	670	40	30	63
Pad Thai Chicken	1 serv	560	35	20	61
Pad Thai Shrimp	1 serv	490	27	17	60
Pei Wei Spicy Beef	1 serv	480	34	26	25
Pei Wei Spicy Chicken	1 serv	330	28	13	25
Pei Wei Spicy Shrimp	1 serv	300	19	11	29
Rice Brown	1 serv	170	4	2	37
Rice Fried	1 serv	260	9	5	44
Rice Sticks	1 cup	130	0	0	33
Rice White	1 serv	200	4	0	44
Spicy Korean Beef	1 serv	490	41	24	26
Spicy Korean Chicken	1 serv	350	15	11	26
Spicy Korean Shrimp	1 serv	280	26	9	24
Spicy Korean Vegetables & Tofu	1 serv	240	15	9	27
Spring Rolls	2	90	2	5	11
Sweet & Sour Chicken	1 serv	440	21	13	61
Sweet & Sour Shrimp	1 serv	390	14	11	59
Thai Coconut Curry Beef	1 serv	550	36	37	20
Thai Coconut Curry Chicken	1 serv	380	30	19	23
Thai Coconut Curry Shrimp	1 serv	300	21	17	18
Thai Coconut Curry Vegetables & Tofu	1 serv	220	8	14	19
Thai Dynamite Chicken	1 serv	390	33	19	20
Thai Dynamite Shrimp	1 serv	280	15	16	20
Thai Dynamite Vegetables & Tofu	1 serv	220	6	16	15
Wontons Crab	4	190	8	13	9
SALAD DRESSINGS AND SAUCES					
Dressing Sesame Ginger	1 serv (2 oz)	170	1	16	5
Lime Vinaigrette	1 serv (2 oz)	230	0	20	13
Sauce Lettuce Wrap	1 serv (2 oz)	70	4	5	2
Sauce Sweet Chili	1 serv (2 oz)	140	0	0	34
Sauce Thai Peanut	1 serv (2 oz)	168	5	11	15
SALADS					
Asian Chopped Chicken w/ Dressing	1 serv	280	24	15	13
Asian Chopped Chicken w/o Dressing	1 serv	200	23	8	10

FOOD	PORTION	CALS	PROT	FAT	CARB
Pei Wei Spicy Chicken w/ Dressing	1 serv	350	22	16	28
Pei Wei Spicy Chicken w/o Dressing	1 serv	210	22	3	23
Vietnamese Chicken Salad Rolls	3	53	3	3	5

P.F. CHANG'S CHINA BISTRO
DESSERTS

FOOD	PORTION	CALS	PROT	FAT	CARB
Banana Spring Rolls	1 serv	814	12	37	130
Cake The Great Wall Of Chocolate	1 serv	2237	20	90	376
Flourless Chocolate Dome Gluten Free	1 serv	572	8	26	84
Ice Cream Pineapple Coconut	1 serv	111	4	12	25
Mini Dessert Apple Pie	1	170	1	4	34
Mini Dessert Banana Split	1	167	1	6	28
Mini Dessert Carrot Cake	1	295	2	14	42
Mini Dessert Creamy Strawberry Cheesecake	1	239	3	20	14
Mini Dessert Great Wall Of Chocolate	1	336	1	26	24
Mini Dessert S'mores	1	323	3	12	50
Mini Dessert Tiramisu	1	202	3	14	15
Mini Dessert Tres Leche Lemon Dream	1	216	4	8	32

MAIN MENU SELECTIONS

FOOD	PORTION	CALS	PROT	FAT	CARB
Almond & Cashew Chicken	1 serv	815	81	30	63
Asian Marinated New York Strip	1 serv	1432	92	86	68
Asian Slaw	1 serv	585	5	57	19
Beef A La Sichuan	1 serv	1172	86	64	56
Beef w/ Broccoli	1 serv	1118	93	65	38
Buddha's Feast Steamed	1 serv	137	8	1	29
Buddha's Feast Stir Fried	1 serv	367	25	5	66
Calamari Salt & Pepper	1 serv	720	33	11	118
Cantonese Chow Fun w/ Beef	1 serv	1212	69	38	142
Cantonese Chow Fun w/ Chicken	1 serv	1045	60	23	146
Cantonese Scallops	1 serv	408	39	16	26
Cantonese Shrimp	1 serv	330	33	12	21
Chang's Spicy Chicken	1 serv	923	56	37	88
Chengdu Spiced Lamb	1 serv	1056	62	75	34

FOOD	PORTION	CALS	PROT	FAT	CARB
Chicken w/ Black Bean Sauce	1 serv	678	76	23	33
Chow Fun Vegetable	1 serv	878	22	8	181
Chow Mein Combo	1 serv	912	61	34	86
Chow Mein w/ Beef	1 serv	793	54	26	84
Chow Mein w/ Chicken	1 serv	689	49	16	84
Chow Mein w/ Pork	1 serv	898	61	34	83
Chow Mein w/ Shrimp	1 serv	625	41	13	84
Citrus Soy Salmon w/ Brown Rice	1 serv	1000	69	59	42
Citrus Soy Salmon w/ White Rice	1 serv	1025	70	58	49
Coconut Curry Vegetables	1 serv	686	30	46	48
Crispy Green Beans	1 serv	507	8	28	59
Crispy Honey Chicken	1 serv	867	53	11	121
Crispy Honey Shrimp	1 serv	1061	35	44	118
Dali Chicken	1 serv	1091	91	52	53
Double Pan Fried Noodles Combo	1 serv	1384	68	69	118
Double Pan Fried Noodles w/ Beef	1 serv	1186	53	56	112
Double Pan Fried Noodles w/ Chicken	1 serv	1072	42	47	115
Double Pan Fried Noodles w/ Pork	1 serv	1208	50	60	114
Double Pan Fried Noodles w/ Shrimp	1 serv	1031	37	46	115
Dumplings Peking Pan Fried	1 serv	367	18	23	21
Dumplings Peking Steamed	1 serv	327	18	18	21
Dumplings Shrimp Pan Fried	1 serv	305	21	13	25
Dumplings Shrimp Steamed	1 serv	265	21	8	25
Dumplings Vegetable Pan Fried	1 serv	307	9	11	43
Dumplings Vegetable Steamed	1 serv	267	9	7	43
Eggplant Stir Fried	1 serv	590	10	34	64
Fried Rice Combo	1 serv	1539	68	69	154
Fried Rice w/ Beef	1 serv	1228	58	40	150
Fried Rice w/ Chicken	1 serv	1208	47	44	151
Fried Rice w/ Pork	1 serv	1360	55	57	150
Fried Rice w/ Shrimp	1 serv	1154	40	41	149
Garlic Noodles	1 serv	612	18	11	111
Garlic Snap Peas	1 sm	129	4	7	13

FOOD	PORTION	CALS	PROT	FAT	CARB
Ginger Chicken w/ Broccoli	1 serv	656	60	26	45
Ginger Chicken w/ Broccoli Gluten Free	1 serv	677	61	30	43
Ground Chicken & Eggplant	1 serv	792	33	40	73
Harvest Spring Rolls	1 serv	287	6	15	30
Hot Fish	1 serv	1338	60	71	111
Kung Pao Chicken	1 serv	1228	74	79	58
Kung Pao Scallops	1 serv	1136	87	57	66
Kung Pao Shrimp	1 serv	977	60	58	58
Lemon Pepper Shrimp	1 serv	701	36	36	59
Lemon Scallops	1 serv	952	60	28	100
Lemongrass Prawns	1 serv	907	34	58	65
Lettuce Wraps Chicken	1 serv	377	28	12	35
Lettuce Wraps Gluten Free Chicken	1 serv	477	31	12	63
Lettuce Wraps Vegetarian	1 serv	281	25	4	37
Lo Mein Combo	1 serv	1409	66	83	98
Lo Mein w/ Beef	1 serv	1374	67	80	94
Lo Mein w/ Chicken	1 serv	1198	51	67	97
Lo Mein w/ Pork	1 serv	1400	63	54	95
Lo Mein w/ Shrimp	1 serv	1134	43	64	97
Lunch Bowl Almond & Cashew Chicken w/ White Rice	1	955	63	26	112
Lunch Bowl Beef w/ Broccoli w/ Brown Rice	1	844	58	27	87
Lunch Bowl Beef w/ Broccoli w/ White Rice	1	890	59	26	99
Lunch Bowl Buddha's Feast w/ Brown Rice	1	541	23	8	101
Lunch Bowl Buddha's Feast w/ White Rice	1	587	24	6	113
Lunch Bowl Citrus Soy Salmon w/ Brown Rice	1	1047	48	63	67
Lunch Bowl Citrus Soy Salmon w/ White Rice	1	1093	49	62	79
Lunch Bowl Crispy Honey Chicken w/ Brown Rice	1	943	61	13	126
Lunch Bowl Crispy Honey Chicken w/ White Rice	1	989	62	12	138

FOOD	PORTION	CALS	PROT	FAT	CARB
Lunch Bowl Moo Goo Gai Pan w/ Brown Rice	1	545	40	8	76
Lunch Bowl Moo Goo Gai Pan w/ White Rice	1	591	41	6	88
Lunch Bowl Pepper Steak w/ Brown Rice	1	820	54	28	82
Lunch Bowl Pepper Steak w/ White Rice	1 serv	968	55	39	94
Lunch Bowl Shrimp w/ Lobster Sauce w/ Brown Rice	1	686	37	25	75
Lunch Bowl Shrimp w/ Lobster Sauce w/ White Rice	1	732	38	23	87
Mongolian Beef	1 serv	1178	96	73	29
Moo Goo Gai Pan	1 serv	661	54	34	32
Mu Shu Chicken	1 serv	715	47	38	49
Mu Shu Pork	1 serv	871	57	50	50
Noodles Dan Dan	1 serv	1087	51	30	145
Noodles Tam's	1 serv	1678	58	93	144
Oolong Marinated Sea Bass	1 serv	521	64	12	40
Orange Peel Beef	1 serv	1568	88	85	115
Orange Peel Chicken	1 serv	1151	61	46	127
Orange Peel Shrimp	1 serv	1010	47	41	118
Pepper Steak	1 serv	971	95	48	32
Philip's Better Lemon Chicken	1 serv	1051	58	42	113
Rice Brown	1 cup	254	5	2	53
Rice Sticks	1 serv	135	0	0	33
Rice White	1 cup	295	6	1	64
Salt & Pepper Prawns	1 serv	844	45	50	55
Seared Ahi Tuna	1 serv	210	26	9	9
Shanghai Cucumbers	1 serv	124	10	6	8
Shrimp w/ Candied Walnuts	1 serv	1225	60	80	74
Shrimp w/ Lobster Sauce	1 serv	480	42	22	24
Sichuan Asparagus	1 sm	97	6	3	16
Sichuan Chicken Flatbread	1 serv	1160	52	80	56
Sichuan From The Sea Calamari	1 serv	1078	69	36	118
Sichuan From The Sea Scallops	1 serv	1030	70	36	98
Sichuan From The Sea Shrimp	1 serv	728	44	37	55
Singapore Street Noodles	1 serv	572	28	16	81
Singapore Street Noodles Gluten Free	1 serv	566	28	15	81

FOOD	PORTION	CALS	PROT	FAT	CARB
Spare Ribs Chang's	1 serv	1356	93	89	43
Spare Ribs Northern Style	1 serv	720	49	54	6
Spicy Green Beans	1 sm	234	7	13	23
Spinach w/ Garlic Stir Fried	1 sm	77	7	3	9
Sweet & Sour Chicken	1 serv	764	40	20	107
Sweet & Sour Pork	1 serv	1095	61	46	106
Vegetarian Ma Po Tofu	1 serv	537	40	19	51
Wild Alaskan Sockeye Salmon Steamed w/ Ginger	1 serv	646	60	36	23
Wild Aslaskan Sockeye Salmon Steamed w/ Ginger Gluten Free	1 serv	672	60	36	30
Wok Charred Beef	1 serv	941	63	63	33
Wok Seared Lamb	1 serv	1081	62	80	29
Wontons Crab	1 serv	440	19	25	32
SALAD DRESSINGS AND SAUCES					
Dressing Creamy Wedge	1 serv	443	3	43	8
Dressing Signature Ginger	1 serv	483	1	48	9
Sauce Chili Bean	1 serv	81	3	1	12
Sauce Crispy Green Bean	1 serv	451	0	48	5
Sauce Potsticker	1 serv	36	2	1	6
Sauce Shrimp Dumpling	1 serv	24	3	0	1
Sauce Special	1 serv	55	2	1	9
Sauce Spicy Plum	1 serv	110	0	0	28
Sauce Sweet & Sour	1 serv	57	0	0	15
Vinaigrette Mustard	1 serv	66	4	2	7
Vinaigrette Watermelon Citrus	1 serv	240	1	23	7
SALADS					
Bikini Shrimp w/o Dressing	1 serv	192	8	6	30
Chang's Wedge w/ Chicken w/o Dressing	1 serve	595	57	35	12
Chang's Wedge w/o Dressing	1 serv	244	8	19	12
Chopped Chicken w/o Dressing	1 serv	401	47	14	21
SOUPS					
Chicken Noodle	1 bowl	512	64	13	30
Egg Drop	1 cup	48	1	2	7
Hot & Sour	1 cup	85	5	2	11
Wonton	1 bowl	354	21	10	44
PINKBERRY					
Frozen Yogurt Coffee	½ cup	90	4	0	24

FOOD	PORTION	CALS	PROT	FAT	CARB
Frozen Yogurt Green Tea	½ cup	50	3	0	10
Frozen Yogurt Original	½ cup	70	3	0	14

PIZZA FUSION
DESSERTS

FOOD	PORTION	CALS	PROT	FAT	CARB
Brownies Gluten Free	½ serv	232	1	16	27
Calzone Chocolate	½	209	5	9	30
Cookies Chocolate Chip	⅓ serv	250	4	13	33
Pastry Strawberry Cheese	1 serv	338	9	10	54

PIZZA

FOOD	PORTION	CALS	PROT	FAT	CARB
BBQ Chicken	1 slice	181	8	4	26
Big Kahuna	1 slice	236	12	9	26
Bruschetta	1 slice	159	8	4	23
Cheese	1 slice	167	7	5	23
Eggplant & Mozzarella	1 slice	181	7	6	24
Farmer's Market	1 slice	190	9	6	25
Founder's Pie	1 slice	201	8	7	25
Four Cheese & Sundried Tomato	1 slice	175	8	5	26
Greek	1 slice	204	9	7	25
Pepperoni	1 slice	220	10	9	23
Personal BBQ Chicken	½ pie	272	11	6	43
Personal Big Kahuna	½ pie	365	18	13	39
Personal Bruschetta	½ pie	234	10	5	37
Personal Cheese	½ pie	233	10	6	35
Personal Eggplant & Mozzarella	½ pie	304	12	11	39
Personal Farmer's Market	½ pie	279	12	8	40
Personal Founder's Pie	½ pie	347	14	14	41
Personal Four Cheese & Sundried Tomato	½ pie	262	12	7	39
Personal Greek	½ pie	299	12	11	39
Personal Pepperoni	½ pie	359	17	15	37
Personal Philly Steak	½ pie	358	19	14	42
Personal Sausage & Tri-Peppers	½ pie	323	15	12	39
Personal Spinach & Artichoke	½ pie	270	12	7	41
Personal Very Vegan	½ pie	321	9	15	41
Philly Steak	1 slice	220	11	8	26
Sausage & Tri-Peppers	1 slice	212	10	8	25
Spinach & Artichoke	1 slice	184	9	5	25
Very Vegan	1 slice	195	6	8	27

FOOD	PORTION	CALS	PROT	FAT	CARB
SALADS					
Caesar & Roasted Chicken	½ serv	358	9	21	28
Chicken Bruschetta	½ serv	331	11	22	22
Fusion	½ serv	244	5	8	20
Pan Roasted Steak	½ serv	388	18	26	22
Pear & Gorganzola	½ serv	380	12	34	12
Roasted Beet & Feta	½ serv	320	8	25	19
Side Salad Arugula	1 serv	48	1	4	1
SANDWICHES					
Philly Phusion	½	473	28	23	39
Portabello Grill	½	380	14	20	38
Roasted Chicken	½	357	17	14	41
Roasted Turkey	½	417	26	19	35
STARTERS					
Flatbread	1 (2 serv)	198	14	2	76
Stuffed Portobello Mushroom	½ serv	140	5	11	9
Trio Of Dips	⅓ serv	191	6	11	30
PRETZELMAKER					
Bites	1 sm (5.3 oz)	450	9	11	80
Bites	1 med (7.4 oz)	640	13	16	112
Bites Cinnamon Sugar	1 serv (5.8 oz)	520	9	12	95
Breezer Coffee	1 (20 oz)	640	6	21	107
Breezer Mocha	1 (20 oz)	620	6	20	106
Breezer Peach	1 (20 oz)	650	6	20	117
Breezer Raspberry	1 (20 oz)	650	6	20	117
Breezer Strawberry Banana	1 (20 oz)	650	6	20	115
Caramel Nut	1 (4.5 oz)	390	7	7	74
Cinnamon Sugar	1 (4.3 oz)	370	7	8	68
Cream Cheese	1 serv (1.5 oz)	200	2	20	4
Diet Coke	1 sm (20 oz)	0	0	0	0
Garlic	1 (4.1 oz)	350	7	7	64
Icing Cream Cheese	1 serv (1.5 oz)	180	1	9	22
Ketchup	2 pkg (0.6 oz)	20	0	0	4
Lemonade	1 sm (20 oz)	160	0	0	92
Mustard	2 pkg (0.4 oz)	5	0	0	1
Original	1 (4 oz)	340	7	7	61
Parmesan	1 (4.2 oz)	360	9	9	61
Plain	1 (4 oz)	209	7	2	61
PT Pretzel Dog	1 (6 oz)	440	15	27	34
Ranch	1 (4.1 oz)	240	7	7	63
Sauce Caramel	1 serv (1.5 oz)	140	1	0	35

FOOD	PORTION	CALS	PROT	FAT	CARB
Sauce Cheddar Cheese	1 serv (1.5 oz)	70	1	5	6
Sauce Nacho Cheese	1 serv (1.5 oz)	80	1	5	7
Sauce Pizza	1 serv (1.5 oz)	30	1	1	6

QUIZNO'S
COOKIES

FOOD	PORTION	CALS	PROT	FAT	CARB
Dark Chocolate Chunk	1	380	5	15	58
Double Chocolate Chip	1	370	5	15	58
Oatmeal Raisin	1	340	5	11	59
Snickerdoodle	1	400	3	16	59

SANDWICHES

FOOD	PORTION	CALS	PROT	FAT	CARB
Breakfast Bacon Egg Cheddar	1	380	21	21	36
Breakfast Black Angus Steak & Cheddar	1 sm	330	26	13	36
Breakfast Egg & Cheddar	1	240	12	11	35
Breakfast Garden Vegetable Cheddar	1	250	13	11	38
Breakfast Ham Egg Cheddar	1	290	19	12	37
Deli Honey Ham & Swiss	1	260	17	4	38
Deli Oven Roasted Turkey & Cheese	1	250	15	4	39
Deli Roast Beef & Cheddar	1	230	13	4	37
Deli Tuna Melt	1	500	14	33	37
Sammie Alpine Chicken	1	200	13	6	24
Sammie Balsamic Chicken	1	170	11	4	24
Sammie Bistro Steak Melt	1	180	11	4	25
Sammie Black Angus Steak	1	180	11	4	24
Sammie Italiano	1	240	10	11	24
Sammie Sonoma Turkey	1	160	8	4	25
Sub Baja Chicken w/ Bacon	1 sm	320	25	9	37
Sub Black Angus Steak On Rosemary Parmesan	1 sm	380	30	8	46
Sub Chicken Carbonara w/ Bacon	1 sm	360	26	10	42
Sub Classic Club w/ Bacon	1 sm	320	21	9	39
Sub Classic Italian	1 sm	360	18	15	38
Sub Honey Bacon Club	1 sm	320	21	9	39
Sub Honey Bourbon Chicken	1 sm	260	28	4	38
Sub Honey Mustard Chicken w/ Bacon	1 sm	330	25	9	38
Sub Mesquite Chicken w/ Bacon	1 sm	330	25	9	38

FOOD	PORTION	CALS	PROT	FAT	CARB
Sub Prime Rib Cheesesteak	1 sm	360	24	11	40
Sub Prime Rib & Peppercorn	1 sm	380	30	8	46
Sub Steakhouse Beef Dip	1 sm	260	13	6	37
Sub The Traditional	1 sm	260	16	5	39
Sub Turkey Bacon Guacamole	1 sm	360	21	12	43
Sub Turkey Ranch & Swiss	1 sm	250	16	4	39
Sub Tuscan Turkey On Rosemary Parmesan	1 sm	300	17	5	47
Sub Veggie	1 sm	270	10	8	41
SOUPS					
Bread Bowl Country French	1 serv	720	28	22	100
Bread Bowl Chili	1 serv	730	31	22	104
Broccoli Cheese	1 cup	150	7	10	10
Chicken Noodle	1 cup	130	6	3	18
Chili	1 cup	140	9	7	12

RANCH 1
BEVERAGES

FOOD	PORTION	CALS	PROT	FAT	CARB
Barq's Root Beer	1 sm (16 oz)	167	0	0	45
Coca-Cola	1 sm (16 oz)	150	0	0	40
Diet Coke	1 sm (16 oz)	2	0	0	0
Sprite	1 sm (16 oz)	150	0	0	40
CHILDREN'S MENU SELECTIONS					
Kids Meal Chicken Tenders	1 (2 oz)	111	10	4	9
Kids Meal Fries	1 serv (4 oz)	279	4	15	31
Kids Meal Popcorn Chicken	1 (2 oz)	112	9	4	10
MAIN MENU SELECTIONS					
Bowl Chicken Teriyaki	1 (19.3 oz)	504	34	7	78
Chicken Crispy (5 oz)	1 serv	326	27	15	22
Chicken Grilled (3.9 oz)	1 serv	146	24	6	0
Chicken On Mixed Greens	1 serv (21 oz)	340	29	19	17
Chicken Popcorn	1 serv (5.5 oz)	325	27	12	30
Chicken Tenders	1 serv (5.6 oz)	387	35	14	32
Fajita Mix Tomatoes Onion & Carrot	1 serv (3.2 oz)	20	1	0	5
Fajitas Chicken	1 serv (10 oz)	540	30	24	53
Fries	1 med	381	6	21	43
Fries Cheese	1 reg	493	8	27	54
Green Mix For Sandwiches	1 serv (2.5 oz)	31	1	2	2
Peppers & Onions	1 serv (1.6 oz)	27	0	2	3
Platter Chicken Rice	1 (10.9 oz)	273	28	6	28

FOOD	PORTION	CALS	PROT	FAT	CARB
Popcorn Chicken	1 sm	325	27	12	30
Rice	1 serv (4 oz)	97	3	0	21
Sandwich Chicken & Cheese	1 (11.2 oz)	389	33	12	39
Sandwich Chicken Philly	1 (9.2 oz)	410	36	13	40
Sandwich Crispy Chicken	1 (11.4 oz)	711	33	39	60
Sandwich Crispy Spicy Chicken	1 (11.4 oz)	543	34	17	68
Sandwich Grilled Spicy Chicken	1 (10.3 oz)	363	31	7	46
Sandwich Ranch 1 Classic	1 (9.4 oz)	683	29	47	37
Steamed Vegetables	1 serv (3 oz)	27	2	0	6
Wrap Grilled Chicken Caesar	1 (13.2 oz)	746	44	41	55
SALAD DRESSINGS AND SAUCES					
Dressing Balsamic Vinaigrette	1 oz	71	0	8	1
Dressing Classic Caesar	1 oz	103	1	11	1
Dressing Salad	1 oz	201	0	22	0
Sauce Ancho Chili Pepper	1 oz	134	1	14	1
Sauce BBQ	1 oz	84	0	4	12
Sauce Honey Mustard	1 oz	110	0	8	9
Sauce Pepper & Onion Saute	1 oz	143	0	16	1
Sauce Roasted Red Pepper	1 oz	232	0	26	0
Sauce Teriyaki	1 oz	24	1	0	5
SALADS					
Caesar	1 (7 oz)	34	2	1	7
Caesar Grilled Chicken	1 (11.3 oz)	223	28	8	13
Crispy Chicken Club	1 (13.6 oz)	495	30	26	29
Mandarin Chicken	1 (14.5 oz)	553	15	31	62
Mixed Greens w/o Cheese	1 (17 oz)	194	5	14	17
Salad Blend	1 serv (10.3 oz)	45	3	1	9
Southwest Chicken Chop	1 (17.6 oz)	681	33	43	44
RED MANGO					
Blenders Blueberry Moon	1 cup	150	3	2	33
Blenders Captain Berry	1 cup	140	4	1	31
Blenders Green Tea Blueberry	1 cup	130	3	0	29
Blenders Green Tea Honeydew	1 cup	130	3	0	29
Blenders Mango Island	1 cup	150	3	2	31
Blenders Pina Colada	1 cup	160	4	3	30
Blenders Tri-Berry	1 cup	130	3	0	30
Blenders Watermelon Breeze	1 cup	130	3	0	29
Frozen Yogurt All Flavors	½ cup	90	3	0	19

FOOD	PORTION	CALS	PROT	FAT	CARB
ROBEKS					
FREEZES AND SHAKES					
800 Lb Gorilla	12 oz	375	26	9	50
Freeze Lemon	12 oz	279	2	2	60
Freeze Orange	12 oz	242	9	0	56
Shake Bananasplit	12 oz	302	11	0	69
Shake P-Nut Power	12 oz	422	17	18	52
SMOOTHIES					
Acai Energizer	12 oz	167	2	1	36
Awesome Acai	12 oz	183	34	1	42
Banzai Blueberry	12 oz	175	31	1	38
Berry Brilliance	12 oz	194	30	1	45
Big Wednesday	12 oz	172	1	1	40
Cardio Cooler	12 oz	215	9	1	44
Citrus Stinger	12 oz	194	56	1	40
Cranberry Quest	12 oz	173	24	0	40
Dr. Robeks	12 oz	181	3	1	40
Guava Lava	12 oz	180	20	1	42
Hummingbird	12 oz	185	2	1	44
Infinite Orange	12 oz	181	4	0	42
Mahalo Mango	12 oz	174	2	1	42
Malibu Peach	12 oz	153	3	0	36
Outrageous Raspberry	12 oz	174	2	1	39
Passionfruit Cove	12 oz	168	2	1	38
Pina Koolada	12 oz	261	39	8	46
Polar Pineapple	12 oz	164	13	1	38
Pomegranate Passion	12 oz	196	4	0	48
Pomegranate Power	12 oz	211	3	0	50
Pro Arobek	12 oz	265	15	1	54
Raspberry Romance	12 oz	172	4	0	42
Robeks MuscleMax	12 oz	202	11	1	38
Robeks Rejuvenator	12 oz	193	5	1	43
South Pacific Squeeze	12 oz	188	2	1	42
Strawnana Berry	12 oz	179	3	0	44
Venice Burner	12 oz	231	9	1	46
Zen Berry	12 oz	190	3	1	45
SAMURAI SAM'S					
BOWLS					
Low Carb	1 reg	230	33	4	16
Spicy Beef 'N Broccoli	1 reg	620	26	13	97

FOOD	PORTION	CALS	PROT	FAT	CARB
Spicy Beef 'N Broccoli Brown Rice	1 reg	580	26	14	85
Sumo Brown Rice	1	1022	81	23	111
Sumo White Rice	1	1083	81	21	128
Sweet & Sour Dark Chicken	1 reg	610	32	10	96
Sweet & Sour Dark Chicken Brown Rice	1 reg	570	32	12	84
Sweet & Sour White Chicken	1 reg	580	37	5	96
Sweet & Sour White Chicken Brown Rice	1 reg	540	37	6	85
Teriyaki Dark Chicken	1 reg	540	31	10	79
Teriyaki Dark Chicken Brown Rice	1 reg	500	31	11	68
Teriyaki Dark Chicken & Shrimp	1 reg	492	29	6	78
Teriyaki Dark Chicken & Shrimp Brown Rice	1 reg	451	29	7	67
Teriyaki Dark Chicken & Steak	1 reg	540	27	9	83
Teriyaki Dark Chicken & Steak Brown Rice	1 reg	490	27	10	71
Teriyaki Salmon	1 reg	643	33	3	121
Teriyaki Shrimp Brown Rice	1 reg	407	28	3	65
Teriyaki Steak	1 reg	530	23	8	86
Teriyaki Steak Brown Rice	1 reg	490	23	9	74
Teriyaki Steak & Shrimp	1 reg	483	26	5	77
Teriyaki Steak & Shrimp Brown Rice	1 reg	442	25	6	66
Teriyaki Veggie	1 reg	363	8	1	81
Teriyaki Veggie Brown Rice	1 reg	323	8	2	69
Teriyaki White Chicken	1 reg	520	37	4	79
Teriyaki White Chicken Brown Rice	1 reg	470	36	5	68
Teriyaki White Chicken & Shrimp	1 reg	478	32	2	78
Teriyaki White Chicken & Shrimp Brown Rice	1 reg	437	32	4	67
Teriyaki White Chicken & Steak	1 reg	520	30	6	83
Teriyaki White Chicken & Steak Brown Rice	1 reg	480	30	7	71
Yakisoba Dark Chicken	1	842	60	24	114
Yakisoba Dark Chicken & Steak	1	825	54	22	113

FOOD	PORTION	CALS	PROT	FAT	CARB
Yakisoba Shrimp	1	677	55	10	110
Yakisoba Steak	1	809	48	20	112
Yakisoba Veggie	1	509	19	8	110
Yakisoba White Chicken	1	794	70	14	114
Yakisoba White Chicken & Steak	1	801	59	17	113
SALADS AND SIDES					
Crab Rangoon	1 serv	210	7	12	20
Dressing Chinese	1 serv (3.5 oz)	230	0	7	44
Dressing Chinese Ginger	1 serv (1 oz)	85	0	5	9
Dressing Oriental	1 serv (1 oz)	70	0	2	12
Egg Roll Grilled Chicken	1	150	7	7	17
Salad Oriental Chicken	1 serv	220	36	4	9
Salad Side	1	10	1	1	2
Salad Toss Sesame Chicken	1	490	41	13	57
Soup Asian Noodle	1 serv	89	5	2	14
Teriyaki Sauce	1 serv (1 oz)	40	1	0	9
WRAPS					
Teriyaki Dark Chicken	1	670	34	16	95
Teriyaki Dark Chicken Brown Rice	1	650	34	17	90
Teriyaki Steak	1	650	27	14	101
Teriyaki Steak Brown Rice	1	630	27	15	95
Teriyaki Veggie	1	510	14	8	94
Teriyaki Veggie Brown Rice	1	490	13	9	89
Teriyaki White Chicken	1	640	39	11	96
Teriyaki White Chicken Brown Rice	1	620	39	12	90
Teriyaki White Chicken & Steak	1	649	33	13	95
Teriyaki White Chicken & Steak Brown Rice	1	628	33	13	89

SCHLOTZSKY'S DELI
CHILDREN'S MENU SELECTIONS

FOOD	PORTION	CALS	PROT	FAT	CARB
Pizza Cheese	1 serv	479	18	13	73
Pizza Pepperoni	1 serv	523	20	17	73
Sandwich Cheese	1	394	17	15	48
Sandwich Ham & Cheese	1	424	21	16	49
Sandwich Turkey	1	300	13	5	49
DESSERTS					
Carrot Cake	1 serv	717	7	42	80
Cookie Chocolate Chip	1	160	2	8	22

FOOD	PORTION	CALS	PROT	FAT	CARB
Cookie Fudge Chocolate Chip	1	160	2	8	22
Cookie Oatmeal Raisin	1	150	2	6	22
Cookie Sugar	1	160	2	7	22
Cookie White Chocolate Macadamia	1	170	2	9	21
MAIN MENU SELECTIONS					
Salad Caesar	1 serv	103	6	5	10
Salad Garden	1 serv	51	3	1	12
Salad Grilled Chicken Caesar	1 serv	221	53	8	12
Salad Turkey Chef	1 serv	309	26	18	14
Sandwich Angus Roast Beef & Cheese	1 sm	534	33	22	50
Sandwich Chicken Breast	1 sm	342	39	4	52
Sandwich Fresh Veggie	1 sm	342	19	10	50
Sandwich Ham & Cheese	1 sm	508	31	19	54
Sandwich Smoked Turkey Breast	1 sm	353	20	6	52
Sandwich The Original	1 sm	559	28	26	52
Sandwich Turkey	1 sm	602	34	27	54
Sandwich Turkey Bacon Club	1 sm	561	32	25	51
Wraps Asian Chicken	1	537	56	12	80
Wraps Parmesan Chicken Caesar	1	556	61	21	61

SONIC DRIVE-IN
ADD-ONS

FOOD	PORTION	CALS	PROT	FAT	CARB
Bacon	1 serv (0.5 oz)	70	4	5	0
Cheese	1 serv (0.7 oz)	60	3	5	2
Chili	1 serv (1.2 oz)	50	3	4	2
Green Chilies	1 serv (1 oz)	5	0	0	1
Grilled Onions	1 serv (1 oz)	25	0	2	2
Jalapenos	1 serv (0.7 oz)	5	0	0	1
Slaw	1 serv (1 oz)	45	0	3	4
BEVERAGES					
Barq's Root Beer	1 sm (14 oz)	160	0	0	43
Coca Cola	1 sm (14 oz)	140	0	0	39
Cream Pie Shake Banana	1 reg (14 oz)	590	7	19	98
Cream Pie Shake Chocolate	1 reg (14 oz)	660	7	19	114
Cream Pie Shake Coconut Cream	1 reg (14 oz)	580	7	20	93
CreamSlush Blue Coconut	1 reg (14 oz)	430	5	13	76

FOOD	PORTION	CALS	PROT	FAT	CARB
CreamSlush Cherry	1 reg (14 oz)	440	5	13	77
CreamSlush Grape	1 reg (14 oz)	430	5	13	76
CreamSlush Orange	1 reg (14 oz)	430	5	13	77
CreamSlush Strawberry	1 reg (14 oz)	450	5	12	84
CreamSlush Watermelon	1 reg (14 oz)	440	5	13	77
Diet Coke	1 reg (14 oz)	0	0	0	0
Dr Pepper	1 reg (14 oz)	130	0	0	37
Float Barq's Root Beer	1 reg (14 oz)	300	3	8	56
Float Coca Cola	1 reg (14 oz)	290	3	8	54
Float Dr Pepper	1 reg (14 oz)	310	3	8	58
Limeade	1 sm (14 oz)	140	0	0	38
Limeade Cherry	1 sm (14 oz)	170	0	0	45
Limeade Strawberry	1 sm (14 oz)	170	0	0	45
Malt Banana	1 reg (14 oz)	490	7	17	78
Malt Caramel	1 reg (14 oz)	550	7	18	90
Malt Chocolate	1 reg (14 oz)	550	7	17	91
Malt Hot Fudge	1 reg (14 oz)	580	7	22	87
Malt Peanut Butter	1 reg (14 oz)	870	11	36	78
Malt Peanut Butter Fudge	1 reg (14 oz)	620	9	29	83
Malt Pineapple	1 reg (14 oz)	510	7	17	82
Malt Strawberry	1 reg (14 oz)	520	7	17	85
Malt Vanilla	1 reg (14 oz)	480	7	18	72
Milk 1%	8.5 oz	110	8	3	13
Milk Chocolate 1%	8.5 oz	160	8	3	27
Shake Banana	1 reg (14 oz)	470	7	16	76
Shake Chocolate	1 reg (14 oz)	540	6	16	89
Shake Hot Fudge	1 reg (14 oz)	570	6	21	85
Shake Peanut Butter	1 reg (14 oz)	640	10	34	75
Shake Peanut Butter Fudge	1 reg	610	8	28	81
Shake Pineapple	1 reg (14 oz)	500	6	16	80
Shake Strawberry	1 reg (14 oz)	510	7	16	83
Shake Vanilla	1 reg (14 oz)	470	7	17	71
Sonic Blast Butterfinger	1 reg (14 oz)	580	8	22	88
Sonic Blast M&M's	1 reg (14 oz)	600	8	24	88
Sonic Blast Oreo	1 reg (14 oz)	540	7	21	80
Sonic Blast Reese's Peanut Butter Cup	1 reg (14 oz)	560	9	19	89
Sprite	1 sm (14 oz)	104	0	0	37
Sprite Zero	1 sm (14 oz)	5	0	0	0

FOOD	PORTION	CALS	PROT	FAT	CARB
BREAKFAST SELECTIONS					
Breakfast Burrito Jr.	1 (4.1 oz)	330	13	21	25
Breakfast Burrito Sausage Egg Cheese	1 (5.9 oz)	480	18	31	38
Breakfast Toaster Bacon Egg Cheese	1 (5.6 oz)	530	20	32	40
Breakfast Toaster Ham Egg Cheese	1 (6.5 oz)	490	24	26	40
Breakfast Toaster Sausage Egg Cheese	1 (6.8 oz)	620	20	42	40
CroisSonic Bacon	1 (5.3 oz)	510	18	36	29
CroisSonic Sausage	1 (6.2 oz)	600	19	46	29
DESSERTS					
Apple Slice w/ Fat Free Caramel Dipping Sauce	1 serv (3.4 oz)	120	0	0	27
Apple Slices	1 serv (2.4 oz)	35	0	0	9
Banana Split	1 (10.8 oz)	420	4	9	80
Cone Vanilla	1 (4.7 oz)	180	2	6	30
Dish Vanilla	1 (6.5 oz)	240	3	9	36
Sundae Chocolate	1 (8.9 oz)	410	4	13	67
Sundae Hot Fudge	1 (8.9 oz)	440	4	18	63
Sundae Pineapple	1 (8.8 oz)	370	4	13	58
Sundae Strawberry	1 (8.8 oz)	380	4	13	61
MAIN MENU SELECTIONS					
California Cheeseburger	1 (9.3 oz)	690	29	39	57
Ched 'R' Bites	12 (3 oz)	280	13	15	22
Ched 'R' Peppers	4 (4.2 oz)	330	8	17	36
Chicken Strip Dinner	1 serv (13.5 oz)	930	36	43	100
Chicken Strips	2 (2.5 oz)	200	14	11	10
Chili Cheeseburger	1 (7.9 oz)	660	31	35	56
Coney Extra Long Chili Cheese	1 (9 oz)	660	28	39	55
Coney Regular	1 (5.2 oz)	390	17	23	32
Corn Dog	1 (2.6 oz)	210	6	11	23
Crispy Chicken Bacon Ranch	1 serv (8.9 oz)	610	30	34	48
French Fries	1 sm (2.5 oz)	200	2	8	30
French Fries w/ Cheese	1 sm (3 oz)	270	5	13	32
French Fries w/ Chili & Cheese	1 sm (4.1 oz)	300	8	16	33
Fritos Chili Pie	1 med (4.8 oz)	470	13	32	36
Green Chili Cheeseburger	1 (10 oz)	630	29	31	56

FOOD	PORTION	CALS	PROT	FAT	CARB
Grilled Chicken Bacon Ranch	1 serv (8.9 oz)	470	35	22	35
Hickory Cheeseburger	1 (8.3 oz)	640	28	31	61
Jalapeno Burger	1 (7.6 oz)	550	25	26	53
Jalapeno Cheeseburger	1 (8.3 oz)	620	28	31	54
Jr. Bacon Cheeseburger	1 (5 oz)	410	20	23	31
Jr. Burger	1 (4.1 oz)	310	15	15	30
Jr. Burger Deluxe	1 (4.7 oz)	350	15	20	28
Jr. Double Cheeseburger	1 (6.7 oz)	570	30	35	33
Jumbo Popcorn Chicken	1 sm (4 oz)	380	18	22	27
Mozzarella Sticks	1 serv (5 oz)	440	19	22	40
Onion Rings Onion Rings	1 med (5.5 oz)	440	6	21	55
Pickle-O's	1 serv (4 oz)	310	5	16	36
Sandwich Breaded Pork Fritter	1 (8.5 oz)	640	22	33	66
Sandwich Crispy Chicken	1 (7.9 oz)	550	22	32	46
Sandwich Fish	1 (8.6 oz)	650	22	31	71
Sandwich Grilled Cheese	1 (3.9 oz)	380	12	20	39
Sandwich Grilled Chicken	1 (7.8 oz)	400	28	19	32
Sonic Bacon Cheeseburger w/ Mayonnaise	1 (9.8 oz)	780	33	48	57
Sonic Cheeseburger w/ Ketchup	1 (9.3 oz)	630	29	31	59
Sonic Cheeseburger w/ Mayonnaise	1 (9.3 oz)	720	29	42	56
Sonic Cheeseburger w/ Mustard	1 (9.1 oz)	620	29	31	55
Sonic Burger w/ Ketchup	1 (8.7 oz)	560	26	26	57
Sonic Burger w/ Mayonnaise	1 (8.7 oz)	650	26	37	55
Sonic Burger w/ Mustard	1 (8.5 oz)	560	26	26	54
SuperSonic Cheeseburger w/ Ketchup	1 (12 oz)	900	46	53	60
SuperSonic Cheeseburger w/ Mayonnaise	1 (12 oz)	980	46	64	58
SuperSonic Cheeseburger w/ Mustard	1 (11.8 oz)	890	46	53	57
Thousand Island Burger	1 (8.7 oz)	610	26	32	56
Toaster Sandwich Bacon Cheeseburger	1 (8.5 oz)	670	29	39	52
Toaster Sandwich BLT	1 (5.2 oz)	500	17	29	45
Toaster Sandwich Chicken Club	1 (9 oz)	740	29	46	55
Toaster Sandwich Country Fried Steak	1 (8.5 oz)	670	14	37	71
Tots	1 sm (1.5 oz)	130	1	8	13

FOOD	PORTION	CALS	PROT	FAT	CARB
Tots w/ Cheese	1 sm (2.2 oz)	190	4	13	14
Tots w/ Chili & Cheese	1 sm (3.2 oz)	220	7	16	16
Wrap Crispy Chicken	1 (8.2 oz)	490	21	23	49
Wrap Fritos Chili Cheese	1 (8.5 oz)	670	21	39	66
Wrap Grilled Chicken	1 (8.8 oz)	390	28	14	39
SALAD DRESSINGS AND SAUCES					
Dressing Honey Mustard	1 serv (1.5 oz)	180	1	16	10
Dressing Original Ranch	1 serv (1.5 oz)	190	1	20	2
Dressing Original Ranch Light	1 serv (1.5 oz)	110	3	5	14
Dressing Thousand Island	1 serv (1.5 oz)	190	1	19	7
Italian Fat Free	1 serv (1.5 oz)	40	0	0	10
Sauce BBQ	1 serv (1 oz)	45	0	0	11
Sauce Honey Mustard	1 serv (1 oz)	90	0	7	7
Sauce Marinara	1 serv (1 oz)	15	0	0	3
Sauce Ranch	1 serv (1 oz)	140	0	16	1
SALADS					
Crispy Chicken	1 serv (11.4 oz)	340	20	19	24
Grilled Chicken	1 serv (12 oz)	250	29	10	12
SOUPER SALAD					
BEVERAGES					
Lemonade	1 (24 oz)	190	0	0	49
Lemonade Mango	1 (24 oz)	220	0	0	58
Lemonade Raspberry	1 (24 oz)	220	0	0	58
Lemonade Strawberry	1 (24 oz)	220	0	0	57
Smoothie Mango	1 tall	250	0	0	64
Smoothie Peach	1 tall	230	0	0	62
Smoothie Raspberry	1 tall	230	0	0	62
Smoothie Strawberry	1 tall	230	0	0	60
DESSERTS					
Blueberry Bread	1 piece	150	3	3	29
Brownies	2 pieces	120	1	5	21
Cornbread	1 piece	170	3	5	30
Cottage Cheese	½ cup	90	13	2	5
Gingerbread	1 piece	180	2	6	30
Peaches	½ cup	70	0	0	17
Pineapple Tidbits	¼ cup	60	0	0	15
Pudding Banana	½ cup	160	2	6	26
Pudding Chocolate	½ cup	170	2	5	30
Soft Serve Cone Chocolate	1	120	1	2	22

FOOD	PORTION	CALS	PROT	FAT	CARB
Soft Serve Cone Vanilla	1	120	0	3	22
Sponge Cake	4 pieces	80	1	2	14
Strawberry Parfait	½ cup	100	2	2	19
Vanilla Wafers	4	70	1	2	13
Whipped Topping	½ cup	100	0	8	8
PASTA AND PIZZA					
Chicken Alfredo	1 cup	320	19	9	40
Macaroni & Cheese	1 cup	380	15	18	38
Pizza Slice Cheese	1	70	4	3	8
Pizza Slice Garden	1	80	4	3	9
Pizza Slice Pepperoni	1	90	5	4	8
Pizza Slice Sausage	1	80	4	4	9
Spaghetti & Meatballs	1 cup	280	11	9	38
SALAD DRESSINGS AND SAUCES					
Balsamic Vinegar	1 oz	60	0	0	15
Bleu Cheese	2 oz	220	2	23	1
Caesar	2 oz	280	4	30	4
Chipotle Ranch	2 oz	280	0	28	8
Fat Free French	2 oz	60	0	0	18
Fat Free Italian w/ Cheese	2 oz	30	0	0	6
Green Goddess	2 oz	260	2	24	4
Honey Mustard	2 oz	240	0	26	2
Mayonnaise	2 tbsp	200	0	22	20
Olive Oil	1 oz	240	0	28	0
Peppercorn Ranch	2 oz	220	1	23	2
Pesto Basil	1 tbsp	45	1	5	0
Ranch	2 oz	220	1	23	2
Reduced Calorie Ranch	2 oz	120	2	11	3
Sauce Alfredo	1½ tbsp	45	2	4	2
Sauce Chipotle Pepper	¼ tsp	0	0	0	0
Sauce Cholula Hot	¼ tsp	0	0	0	0
Sauce Jalapeno Cheese	1 serv (2 oz)	35	1	2	5
Sauce Marinara	1½ tbsp	10	0	0	2
Sauce Meaty Marinara	1½ tbsp	40	1	1	2
Sauce Sriracha Hot	¼ tsp	0	0	0	0
Sour Cream Light	2 tbsp	40	1	3	3
Tangy Oriental	2 oz	160	0	12	10
Thousand Island	1 oz	300	0	30	6
Vinaigrette Cranberry	2 oz	100	0	0	24
Vinaigrette House	2 oz	220	0	22	4

FOOD	PORTION	CALS	PROT	FAT	CARB
SALADS					
Apple Walnut	1 cup	130	3	11	7
Asian Chicken	1 cup	80	3	3	10
Asian Shrimp	1 cup	100	4	4	13
Buffalo Chicken	1 cup	70	3	6	3
Caesar Chicken	1 cup	90	5	7	4
Caesar Chicken Salsa	1 cup	80	4	5	4
Caesar Shrimp	1 cup	90	4	7	3
California Chicken Salad	⅓ cup	80	5	6	4
Capri	1 cup	50	1	2	8
Chicago Chopped	1 cup	120	4	10	3
Chickpea	⅓ cup	110	3	6	11
Cobb	1 cup	100	4	8	2
Coleslaw Broccoli	⅓ cup	80	1	6	6
Edamame	⅓ cup	70	4	5	4
Fisherman's Kettle Shrimp & Crab	⅓ cup	120	3	8	15
Gazpacho	⅓ cup	30	0	3	3
Green Goddess Crab	1 cup	70	2	5	4
Italian Antipasto	1 cup	70	2	5	3
Mango Berry	1 cup	110	1	6	13
Marinated Mushrooms	⅓ cup	60	1	7	1
Marinated Oriental Cucumber	⅓ cup	10	0	0	2
Marinated Tomato	1 cup	60	1	2	11
Melon Couscous	⅓ cup	50	1	1	10
Mustard Potato	⅓ cup	80	1	5	7
Paco's Taco	⅓ cup	100	3	5	12
Pasta De Garden	⅓ cup	80	1	5	8
Pasta Fettuccine	⅓ cup	100	2	5	11
Pasta Primavera	⅓ cup	45	1	3	4
Pasta Thai Chicken	⅓ cup	100	3	5	11
Pasta Tuna Skroodle	⅓ cup	130	3	9	10
Red Potato	⅓ cup	50	1	4	5
Rice Florentine	⅓ cup	90	1	5	11
Roasted Mushrooms & Artichokes w/ Feta Cheese	⅓ cup	40	1	3	3
Roasted Vegetables	⅓ cup	20	0	2	2
Salad Of The Sea	⅓ cup	50	2	2	6
Salmon Medley	1 cup	70	4	2	10
Santa Fe Corn	⅓ cup	100	4	4	13

FOOD	PORTION	CALS	PROT	FAT	CARB
Shrimp & Crab Louie	1 cup	130	5	10	5
Southwest Chicken Chipotle	1 cup	90	3	7	4
Sweet Garden Slaw	⅓ cup	35	0	2	4
Tropical Tuxedo	⅓ cup	60	1	3	7
Tuna Fish	⅓ cup	70	6	5	1
SOUPS					
Adobe Rice & Chicken	1 (5 oz)	100	3	5	10
Alaskan Salmon Chowder	1 (5 oz)	70	3	2	9
Beef Mushroom Barley	1 (5 oz)	80	4	2	11
Beef Noodle	1 (5 oz)	80	4	3	10
Beef Shellini	1 (5 oz)	90	5	3	11
Beef Stroganoff	1 (5 oz)	120	5	5	13
Black Bean	1 (5 oz)	80	8	2	20
Broccoli Cheese	1 (5 oz)	70	2	2	10
Cajun Gumbo	1 (5 oz)	110	5	4	13
Cauliflower Cheese	1 (5 oz)	70	2	2	11
Cheddar Chicken Broccoli Stew	1 (5 oz)	140	6	6	15
Cherokee Joe Cornbread	1 (5 oz)	70	2	2	13
Chicken Creole	1 (5 oz)	100	5	4	12
Chicken Enchilada	1 (5 oz)	180	6	12	13
Chicken Gumbo	1 (5 oz)	90	4	4	10
Chicken Mushroom Barley	1 (5 oz)	80	5	3	9
Chicken Noodle	1 (5 oz)	80	5	3	9
Chicken Tetrazini	1 (5 oz)	120	6	5	13
Chicken Tortilla	1 (5 oz)	60	4	2	7
Cream Of Asparagus	1 (5 oz)	140	2	10	7
Cream Of Broccoli	1 (5 oz)	60	2	2	9
Cream Of Cauliflower	1 (5 oz)	60	2	2	10
Cream Of Chicken	1 (5 oz)	100	5	5	9
Cream Of Mushroom	1 (5 oz)	80	2	4	10
Holiday Harvest	1 (5 oz)	90	3	6	5
Vegan Split Pea	1 (5 oz)	90	4	1	16
Vegetable Beef	1 (5 oz)	80	4	3	11
Vegetable Cheese	1 (5 oz)	80	2	3	12
Vegetable Lentil	1 (5 oz)	70	5	0	16
Vegetarian Butter Bean	1 (5 oz)	70	6	0	21
Vegetarian Vegetable	1 (5 oz)	50	2	1	11

STARBUCKS
BAKED SELECTIONS

FOOD	PORTION	CALS	PROT	FAT	CARB
Apple Fritter	1	480	4	22	64

FOOD	PORTION	CALS	PROT	FAT	CARB
Bagel French Toast	1	280	8	1	62
Bagel Multigrain	1	280	10	3	60
Bagel Plain	1	280	10	0	62
Bar Cranberry Bliss	1	320	3	16	41
Bar Toffee Almond	1	400	4	19	53
Brownie Espresso	1	340	4	19	40
Cinnamon Roll	1	470	6	26	56
Cocoa Crispy Square	1	420	5	17	66
Cookie Chocolate Chunk	1	420	7	20	56
Cookie Coffee Ginger	1	470	6	18	70
Cookie Penguin	1	370	4	18	50
Cookie Rainbow	1	420	5	19	61
Cookies Mini Black & White	2	240	2	12	32
Croissant Butter	1	370	5	23	35
Dougnut Glazed	1	490	4	23	65
Loaf Banana Nut	1 serv	470	7	24	56
Loaf Iced Lemon	1 serv	500	7	18	78
Loaf Marble	1 serv	410	6	22	52
Loaf Pumpkin	1 serv	380	5	14	59
Mallorca Sweet Bread	1	420	7	24	43
Muffin Blueberry	1	310	5	11	55
Muffin Pumpkin Cream Cheese	1	490	6	24	63
Muffin Reduced Fat Chocolate	1	290	6	5	53
Muffin Walnut Bran	1	430	8	18	62
Reduced Fat Coffee Cake Banana Chocolate Chip	1	390	5	8	76
Reduced Fat Coffee Cake Blueberry	1 serv	320	4	6	54
Reduced Fat Coffee Cake Cinnamon Swirl	1 serv	290	4	4	52
Reduced Fat Coffee Cake Pumpkin Chocolate Chip	1	300	5	6	58
Rustic Apple Tart	1	190	1	5	37
Scone Blueberry	1	480	7	22	64
Scone Cran Apple Crumb	1	490	7	20	74
Scone Raspberry	1	470	7	21	64
BEVERAGES					
Apple Juice	1 grande	250	0	0	64
Cafe Americano	1 grande	15	1	0	3
Cafe Au Lait Nonfat Milk	1 grande	70	7	0	10

FOOD	PORTION	CALS	PROT	FAT	CARB
Caffe Mocha No Whip Nonfat Milk	1 grande	220	13	3	42
Caffe Mocha Whip Nonfat Milk	1 grande	290	13	10	44
Cappuccino Nonfat Milk	1 grande	80	8	0	12
Caramel Apple Cider Whip	1 grande	380	0	8	76
Caramel Apple Spice No Whip	1 grande	310	0	tr	74
Caramel Macchiato Nonfat Milk	1 grande	190	11	1	35
Chocolate Milk Nonfat	1 grande	280	18	3	53
Cinnamon Dolce Creme No Whip Nonfat Milk	1 grande	220	12	0	41
Cinnamon Dolce Whip Nonfat Milk	1 grande	290	13	7	43
Coffee Of The Week	1 grande	5	1	tr	0
Coffee Of The Week Decaf	1 grande	5	1	0	0
Frappuccino Blended Coffee Cafe Vanilla Whip Nonfat Milk	1 grande	430	6	14	70
Frappuccino Blended Coffee Cafe Vanilla Whip Soy	1 grande	430	6	14	70
Frappuccino Blended Coffee Cafe Vanilla No Whip Soy	1 grande	310	5	3	67
Frappuccino Blended Coffee Caffe Vanilla No Whip Nonfat Milk	1 grande	310	5	3	67
Frappuccino Blended Coffee Caramel No Whip Nonfat Milk	1 grande	270	5	4	53
Frappuccino Blended Coffee Caramel No Whip Soy	1 grande	270	5	4	53
Frappuccino Blended Coffee Caramel Whip Soy	1 grande	380	6	15	57
Frappuccino Blended Coffee Cinnamon Dolce No Whip Nonfat Milk	1 grande	260	5	3	52
Frappuccino Blended Coffee Cinnamon Dolce No Whip Soy	1 grande	260	5	3	52
Frappuccino Blended Coffee Cinnamon Dolce Whip Soy	1 grande	370	6	14	55
Frappuccino Blended Coffee Espresso Nonfat Milk	1 grande	190	4	3	38

FOOD	PORTION	CALS	PROT	FAT	CARB
Frappuccino Blended Coffee Java Chip No Whip Nonfat Milk	1 grande	340	7	8	64
Frappuccino Blended Coffee Java Chip No Whip Soy	1 grande	190	4	3	38
Frappuccino Blended Coffee Java Chip Whip Nonfat Milk	1 grande	460	7	19	67
Frappuccino Blended Coffee Java Chip Whip Soy	1 grande	460	7	19	67
Frappuccino Blended Coffee Mocha No Whip Nonfat Milk	1 grande	260	6	4	54
Frappuccino Blended Coffee Mocha No Whip Soy	1 grande	260	6	4	54
Frappuccino Blended Coffee Mocha Whip Nonfat Milk	1 grande	380	6	15	57
Frappuccino Blended Coffee Pumpkin Spice No Whip Nonfat Milk	1 grande	290	6	4	59
Frappuccino Blended Coffee Pumpkin Spice No Whip Soy	1 grande	290	6	4	59
Frappuccino Blended Coffee Pumpkin Spice Whip Nonfat Milk	1 grande	400	7	15	62
Frappuccino Blended Coffee Pumpkin Spice Whip Soy	1 grande	400	7	15	62
Frappuccino Blended Coffee Whip Nonfat Milk	1 grande	370	6	14	55
Frappuccino Blended Coffee White Chocolate Mocha No Whip Nonfat Milk	1 grande	300	6	5	59
Frappuccino Blended Coffee White Chocolate Mocha No Whip Soy	1 grande	300	6	5	59
Frappuccino Blended Coffee White Chocolate Mocha Whip Nonfat Milk	1 grande	410	7	16	62
Frappuccino Blended Coffee White Chocolate Mocha Whip Soy	1 grande	410	7	16	62
Frappuccino Blended Creme Tazo Chai No Whip Nonfat Milk	1 grande	330	10	2	67

FOOD	PORTION	CALS	PROT	FAT	CARB
Frappuccino Blended Creme Tazo Chai Whip Nonfat Milk	1 grande	570	12	15	95
Frappuccino Blended Creme Vanilla Bean No Whip Nonfat Milk	1 grande	350	11	3	72
Frappuccino Blended Creme Vanilla Bean Whip Nonfat Milk	1 grande	470	12	14	75
Frappuccino Light Blended Coffee Cafe Vanilla Nonfat Milk	1 grande	190	6	1	42
Frappuccino Light Blended Coffee Caramel	1 grande	160	5	2	30
Frappuccino Light Blended Coffee Cinnamon Dolce Nonfat Milk	1 grande	140	5	1	29
Frappuccino Light Blended Coffee Java Chip Nonfat Milk	1 grande	200	6	5	36
Frappuccino Light Blended Coffee Mocha Nonfat Milk	1 grande	140	6	1	29
Frappuccino Light Blended Coffee Nonfat Milk	1 grande	130	5	1	25
Frappuccino Light Blended Coffee Pumpkin Spice Nonfat Milk	1 grande	150	6	1	31
Frappuccino Light Blended Creme Double Chocolaty Chip Whip Nonfat Milk	1 grande	510	14	19	78
Frappuccino Light Blended Creme Pumpkin Spice No Whip Nonfat Milk	1 grande	360	12	3	71
Frappuccino Light Blended Creme Pumpkin Spice Whip Nonfat Milk	1 grande	470	13	13	74
Frappuccino Light Blended Creme Tazo Green Tea No Whip Nonfat Milk	1 grande	380	11	3	78
Frappuccino Light Blended Creme Tazo Green Tea Whip Nonfat Milk	1 grande	440	11	13	71

FOOD	PORTION	CALS	PROT	FAT	CARB
Frappuccino Light Blended Creme Tazo Green Tea Whip Nonfat Milk	1 grande	490	12	14	82
Frappuccino Light Blended Creme White Chocolate No Whip Nonfat Milk	1 grande	480	15	7	89
Frappuccino Light Blended Creme White Chocolate Whip Nonfat Milk	1 grande	610	15	19	92
Frappuccino Light Espresso Nonfat Milk	1 grande	110	5	1	20
Hot Chocolate No Whip Nonfat Milk	1 grande	240	14	3	48
Hot Chocolate Whip Nonfat Milk	1 grande	320	14	10	50
Iced Brewed Coffee	1 grande	90	0	0	21
Iced Cafe Mocha Whip Nonfat Milk	1 grande	290	9	14	39
Iced Caffe Americano	1 grande	15	1	0	3
Iced Caffe Latte Nonfat Milk	1 grande	90	8	0	13
Iced Caffe Mocha No Whip Nonfat Milk	1 grande	170	9	3	36
Iced Caramel Macchiato Nonfat Milk	1 grande	190	10	2	34
Iced Latte Pumpkin Spice No Whip Nonfat Milk	1 grande	220	10	0	44
Iced Latte Pumpkin Spice Whip Nonfat Milk	1 grande	330	11	11	48
Iced Latte Skinny Cinnamon Dolce No Whip Nonfat Milk	1 grande	80	7	0	12
Iced Latte Sugar Free Flavored Syrup Nonfat Milk	1 grande	80	7	0	12
Iced Latte Syrup Flavored Nonfat Milk	1 grande	160	7	0	31
Iced Latte Vanilla Nonfat Milk	1 grande	160	7	0	31
Iced Peppermint White Chocolate Mocha No Whip Nonfat Milk	1 grande	370	10	6	72
Iced Peppermint White Chocolate Mocha Whip Nonfat Milk	1 grande	490	10	17	75

FOOD	PORTION	CALS	PROT	FAT	CARB
Iced Tazo Latte Black Tea Nonfat Milk	1 grande	170	8	0	35
Iced Tazo Latte Black Tea Soy	1 grande	200	6	3	38
Iced Tazo Latte Chai Nonfat Milk	1 grande	200	8	0	44
Iced Tazo Latte Green Tea Nonfat Milk	1 grande	220	10	5	45
Iced Tazo Latte Green Tea Soy	1 grande	260	7	4	48
Iced Tazo Latte Red Tea	1 grande	200	6	3	38
Iced Tazo Latte Red Tea Nonfat Milk	1 grande	170	8	0	35
Iced White Chocolate Mocha No Whip Nonfat Milk	1 grande	310	11	6	55
Iced White Chocolate Mocha Whip Nonfat Milk	1 grande	430	11	17	59
Latte Caffe Nonfat Milk	1 grande	130	13	5	19
Latte Cinnamon Dolce No Whip Nonfat Milk	1 grande	210	11	0	41
Latte Cinnamon Dolce w/ Sugar Free Syrup Nonfat Milk	1 grande	130	12	0	19
Latte Cinnamon Dolce Whip Nonfat Milk	1 grande	280	12	7	43
Latte Pumpkin Spice No Whip Nonfat Milk	1 grande	260	14	0	50
Latte Pumpkin Spice Whip Nonfat Milk	1 grande	330	14	7	52
Latte Skinny Caramel No Whip Nonfat Milk	1 grande	130	12	0	19
Latte Skinny Cinnamon Dolce No Whip Nonfat Milk	1 grande	130	12	0	19
Latte Skinny Cinnamon Dolce No Whip Nonfat Milk	1 grande	130	12	0	19
Latte Skinny Hazelnut No Whip Nonfat Milk	1 grande	130	12	0	19
Latte Skinny Vanilla No Whip Nonfat Milk	1 grande	130	12	0	19
Latte Syrup Flavored Nonfat Milk	1 grande	200	12	0	37
Milk Nonfat	1 grande	180	18	0	26

FOOD	PORTION	CALS	PROT	FAT	CARB
Peppermint White Chocolate Mocha No Whip Nonfat Milk	1 grande	420	14	6	78
Peppermint White Chocolate Mocha Whip Nonfat Milk	1 grande	490	14	13	80
Pumpkin Spice Creme No Whip Nonfat Milk	1 grande	270	15	0	51
Pumpkin Spice Creme Whip Nonfat Milk	1 grande	340	15	7	53
Shaken Black Iced Tea & Lemonade	1 grande	130	0	0	33
Shaken White Iced Tea Blueberry	1 grande	80	0	0	21
Steamed Apple Juice	1 grande	230	0	0	56
Tazo Black Shaken Iced Tea & Lemonade	1 grande	130	0	0	33
Tazo Chai Latte Iced Tea Soy	1 grande	230	6	3	47
Tazo Chai Latte Nonfat Milk	1 grande	200	8	0	44
Tazo Chai Latte Soy	1 grande	230	5	3	47
Tazo Latte Black Tea Nonfat Milk	1 grande	170	7	0	34
Tazo Latte Black Tea Soy	1 grande	190	5	3	36
Tazo Latte Green Tea Nonfat Milk	1 grande	200	8	0	42
Tazo Latte Green Tea Soy	1 grande	220	6	3	44
Tazo Latte Red Tea Nonfat Milk	1 grande	170	7	0	34
Tazo Latte Red Tea Soy	1 grande	190	5	3	36
Tazo Shaken Iced Tea Green	1 grande	80	0	0	21
Tazo Shaken Iced Tea Green & Lemonade	1 grande	130	0	0	33
Tazo Shaken Iced Tea Orange Passion	1 grande	70	0	0	19
Tazo Shaken Iced Tea Passion	1 grande	80	0	0	21
Tazo Shaken Iced Tea Passion & Lemonade	1 grande	130	0	0	33
Tazo Tea	1 grande	0	0	0	0
Vanilla Creme Whip Nonfat Milk	1 grande	270	13	7	39
Vanilla Creme No Whip Nonfat Milk	1 grande	200	12	0	37
Vivanno Blend Banana Chocolate	1 grande (20 oz)	270	21	2	44

FOOD	PORTION	CALS	PROT	FAT	CARB
Vivanno Blend Orange Mango Banana	1 grande (20 oz)	250	16	2	47
White Chocolate Mocha No Whip Nonfat Milk	1 grande	360	16	6	62
White Chocolate Mocha Whip Nonfat Milk	1 grande	430	16	13	64
SALADS					
Fiesta	1 (9.4 oz)	320	16	10	44
Fruit & Cheese Plate	1 (8.6 oz)	400	14	20	44
Vegetable Vinaigrette	1 (10.7 oz)	310	8	15	40
SANDWICHES					
Club Chicken Cheddar Bacon w/ Mayo	1	480	31	18	48
Club Turkey & Avocado	1	390	26	19	33
Egg Salad On Multigrain	1	470	19	21	53
Turkey & Swiss w/ Mayo	1	310	26	13	26
TOPPINGS					
Caramel	1 tbsp	15	0	1	2
Chocolate	1 tsp	5	0	0	1
Flavored Sugar Free Syrup	1 pump	0	0	0	0
Flavored Syrup	1 pump	20	0	0	5
Mocha Syrup	1 pump	25	1	1	5
Sprinkles	1 serv	0	0	0	0

SUBWAY
ADD-ONS AND SALAD DRESSINGS

FOOD	PORTION	CALS	PROT	FAT	CARB
American Cheese	1 serv (0.4 oz)	40	2	4	1
Bacon Strips	2	45	3	4	0
Banana Pepper Slices	3	0	0	0	0
Cheddar	1 serv (0.5 oz)	60	4	5	0
Fat Free Italian	1 serv (2 oz)	35	1	0	7
Fat Free Red Wine Vinaigrette	1 serv (0.7 oz)	30	0	0	6
Jalapeno Pepper Slices	3	<5	0	0	0
Mayonnaise	1 tbsp	110	0	12	0
Mayonnaise Light	1 tbsp	50	0	5	tr
Monterey Cheddar Shredded	1 serv (0.5 oz)	50	3	5	1
Mustard Yellow or Deli	2 tsp	5	0	0	tr
Olive Oil Blend	1 tsp	45	0	5	0
Pepperjack Cheese	1 serv (0.5 oz)	50	3	4	0
Provolone	1 serv (0.5 oz)	50	4	4	0
Ranch Low Fat	1.5 tbsp	120	0	13	1

FOOD	PORTION	CALS	PROT	FAT	CARB
Ranch	1 serv (2 oz)	320	0	35	3
Red Wine Vinaigrette	1 serv (2 oz)	80	1	1	17
Sauce Chipotle Southwest	1.5 tbsp	100	0	10	1
Sauce Fat Free Honey Mustard	1.5 tbsp	30	0	0	7
Sauce Fat Free Sweet Onion	1.5 tbsp	40	0	0	9
Swiss	1 serv (0.5 oz)	50	4	5	0
Vinegar	1 tsp	0	0	0	0
BREADS					
Hearty Italian	6 inch	220	8	2	41
Honey Oat	6 inch	250	10	4	48
Italian	6 inch	200	7	2	38
Italian Herb & Cheese	6 inch	250	10	5	40
Italian White	1 mini	140	5	2	26
Monterey Cheddar	6 inch	240	10	5	39
Parmesan Oregano	6 inch	220	8	3	40
Wheat	1 mini	140	6	2	27
Wheat	6 inch	200	8	3	40
Wrap	1	190	6	5	33
DESSERTS					
Apple Slices	1 pkg	35	0	0	9
Cookie Chocolate Chip	1	210	2	10	30
Cookie Chocolate Chip w/ M&M's	1 (1.6 oz)	210	2	10	32
Cookie Chocolate Chunk	1	220	2	10	30
Cookie Double Chocolate Chip	1 (1.6 oz)	210	2	10	30
Cookie Oatmeal Raisin	1	200	3	8	30
Cookie Peanut Butter	1	220	4	12	26
Cookie Sugar	1	220	2	12	28
Cookie White Chip Macadamia Nut	1	220	2	11	29
Raisins	1 pkg	150	2	0	33
SALADS					
Ham w/o Dressing & Croutons	1 serv	120	12	3	14
Oven Roasted Chicken Breast w/o Dressing & Croutons	1 serv	140	19	3	11
Roast Beef w/o Dressing & Croutons	1 serv	120	13	3	12
Subway Club w/o Dressing & Croutons	1 serv	150	18	4	14

FOOD	PORTION	CALS	PROT	FAT	CARB
Sweet Onion Chicken Teriyaki w/o Dressing & Croutons	1 serv	210	20	3	26
Turkey Breast	1 serv	110	12	3	13
Turkey Breast & Ham w/o Dressing & Croutons	1 serv	120	14	3	14
Veggie Delight w/o Dressing & Croutons	1 serv	60	3	1	11
SANDWICHES					
6 Inch Chicken & Bacon Ranch	1	580	36	30	47
6 Inch Cold Cut Combo	1	410	21	17	47
6 Inch Double Stacked Cold Cut Combo	1	550	31	28	49
6 Inch Double Stacked Italian BMT	1	630	34	35	49
6 Inch Double Stacked Steak & Cheese	1	540	46	18	49
6 Inch Double Stacked Subway Club	1	420	39	8	50
6 Inch Double Stacked Sweet Onion Chicken Teriyaki	1	480	43	7	65
6 Inch Double Stacked Turkey Breast	1	330	28	5	48
6 Inch Ham	1	290	18	5	47
6 Inch Italian BMT	1	450	23	21	47
6 Inch Meatball Marinara	1	560	24	24	63
6 Inch Oven Roasted Chicken Breast	1	310	24	5	48
6 Inch Roast Beef	1	290	19	5	45
6 Inch Spicy Italian	1	480	21	25	45
6 Inch Steak & Cheese	1	400	29	12	48
6 Inch Subway Club	1	320	24	6	47
6 Inch Subway Melt	1	380	25	12	48
6 Inch Sweet Onion Chicken Teriyaki	1	370	26	5	59
6 Inch Tuna	1	530	22	31	44
6 Inch Turkey Breast	1	280	18	5	46
6 Inch Turkey Breast & Ham	1	290	20	5	47
6 Inch Veggie Delite	1	230	9	3	44
Mini Sub Ham	1	180	11	3	30
Mini Sub Roast Beef	1	190	13	4	30

FOOD	PORTION	CALS	PROT	FAT	CARB
Mini Sub Tuna w/ Cheese	1	320	13	18	30
Mini Sub Turkey Breast	1	190	12	3	30
Softwich Santa Fe Turkey	1	520	33	10	78

TACO BELL

FOOD	PORTION	CALS	PROT	FAT	CARB
Border Bowl Southwest Steak	1 serv	600	28	24	68
Border Bowl Zesty Chicken	1 serv	640	22	35	60
Border Bowl Zesty Chicken w/o Dressing	1 serv	440	21	15	57
Burrito 7 Layer	1	490	17	18	65
Burrito Bean	1	350	13	9	54
Burrito Chili Cheese	1	370	16	16	40
Burrito Grilled Stuft Chicken	1	640	34	23	73
Burrito Supreme Beef	1	420	17	17	51
Burrito ½ Lb Beef & Potato	1	530	15	23	68
Burrito ½ Lb Combo Beef	1	440	21	18	51
Burrito Fiesta Chicken	1	360	18	10	47
Burrito Fiesta Steak	1	370	14	13	49
Burrito Stuft Grilled Stuft Steak	1	630	30	25	72
Burrito Supreme Chicken	1	400	20	13	49
Burrito Supreme Steak	1	390	18	14	49
Chalupa Baja Beef	1	410	13	27	30
Chalupa Baja Chicken	1	390	17	23	29
Chalupa Baja Steak	1	390	15	24	28
Chalupa Nacho Cheese Beef	1	370	12	22	32
Chalupa Nacho Cheese Chicken	1	360	16	18	30
Chalupa Nacho Cheese Steak	1	340	14	19	30
Chalupa Supreme Beef	1	380	14	20	30
Chalupa Supreme Chicken	1	360	17	20	29
Chalupa Supreme Steak	1	360	15	21	28
Cheesy Fiesta Potatoes	1 serv	290	4	17	29
Cinnamon Twists	1 serv	170	1	7	26
Crunchwrap Supreme	1	560	17	24	68
Crunchwrap Supreme Spicy Chicken	1	540	19	24	67
Crunchy Taco	1	170	8	25	13
Crunchy Taco Supreme	1	210	9	10	15
Empanada Caramel Apple	1	290	3	14	37
Enchirito Beef	1	360	18	17	34
Enchirito Chicken	1	340	22	13	33

FOOD	PORTION	CALS	PROT	FAT	CARB
Fresco Border Bowl Zesty Chicken w/o Dressing	1 serv	350	19	8	51
Fresco Burrito Bean	1 (7.5 oz)	340	12	8	56
Fresco Burrito Fiesta Chicken	1	330	16	8	48
Fresco Burrito Supreme Chicken	1 (8.5 oz)	340	18	8	50
Fresco Burrito Supreme Steak	1 (8.5 oz)	330	16	8	49
Fresco Crunchy Taco	1 (3.2 oz)	150	7	7	13
Fresco Soft Taco Beef	1 (4 oz)	180	8	7	22
Fresco Soft Taco Grilled Steak	1 (4.5 oz)	160	9	4	21
Fresco Soft Taco Ranchero Chicken	1 (4.7 oz)	170	12	4	22
Gordita Baja Beef	1	340	13	19	29
Gordita Baja Chicken	1	320	17	16	28
Gordita Baja Steak	1	320	15	17	27
Gordita Nacho Cheese Beef	1	300	12	14	31
Gordita Nacho Cheese Chicken	1	280	16	11	29
Gordita Nacho Cheese Steak	1	270	14	12	29
Gordita Supreme Beef	1	310	14	16	29
Gordita Supreme Chicken	1	290	17	12	28
Gordita Supreme Steak	1	290	15	13	28
Guacamole Side	1 serv	70	1	5	5
Mexican Pizza	1	530	20	30	46
Mexican Rice	1 serv	180	6	7	23
MexiMelt	1 serv	260	15	14	22
Nacho Supreme	1 serv	440	12	26	41
Nachos	1 serv	330	4	21	32
Nachos Bellgrande	1 serv	770	19	44	77
Pintos 'n Cheese	1 serv	160	9	6	19
Quesadilla Cheese	1	470	19	26	39
Quesadilla Chicken	1	520	28	28	40
Quesadilla Steak	1	520	26	28	39
Salsa Side	1 serv	15	0	0	3
Soft Taco Grande	1	430	19	20	43
Soft Taco Grilled Steak	1	270	12	16	20
Soft Taco Ranchero Chicken	1	270	14	14	21
Soft Taco Supreme Beef	1	250	11	13	23
Sour Cream Side	1 serv	80	1	7	3
Taco Double Decker	1	320	14	13	38
Taco Double Decker Supreme	1	370	14	17	40

FOOD	PORTION	CALS	PROT	FAT	CARB
Taco Spicy Chicken	1	170	10	8	20
Taco Salad Express	1	610	25	32	56
Taco Salad Fiesta	1	840	30	45	80
Taco Salad Fiesta w/o Shell	1	470	23	24	41
Taco Salad Fiesta Chicken	1	790	37	38	77
Taco Salad Fiesta Chicken w/o Shell	1	430	30	18	38
Taquitos Chicken Grilled	1 serv	310	18	11	37
Taquitos Steak Grilled	1 serv	310	16	11	36
Tostada	1	240	11	10	27

TACO BUENO
MAIN MENU SELECTIONS

FOOD	PORTION	CALS	PROT	FAT	CARB
Bueno Chilada Beef	1 (7.9 oz)	523	24	32	42
Bueno Chilada Beef w/o Chili	1 (5.5 oz)	412	19	26	29
Bueno Chilada Beef w/o Queso	1 (5.6 oz)	337	14	18	36
Bueno Chilada Chicken	1 (7.4 oz)	477	24	26	43
Bueno Chilada Chicken w/o Chili	1 (5 oz)	366	19	20	30
Bueno Chilada Chicken w/o Queso	1 (5.1 oz)	290	14	12	30
Burrito Bean	1 (6.4 oz)	490	15	29	45
Burrito Bean w/o Cheddar Cheese	1 (5.9 oz)	412	11	23	44
Burrito Bean w/o Chili	1 (5.2 oz)	434	13	26	39
Burrito Beef	1 (6.9 oz)	510	23	29	41
Burrito Beef Potato	1 (4.8 oz)	350	11	21	32
Burrito Beef Potato w/o Queso	1 (4.1 oz)	305	9	17	30
Burrito Beef Potato w/o Sour Cream	1 (4.3 oz)	330	11	18	31
Burrito Beef w/o Cheddar Cheese	1 (6.4 oz)	432	19	22	40
Burrito Beef w/o Chili	1 (5.7 oz)	455	20	25	36
Burrito Big Ol' Beef	1 (10.6 oz)	772	33	46	57
Burrito Big Ol' Beef w/o Cheddar Cheese	1 (9.6 oz)	615	24	33	56
Burrito Big Ol' Beef w/o Chili	1 (9.4 oz)	716	31	43	51
Burrito Big Ol' Beef w/o Sour Cream	1 (9.6 oz)	715	32	40	55
Burrito Big Ol' Chicken	1 (8.4 oz)	607	31	30	53

FOOD	PORTION	CALS	PROT	FAT	CARB
Burrito Big Ol' Chicken w/o Cheddar Cheese	1 (7.4 oz)	450	22	17	52
Burrito Big Ol' Chicken w/o Sour Cream	1 (7.4 oz)	551	30	24	51
Burrito Chicken Potato	1 (4.5 oz)	327	11	18	33
Burrito Chicken Potato w/o Queso	1 (3.8 oz)	274	9	14	31
Burrito Chicken Potato w/o Sour Cream	1 (4 oz)	299	11	15	32
Burrito Combination	1 (6.8 oz)	507	19	29	43
Burrito Combination w/o Cheddar Cheese	1 (6.3 oz)	429	15	23	42
Burrito Combination w/o Chili	1 (5.6 oz)	452	17	26	37
Burrito Combination w/o Refried Beans	1 (5.7 oz)	440	18	23	40
Burrito Party	1 (4 oz)	298	9	18	29
Burrito Party w/o Cheddar Cheese	1 (3.8 oz)	259	7	14	29
Chimichanger Cheesecake	1 (2 oz)	210	4	11	24
Cinnamon Chips (4.5 oz)	1 serv	676	8	31	95
Corn Tortilla Chips	1 serv (1.5 oz)	219	3	11	27
Guacamole	1 serv (0.9 oz)	55	1	5	2
Jalapenos	1 serv (0.7 oz)	3	0	0	1
Mexican Rice	1 serv (4.2 oz)	469	10	12	83
Muchaco Beef	1 (5.2 oz)	449	15	25	40
Muchaco Beef w/o Cheddar Cheese	1 (4.9 oz)	410	13	22	40
Muchaco Beef w/o Refried Beans	1 (4.2 oz)	392	14	20	38
Muchaco Chicken	1 (4.6 oz)	387	17	18	40
Muchaco Chicken w/o Cheddar Cheese	1 (4.4 oz)	348	15	14	39
Nachos Cheese	1 serv (5.5 oz)	572	18	35	47
Quesadilla Beef	1 (8.5 oz)	823	38	51	49
Quesadilla Cheese	1 (6.5 oz)	709	30	42	48
Quesadilla Chicken	1 (7.9 oz)	761	38	44	50
Quesadilla Kids Cheese	1 (2.2 oz)	219	8	11	23
Quesadilla Mini Cheese	1 (2.7)	274	11	15	23
Refried Beans Powdered	1 serv (6.3 oz)	406	12	34	17

FOOD	PORTION	CALS	PROT	FAT	CARB
Refried Beans w/o Cheddar Cheese	1 serv (5.8 oz)	327	8	28	16
Refried Beans w/o Chili	1 serv (5.1 oz)	360	9	31	11
Salsa Red	1 serv (2 oz)	14	1	0	3
Soup Tortilla	1 bowl	237	20	11	19
Soup Tortilla w/o Tortilla Strips & Cheese	1 bowl	148	17	6	11
Sour Cream	1 serv (1 oz)	57	1	6	2
Taco Party	1 (1.9 oz)	143	7	10	5
Taco w/o Cheddar Cheese	1 (1.5 oz)	104	4	7	5
Taco Crispy Beef	1 (2.6 oz)	200	10	14	7
Taco Crispy Chicken	1 (1.9 oz)	140	9	7	8
Taco Crispy Chicken w/o Cheddar Cheese	1 (1.7 oz)	100	7	4	7
Taco Crispy w/o Cheddar Cheese	1 (2.4 oz)	161	7	11	6
Taco Soft Beef	1 (3.5 oz)	245	11	14	18
Taco Soft Beef w/o Cheddar Cheese	1 (3.2 oz)	206	9	11	17
Taco Soft Chicken	1 (2.9 oz)	184	10	8	19
Taco Soft Chicken w/o Cheddar Cheese	1 (2.5 oz)	145	8	5	18
Tostada	1 (4.1 oz)	324	11	24	18
Tostada w/o Cheddar Cheese	1 (3.3 oz	207	5	15	17
Tostada w/o Chili	1 (2.9 oz)	269	9	21	12
Tostada w/o Refried Beans	1 (2.5 oz)	234	10	16	15
SALADS					
Nacho Beef	1 (9.3 oz)	759	28	48	58
Nacho Beef w/o Cheddar Cheese	1 (8.8 oz)	681	24	42	57
Nacho Beef w/o Chili	1 (6.9 oz)	648	24	41	45
Nacho Chicken	1 (8.9 oz)	713	28	43	59
Nacho Chicken w/o Cheddar Cheese	1 (8.4 oz)	634	24	37	58
Nacho Chicken w/o Chili	1 (6.5 oz)	601	24	36	46
Taco Beef	1 (12.7 oz)	1043	36	75	58
Taco Beef w/o Cheddar Cheese	1 (11.7 oz)	886	27	62	56
Taco Beef w/o Chili	1 (11.5 oz)	987	33	72	51
Taco Beef w/o Guacamole	1 (11.7 oz)	988	35	70	56

FOOD	PORTION	CALS	PROT	FAT	CARB
Taco Beef w/o Sour Cream	1 (11.7 oz)	986	35	70	56
Taco Beef w/o Tortilla Bowl	1 (9.7 oz)	564	28	45	15
Taco Chicken	1 (9.6 oz)	838	30	57	53
Taco Chicken w/o Cheddar Cheese	1 (8.6 oz)	680	21	44	52
Taco Chicken w/o Guacamole	1 (8.6 oz)	783	29	52	51
Taco Chicken w/o Sour Cream	1 (8.6 oz)	781	29	51	51
Taco Chicken w/o Tortilla Bowl	1 (6.6 oz)	359	22	26	10

TACOTIME
DESSERTS

FOOD	PORTION	CALS	PROT	FAT	CARB
Churro Plain	1 (1.5 oz)	205	2	15	16
Churro w/ Cinnamon & Sugar	1 (2 oz)	245	2	15	26
Crustos	1 serv	294	6	6	58
Empanada Apple	1 (4 oz)	234	4	7	40
Empanada Cherry	1 (4 oz)	240	4	7	41
Empanada Pumpkin	1 (4 oz)	256	6	8	42

MAIN MENU SELECTIONS

FOOD	PORTION	CALS	PROT	FAT	CARB
Burrito Big Juan Chicken	1 (13 oz)	594	35	19	68
Burrito Big Juan Seasoned Ground Beef	1 (13 oz)	651	30	28	71
Burrito Big Juan Shredded Beef	1 (13 oz)	633	33	25	67
Burrito Casita Chicken	1 (12 oz)	494	34	18	43
Burrito Casita Seasoned Ground Beef	1 (12 oz)	552	29	25	46
Burrito Casita Shredded Beef	1 (12 oz)	533	31	25	42
Burrito Chicken & Black Bean	1 (10 oz)	478	30	16	51
Burrito Chicken BLT	1 (10 oz)	721	41	41	44
Burrito Chicken Ranchero	1 (10.8 oz)	654	36	32	52
Burrito Crisp Chicken	1 (5.5 oz)	336	27	10	32
Burrito Crisp Meat	1 (5.8 oz)	450	23	22	36
Burrito Crisp Pinto Bean	1 (6 oz)	394	13	16	50
Burrito Soft Meat	1 (6.7 oz)	426	23	16	43
Burrito Soft Pinto Bean	1 (6.7 oz)	377	14	11	54
Burrito Veggie	1 (11 oz)	534	18	18	74
Cheddar Fries	1 sm (6 oz)	374	8	26	29
Cheddar Melt	1 (2.8 oz)	250	11	12	25
Mexi-Fries	1 sm (5 oz)	290	3	19	29
Mexi-Rice	1 serv (4 oz)	87	2	1	19
Nachos Grande	1 serv (16.5 oz)	1132	39	57	114

FOOD	PORTION	CALS	PROT	FAT	CARB
Refritos w/ Chips	1 serv (7 oz)	304	14	11	35
Refritos w/o Chips	1 serv (6.7 oz)	285	13	11	32
Stuffed Fries	1 sm (5 oz)	321	7	7	29
Taco Crisp Seasoned Ground Beef	1 (4.3 oz)	225	15	12	12
Taco Super Soft Chicken	1 (11 oz)	540	35	18	56
Taco Super Soft Seasoned Ground Beef	1 (11 oz)	598	30	25	59
Taco Super Soft Shredded Beef	1 (11 oz)	579	32	25	55
Taco Value Soft	1 (5.3 oz)	314	18	13	28
Taco ½ Lb Shredded Beef	1 (9 oz)	440	28	18	42
Taco ½ Lb Soft Chicken	1 (9 oz)	401	30	11	43
Taco ½ Lb Soft Seasoned Ground Beef	1 (9 oz)	459	25	18	46
Taco Chips	1 serv (2 oz)	150	3	3	27
SALAD DRESSINGS AND TOPPINGS					
Cheddar Cheese	1 serv (2 oz)	223	14	18	1
Dressing Chipotle Ranch	1 serv (1 oz)	165	1	18	1
Dressing Ranch	1 serv (1 oz)	181	1	20	1
Dressing Thousand Island	1 serv (1 oz)	132	0	12	5
Guacamole	1 serv (1 oz)	50	0	5	2
Salsa Nuevo	1 serv (1 oz)	8	0	0	2
Salsa Verde	1 serv (1 oz)	6	0	0	2
Sour Cream	1 serv (1.5 oz)	85	1	7	1
SALADS					
Taco Chicken	1 reg (9.2 oz)	351	27	15	24
Taco Seasoned Ground Beef	1 reg (7.8 oz)	396	22	23	24
Taco Shredded Beef	1 reg (7.8 oz)	377	25	22	21
Tostada Delight Chicken	1 (10.5 oz)	565	37	29	36
Tostada Delight Seasoned Ground Beef	1 (10.5 oz)	623	32	36	39
Tostada Delight Shredded Beef	1 (10.5 oz)	604	35	36	35

TCBY

FROZEN YOGURT AND SORBET

FOOD	PORTION	CALS	PROT	FAT	CARB
Hand Scooped Butter Pecan Perfection	½ cup	110	4	5	14
Hand Scooped Chocolate Chocolate Swirl	½ cup	120	4	4	19
Hand Scooped Chocolate Chunk Cookie Dough	½ cup	160	3	6	24

FOOD	PORTION	CALS	PROT	FAT	CARB
Hand Scooped Cookies & Cream	½ cup	140	3	4	22
Hand Scooped Cotton Candy	½ cup	120	3	4	20
Hand Scooped Mint Chocolate Chunk	½ cup	140	3	5	22
Hand Scooped Mocha Almond	½ cup	150	3	5	22
Hand Scooped No Sugar Added Chocolate Chocolate Swirl	½ cup	90	4	1	23
Hand Scooped No Sugar Added Vanilla	½ cup	80	4	1	19
Hand Scooped No Sugar Added Vanilla Fudge Brownie	½ cup	100	4	2	22
Hand Scooped Pralines & Cream	½ cup	140	3	5	23
Hand Scooped Psychedelic Sorbet	½ cup	290	0	0	75
Hand Scooped Rainbow Cream	½ cup	120	3	4	20
Hand Scooped Rocky Road	½ cup	220	3	7	36
Hand Scooped Strawberries & Cream	½ cup	120	2	3	21
Hand Scooped Vanilla Chocolate Chunk	½ cup	140	3	5	22
Hand Scooped Vanilla Bean	½ cup	120	3	4	19
Soft Serve Frozen Yogurt All Flavors 96% Fat Free	½ cup	140	4	3	23
Soft Serve Frozen Yogurt All Flavors Low Carb	½ cup	110	3	7	16
Soft Serve Frozen Yogurt All Flavors Nonfat	½ cup	110	4	0	23
Soft Serve Frozen Yogurt All Flavors Nonfat No Sugar Added	½ cup	90	4	0	20
Soft Serve Sorbet All Flavors Nonfat Nondairy	½ cup	100	0	0	24
SMOOTHIES					
Berrylicious	1 (16 oz)	290	3	3	65
Black 'N Blueberry	1 (16 oz)	280	3	3	63
Mango Tango	1 (16 oz)	330	2	3	76
Mangolada	1 (16 oz)	340	3	6	70
Mondo Mango	1 (16 oz)	310	3	3	70

FOOD	PORTION	CALS	PROT	FAT	CARB
Pina Paradise	1 (16 oz)	350	3	12	58
Pink Pineapple	1 (16 oz)	340	3	9	63
Straight Up Strawberry	1 (16 oz)	280	3	4	44
Strawberry Bonanza	1 (16 oz)	320	3	4	74
Strawberry Fling	1 (16 oz)	340	3	3	78

TIM HORTONS
BAKED SELECTIONS

FOOD	PORTION	CALS	PROT	FAT	CARB
Bagel Blueberry	1	270	10	1	55
Bagel Cinnamon Raisin	1	270	10	1	55
Bagel Everything	1	280	10	2	53
Bagel Flax Seed	1	290	10	5	53
Bagel Onion	1	260	9	2	53
Bagel Plain	1	260	9	2	52
Bagel Poppy Seed	1	270	9	2	53
Bagel Sesame Seed	1	270	9	3	53
Bagel Sun Dried Tomato	1	310	9	4	59
Bagel Twelve Grain	1	330	10	9	52
Cinnamon Roll Frosted	1	470	4	25	57
Cinnamon Roll Glazed	1	420	4	23	50
Cookie Caramel Chocolate Pecan	1	230	3	11	32
Cookie Chocolate Chip	1	230	3	9	34
Cookie Oatmeal Raisin Spice	1	220	3	8	35
Cookie Peanut Butter Chocolate Chunk	1	260	5	15	28
Cookie Triple Chocolate	1	250	3	13	31
Cookie White Chocolate Macadamia Nut	1	240	3	12	31
Croissant Butter	1	340	7	18	38
Croissant Cheese	1	370	9	20	37
Danish Cherry Cheese	1	330	5	13	46
Danish Chocolate	1	430	4	24	51
Danish Maple Pecan	1	380	4	20	46
Donut Apple Fritter	1	300	4	11	49
Donut Chocolate Dip	1	210	4	9	30
Donut Chocolate Glazed	1	260	4	10	39
Donut Honey Dip	1	210	4	8	33
Donut Maple Dip	1	210	4	8	31
Donut Old Fashion Glazed	1	320	3	19	35
Donut Old Fashion Plain	1	260	3	19	20

FOOD	PORTION	CALS	PROT	FAT	CARB
Donut Sour Cream Plain	1	270	3	17	27
Donut Walnut Crunch	1	360	4	23	35
Donut Filled Angel Cream	1	310	4	13	46
Donut Filled Blueberry	1	230	4	8	36
Donut Filled Boston Cream	1	250	4	9	38
Donut Filled Canadian Maple	1	260	4	9	41
Donut Filled Strawberry	1	230	4	8	36
Honey Cruller	1	320	1	19	37
Muffin Blueberry	1	330	4	11	54
Muffin Blueberry Bran	1	300	6	10	53
Muffin Carrot Wheat	1	400	6	19	55
Muffin Chocolate Chip	1	430	5	16	69
Muffin Cranberry Blueberry Bran	1	290	5	10	51
Muffin Cranberry Fruit	1	350	4	12	59
Muffin Fruit Explosion	1	360	4	11	61
Muffin Raisin Bran	1	360	6	10	65
Muffin Strawberry Sensation	1	350	4	11	61
Muffin Low Fat Blueberry	1	290	4	3	62
Muffin Low Fat Cranberry	1	290	4	3	62
Tea Biscuit Plain	1	250	5	9	35
Tea Biscuit Raisin	1	290	6	10	45
Timbits Apple Fritter	1	50	1	2	9
Timbits Chocolate Glazed	1	70	1	3	10
Timbits Honey Dip	1	60	1	2	9
Timbits Old Fashion Plain	1	70	1	5	5
Timbits Filled Banana Cream	1	60	1	2	9
Timbits Filled Lemon	1	60	1	2	9
Timbits Filled Strawberry	1	60	1	2	10
BEVERAGES					
Cafe Mocha	1 (10 oz)	160	1	7	25
Cappuccino Iced	1 (12 oz)	300	0	15	41
Coffee Decaffeinated Sugar & Cream	1 (10 oz)	75	1	4	9
Coffee Sugar & Cream	1 (10 oz)	75	1	4	9
English Toffee	1 (10 oz)	220	3	6	40
Flavor Shot	1 serv	5	0	0	1
French Vanilla	1 (10 oz)	240	4	7	39
Hot Chocolate	1 (10 oz)	240	2	6	45
Hot Smoothie	1 (10 oz)	260	5	10	39

FOOD	PORTION	CALS	PROT	FAT	CARB
Iced Cappuccino w/ Milk	1 (12 oz)	180	3	2	39
Tea Sugar & Milk	1 (10 oz)	50	1	1	10
CREAM CHEESE					
Garden Vegetable	1.5 oz	120	2	11	3
Light Plain	1.5 oz	60	4	5	3
Plain	1.5 oz	130	2	12	2
Strawberry	1.5 oz	120	6	10	6
SANDWICHES					
B.L.T.	1	450	18	18	53
Breakfast Bacon Egg Cheese	1	410	16	25	31
Breakfast Egg Cheese	1	360	13	21	30
Breakfast Sausage Egg Cheese	1	520	19	37	30
Chicken Salad Salad	1	380	21	9	55
Egg Salad	1	390	17	13	52
Ham & Swiss	1	440	28	12	56
Toasted Chicken Club	1	460	30	7	70
Turkey Breast	1	390	27	5	59
SOUPS					
Beef Stew	1 serv (10 oz)	236	17	8	25
Chicken Noodle	1 serv (10 oz)	120	5	2	18
Chili	1 serv (10 oz)	300	21	16	18
Country Field Mushroom	1 serv (10 oz)	150	3	3	28
Cream Of Broccoli	1 serv (10 oz)	160	6	9	16
Hearty Vegetable	1 serv (10 oz)	70	4	0	14
Minestrone	1 serv (10 oz)	120	4	3	24
Potato Bacon	1 serv (10 oz)	180	3	6	30
Split Pea w/ Ham	1 serv (10 oz)	150	8	3	27
Turkey Rice	1 serv (10 oz)	120	3	2	21
Vegetable Beef Barley	1 serv (10 oz)	110	4	2	21
YOGURT					
Low Fat Creamy Vanilla w/ Berries	1 (6 oz)	160	4	3	32
Low Fat Strawberry w/ Berries	1 (6 oz)	150	4	3	28
TJ CINNAMONS					
Chocolate Twist	1	250	4	12	34
Cinnamon Twist	1	280	3	14	33
Mocha Chill w/ Whipped Cream	1 (12.5 oz)	306	11	7	48
Mocha Chill w/o Whipped Cream	1 (12.5 oz)	264	11	4	48
Original Roll w/o Icing	1	507	10	10	73

FOOD	PORTION	CALS	PROT	FAT	CARB
Pecan Sticky Bun	1	688	12	22	91
TJ Icing	1 serv (1 oz)	117	1	5	18

TOGO'S
SALAD DRESSINGS

FOOD	PORTION	CALS	PROT	FAT	CARB
Asian	1 serv (2.5 oz)	380	0	33	19
Blue Cheese	1 serv (2.5 oz)	260	2	26	3
Buttermilk Ranch	1 serv (2.5 oz)	250	2	26	3
Caesar	1 serv (2.5 oz)	150	2	12	8
Fat Free Serano Grape Vinaigrette	1 serv (2.5 oz)	90	1	0	23
Low Fat Basalmic Vinaigrette	1 serv (2.5 oz)	90	0	4	16

SALADS

FOOD	PORTION	CALS	PROT	FAT	CARB
Asian Chicken w/o Dressing	1 full serv	200	21	9	17
Chicken Caesar w/o Dressing	1 full serv	210	24	6	17
Cobb w/o Dressing	1 full serv	330	29	20	12
Santa Fe Chicken w/o Dressing	1 full serv	370	27	16	33
Taco w/o Dressing	1 full serv	600	26	39	36

SANDWICHES

FOOD	PORTION	CALS	PROT	FAT	CARB
Albacore Tuna	1 reg	660	30	28	73
Avocado & Cucumber	1 reg	560	13	25	75
Black Forest Ham & Cheese	1 reg	670	35	31	67
Capicolla Dry Salami & Provolone	1 reg	1080	73	59	69
Cheese	1 reg	800	34	45	68
Chef's Creations Pacific Cobb	1 reg	710	34	36	68
Chef's Creations Pastrami Reuben	1 reg	990	52	55	67
Chicken Salad	1 reg	650	26	29	74
Egg Salad & Cheese	1 reg	750	31	39	70
Hot BBQ Beef	1 reg	670	40	19	85
Hot Meatball	1 reg	690	33	27	78
Hot Pastrami	1 reg	750	43	33	69
Hot Roast Beef	1 reg	730	58	25	67
Hummus	1 reg	650	19	27	90
Salami & Cheese	1 reg	1100	87	53	73
Turkey & Cranberry	1 reg	670	34	19	95
Turkey & Avocado	1 reg	640	36	26	74
Turkey & Cheese	1 reg	670	42	28	68
Turkey Bacon Club	1 reg	680	35	32	68

FOOD	PORTION	CALS	PROT	FAT	CARB
Turkey Ham & Cheese	1 reg	690	42	29	68

WHATABURGER
BEVERAGES

FOOD	PORTION	CALS	PROT	FAT	CARB
Barq's Root Beer	1 sm (16 oz)	220	0	0	61
Cherry Coke	1 sm (16 oz)	210	0	0	56
Coca Cola	1 sm (16 oz)	207	0	0	56
Coffee	1 sm (8 oz)	5	0	0	1
Coffee Decafe	1 sm (8 oz)	5	0	0	1
Diet Coke	1 sm (16 oz)	0	0	0	0
Dr Pepper	1 sm (16 oz)	190	0	0	51
Fanta Orange	1 sm (16 oz)	210	0	0	56
Fanta Strawberry	1 sm (16 oz)	230	0	0	61
Iced Tea Sweetened	1 (34 oz)	430	0	0	114
Iced Tea Unsweetened	1 sm (19 oz)	0	0	0	0
Lemonade Hi-C Poppin' Pink	1 sm (16 oz)	200	0	0	51
Malt Chocolate	1 sm (16 oz)	670	13	15	123
Malt Strawberry	1 sm (16 oz)	670	12	15	123
Malt Vanilla	1 sm (16 oz)	600	13	17	98
Milk Reduced Fat	8 oz	120	8	5	11
Orange Juice Tropicana	1 (10 oz)	140	3	0	33
Powerade Fruit Punch	1 sm (16 oz)	130	0	0	33
Shake Chocolate	1 sm (16 oz)	630	14	16	111
Shake Strawberry	1 sm (16 oz)	630	13	16	111
Shake Vanilla	1 sm (16 oz)	560	14	17	87
Sprite	1 sm (16 oz)	200	0	0	51

CHILDREN'S MENU SELECTIONS

FOOD	PORTION	CALS	PROT	FAT	CARB
Kid's Meal Chicken Strips	1 serv	770	22	51	53
Kid's Meal Justaburger	1 serv	570	19	29	60

DESSERTS

FOOD	PORTION	CALS	PROT	FAT	CARB
Apple Pie A La Mode	1 serv	520	10	20	75
Apple Pie Hot	1	230	3	11	29
Cinnamon Roll	1	400	6	7	80
Cookie Chocolate Chunk	1 (2 oz)	230	2	11	33
Cookie White Chocolate Chunk Macadamia	1 (2 oz)	250	3	14	30
Peach Pie A La Mode	1 serv	570	10	23	82

MAIN MENU SELECTIONS

FOOD	PORTION	CALS	PROT	FAT	CARB
Biscuit	1	300	5	17	32

FOOD	PORTION	CALS	PROT	FAT	CARB
Biscuit Sandwich Bacon Egg & Cheese	1	500	16	32	33
Biscuit Sandwich Egg & Cheese	1	450	13	28	33
Biscuit Sandwich Honey Butter Chicken	1	610	14	38	51
Biscuit Sandwich Sausage Egg & Cheese	1	690	26	49	33
Biscuit w/ Bacon	1	355	8	20	32
Biscuit w/ Gravy	1	530	9	36	52
Biscuit w/ Sausage	1	540	18	37	32
Breakfast Platter w/ Bacon	1 serv	730	24	45	53
Breakfast Platter w/ Sausage	1 serv	930	34	62	53
Breakfast On A Bun w/ Bacon	1	380	17	22	29
Breakfast On A Bun w/ Sausage	1	570	27	39	29
Chicken Strips	1	200	9	12	11
Chicken Strips w/ Gravy	4	840	37	54	53
French Fries	1 sm	260	4	13	31
Gravy White Peppered	1 serv	60	0	5	8
Hashbrown Sticks	4	200	2	12	20
Justaburger	1	329	15	16	30
Onion Rings	1 med	420	5	28	36
Pancakes Plain	1 serv	580	17	8	112
Pancakes w/ Bacon	1 serv	630	20	12	112
Pancakes w/ Sausage	1 serv	820	30	20	112
Sandwich Chicken Strip Honey BBQ	1	1110	45	59	102
Sandwich Chicken Strip Junior Honey BBQ	1	720	30	41	59
Sandwich Egg	1	330	14	18	29
Sandwich Grilled Chicken	1	450	33	18	45
Taquito w/ Bacon & Egg	1	370	17	21	27
Taquito w/ Bacon Egg & Cheese	1	420	19	24	27
Taquito w/ Potato & Egg	1	430	15	23	37
Taquito w/ Potato Egg & Cheese	1	470	17	27	37
Taquito w/ Sausage & Egg	1	410	17	24	27
Taquito w/ Sausage Egg & Cheese	1	450	19	28	27
Texas Toast	1 slice	180	4	8	25
Whataburger	1	640	30	32	61
Whataburger Double Meat	1	890	47	51	61

FOOD	PORTION	CALS	PROT	FAT	CARB
Whataburger Jr.	1	330	15	16	32
Whataburger Triple Meat	1	1140	65	70	61
Whataburger w/ Bacon & Cheese	1	800	40	45	62
Whatacatch	1	480	17	30	42
Whatacatch Dinner	1 serv	1095	29	92	161
Whatachick'n	1	530	32	20	61
SALADS					
Chicken Strips	1 serv	570	21	38	34
Garden Salad	1	60	3	0	12
Grilled Chicken	1 serv	230	23	7	19
WHITE CASTLE					
BEVERAGES					
Barq's Red Cream Soda	1 sm (21 oz)	260	0	0	69
Barq's Root Beer	1 sm (21 oz)	250	0	0	68
Coca Cola	1 sm (21 oz)	220	0	0	61
Coffee Black	1 sm (12 oz)	<5	0	0	1
Crave Cooler Coke	1 sm (21 oz)	150	0	0	41
Diet Coke	1 sm (21 oz)	0	0	0	0
Fanta Orange	1 sm (21 oz)	240	0	0	64
Hi-C Flashing Fruit Punch	1 sm (21 oz)	240	0	0	63
Hot Chocolate	1 sm (12 oz)	220	1	6	40
Hot Tea	1 sm (12 oz)	0	0	0	0
Iced Tea Sweetened w/ Lemon	1 sm (21 oz)	170	0	0	46
Iced Tea Unsweetened	1 sm (21 oz)	0	0	0	0
Lemonade Raspberry	1 sm (21 oz)	290	0	0	78
Pibb Xtra	1 sm (21 oz)	220	0	0	59
Powerade Mountain Blast	1 sm (21 oz)	140	0	0	38
Sprite	1 sm (21 oz)	220	0	0	59
MAIN MENU SELECTIONS					
Cheeseburger	1	170	7	9	15
Cheeseburger Bacon	1	200	10	11	15
Cheeseburger Bacon Double	1	370	19	22	23
Cheeseburger Double	1	300	14	17	23
Cheeseburger Jalapeno	1	180	8	10	15
Cheeseburger Jalapeno Double	1	320	15	19	23
Chicken Rings	6	210	18	23	15
Clam Strips	1 reg	250	8	22	5
Fish Nibblers	1 reg	280	19	16	24
French Fries	1 reg	310	4	15	39

FOOD	PORTION	CALS	PROT	FAT	CARB
Mozzarella Cheese Sticks	3	250	10	14	22
Onion Chips	1 reg	480	7	23	62
Sandwich Chicken Breast w/ Cheese	1	200	12	8	21
Sandwich Chicken Ring	1	180	7	8	19
Sandwich Chicken Ring w/ Cheese	1	200	8	10	19
Sandwich Fish w/ Cheese	1	180	9	8	19
White Castle	1	140	6	7	14
White Castle Double	1	250	11	13	22
SAUCES AND SPREADS					
Dressing Ranch	1 serv (1 oz)	150	0	17	0
Ketchup	1 pkg	10	0	0	3
Lemon Juice	1 pkg	0	0	0	0
Mayonnaise	1 pkg	60	0	7	0
Sauce BBQ	1 serv (1 oz)	35	0	1	8
Sauce Hot	1 pkg	0	0	0	0
Sauce Marinara	1 serv (1 oz)	15	0	0	4
Sauce Seafood	1 serv (1 oz)	30	0	0	7
Sauce Tartar	1 pkg	30	0	3	2
Sauce Zesty Zing	1 serv (1 oz)	110	0	11	3
Sauce Fat Free Honey Mustard	1 serv (1 oz)	50	0	0	12

WINCHELL'S DONUTS

FOOD	PORTION	CALS	PROT	FAT	CARB
Chocolate Bar	1	240	4	16	29
Chocolate Round	1	240	4	16	29
Chocolate Twist	1	240	4	16	29
Croissant	1	260	5	17	28
Glazed Round	1	230	2	15	27
Glazed Twist	1	230	2	15	27
Iced Chocolate	1	230	2	15	28
Traditional	1	215	2	14	26

WORLD WRAPPS
CHILDREN'S MENU SELECTIONS

FOOD	PORTION	CALS	PROT	FAT	CARB
Kid's Bean & Cheese	1	332	18	11	36
Kid's Chicken & Cheese	1	229	15	4	25
Kid's Quesadilla	1	410	19	20	39
Kid's Teriyaki Chicken	1	407	25	6	52
SALADS					
BBQ Ranch Chicken	1 serv	633	29	48	43

FOOD	PORTION	CALS	PROT	FAT	CARB
Caesar Blackened Salmon	1 serv	612	27	54	9
Caesar Classic	1 serv	417	9	41	7
California Cobb	1 serv	636	29	62	16
Garden Veggie	1 serv	492	4	51	12
Thai Asian Chicken	1 serv	613	36	36	41
SIDES AND SOUPS					
Chips & Mango Salsa	1 serv	224	3	8	34
Chips & Tomato Corn Salsa	1 serv	184	2	8	82
Potstickers	3	170	8	4	24
Soup Thai Lemongrass	1 cup	256	32	8	14
Soup Tortilla	1 cup	191	8	7	26
Yogurt Parfait	1 serv	281	19	5	41
SMOOTHIES					
Black & Blue	1 (16 oz)	319	2	tr	77
Blue Mango Boost	1 (16 oz)	295	4	1	70
Caribbean C	1 (16 oz)	276	3	1	64
Georgia Peach	1 (16 oz)	343	1	tr	86
Peanut Butter Banana	1 (16 oz)	502	18	17	69
Strawberry Orange Banana	1 (16 oz)	268	3	1	61
Triathlete	1 (16 oz)	341	5	1	80
Tropical Storm	1 (16 oz)	309	6	3	72
WRAPS					
Baja Veggie w/ Cheese Sour Cream Avocados	1 sm	541	18	13	89
Barcelona	1 sm	460	24	11	65
Bean & Cheese	1 sm	452	16	13	67
Bombay Curry Veggie	1 sm	495	12	14	81
Buffalo w/ Shrimp	1 sm	422	18	10	65
Burrito w/ Chicken Cheese Sour Cream Avocado	1 sm	576	26	21	66
Burrito w/ Steak Cheese Sour Cream Avocado	1 sm	573	34	20	66
Caribbean Sole	1 sm	523	23	14	80
Chicken Caesar	1 sm	547	25	30	44
Chicken Parmesan	1 sm	495	32	16	53
Portabello & Goat Cheese	1 sm	391	13	13	55
Samurai Salmon	1 sm	543	22	22	65
Spicy Southwest Shrimp	1 sm	460	22	8	75
Tequila Lime Shrimp	1 sm	422	18	10	65
Teriyaki Chicken	1 sm	482	25	10	73

FOOD	PORTION	CALS	PROT	FAT	CARB
Teriyaki Steak	1 sm	497	30	10	69
Teriyaki Tofu & Mushroom	1 sm	387	11	6	58
Texas Roadhouse BBQ Chicken	1 sm	512	27	17	64
Texas Roadhouse BBQ Steak	1 sm	569	28	23	64
Thai Chicken	1 sm	508	30	17	58

YOGEN FRUZ

FOOD	PORTION	CALS	PROT	FAT	CARB
Blend It No Sugar Added Vanilla	1 sm	110	4	0	24
Blend It Probiotic Low Fat Chocolate	1 sm	121	3	2	22
Blend It Probiotic Low Fat Vanilla	1 sm	121	4	2	22
Blend It Probiotic Non Fat Vanilla	1 sm	110	4	0	24
Smoothie Dairy Blueberry Breeze	1 sm	180	3	0	45
Smoothie Dairy Peach Berry Sunset	1 sm	150	3	0	36
Smoothie Dairy Strawberry Banana	1 sm	180	3	0	42
Smoothie Non Dairy Raspberry Blast	1 sm	208	2	0	51
Smoothie Non Dairy Tropical Storm	1 sm	224	2	0	56
Smoothie Non Dairy Very Berry	1 sm	192	0	0	50
Top It Probiotic Soft Serve	1 sm	132	5	0	28

YOGURTLAND

FOOD	PORTION	CALS	PROT	FAT	CARB
Arctic Vanilla	½ cup (3 oz)	108	3	0	24
Blueberry Tart	½ cup (3 oz)	127	7	0	16
Cafe Con Leche	½ cup (3 oz)	108	3	0	24
Chocolate Mint	½ cup (3 oz)	100	2	0	23
Double Cookies & Cream	½ cup (3 oz)	121	3	0	27
Dutch Chocolate	½ cup (3 oz)	118	3	0	27
Fresh Strawberry	½ cup (3 oz)	108	3	0	24
Green Tea	½ cup (3 oz)	107	3	tr	24
Heath Bar	½ cup (3 oz)	132	3	3	25
Mango	½ cup (3 oz)	96	2	0	22
Mango Tart	½ cup (3 oz)	127	7	0	16
No Sugar Added French Vanilla	½ cup (3 oz)	89	6	0	19
NY Cheesecake	½ cup (3 oz)	100	3	0	23

FOOD	PORTION	CALS	PROT	FAT	CARB
Peach	½ cup (3 oz)	100	2	0	23
Peach Tart	½ cup (3 oz)	127	7	0	16
Peanut Butter	½ cup (3 oz)	119	3	3	24
Pineapple Tart	½ cup (3 oz)	127	7	0	16
Pistachio	½ cup (3 oz)	100	3	0	22
Plain Tart	½ cup (3 oz)	108	8	0	19
Strawberry Tart	½ cup (3 oz)	127	7	0	16
Taro	½ cup (3 oz)	102	2	0	23

ZOUP!
DESSERTS

FOOD	PORTION	CALS	PROT	FAT	CARB
Cookie Chocolate Chunk	1	410	4	19	57
Cookie Peanut Butter	1	420	6	21	43

SANDWICHES

FOOD	PORTION	CALS	PROT	FAT	CARB
Grilled Turkey Club	½	470	29	28	22
Panini Italian Chicken	½	370	22	21	22
Pesto Three Cheese	1	720	44	42	42
Tuna Melt	1	600	50	23	42
Wrap American Farm	½	435	13	29	30
Wrap Asian	½	615	28	33	54
Wrap Chicken Caesar w/o Dressing	½	505	38	19	43
Wrap Greek w/o Dressing	½	485	15	33	33
Wrap Sonoma	½	595	18	37	38
Wrap Tuna	½	365	28	13	35
Zesty Southwest Turkey	½	310	19	16	22

SOUPS

FOOD	PORTION	CALS	PROT	FAT	CARB
Chicken & Dumplings	1 (8 oz)	130	11	3	22
Chicken Potpie	1 (8 oz)	200	13	8	21
Italian Wedding w/ Turkey Meatballs	1 (8 oz)	120	10	4	13
Jamaican Bay Gumbo	1 (8 oz)	140	12	3	20
Lobster Bisque	1 (8 oz)	260	11	18	14
Pepper Steak	1 (8 oz)	160	11	6	19
Potato Cheddar	1 (8 oz)	210	11	13	16
Sesame Noodle Bowl	1 (8 oz)	80	6	3	7
Shrimp & Crawfish Etouffee	1 (8 oz)	130	10	4	17
Sicilian Pizza	1 (8 oz)	150	6	7	18
Spicy Crab & Rice	1 (8 oz)	110	7	2	21
Turkey Chili	1 (8 oz)	120	11	2	19
Wild Mushroom Barley	1 (8 oz)	108	3	3	18